Test Success

Test-Taking Techniques for Beginning Nursing Students

Seventh Edition

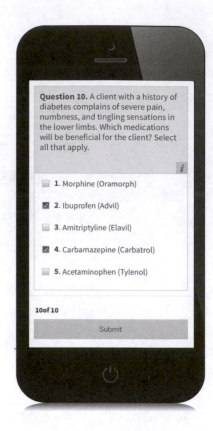
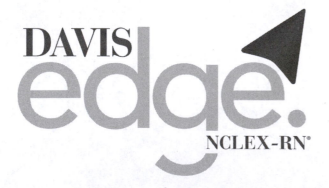

Test **Success**

Test-Taking Techniques for Beginning Nursing Students

Seventh Edition

Patricia M. Nugent, RN, MA, MS, EdD
Professor Emeritus
Adjunct Professor
Nassau Community College
Garden City, New York
Private Practice—President of Nugent Books, Inc.

Barbara A. Vitale, RN, MA
Professor Emeritus
Nassau Community College
Garden City, New York
Private Practice—Professional Resources for Nursing

F.A. Davis Company • Philadelphia

F. A. Davis Company
1915 Arch Street
Philadelphia, PA 19103
www.fadavis.com

Printed in the United States of America

Last digit indicates print number: 10 9 8 7 6 5 4 3 2

Publisher, Nursing: Terri Wood Allen
Content Project Manager: Julia L. Curcio
Electronic Project Editor: Sandra A. Glennie
Design and Illustrations Manager: Carolyn O'Brien

As new scientific information becomes available through basic and clinical research, recommended treatments and drug therapies undergo changes. The author(s) and publisher have done everything possible to make this book accurate, up to date, and in accord with accepted standards at the time of publication. The author(s), editors, and publisher are not responsible for errors or omissions or for consequences from application of the book, and make no warranty, expressed or implied, in regard to the contents of the book. Any practice described in this book should be applied by the reader in accordance with professional standards of care used in regard to the unique circumstances that may apply in each situation. The reader is advised always to check product information (package inserts) for changes and new information regarding dose and contraindications before administering any drug. Caution is especially urged when using new or infrequently ordered drugs.

ISBN: 978-0-8036-4418-2

It is with great pleasure that we dedicate Test Success *to our publisher and friend*
ROBERT MARTONE
Here are a few words that we believe capture your essence: ethical,
innovative, inspired, dedicated, informed, instinctive, knowledgeable,
enthusiastic, exceptional, and in our eyes incomparable and unreplaceable!

We thank you for touching our lives in innumerable ways these past 23 years.
We are indebted to you for inspiring and encouraging us.
We appreciated your trust in our ability to meet expectations.
We are grateful you gave us the opportunity to tackle new titles.
We value our collegial relationship and most importantly your friendship.

We wish you a happy retirement as you move into the next chapter of your life
with your family and especially with your two little grandchildren.
You will be missed!

Preface

Why This Book Is Necessary

- Nursing information and technology are accelerating at a breathtaking rate. Student nurses must learn how to function successfully within nursing programs that have strenuous academic demands.
- The role of the nurse is evolving as the delivery of health care is changing. Student nurses must develop critical-thinking skills and become empowered.
- Beginning nursing students have multiple educational needs (e.g., students who have been out of secondary education for several years, single parents juggling numerous roles within the family, and students who speak English as a second language). Student nurses must learn how to study, manage their time effectively, and develop a positive mental attitude.
- Society is requiring higher educational standards within the professions that provide health-care services. Student nurses must maximize their acquisition of information in the affective, cognitive, and psychomotor domains to increase their success on standardized nursing examinations that require not merely the regurgitation of information but also the comprehension, application, or analysis of information.

Who Should Use This Book

- Students entering a nursing program
- Students who are preparing to take tests at the end of a unit of instruction in nursing or at the completion of a course in fundamentals of nursing
- Students in licensed practical nurse programs who are preparing for class tests, the NCLEX-PN examination, or advanced-standing examinations for entry into a registered nurse program
- Students preparing for the NCLEX-RN examination for licensure
- Licensed professional nurses preparing for a certification examination
- Nursing faculty members who are helping beginning nursing students achieve success in a nursing program
- Nursing faculty members who are designing a test-taking workshop for student nurses

Content in *Test Success* That Helps Students Maximize Success

Chapters 1 through 10 contain information designed to maximize success by helping students to:

- Develop a positive mental attitude
- Understand how critical thinking supports clinical reasoning
- Manage their time
- Study and learn more effectively
- Become test-wise by using the nursing process and test-taking techniques
- Explore all testing formats, specifically multiple-choice and alternate format questions (e.g., multiple response, hot spot, graphic illustration, exhibit, fill-in-the-blank, drag and drop [also called ordered response], audio, and video)
- Appreciate computer applications in nursing education and evaluation

    Chapter 11 contains 500 questions (over 230 alternate format items and more than 260 multiple-choice items) divided into 14 content areas common to nursing practice. The questions in each content area can be answered by a student at the completion of equivalent content in a nursing program.

    Chapter 12 contains a 100-question Comprehensive Final Book Exam. This test includes information from all 14 content areas addressed in Chapter 11. This test can be taken at the completion of a course in fundamentals of nursing. This test contains over 30 alternate format items and more than 60 multiple-choice items.

Every question in the book has rationales for the correct and incorrect options. These rationales should help the learner review some of the basic content in nursing theory as well as practice and contribute to the mastery of answering questions. In addition, the questions include a Test-Taking Tip, when appropriate, to emphasize one or more of the test-taking techniques presented in Chapter 7.

Terminology Used in the Text

- Throughout the book, "patient" is used to indicate the consumer of health care; "client" is used occasionally in questions related to community-based care; and "resident" is used occasionally for the consumer of care in the nursing home setting.
- "Nurse" is used consistently to indicate a licensed nurse. This individual may also be referred to by other titles such as "patient care coordinator" or "nurse manager."
- "Nurse's aide" and "nursing assistant" are used consistently to indicate credentialed or uncredentialed supportive nursing staff members. These individuals are sometimes referred to by other titles such as "patient care assistant," "nurse technician," or "comfort care associate."
- "Primary health-care provider" indicates health-care professionals with prescriptive privileges (e.g., nurse practitioners, physician's assistants, podiatrists, and dentists).

Self-Assessment Tools to Explore Personal Performance

Many tools are included to allow the student to perform self-assessments and ultimately improve time management, studying, and testing performance.

- **Chapter 3** presents three tools and an individualized corrective action plan to maximize productivity:
  - Assessment of Inconsistencies Between Values and Behavior
  - Personal Time/Activity Journal
  - Self-Assessment of Barriers to Productivity
  - Corrective Action Plan to Maximize Your Productivity
- **Chapter 10** presents two tools and an individualized corrective action guide:
  - Information-Processing Analysis
    - Processing Errors
    - Personal Performance Trends
  - Knowledge Analysis
  - Corrective Action Guide for Information Processing Analysis

DavisPlus

Visit http://www.davisplus.com to access **two additional 75-item Comprehensive Course Exit Exams**. The questions on these tests reflect information from the content areas presented in Chapter 11. Each 75-item test contains about 25 alternate format items and close to 50 multiple-choice items. These provide students with simulated comprehensive examinations on the computer. The earlier that nursing students practice taking comprehensive computerized tests, the better prepared they will be for the NCLEX examinations.

New Additions to *Test Success*, Seventh Edition

When the First Edition of *Test Success* was introduced, it was the only book that presented information to maximize the educational and testing performance of students in fundamentals of nursing courses. Most nursing examinations were paper-and-pencil tests and contained only multiple-choice questions. As nursing examinations changed, subsequent editions of *Test Success* evolved to be consistent with them. This edition continues this pattern. The Seventh Edition of *Test Success* is enriched by the following inclusions.

- Revision of questions to reflect the NCLEX examination questions with stems that ask a question, ending with a question mark (?).

- Every question in Chapter 11, Chapter 12, and the 2 Exit Exams on Davis*Plus*, when appropriate, contain a Test-Taking Tip.
- There are a total of 933 questions in the 7th edition of Test Success. Of the 933 questions, over 200 questions (28%) are new to reflect changes in standards of practice, CPR, and obstruction of the airway; higher cognitive–level questions; and alternate format items.
- 35.6% of the questions are alternate format items including approximately 25 hot spot, 30 drag and drop/ordered response, 170 multiple response, 20 graphic, 30 illustration, 30 fill-in-the-blank calculation, and 20 exhibit items.
- The Comprehensive Final Book Exam now contains 35 alternate format items and 65 multiple-choice items.
- Each 75 item Comprehensive Course Exit Exam now contains over 25 alternate format items and close to 50 multiple-choice items.

Contributors

Item Writers

Mary Ann Hellmer Saul, PhD, RN, CNE
Professor
Nassau Community College
Garden City, New York

Medical Consultant

Joanne M. Vitale, RPA-C
Physician Assistant
Romanelli Cosmetic Surgery
Huntington, New York
Huntington Hospital
North Shore LIJ Health System

Michael W. Mangino, Jr., RN, NP-Psychiatry
Associate Professor
Suffolk County Community College
Selden, New York

Reviewers

Carol Alexander
Palm Beach State College
Lake Worth, Florida

Billie Blake
St. Johns River State College
Orange Park, Florida

Laura Brennan
Elmhurst College
Elmhurst, Illinois

Pat Cannon
South University
Columbia, South Carolina

Cindi Eads
Holmes Community College
Ridgeland Campus
Ridgeland, Mississippi

Cris Finn
Regis University
Denver, Colorado

Elizabeth Kawecki
South University
Royal Palm Beach, Florida

Maxine Kron
Hinds Community College
Jackson, Mississippi

Margie Lafferty
Northampton Community College
Bethlehem, Pennsylvania

Beth Phillips
Duke University
Durham, North Carolina

Anita Reinhardt
New Mexico State University
Las Cruces, New Mexico

Amy Shennum
College of the Canyons
Santa Clarita, California

Becky Weatherly
Greenville Technical College
Greenville, South Carolina

Acknowledgments

Many people were essential to production of this revision. We want to give special thanks to Bob Martone, Publisher for Nursing, who has guided and supported us through the publication process, always being innovative and challenging us with new ideas. Our association has spanned over 23 years, and we value him not only as a colleague but also, most importantly, as a friend. We thank Terri Wood Allen, Acquisitions Editor, for her support and encouragement. We thank Jacalyn Clay and Julia Curcio, Content Project Managers, and Lisa Thompson, Production Editor, for their enthusiasm, competence, quick response to our questions, support, and for keeping the project on task. In addition, we appreciated the collaborative efforts of the expert and professional F.A. Davis team who ensured that this project progressed from a manuscript to a book, especially Holly Lukens (Copy Editor), Daniel Domzalski (Illustration Coordinator), Bob Butler (Production Manager), and Kristin Testa, Marketing Manager.

Special recognition goes to all the nursing students and faculty who participated in focus groups for their commitment to excellence and generosity in sharing their time, energy, and intellect. We thank our item writers, Dr. Mary Ann Hellmer Saul and Michael Mangino, for their contributions, Joanne Vitale for her expert review of the medical/surgical content, and all the reviewers for their expertise in examining the manuscript.

We give special thanks to our children and their spouses— Kelly and John Dall, and Heather and James McCormack, Joseph and Nicole Vitale, John and JoAnne Vitale, and Christopher and Whitney Vitale—for their love and support. We give particular thanks to our grandchildren, Sean, Ava, and Elle Dall; Aidan, Cade, and Ronan McCormack; and Joseph, Andie Grace, Andrew, Nathan, Alex, William, and James Vitale, who are the best stress reducers. They make our day.

Lastly we thank our husbands, Neil Nugent and Joseph Vitale, for their love, sense of humor, enthusiasm for life, and their attempts to keep our compulsive natures under control. Their support was critical to the completion of this revision, and they are loved and appreciated by us.

Patricia M. Nugent
Barbara A. Vitale

Contents

How to Use This Book to Maximize Success

It is amazing what **you** can achieve when **you** are tenacious, organized, and determined to attain a goal. By purchasing this book, **you** have demonstrated a beginning commitment to do what **you** have to do to improve your success in nursing examinations. This book is designed to introduce **you** to various techniques that can contribute to a positive mental attitude, promote the development of critical-thinking skills, and help **you** become test-wise. If you are beginning to get the feeling that **"you"** is an important word, **"you"** are right! Learning requires you to be an active participant in your own learning. Your ultimate success can be maximized if you progress through this book in a planned and organized fashion and are willing to practice the techniques suggested. Effort is directly correlated with the benefits you will derive from this book. After you have determined that you are eager and motivated to learn, you are ready to begin.

Chapter content is organized in a specific order to provide you with skills that will contribute to your success when taking a nursing examination.

Chapter 1: Empowerment—Develop a positive mental attitude.

Chapter 2: Critical Thinking—Maximize your critical-thinking abilities.

Chapter 3: Time Management—Use self-assessment tools to maximize your use of time.
- Assessment of Inconsistencies Between Values and Behavior
- Personal Time/Activity Journal
- Self-Assessment of Barriers to Productivity
- Corrective Action Plan to Maximize Your Productivity

Chapter 4: Study Techniques—Use general and specific study techniques to increase your ability to recall, understand, apply, and analyze information when answering nursing examination questions.

Chapter 5: The Multiple-Choice Question—Improve your understanding of the components of a multiple-choice question: the first part that asks a question (stem) and the second part that presents potential answers (options).

Chapter 6: The Nursing Process—Expand your ability to identify the focus of a nursing examination question within the framework of the nursing process to better understand what the question is asking.

Chapter 7: Test-Taking Techniques—Learn to use specific test-taking techniques to critically analyze the stem and options in a multiple-choice question.

Chapter 8: Testing Formats Other Than Multiple-Choice Questions—Increase your ability to analyze and answer alternate format items (fill-in-the-blank calculation, hot spot, graphic and illustration, drag and drop/ordered response, multiple response, exhibit) that appear on the NCLEX examination.

Chapter 9: Computer Applications in Education and Evaluation—Increase your understanding that you must become an active participant in the use of computers in education, evaluation, and the clinical setting.

Chapter 10: Analyze Your Test Performance—Use self-assessment tools to identify what you know, what you need to know, your information processing errors, your personal performance trends, and how you can correct information-processing errors.
- Information Process Analysis
  - Processing Errors
  - Personal Performance Trends
- Knowledge Analysis
- Corrective Action Guide for Information-Processing Errors

Chapter 11: Practice Questions With Answers and Rationales—Practice answering 500 nursing questions, 46% (232 items) of which are alternate format items reflective of the NCLEX examination. The questions are divided into 14 content areas common to fundamentals of nursing practice. Every question has the rationale for the correct answer and the incorrect options to reinforce fundamentals of nursing theory and principles. The majority of questions have one or more Test-Taking Tips identical to the tips presented in Chapter 7.

Chapter 12: Comprehensive Final Book Exam—Practice taking a comprehensive 100-item test, 35% (35 items) of which are alternate format items reflective of the NCLEX examination. This test incorporates information from the 14 content areas in Chapter 11. Every question has the rationale for the correct answer and the incorrect options to reinforce fundamentals of nursing theory and principles. The majority of questions have one or more Test-Taking Tips identical to the tips presented in Chapter 7.

DavisPlus: Comprehensive Course Exam I and II—Practice taking two 75-item comprehensive examinations that incorporate information from the 14 content areas in Chapter 11; 36% (27 items) of each 75-item exam includes alternate format items reflective of the NCLEX examination. Every question has the rationale for the correct answer and the incorrect options to reinforce fundamentals of nursing theory and principles. The majority of questions have one or more Test-Taking Tips identical to the tips presented in Chapter 7.

To use this book to its best advantage, read Chapters 1 through 10. Then answer the questions in Chapter 11. Be sure to study the rationales, because this information will review and reinforce the material you are learning in your fundamentals of nursing course. To maximize learning, it is suggested that you answer the questions in the specific categories in Chapter 11 after you have learned the content in class. Then take the Comprehensive Course Exit Exam I on DavisPlus. Immediately after taking the exam, evaluate your performance using the tools presented in Chapter 10. This analysis will help you identify information-processing errors, personal performance trends, and knowledge deficits, and provide suggestions for corrective action. After you have followed your individualized corrective action plan to maximize your strengths and minimize your weaknesses, take the Comprehensive Course Exit Exam II on DavisPlus. Again, evaluate your performance using the self-assessment tools in Chapter 10. By this time, you should have expanded your knowledge and abilities, and your performance should have improved. Although it is suggested that you take Exam I and Exam II in sequence, the order in which you take them does not matter. Finally, take the Comprehensive Final Book Exam in Chapter 12. Again, evaluate your performance using the self-assessment tools in Chapter 10, and use the corrective action plan to focus your study. The self-assessment tools should be used not only in conjunction with this book but also to analyze your performance after every test you take in your nursing course.

You should be commended for your efforts to achieve success. It is hard work to take responsibility for your own learning. The magnitude of your learning will be in direct proportion to the amount of energy you are willing to expend in the effort to improve your skills. You will become a more successful test taker when you:

- Function from a position of strength
- Think critically
- Manage your time
- Study more effectively
- Become test-wise
- Are able to apply the nursing process to determine what the question is asking
- Practice test taking
- Analyze your test performance

MUCH SUCCESS ON YOUR NURSING EXAMINATIONS!

Empowerment

DEVELOP A POSITIVE MENTAL ATTITUDE

A positive mental attitude can help you control test anxiety by limiting anxious responses so that you can be a more successful test taker. A positive mental attitude requires you to function from a position of strength. This does not imply that you have to be powerful, manipulative, or dominant. What it does require is that you develop techniques that put you in control of your own thoughts and behavior. To be in control of yourself, you should operate from a position of positive self-worth with a feeling of empowerment. This begins with self-assessment.

You have both strengths and weaknesses. Both should be identified to maximize your potential. Strengths are easy to focus on because you feel safe and nonthreatened. Weaknesses are more difficult to focus on because you may feel inadequate and uncomfortable. When performing a self-assessment, be honest with yourself. You must separate your ego from your assessment. Only you will know the result. Remember, few people are perfect! Have the courage to be honest with yourself and identify your imperfections. You can have weaknesses and imperfections and still have a positive self-concept.

To develop self-worth, you must be willing to look within yourself and appreciate that you are valuable. Acting from a position of strength requires you to start saying and believing that you are worthwhile. Self-worth increases when you believe, down to your very core, that you are important.

A feeling of empowerment increases when you are able to use all your available resources and learned strategies to achieve your goals. To achieve empowerment, you need to develop techniques and skills that not only make you feel in control but actually position you in control. When you are in control, you function from a position of strength.

To achieve a sense of self-worth and a feeling of empowerment that will help you succeed in test taking, you must learn various techniques that should be practiced before taking the test. These techniques will help you to control stressful situations, reduce anxious responses, and enhance concentration, thereby improving your analytical and problem-solving abilities and strengthening your test performance. By learning and practicing the following techniques, you will have a foundation on which to operate from a position of strength.

Establish a Positive Internal Locus of Control

Henry Ford once said, "Whether you think you can, or think you can't . . . you're right." In other words, what you *think* can be a self-fulfilling prophecy. The way you talk to yourself influences the way you think about yourself. The content of what you say indicates how you feel about the control of your behavior and your life. "I was lucky to pass that test." "I could not help failing because the teacher is hard." "I got test anxiety, and I just became paralyzed during the test." Each of these internal dialogues indicates that you see yourself as powerless. When you say these things, you fail to take control.

Identify your pattern of talking to yourself. Do you blame others, attribute failure to external causes, and use the words "I couldn't," "I should," "I need," or "I have to"? If you do, then you are using language that places you in a position of impotence, dependence, defenselessness, and hopelessness. YOU MUST ESTABLISH A POSITIVE INTERNAL LOCUS OF CONTROL. You do this by replacing this language with language that reflects control and strength. You must say, "I want," "I can," and "I will." When you use these words, you imply that you are committed to a task until you succeed. Place index cards around your environment with "I WANT," "I CAN," and "I WILL" on them to cue you into a positive pattern of talking to yourself.

Challenge Negative Thoughts

Your value as an individual should not be linked to how well you do on an examination. Your self-worth and your test score are distinctly isolated entities. If you believe that you are good when you do well on a test and bad when you do poorly, you must alter your thinking. You need to work at recognizing that this is illogical thinking. Illogical or negative thinking is self-destructive. Negative thoughts must be changed into positive thoughts to build confidence and self-worth. As confidence and self-worth increase, anxiety can be controlled and minimized.

Positive thinking focuses your attention on your desired outcomes. If you think you can do well on a test, you are more likely to fulfill this prophecy. It is critical that you control negative thoughts by developing a positive mental attitude. When you say to yourself, "This is going to be a hard test. I'll never pass," CHALLENGE THIS STATEMENT. Instead, say to yourself, "This is a ridiculous statement. Of course I can pass this test. All I have to do is study hard!" It is crucial that you challenge negative thoughts with optimistic thoughts. Optimistic thoughts are valuable because they can be converted into positive actions and feelings, thus placing you in a position of control.

For this technique to work, you must first stop negative thoughts. To use the technique called ARREST NEGATIVE THOUGHTS, you should identity the pattern of negative thinking that you use to defend yourself. After you identify a negative thought, envision a police car with flashing lights that signifies ARREST NEGATIVE THOUGHTS. You can even place pictures of police cars around your environment to cue you to ARREST NEGATIVE THOUGHTS. After you identify negative thoughts, handcuff them and lock them away so that they will no longer be a threat. Actually envision negative thoughts locked up in a cell with bars and yourself throwing away the key.

After you stop a negative thought, replace it with a POSITIVE THOUGHT. If you have difficulty identifying a positive thought, praise yourself or give yourself a compliment. Tell yourself, "Wow! I am really working hard to pass this test." "Congratulations! I was able to arrest that negative thought and be in control." To increase control, make an inventory of the things you can do, the things you want to achieve, and the feelings you want to feel that contribute to a positive mental attitude. Throughout the day take an "attitude inventory." Identify the status of your mental attitude. If it is not consistent with your list of the feelings you want to feel or the positive image you have of yourself, CHALLENGE YOUR ATTITUDE. Compose statements that support the feelings that you want to feel and read them over and over. Such statements might include "I can pass this test!" or "I am in control of my attitudes, and my attitudes are positive!" Make sure that you end the day with a positive thought, and even identify something that you want to accomplish the next day. Forecasting positive events establishes a positive direction in which you can focus your attention.

Use Controlled Breathing (Diaphragmatic Breathing)

An excellent way to reduce feelings of anxiety is to use the technique of controlled breathing. When you control your breathing, you can break the pattern of shallow short breaths associated with anxious feelings. Abdominal or diaphragmatic breathing enhances the relaxation response. When a person exhales, tense muscles tend to relax. You probably do this now unconsciously. Most people take a deep breath and exhale (sigh) several times an hour.

When you "sigh," it is a form of diaphragmatic breathing. Diaphragmatic breathing causes the diaphragm to flatten and the abdomen to expand outward on inspiration. On exhalation, the abdominal muscles contract. As you slowly let out this deep breath, the other muscles of the body tend to "let go" and relax. This technique enables you to breathe more deeply than if you just inflate your chest on inspiration. Controlled breathing can be helpful to reduce anxious responses that occur at the beginning of a test, when you are stumped by a tough question, or when you are nearing the end of the test. During these critical times you can use controlled breathing to induce the relaxation response.

When practicing diaphragmatic breathing, place your hands lightly over the front of the lower ribs and upper abdomen so that you can monitor the movement you are trying to achieve. As you become accomplished in this technique, you will not need to position your hands on your body. Practice the following steps:

1. Gently position your hands over the front of your lower ribs and upper abdomen.
2. Exhale gently and fully. Feel your ribs and abdomen sink inward toward the middle of your body.
3. Slowly inhale, taking a deep breath through your nose and expanding your abdomen first and then your chest. Do this as you slowly count to four.
4. Hold your breath at the height of inhalation as you count to four.
5. Exhale fully by contracting your abdominal muscles and then your chest. Let out all the air slowly and smoothly through your mouth as you count to eight.

Monitor the pace of your breathing. Notice how your muscles relax each time you exhale. You may feel warm, tingly, and relaxed. Enjoy the feeling as you breathe deeply and evenly. You should practice this technique so that controlled breathing automatically induces the relaxation response after several breaths. After you are able to induce the relaxation response with controlled breathing, you can effectively draw on this strategy when you need to be in control.

It is important not to do this exercise too forcefully or too rapidly because it can cause you to hyperventilate. Hyperventilation may cause dizziness and light-headedness. If either of these occurs, cup your hands over your nose and mouth and slowly rebreathe your exhaled air. These symptoms should subside. Then you can continue the exercise less vigorously. Always monitor your responses throughout the exercise.

Desensitize Yourself to the Fear Response

Individuals generally connect a certain feeling with a specific situation. To learn to control your feelings, you must first recognize how you consider and visualize events. It is not uncommon to connect a feeling of fear with an event. In a testing situation, the examination is the event and the response of fear is the feeling. If this happens to you, then you must interrupt this fear response. You have the ability to control how you respond to fear. When you are able to separate the event from the feeling, you will establish control and become empowered. However, establishing control does not happen automatically. You need to desensitize yourself to the event to control the fear response.

Desensitization involves repeatedly exposing yourself to the identified emotionally distressing event in a limited and/or controlled setting until the event no longer precipitates the feeling of fear. Desensitization is dependent on associating relaxation with the fear response. To achieve this response, you should practice the following routine:

First, you must practice a relaxation response. Controlled breathing, an excellent relaxation technique, has already been described. After you are comfortable with the technique of controlled breathing, you can use it in the desensitization routine.

Second, you should make a list of five events associated with a testing situation that cause fear and rank them, starting with the one that causes the most anxiety and progressing to the one that causes the least anxiety. The following is an example:

1. Taking an important examination on difficult material
2. Taking an important examination on material you know well

3. Taking a small quiz on difficult material
4. Taking a small quiz on material you know well
5. Taking a practice test that does not count

Event number 5 should evoke the least amount of fear.
Third, you should practice the following routine:

1. Practice controlled breathing and become relaxed.
2. Now imagine event number 5. If you feel fearful, turn off the scene and go back to controlled breathing for about 30 seconds.
3. After you are relaxed, again imagine scene number 5. Try to visualize the event for 30 seconds without becoming uncomfortable.
4. After you have accomplished the previous step, move up the list of events until you are able to imagine event number 1 without feeling uncomfortable.

When you are successful in controlling the fear response in an imagined situation, you can attempt to accomplish the same success in simulated tests at home. After you are successful in controlling the fear response in simulated tests at home, you can take some simulated tests in a classroom setting. Continue practicing desensitization until you have a feeling of control in an actual testing situation. This may take practice. It will not be accomplished in one practice session.

Another way you can use the concept of desensitization is to practice positive dialogue within yourself. For example, imagine the following internal dialogue within yourself:

"How am I feeling about the examination today?"	"A little uncomfortable and fearful."
"Do I want to feel this way?"	"Absolutely not!"
"How do I want to feel?"	"I want to feel calm, in control, and effective."
"What am I going to do to achieve that feeling?"	"I am going to practice relaxation and controlled breathing."

You might be saying to yourself, "I don't see myself doing this. This is silly." The resilient and tenacious individual who is flexible and willing to try new techniques is in a position of control. If your goal is to be empowered, then you have only to be open and willing to learn.

Perform Muscle Relaxation

The muscle relaxation technique involves learning how to tense and relax each muscle group of your body until all of your muscle groups are relaxed. This technique requires practice. Initially you must assume a comfortable position and then sequentially contract and relax each muscle group in your body from your head to your toes. When a muscle group is tensed and then released, the muscles relax. It is not a technique that can be quickly described in a short paragraph. However, the following brief exercise is included as an example:

Find a comfortable chair in a quiet place. Close your eyes and use diaphragmatic breathing, taking several deep breaths to relax. You are now ready to begin progressive muscle relaxation. Sequentially, move from one muscle group in the body to another, contracting and relaxing each for 10 seconds. After each muscle group is tensed and then relaxed, take a deep, slow breath using diaphragmatic breathing. As you are relaxing, observe how you feel. Experience the sensation. You may want to reinforce the feeling of relaxation by saying, "My muscles are relaxing. I can feel the tension flowing out of my muscles." Remember not to breathe too forcefully to avoid hyperventilation. The following is a sample of muscle groups that should be included in a progressive muscle relaxation routine:

1. Bend your head and try to rest your right ear as close as you can to your right shoulder. Count to 10. Assume normal alignment, relax, and take a deep breath.
2. Bend your head and try to rest your left ear as close as you can to your left shoulder. Count to 10. Assume normal alignment, relax, and take a deep breath.
3. Flex your head and try to touch your chin to your chest. Count to 10. Assume normal alignment, relax, and take a deep breath.
4. Make a fist and tense your right forearm. Count to 10. Relax and take a deep breath.
5. Make a fist and tense your left forearm. Count to 10. Relax and take a deep breath.
6. Tense your right biceps by tightly bending (flexing) the right arm at the elbow. Count to 10. Relax and take a deep breath.

Continue moving from the head to the arms, trunk, and legs by contracting and relaxing each of the muscle groups within these areas of your body. You can understand and master this technique by obtaining a product that is designed to direct and instruct you through the entire routine of tensing and relaxing each muscle group. The muscle relaxation technique should be practiced every day until it becomes natural. After you have mastered this technique, you can use a shortened version of progressive relaxation along with controlled breathing at critical times during a test.

Use Imagery

Using imagery can help you to establish a state of relaxation. When we remember a fearful event, our heart and respiratory rates increase just as they did when the event occurred. Similarly, when we recall a happy, relaxing period, we can regenerate and re-create the atmosphere and feeling that we had during that pleasant event. Using imagery is not a difficult technique to master. Just let go and enjoy the experience.

Position yourself in a comfortable chair, close your eyes, and construct an image in your mind of a place that makes you feel calm, happy, and relaxed. It may be at the seashore or in a field of wildflowers. Let your mind picture what is happening. Observe the colors of the landscape. Notice the soothing sounds of the environment. Notice the smells in the air, the shapes of objects, and movement about you. Recall the positive feelings that flow over you when you are in that scene and relax. You can now open your eyes relaxed, refreshed, and calm.

At critical times during a test, you can take a few minutes to use imagery to induce the relaxation response. To successfully reduce stress, you must position yourself in control. When you are in control, your test performance generally improves.

Overprepare for a Test

One of the best ways to reduce text anxiety is to be overprepared. The more prepared you are to take the test, the more confident you will be. The more confident you are, the more able you are to challenge the fear of being unprepared. Study the textbook, read your notes, take practice tests, and prepare with other students in a study group. Even when you think that you know the information, study the same information again to reinforce your learning. For this technique to be successful, you should plan a significant amount of time for studying. Although it is time-consuming, it does build confidence and reduce anxiety. No one has said that learning is easy. Any worthwhile goal deserves the effort necessary to achieve success. Being overprepared is the BEST way to place yourself in a position of strength.

Consider the following scenario. A student was not doing well in school and asked what she could do to improve her performance. The concept of being overprepared was discussed, and she worked out a study schedule of 2 hours a day for 2 weeks before the next test. After the test, the student said that she thought she did well because the test was easy. It had to be pointed out that she perceived the test as easy because she had attained the knowledge that enabled her to answer the questions correctly. Her eyes lit up as if someone had turned on a lightbulb over her head! When you recognize that you have the opportunity to be in control and take responsibility for your own learning, you become all that you can be.

Exercise Regularly

Exercising regularly helps you to expend nervous energy. Walking, aerobic exercise, swimming, bike riding, or running at least three times a week for 20 minutes is an effective way to maintain or improve your physical and mental status. The most important thing to remember about regular exercise is to slowly increase the degree and duration of the exercise. Your exercise program should not be so rigorous that it leaves you exhausted. It should serve to clear your mind and make you mentally alert and better able to cope with the challenge of a test. Exercise should not be performed just before going to bed because it can interfere with sleep. Regular exercise should become a routine activity in your weekly schedule, not just a response to the tension of an upcoming test. After you establish a regular exercise program, you should experience physical and psychological benefits.

ESTABLISH CONTROL BEFORE AND DURING THE TEST

It is important to maximize your opportunities to feel in control in the testing situation. Additional techniques you can use to establish a tranquil and composed atmosphere require you to take control of your testing equipment, your activities before and during a test, and your immediate physical space. Techniques to help create this atmosphere are reinforced in Chapter 7, Test-Taking Techniques. However, they are also discussed here because they can be used to reduce anxiety and promote empowerment.

Manage Your Daily Routine Before the Test

It is important to maintain your usual daily routine the day of the test. Eat what you usually eat, but avoid food and beverages with caffeine. Caffeine can lessen your attention span and reduce your concentration by overstimulating your metabolism. Avoid the urge to stay up late the night before a test. If you are tired when taking a test, your ability to concentrate and solve problems may be limited. Go to bed at your regular time. Following your usual routines can be relaxing and can contribute to a feeling of control.

Manage Your Study Habits Before the Test

Do not stay up late studying the night before the big test. Squeezing in last-minute studying may increase anxiety and contribute to feelings of powerlessness and helplessness. DO NOT CRAM. If you have implemented a study routine in preparation for the test, then you should have confidence in what you have learned. Establish control by saying to yourself, "I have studied hard for this test and I am well prepared. I can relax tonight because I know the material for the test tomorrow and I will do well." Avoid giving in to the desire to cram. Instead, use the various techniques discussed earlier in this chapter to maintain a positive mental attitude.

Manage Your Travel the Day of the Test

Plan to arrive early the day of the test. It is important to plan for potential events that can delay you, such as traffic jams or a flat tire. The more important the test, the more time you should schedule for travel. If you live a substantial distance from the testing site, you might ask another student who lives closer to allow you to sleep over the night before the test. The midterm or final examination for a course may be held in a different location than the regularly scheduled classroom used for the lecture. If you are unfamiliar with the examination room, make a practice run to locate where it is and note how long it takes to get there. Nothing produces more anxiety than rushing to a test or arriving after the start of a test. A feeling of control reduces tension and the fear response. You can be in control if you manage your travel time with time to spare.

Manage the Supplies You Need for the Test

The more variables you have control over, the more calm and relaxed you will feel. Compose a list of the items to bring with you to the test. Sometimes the supplies that can be used are stipulated by the institution giving the test. They may include pencils, pens, scrap paper, erasers, a ruler, a watch, and even a lucky charm. It is suggested that you collect the items the day before the test. This eliminates a task that you do not have to perform on the day of the test and contributes to your sense of control. Some testing sites do not permit the presence of any personal items. This includes venues for nurse licensure examinations.

Manage Your Personal Comfort

Maslow's Hierarchy of Needs specifies that basic physiological needs must be met before you attempt to meet higher-level needs. Be aware of your own basic needs relating to factors such as nutrition, elimination, and physical comfort. Meet these basic needs before the test because unfulfilled needs will compete for your attention. For example, arrive early so that you can visit the restroom; wear layers of clothing so that you can adjust to various environmental temperatures; and eat a light, balanced meal to maintain your blood glucose level. Once these basic needs are met, then you can progress up the ladder of needs to self-actualization.

Manage the Test Environment

When you arrive early, you generally have the choice of where to sit in the room. This contributes to a feeling of control because you are able to sit where you are most comfortable. You might prefer to sit by a window, near a heat source, or in the back of the room. Generally, it helps to sit near the administrator of the test. Directions may be heard more clearly, and the administrator's attention may be gained more easily if you have a question. It is wise to avoid sitting by a door. The commotion made by people entering or exiting the room can be a distraction and interfere with your ability to concentrate. Take every opportunity to control your environment. Measures that help you feel in control contribute to a positive mental attitude.

Maintain a Positive Mental Attitude

Remind yourself of how hard you worked and how well prepared you are to take this test. ESTABLISH CONTROL by arresting negative thoughts and focusing on the positive. Say to yourself, "I am ready for this test! I will do well on this test! I can get an 'A' on this test!" These statements support a positive mental attitude and enhance a feeling of control.

Manage Your Physical and Emotional Responses

At critical times during the test, you may feel nervous, your breathing may become rapid and shallow, or you may draw a blank on a question. Stop and take a minibreak. Use controlled breathing to induce the relaxation response. You may also use a shortened version of progressive relaxation exercises to induce the relaxation response. Daily practice of breathing and relaxation exercises will enable you to quickly induce the relaxation response during times of stress. After these techniques are implemented, you should feel in control and empowered.

SUMMARY

The techniques described in this chapter are designed to increase your mastery over the stress of the testing situation. When you feel positive about yourself and have a strong self-image and a feeling of self-worth, you will develop a sense of control. When you are able to draw on various techniques that empower you to respond to the testing situation with a sense of calm, you will improve your effectiveness. Use these techniques along with the other skills suggested in this book, practice the questions, and take the simulated practice tests as instructed in the section "How to Use This Book to Maximize Success" at the beginning of this text. These activities will support your self-worth, provide you with a feeling of control, and increase your effectiveness in the testing situation.

Critical Thinking

2

If your ultimate goal is to become a competent nurse, first you have to identify what knowledge base and skills are required to achieve this goal. Study skills, critical-thinking skills, and problem-solving skills are essential to achieve success as a learner. Your goal should be to develop skills that support your ability to use reasoning and not just react by rote (a fixed, routine, mechanical way of doing something). Several chapters in this book are designed to assist you in the journey toward this goal. General and specific study skills are addressed in Chapter 4; the nursing process as a problem-solving process is addressed in Chapter 6; and critical-thinking skills are addressed in this chapter. No one can argue with the statement that a nurse must be a safe, qualified, and technically proficient practitioner. Consumers of nursing care are most aware of the actions (psychomotor skills) that nurses engage in and generally rate the quality of nursing care in relation to the degree to which their expectations are satisfied. However, the quality of nursing care is based on more than just what the nurse does. It also is based on how the nurse thinks (cognitive skills) in relation to how conclusions are drawn, decisions are made, and problems are resolved.

Thinking is the hardest work there is, which is the probable reason why so few engage in it.

—HENRY FORD

The thinking skills that rarely are recognized by the consumer, such as reflecting, clarifying, analyzing, and reasoning, are crucial to the development of a competent nurse. Historically, critical thinking in nursing was associated just with the nursing process (assessment, analysis/diagnosis, planning, implementation, and evaluation). This theoretical framework, which is used to identify and attain solutions to complex problems, is the foundation for nursing education, practice, and research. It is a systematic, orderly, step-by-step progression with a beginning and an end (linear format). Clinical decision making in relation to the nursing process produces a nursing care plan or "product." In Chapter 6 the steps in the nursing process are addressed and many sample items are provided that demonstrate application of information within the context of the nursing process.

Because nursing entails more than just the solving of problems, the concept of critical thinking as a "process" is receiving increasing attention. Various researchers believe that critical thinking in nursing is more than just a behavioral, task-oriented, linear approach demonstrated in problem solving and that critical thinking should be based on an emancipatory model. Emancipatory models embrace the concept of empowerment and autonomous action stemming from critical insights. These models stress critical thinking as a process rather than just a method of producing a product or solution.

DEFINITION OF CRITICAL THINKING

Leaders in the field of nursing do not agree on any one definition of critical thinking. However, the following excerpts may enhance your understanding of the concept. Chaffee (2015) explains that "the process of thinking critically involves thinking for ourselves by carefully examining the way that we make sense of the world." He further explains that as humans we have an ability to reflect back on what we are thinking, doing, or feeling; this reflection makes us more effective thinkers. Alfaro-LeFevre (2009) summarized that critical thinking:

- Entails purposeful, goal-directed thinking
- Aims to make clinical judgments based on evidence (fact) rather than conjecture (guesswork)
- Is based on principles of science and the scientific method
- Requires strategies that maximize *human potential* and compensate for problems caused by *human nature*. Alfaro-LeFevre (2011) further indicated that the word *reasoning* could be used as a synonym for critical thinking because it implies careful, deliberate thought.

The Delphi Research Project characterized the ideal critical thinker as one who is habitually inquisitive, well informed, trustful of reason, open-minded in evaluation, honest in facing personal biases, prudent in making judgments, willing to reconsider, clear about issues, orderly in complex matters, diligent in seeking relevant information, reasonable in the selection of criteria, focused in inquiry, and persistent in seeking results that are as precise as the subject and the circumstances of inquiry permit (American Philosophical Association, 1990).

Brookfield (1991) described four components of critical thinking: identifying and challenging assumptions, becoming aware of the importance of context in creating meaning, imagining and exploring alternatives, and cultivating a reflective skepticism.

Pless (1993) identified these critical-thinking cognitive skills and subskills as essential for critical thinking:

- Interpretation—categorization, decoding significance, and clarifying meaning
- Analysis—examining ideas, identifying arguments, and analyzing arguments
- Evaluation—assessing claims and assessing arguments
- Inference—querying evidence, conjecturing alternatives, and drawing conclusions
- Explanation—stating results, justifying procedures, and presenting arguments
- Self-regulation—self-examination and self-correction

CRITICAL THINKING IN NURSING

Nursing requires not only the learning of facts and procedures but also the ability to evaluate each unique patient situation. In Chapter 4, Study Techniques, a section titled "Specific Study Techniques Related to Cognitive Levels of Nursing Questions" addresses the variety of thinking processes—knowledge, comprehension, application, and analysis—that the nurse uses when managing data and identifying and meeting a patient's needs.

Because these thinking processes are important to both the process and product inherent in nursing care, multiple-choice questions in Chapter 4 are designed to test your knowledge base, comprehension of information, application of theory and principles, and analytical ability. In all but knowledge-type questions, intellectual skills that involve more than just the recall of information are required. In comprehension-type questions, you are required to translate, interpret, and determine the implications, consequences, and corollaries of the effects of information. In application-type questions you are required to use information in a new situation. In analysis-type questions you must interpret a variety of data and recognize the commonalities, differences, and interrelationships among the ideas presented. Numerous sample items in Chapter 4 challenge your analytical abilities, address the cognitive domains, and demonstrate the concepts being presented.

An understanding of the nursing process and the cognitive domains is important; however, critical-thinking skills must be developed if you are going to be a successful thinker and, ultimately, an expert nurse. The first step is to build a foundation of knowledge and information that eventually can be applied in clinical situations.

Both minds and fountain pens will work when filled. but minds, like fountain pens, must first be filled.

—ARTHUR GUITERMAN

Before you can apply knowledge, you need to know what needs to be known and how the knowledge can be applied. Therefore, you must ask yourself serious questions, such as: "What do I know?" "What do I need to know?" "What do I have to do to know it?" This is a new activity for some students. It can be threatening and even anxiety producing. It is not easy to acknowledge the degree of your own lack of knowledge or ignorance, and it can be a sobering experience.

The more I know I know, I know the less.

—ROBERT OWEN

Therefore, to fill voids in your knowledge you need to study. Avoid the pitfall of being a superficial thinker. This type of thinker devotes excessive time to memorization and rote learning. Become a deep thinker.

Many bring rakes but few shovels.

—FRANK C. BROWN

A deep thinker develops a thorough understanding of the material studied. In Chapter 4, Study Techniques, strategies are discussed that will help you answer some of the questions raised in this chapter and study more effectively and efficiently.

After you know basic information, you are better able to recognize the significance of cue data. Nursing questions are carefully designed to test your knowledge and comprehension of information regarding key concepts and your ability to analyze and apply this information in various situations. As you move from being a neophyte to a more experienced student, you are more able to identify the significance of cues and respond readily in all situations, whether in a laboratory setting, in a computer simulation, in a clinical setting, or on a test. In nursing questions, you must recognize the key words and concepts being tested in the question. They require that you ask, "What is happening?" and "What should I do?" Before you can answer these questions, it is helpful to identify the information processing style you use when confronted with a situation that requires a response.

Left-Hemisphere and Right-Hemisphere Brain Information Processing

Taggart and Torrance (1984) explored left- and right-hemisphere information processing and found that individuals who used **left-hemisphere information processing functions** used rational problem-solving strategies and logical sequencing. Rational learners break down situations into components and look for universal rules and approaches that can be applied in all situations. Individuals who used **right-hemisphere information processing functions** looked for main ideas to establish relationships that can be abstracted as the foundation for intuitive problem solving. The intuitive learner first learns from context and experience and then applies and analyzes principles. Additional research in this area demonstrates that, although both the novice and the expert use logical and rational problem-solving strategies, it is the expert who uses a broad range of thinking skills that integrate both logical and intuitive thinking to address facts and feelings to achieve accurate decision making.

Clinical Judgments

Clinical judgments are conclusions or enlightened opinions arrived at after using reasoning or critical thinking. The ability to build a foundation of data, inferences, and hypotheses for nursing decision making is dependent on your ability to use several types of clinical judgments. **Perceptual judgments** are judgments that you make regarding the data you need to collect and the validation of the importance of the data you collect within the context of the situation. **Inferential judgments** are judgments that you make when you determine which data are significant, eliminate data that are insignificant, and identify the relationship that exists among the data collected. **Diagnostic judgments** are judgments that you make when you link clusters of data with patterns affiliated with a specific nursing diagnosis.

Levels of Critical Thinking

As your knowledge of theory and experience increases, you will be constructing a scientific foundation to support critical thinking and clinical decision making. When developing critical-thinking skills, you will advance through three levels of competence: basic, complex, and expert. As a student, you are a basic-level critical thinker. As a **basic-level critical thinker,** you are building a novice's database of information and experiential knowledge. When you are confronted with a situation, initially your response is based on recall and rote memory. You tend to guide your responses by rules and procedures and seek concrete actions. You reduce situations to their distinct and independent parts. For example, when applying a simple dry, sterile dressing for an abdominal wound with approximated edges (healing by primary intention), you may use a procedure book and follow each step as outlined. As you acquire more knowledge and experience, you will advance from a basic-level thinker to a complex-level thinker. As a **complex-level thinker,** you will be guided by the need to explore options based on principles and patterns and an understanding of commonalities and differences. Your response will begin to be based on the ability to identify cue data, analyze clustered information, sort and choose the most appropriate action, and evaluate the patient's response. For example, when performing a sterile dressing for an open wound where the edges are not readily approximated (healing by secondary intention), you may need to modify the procedure. Depending on the situation, you may reposition the patient, use additional sterile equipment, or irrigate the wound. The more knowledge and experience you gain, the more solid the connections between your knowledge base and the application of that knowledge will become. You are now becoming an expert critical thinker. As an **expert critical thinker,** you will develop reasoning based on models, patterns, and standards associated with the "uniqueness" and "wholeness" of each situation. For example, when performing a sterile dressing on a large, gaping wound that is purposely left open (healing by tertiary intention), critical thinking will require a higher level of sophistication. You will need to consider concepts such as dehiscence, evisceration, fistula formation, sinus tracking, undermining, presence of infection, necrosis, factors that impair or facilitate wound healing, and dressing alternatives. The expert views the situation from an entire perspective that can be accomplished only with a broad and deep knowledge base and experience.

All critical thinkers should be asking, "What is wrong?" "Why?" "How?" "What else?" "What if?" and even "So what!" However, at each successive level of critical thinking the degree of sophistication required to explore these questions increases. These questions need to be asked when studying, when faced with a clinical situation (whether simulated or real), and when challenged by a test question. As a beginning nursing student, you are a novice, not an expert! Nursing school is several years long for a purpose. Be realistic with your self-expectations. It takes time to acquire and integrate the knowledge and experience necessary to be an expert critical thinker.

PRACTICE CRITICAL THINKING

You first learned how to turn over, crawl, stand, walk, and then run by practicing balance and building strength and endurance. You also must learn and practice critical-thinking and problem-solving skills until you are proficient in using these skills and can respond accurately and achieve your goal of being an expert critical thinker. For you to be able to tap your critical-thinking skills when taking an examination these skills must be well entrenched in your approach to all professional endeavors.

Strategies to Employ in Critical Thinking

When challenged by any patient situation, you should employ these strategies:

- Identify assumptions.
- Use a method to collect and organize information.
- Validate the accuracy and reliability of collected information.
- Determine the significance of collected information.
- Determine inconsistencies in collected information.
- Identify commonalities and differences.
- Identify patterns of patient responses.
- Identify stressors and common responses to stressors.
- Identify discrepancies or gaps in information.
- Cluster information to determine relationships.
- Make inferences based on collected information.
- Identify actual problems and patients who may be at risk for problems.
- Establish priorities (Maslow's Hierarchy of Needs is an excellent model to use to achieve this goal).
- Formulate specific, patient-centered, realistic, measurable goals with a time frame.
- Identify appropriate nursing actions.
- Evaluate outcomes.
- Evaluate and modify critical-thinking activities.

This list of strategies reflects sophisticated, deep thinking. Critical thinking is a type of highly developed thinking and a learned skill. The learner must be actively involved in the learning process. Critical thinking cannot be memorized; it must be practiced.

Knowledge is a treasure, but practice is the key to it.

—THOMAS FULLER

Activities to Improve Critical Thinking

To develop or refine thinking that can become more critical, it is suggested that you engage in the following activities while incorporating the strategies previously listed.

THINKING ALOUD

The proficient thinker verbalizes thought processes and rationales. The actual expression of thoughts in words helps to clarify and solidify thinking. Thinking aloud can be used while you are engaged in an activity that does not involve a patient or later when you review your performance. Clinical postconferences and individual mentoring experiences in which information is exchanged promote critical thinking.

REVIEW OF PATIENT SCENARIOS

Chart review, grand rounds, and case study approaches when performed in a group provide interdisciplinary exchanges, a variety of different thinking perspectives, and learning from role models. These approaches require a verbal exchange that includes reasoning, interpreting, identifying evidence, deducing, and concluding. In these situations you can examine your viewpoint in relation to the viewpoints of others. This exchange promotes learning and stimulates critical thinking.

WRITTEN ASSIGNMENTS

Written assignments are not just "busy work." Journal writing is an activity that requires you to log and respond to important and meaningful situations. Faculty review of your journal (with comments) and periodic study and review of it by you will enable you to identify your progress and growth. Journal writing involves you in the process of learning. It encourages you to use abstract thinking and to conceptualize, elaborate, generalize, and interpret, all of which promote critical thinking. A term paper is a written assignment in which you are involved not only in the process of writing but also in the development of a product. When this product is reviewed by the instructor, conclusions can be drawn regarding your command of the information and your ability to convey your knowledge to others. Written assignments require organizing, prioritizing, integrating, persuading, proving, and summarizing, all of which require *critical thinking*.

COMPUTER-ASSISTED LEARNING

Computers provide an environment that enhances and challenges critical-thinking skills. Software offers a variety of critical-thinking programs, from a simple lesson presenting content using an interactive linear approach to programs in which the learner is challenged to seek solutions to complex problems following a branching design. Computers allow for thinking and learning in a nonthreatening and safe environment. Refer to Chapter 9, Computer Applications in Education and Evaluation, for more details regarding the valuable use of computers to increase learning.

VIDEOTAPING

Videotaping can be used to record role-playing scenarios or the performance of a skill. Videotaping allows you to engage in an activity and then be able to review your performance. During this review, you, as well as others, can examine, analyze, rationalize, justify, and correct your performance, which can support critical thinking.

CLINICAL PROCESS RECORDS

A clinical process record is a focused writing assignment, similar to a case study that centers on a simulated or specific patient experience. It requires you to use the problem-solving process, examine the scientific reasons for health-care interventions, assess outcomes, and evaluate and modify the plan of care, which all contribute to critical thinking.

EXAMINATIONS

Examinations should be approached as learning opportunities. All examinations must be thoughtfully reviewed. Small groups of four or five students should review and discuss each question. Group members help one another to identify the key concepts being tested and how to best answer the questions "What is happening?" and "What should I do?" When reviewing examination questions, be willing to listen to other people's interpretation of the question. If all of your energy is spent defending your response, then your mind is not open to different perspectives, which limits your learning. Reviewing examinations requires you to integrate information, apply theory and principles, analyze content, compare and contrast information, and rationalize your response, all of which contribute to critical thinking.

APPLY CRITICAL THINKING TO MULTIPLE-CHOICE QUESTIONS

Case (1994) explored the concept of critical thinking as a journey, not a destination. Case stated, "We cannot stand in the same river twice, because water rushes away as new water takes its place and the rushing water changes the river bed. The decisions we make today may not fit circumstances that change tomorrow." This concept applies to clinical situations as well as nursing test questions. Just as no clinical situation will be exactly like a previous experience, no test question will be exactly like a previous question. One different factor in a situation can change the entire landscape of the situation. One different word in a question can change what the question is asking. Practicing critical thinking when answering questions will improve your ability to think critically and be more successful when taking a test.

Identify the Key Concept Being Tested

Each question scenario is different and requires you to identify the key concept being tested and to answer the questions "What is happening?" and "What should I do?" Reframe, critique, and evaluate the stem of each question. Then, try to construct the correct answer before looking at the options. When assessing the options in a multiple-choice question, manipulate the information by cognitive activities such as organizing, correlating, differentiating, reasoning, and evaluating against standards of practice, criteria, and critical elements. Review the following sample item.

SAMPLE ITEM 2-1

A patient has just returned from the operating room with a urinary retention (Foley) catheter, an IV line, and an oral airway and is still unresponsive. Which nursing assessment should be made first?

1. Check the surgical dressing to ensure that it is intact.

2. Confirm the placement of the oral airway.

3. Observe the Foley catheter for drainage.

4. Examine the IV site for infiltration.

First, you need to identify the key concept being tested in the question. The key concept in this question is the **priority care for the unresponsive postoperative patient.** The key words in the question that ask "What is happening?" are **postoperative patient, oral airway,** and **unresponsive.** The key words in the question that ask "What should I do?" are **assessment** and **should be made first.** The question being asked is: **What assessment takes priority when caring for an unresponsive postoperative patient with an oral airway?** Although the IV line, the retention catheter, and surgical dressing are important and must be assessed, it is ensuring the correct placement of the oral airway that takes priority.

To answer this question you need to know: the normal anatomy and physiology associated with the respiratory system and the body's essential need for a continuous exchange of oxygen and carbon dioxide; that a patent airway is essential to the exchange of oxygen and carbon dioxide; the ABCs of life support, which refer to Airway, Breathing, and Circulation, and thus that maintaining an airway takes priority; that a common response to anesthesia is lack of a gag reflex; and that a correctly placed oral airway will contribute to maintaining an open airway.

Another critical-thinking study technique when answering multiple-choice questions is to explore the consequences of each nursing action presented in the alternatives. You can ask many different questions: "Is the action safe or unsafe?" "Is the statement true or false?" "Is it fact or inference?"

Avoid Reading Into the Question

Highly discriminating questions are questions that are answered correctly by the test taker who scored in the top percent of the class versus the test taker who answered the question incorrectly and scored in the bottom percent of the class on the same examination. It is believed that the student who answers a highly discriminating question correctly generally is responding to subtle cues based on more highly developed critical-thinking skills. However, students who come to the testing situation with an in-depth perspective sometimes will "read into" the meaning of the question because of the "context" they bring to the test item. It is often frustrating for students who are sophisticated, deep thinkers to accept lost points on an examination because they "read into" the question. Analyze questions you answer incorrectly and determine "why" by asking questions such as: "Did I add information to the stem?" "Did I have difficulty deciding among the options presented because I would have done something completely different?" "Did I delete an option because my experience was different from the patient situation presented?" "Did I view the question in light of a more sophisticated level of curricular content than that being tested?" "Did I view the patient scenario in more depth and breadth than was necessary?" Multiple-choice questions provide all the information necessary to answer the question. Your job is to use critical thinking to answer the question, not rewrite the question. For additional information see Chapter 10, Analyze Your Test Performance.

Study the Rationales for the Right and Wrong Answers

Every nursing action is based on a standard of practice that has a scientific foundation. When practicing test taking, in your own words, identify the reason why the option you chose is correct and why the options you considered incorrect are wrong. Now compare your rationales with the rationales presented. When you answered a question correctly, review the rationales several times to reinforce your knowledge. When you answered a question incorrectly, identify your faulty thinking by comparing your rationale to the presented rationale. When you identify content that you did not know or cannot apply, review this content in your nursing textbook. An excellent study technique associated with principles is to identify other situations in which the same principle applies and situations in which it is different. See Chapter 10, Analyze Your Test Performance, to design a corrective action plan.

Change the Focus of the Question

A great way to explore additional situations using multiple-choice questions is to change one of the key facts in the stem of a question to alter the focus of the question (see Sample Items 2-2 and 2-3). Also, in a question that expects you to set a priority, you can eliminate the option that is the correct answer (see Sample Items 2-4 and 2-5). This requires you to identify the next best option that answers the question. When the context of the question is altered even slightly, the contour or territory around it changes, which may significantly rearrange the internal structure of the entire question. When a question is altered, the meaning of the situation may require a distinctly different nursing assessment or action.

SAMPLE ITEM 2-2
Which is associated with a physiological need of a patient with a colostomy?
1. Disturbance in body image
2. Inadequate nutrition
3. Lack of knowledge
4. Skin breakdown

The correct answer is option 4. The word "physiological" modifies the word "need" and is a clue in the stem. For study purposes, you can change the focus of this question by changing the word "physiological" to "psychological" in the stem. Now answer this question from this new perspective.

SAMPLE ITEM 2-3

Which is associated with a psychological need of a patient with a colostomy?

1. Disturbance in body image
2. Inadequate nutrition
3. Lack of knowledge
4. Skin breakdown

   The correct answer is option 1. The entire focus of this question has changed. The focus has moved from "physiological" to "psychological." Now the clue in the stem is the word "psychological." By using this technique, you can apply critical thinking to multiple-choice questions and maximize opportunities for learning. This is an effective strategy either when working alone or when working with a study group.

SAMPLE ITEM 2-4

A preoperative patient talks about being afraid of pain because of a previous experience with painful surgery. What should the nurse do *first* to help the patient cope with this fear?

1. Encourage the patient not to be afraid.
2. Teach the patient relaxation techniques.
3. Listen to the patient's concerns about pain.
4. Inform the patient that medication is available.

   The correct answer is option 3. The word "first" is asking you to set a priority. For study purposes, you can change the focus of the question by eliminating the correct answer as a choice and then attempting to answer the question from the remaining three options. Now answer the question from this new perspective.

SAMPLE ITEM 2-5

A preoperative patient talks about being afraid of pain because of a previous experience with painful surgery. What should the nurse do *first* to help the patient cope with this fear?

1. Encourage the patient not to be afraid.
2. Teach the patient relaxation techniques.
3. Inform the patient that medication is available.

   The correct answer is option 2. The technique of eliminating the correct answer and attempting to select the next best action requires you to rank the options presented in order of importance. This strategy works only with questions that require you to set a priority. Key words such as "initially," "first," "best," "priority," and "most" should alert you that the question is a priority question. By using this strategy, you increase opportunities to sharpen your critical-thinking skills.

Study in a Small Group

Studying in groups contributes to building a body of knowledge that increases your perspective and context when the group jointly seeks a solution to a highly discriminating question. This technique is particularly helpful because different people bring different perspectives and thinking styles to the sharing that enrich the learning experience. More perspectives produce a variety of views of the problem and generate more approaches to selecting the most accurate response. Small groups are most effective when the number of members is kept at three to five people. Larger groups tend to have inherent problems such as all members may not express their input, one member may monopolize the discussion, or the activity may progress to a social gathering rather than a focused work group.

Where all think alike, no one thinks very much.

—WALTER LIPPMANN

SUMMARY

In our informational society there is no way you can know or experience everything. With the explosion of knowledge and technology and changes in the role of the nurse within a fluid health-care delivery environment, what is learned today may be obsolete tomorrow. Consequently, an integral part of your continuing education consists of the development and refinement of critical-thinking skills. To be a critical thinker, you must be intellectually humble, able to listen, dissatisfied with the status quo, creative, flexible, self-confident but aware of your limitations, and willing to change. Take time to cultivate your critical-thinking skills because they will be the ultimate tool you bring to patient-care situations—the therapeutic use of self. When you can think critically, you are empowered to maximize your abilities to meet patient needs.

2-1 1. Although checking the surgical dressing is important, it does not involve a life-threatening situation.

2. **Confirming the placement of the oral airway ensures a patent air passage. An oral airway displaces the tongue and prevents obstruction of the trachea, permitting free passage of air to and from the lungs. Oxygen is essential for life, and this action takes priority.**

3. Although observing the Foley catheter for drainage is important, urinary output at this time is less critical than assessing airway, breathing, and circulation.

4. Although examining the IV site is important, an infiltration can be tolerated for a few minutes while higher priority assessments are made.

2-2 1. Concern about body image is a psychological, not physiological, concern.

2. Although inadequate nutrition is a physiological problem, it is not specific to a patient with a colostomy.

3. A knowledge deficit is a cognitive/perceptual problem, not a physiological problem.

4. **Skin breakdown is a common physiological problem associated with the presence of a colostomy because of the digestive enzymes present in feces.**

2-3 1. **Concern about body image is a psychological problem often encountered when a person has surgery that alters the body's structure or function.**

2. Nutrition is a physiological, not a psychological, problem.

3. Knowledge deficit is a cognitive/perceptual problem, not a psychological problem.

4. Skin breakdown is a physiological, not a psychological, problem.

2-4 1. Encouraging the patient not to be afraid denies the patient's fears.

2. Although relaxation techniques may be taught eventually, it is not the priority at this time.

3. **Listening to the patient's concerns about pain supports the patient's need to verbalize fears.**

4. Although medication may be available, this is false reassurance and cuts off communication.

2-5 1. Encouraging the patient not to be afraid denies the patient's fears.

2. **Depending on the relaxation technique used, it can reduce muscle tension, distract the person from the stimulus, and/or limit the physiological response to *fight or flight*, thus reducing pain.**

3. Although medication may be available, this statement is false reassurance and cuts off communication.

Time Management

3

TIME MANAGEMENT EQUALS SELF-MANAGEMENT

Time is an elusive concept that is reflected in countless wise sayings. Time is of the essence! Where did the time go? It's now or never! Never put off until tomorrow what you can do today! Time flies when you are having fun! Time is money! A stitch in time saves nine! Time is on your side! And, finally, the most significant saying, you are the only one who can waste your time!

To achieve your goal to be a nurse, you must progress from being a beginning nursing student (HERE) to graduating and passing a licensing examination (THERE). The major difference between HERE and THERE is the letter T. This T represents Time Management, which equals self-management. How you use your time will reflect directly on how successfully you manage the efforts that will ultimately help you attain your goal. The purpose of this chapter is to help you identify personal values and behaviors that relate to time management and learn ways to maximize your productivity through time-management strategies.

TAKE THE TIME TO ASSESS YOUR TIME-MANAGEMENT ABILITIES

Today many people, particularly students, are attempting to function in a society that stresses the concept of "24/7." They are not running out of time—they are running into it! They are like horses on a merry-go-round that is going faster and faster, and they cannot get off. If you can relate to these people, it is time to take the time to think about time management! The first step in developing a time-management program is to know yourself. It is important to identify how you actually spend your time, identify your personal values, and identify your personal barriers to productivity. Take the time to perform the following three self-assessment tools:

1. Assessment of Inconsistencies Between Values and Behavior
2. Personal Time/Activity Journal
3. Self-Assessment of Barriers to Productivity

Assessment of Inconsistencies Between Values and Behavior

Values are enduring beliefs or attitudes about the worth of a person, object, idea, or action. A **value system** is the organized set of values that is internalized by a person. **Values clarification** is a complex process in which you identify, examine, and develop your own individual values. It is impossible to attempt this process here. However, a simple method will be presented for you to identify inconsistencies (i.e., agreement or disagreement) between what you consider important and how you behave in relation to the delegation of your time.

Make a list of those areas in your life that you value, and then next to it identify the total percent of time during the day (including travel time) you believe you should allocate to each. After you have completed your personal time/activity journal, compare the amount of time you devoted to activities related to the areas you identified as important. Evaluate whether your behavior reflected what you stated you believe is important. When your behavior reflects your values (attitudes and beliefs), you are in harmony. When your behavior does not reflect your values, you are in "value imbalance," and eventually you will experience emotional and physical consequences. Often, when people have a value imbalance, they are reluctant to create change, but change is necessary to promote harmony intrapersonally (within yourself) and interpersonally (with others). Seeking balance is a challenge. However, the challenge can be manageable because it does not have to be outside your value system, nor does it have to be permanent. Adjustments may be necessary just during an academic semester. A colleague of ours used to say, "You can do anything for 16 weeks!" The following is an example of an assessment tool to identify inconsistencies between values and behavior. Modify the areas in your life that you value accordingly to meet your needs.

Assessment of Inconsistencies Between Values and Behavior

Areas in My Life That I Value	Desired Percent of Time	Actual Percent of Time
Self-care (eating, sleeping, grooming)		
Work		
Leisure		
Relationships (family, friends)		
School/studying		
Community activities		
Religion/spiritual		

Personal Time/Activity Journal

Financial consultants who advise on money management recommend to their clients that, for 1 week, they write down every penny they spend. At the end of the week the information is examined to determine where all the money went. The big difference between time and money is that money can be saved but time cannot. How you spend your minutes and hours can make a difference. Therefore, keep track of what you are doing every hour in a journal. At the end of the week, review what you did and next to each entry identify whether it is something that you must do, want to do, or do not need to do. The results of this personal time/activity journal should be compared with the areas you have identified as important in your life. Those activities that do not relate to the necessary activities of daily living or your priorities in life should be curtailed, delegated, or eliminated. The following is an example of an activity journal. Modify it to meet your needs.

Personal Time/Activity Journal

Time	Activity	Must Do	Want to Do	No Need to Do
6-7 AM				
7-8 AM				
8-9 AM				
9-10 AM				
10-11 AM				
11-12 AM				
12-1 PM				
1-2 PM				
2-3 PM				

Personal Time/Activity Journal—cont'd

Time	Activity	Must Do	Want to Do	No Need to Do
3-4 PM				
4-5 PM				
5-6 PM				
6-7 PM				
7-8 PM				
8-9 PM				
9-10 PM				
10-11 PM				

Self-Assessment of Barriers to Productivity

Productivity reflects the amount and quality of outcomes that result from labor. Inherent in this definition are two concepts: amount of outcomes and effectiveness of outcomes. These concepts can be related to studying nursing content in a textbook. If you spend 1 hour studying a chapter in a nursing textbook and at the end of the hour you can define all the significant words, you have numerous concrete results from your studying. If you spend 1 hour studying arterial blood gases and at the end of the hour you are able to understand the interrelationship of the components of acid-base balance, you understand a limited concept. However, you have a quality outcome because this topic is complex. Your effort has been constructive and valuable!

There are many internal and external factors that can affect your productivity. However, they are not as overwhelming as you may think because most people are creatures of habit and there is a pattern to their behavioral responses and performance. With a little honesty and soul-searching, you should be able to identify some of the barriers to your productivity by taking the Self-Assessment of Barriers to Productivity tool that follows. Read each self-assessment statement in relation to yourself and check either the Yes or No column. After you have completed the self-assessment tool, compare your results to the Corrective Action Plan to Maximize Your Productivity.

Self-Assessment of Barriers to Productivity

Self-Assessment Statement	Yes	No
1. I tend to procrastinate.		
2. I expect little help from members of my family.		
3. I lack organization.		
4. I flutter from one task to another.		
5. I tend to be obsessive/compulsive.		
6. I tend to socialize when I should be studying.		
7. I fall behind in my responsibilities.		
8. I have difficulty delegating tasks.		
9. I tend to feel overwhelmed.		
10. I have too many conflicting deadlines.		
11. I set high standards for myself.		
12. I attempt to do too much.		

You have just completed the Self-Assessment of Barriers to Productivity tool. Now look at how you answered each question in the tool. Match each number to which you answered "Yes" to its corresponding number in the Corrective Action Plan to Maximize Your Productivity tool. If your response to one or both of the related questions was a "Yes," review the strategies that relate to the factor that may be interfering with or limiting your productivity.

Corrective Action Plan To Maximize Your Productivity

Question Number*	Self-Assessment Statement	Corrective Action Plan
4	I flutter from one task to another.	Identify Goals, page 24
10	I have too many conflicting deadlines.	Set Priorities, page 25
3	I lack organization.	Get Organized, page 27
9	I tend to feel overwhelmed.	
6	I tend to socialize when I should be studying.	Develop Self-Discipline, page 28
12	I attempt to do too much.	Achieve a Personal Balance, page 32
5	I tend to be obsessive/compulsive.	
11	I set high standards for myself.	Delegate, page 33
2	I expect little help from members of my family.	
8	I have difficulty delegating tasks.	
1	I tend to procrastinate.	Overcome Procrastination, page 34
7	I fall behind in my responsibilities.	

*From: Self-Assessment of Barriers to Productivity on page 23.

MAXIMIZE YOUR PRODUCTIVITY

Now that you have given some thought to what is important to you, how you spend your time, and your barriers to productivity, you need to devise a proactive plan to achieve your goals. To maximize productivity, you need to manage your attitudes and behaviors to use time in a constructive manner to achieve your goals.

Identify Goals

A **goal** is an object or aim you want to attain. Goals can be long-term, intermediate, or short-term.

Long-term goals are related to lifelong journeys that frequently include career aspirations or ambitions. Long-term goals generally address desired outcomes 5 or more years in the future. Two examples of long-term goals might be: "I will earn a bachelor's degree in nursing by the time my children enter high school." "I will be a nurse manager in an acute-care setting within 10 years after graduation from nursing school."

Intermediate goals are related to aims you want to achieve within 1 to 5 years. Appropriately set intermediate goals are the keys to successfully reaching long-term goals. Two examples of intermediate goals are: "I will complete my science prerequisites for the nursing program within 2 years." "I will attend all of my child's soccer games this year."

Short-term goals address desired results that take hours, days, weeks, or months to attain. Some people consider them objectives that must be met to reach intermediate and long-term goals. When short-term goals reflect immediate outcomes, they may end up being just a "To Do" list. Examples of short-term goals are: "I will earn a minimum grade of B in my Fundamentals of Nursing course this semester." "I will read two chapters in my textbook this weekend."

When setting goals, remember that they must contain certain elements to be effective. They must be specific, measurable, and realistic and have a time frame. A goal that is **specific** identifies precisely what is to be attained. A goal that is **measurable** sets a minimum satisfactory level of performance. A goal that is **realistic** has a reasonable chance of being attained. A goal that has a **time frame** states the length of time it will take to attain the goal. Compare these criteria to the goals just stated and to each goal that you write in the future. Work tends to expand in length when there are no guidelines for its performance. Goals are a major way to prevent wasting time in this manner because you know your destination before you begin and you have a time frame in which to get there. There is an old saying that goes something like this: *"If you want to get something done, give it to the busiest person you know."* Effective busy people understand the need to set specific, measurable, realistic goals that can be achieved within a specific time frame.

Most students understand the importance of goals but do not understand how to set them because of the complexity of their lives. One way to begin goal setting is to identify your roles in life. How you identify your roles depends on your frame of reference. For example, you may decide you want to look at your roles in relation to how you relate to people (individual, spouse, parent, friend, coworker) or you may decide you want to look at your roles in relation to what you do (housekeeper, cook, family support person, nurse's aide, Girl Scout leader, Sunday School teacher). After you have defined your roles, identify one or more goals that you want to achieve in each role. They can be short-term, intermediate, or long-term goals, depending on what is important to you. When setting goals, ensure that you take into account the various areas in your life that you considered important when you completed the tool Assessment of Inconsistencies Between Values and Behavior. Your goals need to be in harmony with your values (attitudes and beliefs).

Involve your family members when writing a goal. They will have a vested interest in your attaining your goal when they understand the rationales for the goal. For example, when you earn your license as a Registered Nurse, you can quit your second job, earn more money for vacations, or work the night shift, all of which will allow you to spend more time with them. These are the rewards for attaining your goal. Family-centered goals should be like a pebble dropped in a lake—the ripples of pleasurable rewards should affect all members of the family. Put your goals in writing. It makes them more tangible, and you can review them routinely to remain focused. Share your goals with everyone who will listen. A goal that exists only in your mind is a dream or fantasy and is less likely to become reality. Telling people your goals can be motivating because you create additional emphasis on the need to perform. When you attain goals, reward yourself and family members when appropriate. This will motivate you and recognize the significant others in your life who are helping you to attain your goals.

Goals should be revisited. In our fast-paced society, our roles, responsibilities, and relationships change over time. You must be flexible enough to revise, eliminate, or reset a goal, depending on the factors that change in your life. For example, after taking 12 college credits in one academic semester while working full time, you realize that you are overwhelmed. You may revise your goal of attaining a bachelor's degree in nursing by prolonging the time frame in which to attain this goal. If you have twins while in school, you may decide that taking one course a semester is more realistic than taking three courses a semester. Revising your goals is not a sign of failure but rather a mature recognition of reasonable expectations, which requires you to reset your goals accordingly.

Set Priorities

After students identify their goals, they often ask, "Now what?" Well, now is the time to set priorities! **Setting priorities** is the process of identifying the preferential order of doing something. In other words, what requires your attention first? It is helpful to have criteria for classifying activities so that you can prioritize with less difficulty. For example, you can classify things to do into four categories:

1. **Pressing/Important Tasks**—Tasks that are pressing and important insist on your immediate attention and relate to activities that you consider vital or valuable. Important activities relate to your values and your stated goals. Pressing activities relate to tasks that have to be accomplished in the short term, such as hours or days. These activities must be tackled first. Examples are reviewing class notes for an examination the next day, taking care of a sick child, and finishing writing an assignment that has to be submitted tomorrow. We all have urgent or unexpected activities that must be addressed, but this should not become a standard method of functioning. If you put most of your activities in this category, you are in a crisis management mode because you are dealing with emergencies, problems, or last-minute deadlines. When you constantly function in this mode, you will be anxious, overworked, overwhelmed, and speeding toward burnout.

2. **Not Pressing/Important Tasks**—Tasks that are not pressing but are important also relate to activities that you consider vital and valuable. However, you have several days or weeks before they need to be completed. Although you have the luxury of time, you must be self-directed and proactive to take the initiative to complete them. Most of your life's activities, including academically related tasks, can be placed in this category. Examples are paying monthly bills, playing with your children, and reading the textbook for an examination in 2 weeks. If you put most of your activities in this category, you are probably self-directed and an effective manager of your time. However, if you delay or ignore activities in this category, the pressure to accomplish the task increases until it must be reclassified into the pressing/important category. Attention to details in this category is like preventive maintenance on a car. It gets accomplished before the car breaks down and becomes a crisis. When you function in this category, you are in control and anxiety is kept to a minimum.

3. **Pressing/Not Important Tasks**—Tasks that are pressing but are not important compete for your immediate attention, but they relate to activities you do not consider vital or important. Examples are listening to a telephone call from a telemarketer, watching a specific program on television, and doing something that someone else thinks you should do. When setting priorities, you should limit activities in the pressing/not important category because they are not important. If most of your activities are in this category, reacting and responding are your modes of action rather than being proactive. You are responding to urgent stimuli, but more often than not the urgency and importance of the activity are based on the expectations of others. You are meeting other people's needs, not your own.

4. **Not Pressing/Not Important Tasks**—Tasks that are not urgent and not important are small, minor, insignificant activities. They are not competing for your immediate attention, nor do you consider them important. Examples are cleaning the sock drawer, sharpening all the pencils in your desk, and socializing with uninvited visitors. When setting priorities, you need to limit or eliminate activities in the not pressing/not important category. Why get involved with tasks that are insignificant and unimportant? Why waste your time? If you put most of your activities into this category, you may be overwhelmed and trying to escape from the pressing problems or activities in the pressing/important category. Escape may be your only way to obtain relief.

The examples provided may not reflect your values. Obviously, you need to identify those activities that are important and pressing to you. When setting priorities, you are the only person who can decide if something is important. You can make choices that are in harmony with your values and goals. Unfortunately, you may or may not have control over time frames. Emergencies arise that require immediate attention, due dates for school assignments may be indicated weeks in advance, and some deadlines are self-imposed. Some deadlines cannot be altered, but others may be extended without giving up your goals. The ability to set priorities puts you in a position of control because you are the one making the decisions.

Get Organized

When you look at your life, do you feel like a juggler attempting to keep multiple balls aloft all at the same time while walking on a bed of fire? If so, you are on overload. You may be a mother, daughter, father, son, brother, sister, wife, husband, friend, employee, student, social advocate, and so on. Each role has its related responsibilities and stresses. As a result, you may have *multiple-role overload!* In our world, and especially in nursing, the volume of new information is expanding dramatically. Years ago a nursing fundamentals textbook was several hundred pages long. Today a fundamentals textbook is over a thousand pages long. As a result, you may have *information overload!* Today corporations are focusing on increasing productivity. Your place of business may be reorganizing to maximize your work effort. As a result, you may have *work overload!* The explosion in technology has produced voice-mail, call forwarding, e-mail, text messaging, cell phones, Twitter, and Facebook. You are connected and accessible "24/7." As a result, you may have *access overload!* When overloaded for any length of time, you can spiral toward an overload crisis. You must be organized to regain control of the situation.

Being on overload is a problem, and time management may be the solution. There are many ways to manage time, but a simple, concrete method is the use of calendars. If your goal is to graduate from a nursing program in, you should make a master calendar listing the courses you must take each semester to meet the curriculum requirements for graduation. Next, you may need more detailed calendars, such as monthly, weekly, or daily, to provide additional structure. Also, calendars help you to plan for short- and long-range assignments, provide consistency with a regular schedule, identify priorities, and reduce anxiety.

Monthly calendars help control mental clutter. Make monthly calendars for every month within a semester and insert important personal events (e.g., social engagements, doctor's appointments) and school-related requirements (e.g., first and last days of the semester, examinations, special projects, due dates for written assignments). Also, insert school holidays and vacation periods. These reminders provide a broad overview of your monthly activities. After you insert important events in the calendar, do not use mental energy to keep that information in the forefront of your mind. You just need to check your calendar to verify when an event will take place.

Weekly calendars provide an overview of the week and achieve consistency concerning your day-to-day schedule. They should be constructed just before beginning a new week. Block in all of your required commitments on your weekly calendar. Include time for activities of daily living (e.g., sleeping, grooming, food preparation, eating, doing laundry), children-related activities, work, scheduled classes, religious services, and so on. Allocate additional time to those commitments that require travel. After all your required tasks are inserted into the calendar, you can begin deciding how to carve up the remaining time. Factors that must be considered include setting consistent times to study each day, scheduling breaks within study periods, ensuring recreational activities, determining the time of day when you are most productive, deciding how much time you need to study, and so on. There is an old formula that states that you should study 1 to 2 hours a week for every hour you are in class. For example, if you are in school 12 hours a week, you should be studying 12 to 24 hours a week outside of class. Although this is often true, it is a generality. Only you can decide from your past and present performance how much time you require to study or prepare written assignments outside of class to be successful. In addition, when developing a weekly calendar it is essential to establish consistency in activities from one day to the next because it creates a routine that is familiar, and familiarity reduces anxiety. Also, it reduces the need to expend energy to make decisions. You made the decision once at the beginning of the week to study from 7 to 9 p.m. Monday through Friday. Your job now is to implement the plan without the need to use energy to explore the pros and cons of studying or overcome your own objections to studying. You made a commitment to yourself to study, and you must have the integrity to keep your commitment.

Daily calendars organize your activities so that you can achieve your daily goals efficiently and effectively. Design the calendar in the evening for the next day. This helps to reduce anxiety because you have organized your thoughts, identified your goals, and planned a time to accomplish them. Plan a calendar that is simple. Start by slotting in all the personal and school-related special events for the day that appear on your weekly calendar. Do not include routine tasks such as class time, work, or personal activities such as eating or sleeping. Now make a list of all the academic and nonacademic activities that you want to accomplish. Be as specific as you can. Many people call this a "To Do List." Rank each activity on the list in order of priority, that is, items that must get done first, then those that should get done, and finally those you would like to get done. Plot these activities (particularly the tasks that must get done) around your standard tasks, and coordinate the scheduling of activities to take advantage of blocks of available time that are appropriate for the tasks. Also, combine activities so that you can accomplish more than one task at a time. For example, shop at stores that have multiple departments so that school supplies and food for dinner can be bought at one stop; study flash cards while performing a chore, or use a similar topic for assignments in two different courses so that one search of the literature can be used for both assignments. Welcome to "multitasking," a necessity when maintaining a busy schedule! Although you may have a full schedule, every minute of every day does not have to be accounted for. Tasks may take longer than planned, and unexpected situations may occur. Some tasks may not be accomplished by the end of the day, preferably the lower-priority activities. If you have tasks left over, you may have to revise your future daily lists with a more realistic attitude, move an uncompleted task to the next day, delegate the task, or eliminate it entirely.

Obviously, everyone's calendar will be different, depending on family, school, and work-related commitments. Although individualized, calendars should all be simple, realistic, and flexible. They should not be so complex that they become an additional chore. The course of study to become a nurse is demanding and takes time and energy. Energy can be conserved if time is used efficiently. Many people say they do not have the time to design calendars, but a well-thought-out plan that is followed promotes the efficient use of time, resulting in more available time. You need to spend time to save time!

Develop Self-Discipline

When you feel overwhelmed, have you ever said to yourself, "If only there were 25 hours in a day I would get all my work done." If the truth be told, you probably still would not get your work done if you had 26 hours in a day. The reality is there are only 24 hours in a day and only 168 hours in a week. How you manage yourself in relation to that time is the key to feeling in control rather than feeling overwhelmed.

You start by setting your goals and priorities. If you are to be successful and graduate from nursing school, school must be a priority. If you work full time or several days a week, manage a home with children, and are involved in community activities, then the demands on your time and energy may be excessive. Only you can decide what you are capable of doing. Setting realistic demands on your time and energy is difficult. You may be able to do anything you want, but you may not be able to do everything you want. Rarely in life can you have it all. Therefore, to manage your time and responsibilities efficiently and fairly, you may have to make hard decisions. Reducing work hours, sharing household chores, hiring a babysitter, or limiting your social life may be necessary strategies to help you manage your responsibilities in relation to your schoolwork. You may even decide to delay your goal by taking fewer credits per semester or deciding that this is not the best time to be going to school. Sacrifices in and of themselves should not be viewed negatively. Often these sacrifices will promote growth in you and your family.

After you and your family have set your goals and priorities, you must get their help in establishing your weekly calendar. This calendar should set "firm boundaries" for your future behavior, recognizing that it should be flexible to "bend" with emerging or unexpected priorities. With this calendar, you have made a commitment to yourself and others to achieve certain goals within a time frame. In other words, you have made a promise. Now you must keep it! Keeping promises expands your basic habits of personal effectiveness and builds character, but it requires self-discipline.

Self-discipline is orderly conduct in relation to self-imposed constraints. Self-discipline is an internal factor that is influenced only by what you bring to a situation. Self-discipline involves three important abilities: the ability to say "No," the ability to avoid time traps, and the ability to self-motivate.

SAYING "NO"

The word "No" is a small word that can have a big impact on your ability to manage your life. If you are similar to others who enter the helping professions, you usually use the word "Yes" more often than you use the word "No." You want to help and give of yourself and thus put the needs of others before your own. However, when you are going to school, it is the time to make your needs a priority. Learn to say "No." When asked to do something by someone else, you have to ask yourself questions such as:

- Is this consistent with my identified goal/priorities?
- Is this something I must do?
- Is this something I want to do?
- Is this something I have no need to do?
- Is this person able to do this by himself or herself?
- Is there anyone else who can do this task?

Based on your response to these self-directed questions you can respond with a "Yes" or "No" to the person who is asking you to do something. If you are undecided, buy yourself some time with a response such as, "That sounds interesting, but let me think about it overnight and I will get back to you tomorrow." This response allows you an opportunity to consider how much time the activity will demand and to make a decision that is within your value system. If your answer is "No," it gives you time to construct a response.

The most common consequence of saying "No" is the feeling of guilt. Guilt is a self-imposed feeling that occurs when your conscience identifies that something you have done or not done is unacceptable; only you can make yourself feel guilty. You waste energy when you feel guilty; therefore, use the energy of guilt to prevent guilty feelings. You can cope with guilt in several ways:

- Recognize that you may never eliminate feelings of guilt because you are human. However, you can limit feelings of guilt.
- Understand that there is "good guilt" and there is "bad guilt." **Good guilt** is feeling bad about something you have done or not done that you have based on what you identify as ethically or morally important. Use the energy of good guilt to reestablish your goals, priorities, and calendars. For example: "I will schedule time in my calendar to spend an hour a day in the evening playing with my children." **Bad guilt** is feeling bad about something over which you have no control. Do not waste energy on bad guilt, because it is irrational and physically and emotionally draining. For example: "I am a single parent and I must work to put food on the table and a roof over our heads. I am going to school so that I will be able to reach my goals of being a nurse and earning a better living. While I am in school I must spend more time with my studies and less time with my children."
- You can change the belief on which your guilty feelings are based. For example: "It is appropriate for me to meet my needs before someone else's needs; I am not a bad person if I decide not to do what someone else expects of me."
- You can make a weekly calendar that respects your goals and priorities. When studying, you should not feel guilty about not spending time with the family because you have scheduled time to address family needs.
- You can compensate for your behavior. Compensation is repaying yourself or someone else when something is done or not done as expected. It is used when unexpected priorities arise. However, if you are constantly using compensation, you need to revisit your goals, priorities, and calendars. For example: "I want to watch the ball game on TV tonight, so I will study 2 hours more on the weekend." "We had fast food three times this week, so tonight I will make a great home-cooked meal."

Use feelings of guilt to your advantage. This is an opportunity for personal change and growth.

AVOIDING TIME TRAPS

Time traps are interruptions that interfere with your ability to use your time productively. Earlier in this chapter you were advised to complete a personal time/activity journal. A review of your journal should reveal to you how you spent your time and whether it was productive or you got caught in time traps. You were also asked to perform a self-assessment to identify your barriers to productivity, which included procrastination, difficulty with delegation, lack of organization, an inability to set goals and priorities, perfectionism, and lack of self-discipline. Each of these barriers to productivity has time-trap elements, and corrective actions for each are addressed in this chapter. This section will help you identify seemingly unavoidable events that interfere with your use of time. Do not dribble away time when you are out of control or when others control you. Some time traps cannot be completely avoided. However, an awareness of how events are interfering with your use of time and then effective management can help you address most of these events. First, you must identify when you are caught in a time trap and realize how much time is wasted. Second, you need to set limits on yourself and others and regain control of your time. Some events over which you may believe you have little control are:

- Unwanted phone calls or phone calls that involve unimportant conversations (small talk)
- Long-winded conversations that do not get to the point
- Arrival of unwanted guests
- A crowded library or store
- Waiting for others
- Rush-hour traffic
- Excessively researching a topic
- Too much socializing
- Unnecessary meetings
- Assuming the role of listener or counselor to meet the emotional needs of friends

Many of these occur because you are unaware of how much time they waste, you have not organized your day, or you have not set limits on yourself or others. You are not powerless to control these events. However, to limit or eliminate time traps, you must be proactive. Suggested solutions are as follows:

Manage accessibility:

- Turn off your cell phone or use it only for outgoing calls.
- Indicate on your voicemail that you are available only during certain times.
- Make your home phone unlisted.
- Give your e-mail address only to selected individuals.
- Use caller ID to screen phone calls.
- Turn off the ringer or unplug the phone when studying.
- Block out time for study when you absolutely cannot be interrupted.
- Learn to say, "It's nice to hear from you, but I really can't talk right now. I'll catch up with you next week." This generally works. If the other person is persistent, say, "I'm sorry, I really have to go." And then close the door or hang up.
- Put a "Do Not Disturb" sign on your door. (I used this approach when I had a newborn, and I put a picture of a sleeping baby on the sign.)
- Give family members instructions to interrupt you when you are studying only if there is an emergency.

Manage waiting time:

- Set limits on the amount of time you are willing to wait. Your time is as valuable as another's time.
- Capture moments of time and study flash cards or notes.

- Use captured moments of time to get small tasks accomplished. For example, while waiting for an appointment, write a thank-you note for a gift, write a grocery list, review your schedule for the next day, write a check and prepare a bill to be mailed, or brainstorm how you are going to tackle an upcoming assignment.
- Make appointments with primary health-care providers the first or last appointment of the day. Call to ensure that the primary health-care provider is on schedule.

Avoid wasting time:

- Keep a list of what is done and what still needs to be done so that if you stop in the middle of a project you can pick up where you left off.
- Multitask your errands. Go one-stop shopping and use stores that carry food, hardware, clothes, and so forth.
- Simplify shopping. Reduce trips to the store, follow a shopping list, and maintain a full pantry.
- Simplify meals. Cook one-dish meals. Cook double the amount and freeze half for another day.
- Eat out or buy ready-prepared food when short on time.
- Avoid travel during rush hour. Leave earlier or later, and use the saved time to your best advantage. Truck stops are filled with trucks during rush hour. Professional drivers use this time to eat and sleep rather than spend time in "gridlock." Do the same.
- Simplify gift giving. For example, books are a great gift and all your holiday shopping can be done in one store. Each book can be personalized by topic and a personal message inscribed on the inside cover.
- Avoid meetings unless they are absolutely necessary, such as a parent/teacher conference. If a meeting is necessary, set a time limit on each subject to be discussed and the amount of time each person can speak and stick to it. This requires participants to be concise and focused.
- Shop for food when the stores open in the morning or late at night, preferably midweek, because these are the least crowded times.
- Avoid using the library just before midterms and finals. Using the library at these times is generally the sign of a procrastinator.

Manage your own emotions:

- Lower your expectations. For example, you do not have to research every project beyond what is necessary to meet the criteria of the assignment or you do not have to prepare four-course meals every day. Perfection is not necessary to pass a nursing course.
- Recognize when you are experiencing "good guilt" versus "bad guilt" and act accordingly. For more information, see the section on self-discipline in this chapter.
- Avoid accepting the role of counselor for your friends. Listening to other people's problems is a time-consuming and emotionally exhausting process. Listen for a few minutes and then say, "I'm not a counselor. I think you need to talk to someone who is trained to help you with this problem."

MOTIVATING YOURSELF

Motivation is the driving force that encourages you to do something. It is an incentive or bribe that induces you to action. Motivation can come from within. Learning something new, attaining a goal, and being impressed with your performance are examples of internal motivation. You have to be future oriented to use internal motivation to stimulate yourself toward the achievement of a long-term goal. For example, visualize yourself walking up to receive your diploma, wearing your nurse's uniform, or receiving your first paycheck for being a nurse. This can be difficult because you have to delay gratification in the present for a future abstract goal.

Motivation can also come from without. Earning a high grade, obtaining respect from others, and receiving a reward are examples of external motivation. To deal with the present, a break from studying, a candy bar, a walk around the block, a cold drink, or just sitting down and getting started may be motivating.

Each person's motivator is individual. Think about the tasks that you accomplish every day. What payoff do you receive for completing them? When you are able to identify what really spurs you to action, then you can use these same incentives for accomplishing school-related activities. For a further discussion about motivation, see Balance Sacrifices and Rewards in Chapter 4, Study Techniques.

Achieve a Personal Balance

Do you write and rewrite an assignment until it is perfect? Do you always have to get an "A" on every test? Do you think that no one can do as good a job on a particular project as you can? Do you like others to have an image of you that you are superman or superwoman? Do you study constantly to the detriment of your other personal needs? Do you think that you can be all things to all people? Do you think that the office/committee/family will collapse without you? If you answered "Yes" to several of these questions, you may be a perfectionist.

A **perfectionist** is a person who compulsively strives to attain a degree of excellence according to a given standard. In other words, you think you are perfect. Also, a perfectionist tends to have an idealized self-image. That is, he or she displays to the world a self that is expected to be admired, respected, and loved by others. Unfortunately, if you are a perfectionist, then you are striving for the impossible. It is humanly impossible to be perfect, and attempting to maintain an idealized image is irrational, impractical, and self-destructive.

Perfectionism can be physically and emotionally debilitating. Because you can never really achieve perfection, you set yourself up for not performing according to your own imaginary standard of perfection. When this happens, emotionally you shatter your self-image, which can at best be demoralizing and unmotivating and at worst promote feelings of failure. Also, attempting to complete every role (spouse, parent, worker, and student) to perfection can take its toll on your body. A little stress keeps you alert, motivated, and focused However, excessive stress taxes the endocrine, neurological, and cardiovascular systems, which eventually results in physical depletion and exhaustion. Perfectionism, although considered a noble trait by some, can be emotionally and physically self-destructive and should be brought under control.

To conquer obsessive/compulsive, perfectionistic thinking, you must achieve a sense of personal balance. There is a big difference between expecting perfection and striving for excellence! First, you should recognize that no one, including you, is perfect. Then you must alter your frame of reference. You do this by putting the new set of circumstances into the present situation. Examples of some questions you may ask yourself are:

- Will I still graduate if I earn less than an "A" in my nursing courses?
- Is a grade of "A" on a written assignment worth not going to a child's sporting event?
- Will what it takes to earn an "A" in a nursing course negatively affect the other things I think are important in my life?
- Does this task require perfect effort?
- Does dinner really have to be on the table at 6 p.m.?
- Can I afford to have my lawn cut rather than cut it myself?
- Does dust provide a protective barrier for the surface of furniture?

Individualize the questions you ask yourself to reflect your personal and family responsibilities. We are not suggesting that you lower your standards on those things that are most important to you. However, if you are adding a huge commitment into your life (e.g., nursing school), something else in your life has to give. A student once told us that although she picked up around the house every day, she dusted only every other week. One day she saw the following note from her husband written in the dust on a table top. "I love you!" Underneath the note she wrote back, "Ditto!" She said they had a good laugh over the exchange, but she also demonstrated to him that the dust was not one of her priorities and she was not going to be pressured into dusting. One of our male students indicated that he never studied on Saturday night. He and his girlfriend always had a standing date so that they could spend time together. At graduation several graduates have an opportunity to talk to the convocation. Usually at least one graduate will make reference to the fact that there will be more home-cooked meals and less pizza and Chinese food now that they have graduated. One of the examples presented reflects a behavior that addresses an important value (spending time with a significant other). Other examples demonstrate a relaxation of standards of perfection (a dust-free house and home-cooked meals).

Controlling perfectionism and relaxing an idealized self-image are not easy tasks. However, you must remain true to yourself in light of your values and goals. Seek growth and development, not perfection, as you seek balance in your personal life.

Delegate

If you look up the word "delegate" in a dictionary, you will find words such as "surrender," "relinquish," "renounce," and "give up" used to explain its meaning. Unfortunately, this is why many people have difficulty delegating tasks to others. They look at delegation as a loss, giving something up, or yielding control. Delegation does the exact opposite. When you delegate, you transfer a task to another person and you gain, not lose, something. You gain more time and experience less stress! For delegation to achieve desired results and positive feelings for both people involved, you must follow the guidelines in the following paragraphs.

Identify the personal qualities of the people to whom you can delegate. Before you delegate a task to another person you must identify, alone or in conjunction with the other person, whether the person has the capacity to complete the task. Does the person have the appropriate intellectual, physical, and/or attitudinal ability to be successful at the task? The focus here is not on whether this person has ever done this task before but whether the person has the potential to do the task and is the appropriate person for the task. For example, it is inappropriate to expect 5-year-old children to clean a house but it is appropriate to expect them to pick up their own toys.

Identify the outcomes of the task to be accomplished. Explore with the other person the expected result. You should both have a clear, concise, mutual understanding of what is to be accomplished. The focus here is not on how the task will be done but rather on the product or conclusion. For example, if you delegate doing the laundry, the outcome may be that clothing will be clean, dried, and folded every 3 days. You are not focusing on how the clothing got washed or what cleaning products were used.

Identify the resources that are necessary to accomplish the task. For a task to be accomplished, you must consider the human, economic, technical, or organizational resources that may be necessary for the person to accomplish the desired outcome. There may be necessary information or skills that must be practiced before the person becomes successful in performing a new task. The focus here is not on excessive detail but rather on flexibility in the extent of support. For example, to cook dinner, one person may draw on past experiences; another may need a cookbook; and another may require a demonstration with supervised practice.

Relinquish accountability for the task. Accountability exists when a person assumes responsibility for something. When you delegate in your personal life, you transfer the responsibility for the task to another person and that person assumes ownership of his or her actions and the results of those actions. You will not feel free from the burden of a task unless you relinquish accountability for the task. The focus here is not on authoritarian supervision or consequences for tasks not accomplished but rather on the concept of trust. For example, you cannot hover over, breathe down the neck of, or micromanage another person when he or she is working on a delegated task. You must allow the person room to explore, practice, and grow. Occasionally, you may have to wear pink underwear, tolerate dusty baseboards, or eat tasteless meals. Initially, less than perfect outcomes go with the territory of delegation.

Delegation does not occur in isolation. Communicate your needs to family and friends. Have a family meeting and explore what tasks must be done, what people would like to do, and what skills need to be learned. When family members are involved in the decision-making process there is "ownership," which increases the probability of success. This is an opportunity for both you and family members to grow. You will learn the art of delegation, share your needs, recognize that you are interdependent, and reinforce that you must trust in others. Family members, even children, will learn new skills, feel important, develop confidence, and gain independence. Finally, routinely review the plan and evaluate how it is working. Ask questions such as: Are people accountable? Should tasks be rotated? Do people need additional resources? Is someone ready to learn a new skill? Are priorities being met? Change the plan as necessary. Delegation plans must be flexible to meet the needs of both the family as a whole and the individuals within it.

Overcome Procrastination

Procrastination is putting off or postponing something until a future time. It is a protective mechanism to delay having to deal with something that we would rather not deal with. We procrastinate because in the short term it reduces anxiety. However, in the long term, procrastination wastes time and increases anxiety. We all procrastinate to some degree, but when taken to an extreme it can interfere with our ability to complete tasks for which we are responsible. When delaying a project, have you ever said to yourself:

• This is boring.
• This is too hard.
• I do not know where to begin.
• I am not in the mood.
• I am too tired.
• I am angry/annoyed/frustrated that I have to do this.
• I have more important things to do.
• I can do it tomorrow.
• I have plenty of time.
• I work better under pressure.

These are just a few of the ways in which we rationalize our behavior. **Rationalization** is giving socially acceptable reasons or explanations for our behaviors. When rationalization is used in relation to why we did not do something we were expected to do, usually it is an excuse! Sometimes our excuses are so believable that we convince ourselves. To overcome procrastination, you must first realize that you are procrastinating, stop the procrastinating behavior, and then take constructive action to overcome the procrastination.

Breaking the cycle of procrastination requires a new mind-set. When we delay tasks, it is often because we look at them as "chores," routine activities or responsibilities that we may consider demanding or unpleasant. The word "chores" has a negative undertone. Therefore, tasks associated with schoolwork must never be viewed as chores but placed within a positive frame of reference. They are tasks that must be accomplished to reach your goal of becoming a nurse. Now, take the reason that you stated why something should be postponed and challenge the statement with logic or motivating strategies. For example:

• This is boring. "This is not dull and unexciting because it will help prepare me to be a nurse. It has to get done sooner or later, and it might as well be now."
• This is too hard. "I can do this! It may be difficult, but I did not get this far in my education without being able to do what I have to do to pass a course."
• I do not know where to begin. "Yes, I do! I need to review the requirements related to this assignment. I will make an outline on how I should move forward. I will focus on just a small part of the assignment. I will discuss what I finish today with my instructor tomorrow."
• I am not in the mood. "I will never be in the mood to do this assignment. I can divide the assignment into several parts and reward myself when I finish each part."
• I am too tired. "I am always tired. I will break down the job into sections, and I can do at least one section today."

- I am angry/annoyed/frustrated that I have to do this. "I am feeling this way because . . . , but my feelings are standing in the way of my completing this task. I need to *get a grip*. I will deal with my feelings in more depth after finishing what I have to do now."
- I have more important things to do. "Oh, really! Let me list the other things I have to do, and I will put them in order of importance. Which of these things can I eliminate or delegate? This is the most important thing I have to do now."
- I can do it tomorrow. "No, I will think about it right now. I should not put off until tomorrow what I can do today!"
- I have plenty of time. "I never have plenty of time. There is no time like the present!"
- I work better under pressure. "Who am I kidding? When I leave it to the last minute, I get it done because I have no other choice. I can do a much better job now if I give myself enough time to do it right."

These examples of self-challenge statements are not universal responses. Make your own statements. However, each statement should follow these simple guidelines: identify that you are procrastinating, challenge the procrastination with a direct opposing thought, and justify your challenging statement with a logical explanation. Sometimes the explanations to challenge procrastination involve larger changes, such as modifying your priorities or restructuring your activities of daily living. However, more often than not it involves smaller changes, such as using strategies of motivation. You can motivate yourself by setting short-term goals, providing rewards for finished tasks, using positive self-talk, or being a firm self-taskmaster. Procrastination is a behavior that is initiated from within. When you know and manage yourself, you will be in control of your learning instead of the other way around.

SUMMARY

Controlling the use of time to your best advantage depends on your desire and effort to identify and correct negative patterns that waste time. You should be proactive in the control of your time. To be proactive you need to implement the tools presented in this chapter to identify barriers to productivity, identify common time traps, and implement suggested corrective actions. If successful, you will have more time to tackle the tasks that are not pressing but important. When addressing tasks in this category, you will feel more in control and productive and less overwhelmed and anxious. With a little effort and a desire to change, you can be a master of your own time! Using your time productively can maximize the time you have for studying for nursing examinations.

Study Techniques

4

Learning is the activity by which knowledge, attitudes, and/or skills are acquired. Learning is a complex activity that is influenced by various factors such as genetic endowment, level of maturation, experiential background, effectiveness of formal instruction, self-image, readiness to learn, and level of motivation. Although some of these factors are unchangeable, others you can control.

Learning is an active process that takes place within the learner. Therefore, the role of the learner is to participate in or initiate activities that promote learning. Like test taking, learning is an acquired skill. This chapter presents both general and specific study techniques that should increase your ability to learn. The general study techniques presented include skills that facilitate learning regardless of the topic being studied. The specific study techniques are presented in relation to levels of thinking processes that are required to answer questions in nursing: knowledge, comprehension, application, and analysis. Use of these techniques when studying will help you to comprehend more of what you have studied and retain the information for a longer period of time. This information should increase your success in answering test questions.

GENERAL STUDY TECHNIQUES

There are general techniques to improve study skills that can be applied to any subject and a few specific techniques particularly applicable to studying for nursing examinations. Both types are discussed here.

Establish a Routine

Set aside a regular time to study. Learning requires consistency, repetition, and practice. Deciding to sit down to study is the most difficult part of studying. We tend to procrastinate and think of a variety of things we must do instead of studying. By committing yourself to a regular routine, you eliminate the repetitive need to make the decision to study. If you decide that every evening from 7:00 to 8:30 you are going to study, you are using your internal locus of control and establishing an internal readiness to learn. You must be motivated to learn.

Your study schedule must be reasonable and realistic. Shorter, more frequent study periods are more effective than long study periods. For most people, 1- to 3-hour study periods with a 10-minute break each hour are most effective. Periods of learning must be balanced with adequate rest periods because energy, attention, and endurance decrease over time and limit learning efficiency. Physical and emotional rest makes you more alert and receptive to new information.

When planning a schedule, involve significant family members in the decision making. Because a family is an open system, the action of one family member will influence the other family members. If family members are involved in the decision making, they will have a vested interest and probably be more supportive of your need to study.

Set Short- and Long-Term Goals

A goal is an outcome that a person attempts to attain, and it may be long term or short term. A long-term goal is the eventual desired outcome. A short-term goal is a desired outcome that can be achieved along the path leading to the long-term goal. In other words, a long-term goal is your destination, whereas each short-term goal is an objective that must be attained to help you eventually reach your destination. Each long-term goal may have one or more short-term goals. Goals should be formulated to promote learning that is purposeful, to serve as guides for planning action, and to establish standards so that learning can be evaluated. Goals must be specific, measurable, and realistic and must have a time frame. A specific goal states exactly what is to be accomplished. A measurable goal sets a minimum acceptable level of performance. A realistic goal must be potentially achievable. A goal with a time frame states the time parameters in which the goal will be achieved.

A typical long-term goal is "I will correctly answer 85% of the study questions at the end of Chapter 1 in a fundamentals of nursing textbook within 7 hours." Typical short-term goals might be to read and highlight important information in Chapter 1 within 2 hours, to list the principles presented in Chapter 1 within 1 hour, and to compare and contrast information in your class notes with information in the textbook within 2 hours. Each of these short-term goals can be achieved as a step toward attaining the long-term goal. It is wise to break a big task into small, manageable tasks because it is easier to learn small bits of information than large blocks of information. The most effective learning is goal-directed learning because it is planned learning with a purpose. In addition, attainment of goals increases self-esteem and motivation.

Simulate a Testing Environment

There are vast differences in learning styles, and there are many students who are unconventional learners. This discussion is not attempting to imply that there is only one way to learn. However, this textbook is presenting information that will help promote success on an examination. Therefore, to desensitize yourself to the testing environment it is helpful to simulate that environment when studying. When studying for a test, your posture, surroundings, and equipment should be similar to those in the testing environment. Study at a desk or table and chair and ensure adequate lighting. Avoid the temptation to study in a reclining chair, on the couch, or in bed. Keep pets in another room, avoid eating, and mute the ringer on your phone. Attempt to simulate the testing environment when studying for an examination. Remember, the familiar generally is less stressful than the unfamiliar.

Control Internal and External Distractors

Stimuli, both internal and external, must be controlled to eliminate distractions. External stimuli are environmental happenings that interrupt your thinking and should be limited. Select a place to study where you will not be interrupted by family members, phone calls, the doorbell, or family pets. These stimuli compete for your attention when you should be focusing on your work. Internal stimuli are your inner thoughts, feelings, or concerns that interfere with your ability to study. Internal stimuli are often more difficult to control than external stimuli because they involve attitudes. Review the techniques in Chapter 1 that promote a positive mental attitude. By limiting or eliminating internal and external distractors, you should improve your ability to concentrate.

Prepare for Class

To prepare adequately for class, you need to know the content that will be addressed. Look at the course outline or ask your instructor. "If you don't know where you're going, you can't get there!" After you know the topic, identify the appropriate content in your textbook. To "pre-*pare*" for class you must pare down the written information in your textbook. To "pare" means to trim, clip, or cut back. When reviewing textbook material before class, it is not always necessary to read every word.

- **First,** read the chapter headings. This will give you an overview of the topic presented.
- **Second,** look at tables and figures and read their captions. These provide visual cues.
- **Third,** skim the chapter content but read information that is CAPITALIZED, *italicized*, or **boldfaced.** These formats indicate important information; use a highlighting marker to accentuate these terms and other areas of meaningful content.
- **Fourth,** list the questions you may want to ask in class. You are now minimally prepared for class. Finally, to be well prepared, read the chapter thoroughly to gain an in-depth understanding of the content.

Take Class Notes

Taking notes in class is critical. Class notes are valuable because they provide you with a blueprint for study when preparing for an examination. The following are note-taking tips:

- **Stay focused on the topic being presented.** Generally, instructors present material that they believe is important. Compare this information to the material you highlighted in your textbook.
- **Use your notebook creatively.** Open your notebook so that you have facing sheets. Use the page on the left side for class notes. Save the page on the right side for adding information from the textbook or other sources that clarify the class notes.
- **Use an outline format and abbreviations.** There is no way that you can write down every word that comes out of your instructor's mouth. Focus on concepts because you can expand on the content later. For example, if an instructor is talking about abnormal respiratory rates such as apnea, bradypnea, and tachypnea, write these words down and listen to the instructor's presentation. The definitions can be added at a later time to the page on the right side of your notebook.
- **Ask questions to clarify information.** Your goal is not to be a stenographer. Your goal is to understand the information. Ask questions that you have prepared before class or that you may have as a result of the discussion in class. If you have a question, other students probably have the same question. Have the courage to ask questions. Two of the roles of an instructor are to make the information more understandable and clarify misconceptions. Your tuition pays the instructor's salary, so get your money's worth!
- **Review your notes after class.** You should review your notes within 48 hours after class. Reviewing, reorganizing, and rewriting class notes are techniques of reinforcement. Repetition helps commit information to memory. Some instructors allow you to use a recorder in class. Reviewing class recordings is particularly helpful to students who are auditory learners, those who have difficulty grasping complex material the first time, and those for whom English is a second language.

Identify Learning Domains

How we learn is never identical for two different people, nor is it identical for one person in different situations. Over the years you have developed a learning style with which you feel comfortable and that has proved successful. It is in your best interest, however, to be open to a variety of learning approaches.

Learning is the process by which you attain new information (cognitive domain), acquire new physical skills (psychomotor domain), or form new attitudes (affective domain).

COGNITIVE DOMAIN

Cognitive learning is concerned with understanding information acquired through exploring thoughts, ideas, and concepts. It advances from the simple to the complex and progresses from knowing and comprehending information to applying and analyzing information.

New information usually is learned through symbols such as words or pictures. We read them, see them, or hear them. Use all your senses to acquire new information. The more routes information takes to travel to your brain, the greater are the chances that you will learn the information. For example, when reading information about positioning patients, learning is reinforced by viewing pictures of patients in the various positions.

Psychomotor Domain

Psychomotor learning is concerned with the development of skills. It involves perceptual abilities as well as physical abilities related to endurance, strength, and dexterity. Integrated body movements progress from reflexive movements, to basic fundamental movements, to skilled movements.

New skills involve the physical application of information. It is possible for a person to understand all the goals and steps of a procedure and yet not be able to perform the procedure. For information to get from the head to the hands, the learner must do more than read a book, look at pictures, view a video, or watch other people. The learner must become actively involved. Physical skills are not learned by osmosis or diffusion; they are learned by doing. For example, when learning how to change a sterile dressing, the learner can read a book and look at a video, but it is essential that the learner actually practice changing a sterile dressing.

Affective Domain

Affective learning is concerned with the development of attitudes, which includes interests, appreciations, feelings, and values; it progresses from awareness to an increasing internalization or commitment to the attitude.

Learning new attitudes is the most difficult type of learning because attitudes result from lifelong experiences and tend to be well entrenched. For example, a student may know and understand the theory concerning why a person should be nonjudgmental and yet in clinical situations be judgmental toward the patient. The development of new attitudes is best learned in an atmosphere of acceptance by exploring feelings, becoming involved in group discussions, and observing appropriate role models. For example, before providing physical hygiene for a patient for the first time, it is beneficial to explore one's own feelings about invading a patient's personal space.

Capture Moments of Time

Using your spare moments for reviewing information is a method of maximizing your time for constructive study. We all have periods during the day that are less productive than others, such as waiting at a red light or standing in line at a store. Also, there are times when you engage in repetitive tasks such as vacuuming a rug or raking leaves. Capture these moments of time and use them to study. Carry flash cards, a vocabulary list, or categories of information that you can review when you have unexpected time. These captured moments should be in addition to, rather than a replacement for, your regularly scheduled study periods. There is an old saying that states, "Time is on your side." Capture spare moments of time and use them to your advantage. For additional information about time management, review Chapter 3.

Use Appropriate Resources

The theories and principles of nursing practice are complex. They draw from a variety of disciplines (e.g., psychology, sociology, anatomy and physiology, microbiology), use new terminology, and require unique applications to clinical practice. When you study, you will find that your learning will not proceed in a straight line, moving progressively forward. You may experience plateaus, remissions, and/or periods of confusion when dealing with complex material. When your forward progress is slowed, identify your needs and immediately seek help. Your instructor, another student, a study group, or a tutor may be beneficial. When studying with another student, make sure that the person is a source of correct information. When studying in groups, three to five students are ideal because a group of more than five people becomes a "party." The group should be heterogeneous; that is, there should be a variety of academic abilities, attitudes, skills, and perspectives among the members. This variety should enrich the learning experience and provide checks and balances for the sharing of correct information. Remember, you learn not only from the instructor but also from your classmates.

Generally, people do not like to admit that they have learning difficulties because they think it makes them look inadequate in the eyes of others. For this reason, people may be embarrassed to ask for help. This can be self-destructive because it denies you the opportunity to use resources that support growth. Be careful that you do not fall into this trap! To obtain access to the appropriate resources you must be willing to be open to yourself and others. Resources (e.g., extra help sessions; computer labs; reading, writing, and math centers; psychological counseling; and availability of faculty during office hours) are there to be used. Have the courage to acknowledge to yourself and others that you need help. Seeking help is a sign of maturity rather than a sign of weakness. When you ask for help, you are in control because you are solving problems to meet your own needs.

Balance Sacrifices and Rewards

When you decided to enter nursing school, no one promised you a rose garden. Your commitment to become a nurse requires sacrifice. Your time and energy are being diverted from your usual activities related to a job, family members, friends, and pleasurable pastimes. Rigorous activity, whether physical or mental, requires concentration and endurance. However, too much work hinders productivity. You must establish a balance between energy expenditure and rewards for your efforts. Rewards can be internal or external. Internal rewards are stimulated from within the learner and relate to feelings associated with meaningful achievement. Learning something new, achieving a goal, or increasing self-respect are examples of internal rewards. External rewards come from outside the learner. A grade of 100%, respect and appreciation from others, or a present for achieving a goal are examples of external rewards.

Unfortunately, the rewards for studying usually are not immediate but in the extended future. Graduating from nursing school, passing the NCLEX, earning a paycheck, and enjoying the prestige of being a nurse are future-oriented rewards. Therefore, you should be the one to provide immediate rewards for yourself for studying. During study breaks or at the completion of studying, reward yourself by thinking about how much you have learned, reflecting on the good feelings you have about your accomplishments, relaxing with a significant other, having a beverage, watching a favorite television show, calling a friend on the telephone, or taking a weekend off. Short-term rewards promote a positive mental attitude, reinforce motivation, and provide a respite from studying.

SPECIFIC STUDY TECHNIQUES RELATED TO COGNITIVE LEVELS OF NURSING QUESTIONS

The nurse uses a variety of thinking processes when caring for patients. Therefore, nursing examinations must reflect these thinking processes to evaluate effectively the safe practice of nursing. There are four types of thinking processes that may be required to answer questions concerning the delivery of nursing care: **knowledge, comprehension, application,** and **analysis** (for this discussion, analysis includes synthesis and evaluation). These thinking processes are within the cognitive domain and are ordered according to complexity.

That is, a knowledge question requires the lowest level of thinking (recalling information), whereas an analysis question requires the highest level of thinking (comparing and contrasting information).

In this section of the book each cognitive level is discussed and sample multiple-choice items are presented to illustrate the thinking processes involved in answering the item. In addition, specific study techniques are presented to help you to strengthen your critical-thinking abilities.

The correct answers for the sample items in this chapter and the rationales for all the options are at the end of this chapter.

Knowledge Questions

Knowledge questions require you to **recall or remember information.** To answer a knowledge question, you need to commit facts to memory. Knowledge questions expect you to know terminology, specific facts, trends, classifications, categories, criteria, structures, principles, generalizations, and theories. This basic information is the foundation for thinking critically.

SAMPLE ITEM 4-1

Hospice care lies in which level of prevention?

1. Secondary prevention
2. Morbidity prevention
3. Primary prevention
4. Tertiary prevention

To answer this question you need to know the definitions of the various types of prevention as well as what service hospice provides.

SAMPLE ITEM 4-2

A nurse must make an unoccupied bed. Which is the first step of the procedure for making the bed?

1. Cleaning hands
2. Pulling the curtain
3. Collecting clean linen
4. Placing the bottom sheet

To answer this question correctly, you need to know the sequence of steps in the procedure of making an unoccupied bed or the basic principle that your hands must be cleaned before all procedures.

SAMPLE ITEM 4-3

Which is the expected range of a radial pulse for an adult?

1. 50 to 65 beats per minute
2. 70 to 85 beats per minute
3. 90 to 105 beats per minute
4. 110 to 125 beats per minute

To answer this question correctly, you need to know the expected range of a radial pulse for an adult.

STUDY TECHNIQUES TO INCREASE YOUR KNOWLEDGE

Repetition/Memorization

Through repetition, information is committed to the brain for recall at a later date. Repeatedly studying information by reciting it out loud, reviewing it in your mind, or writing it down increases your chances of remembering the information because a variety of senses are used. Memorization can be facilitated by using lists of related facts, flash cards, or learning wheels. For example:

* On an index card you can list the steps of a procedure. This can be carried with you to study when you capture moments of time.
* On the front of an index card you can write a word and on the back define the word. An entire deck of cards can be developed for the terminology within a unit of study. Use flash cards when you have unexpected time to study.
* To make a learning wheel, cut a piece of cardboard into a circle and draw pie-shaped wedges on the front and back. On a front wedge write a unit of measure, such as 30 mL, and on the corresponding back wedge write its conversion to another unit of measure, such as 1 ounce. Then, on individual spring clothespins, write each of the units of measure that appear on the back of the wheel. When you want to study approximate equivalents, mix up the clothespins and attempt to match each one to its corresponding unit of measure. You can turn the wheel over and evaluate your success by determining if the clothespin you attached to the wheel matches the unit of measure on the back of the wheel.

Alphabet Cues

Memorization of information can be facilitated if the information is associated with letters of the alphabet. Each letter serves as a cue that stimulates the recall of information. The most effective alphabet cues are those you make up yourself. They meet a self-identified need, and you must review the information before you can design the alphabet cue. You can use any combination of letters as long as they have meaning for you and your learning. Examples of alphabet cues include:

* The **CABs** of cardiopulmonary resuscitation for health-care providers are: **C**irculation—initiate cardiac compression; **A**irway—assess the airway; **B**reathing—initiate artificial breathing.
* Identify patients at risk for injury through the letters **A, B, C, D, E, F,** and **G: A**ge—the young and very old; **B**lindness—lack of visual perception; **C**onsciousness—decreased level of consciousness; **D**eafness—lack of auditory perception; **E**motional state—reduced perceptual awareness; **F**requency of accidents—history of accidents; and **G**ait—impaired mobility.
* The **Three Ps** for the cardinal signs of diabetes mellitus are: **P**olyuria, **P**olydipsia, and **P**olyphagia.

Acronyms

An acronym is a word formed from the first letters of a series of statements or facts. Each part of the acronym relates to the information it represents. It is useful to learning because each letter of the word jolts the memory to recall information. An acronym is a technique used to retrieve previously learned information. Examples of acronyms include the following:

* The American Cancer Society teaches the early warning signs of cancer by using the word **CAUTION:**

Change in bowel and bladder habits

A sore that does not heal

Unusual bleeding or discharge

Thickening or a lump

Indigestion or difficulty in swallowing

Obvious change in a wart or mole

Nagging cough or hoarseness

- When assessing a patient for indicators of infection, remember the word **INFECT:**
  Increased pulse, respirations, and white blood cell count

Nodes enlarged

Function impaired

Erythema, Edema, Exudate

Complaints of discomfort or pain

Temperature increase—local and/or systemic

Acrostics

An acrostic is a phrase, motto, or verse in which a letter of each word (usually the first letter) prompts the memory to retrieve information. Memorizing information can be difficult and boring. This technique is a creative way to make learning more effective and fun. Examples of acrostics include:

- When studying the fat-soluble vitamins, recall this motto, "**All Dieters Eat Kilocalories.**" This should help you remember that **A, D, E,** and **K** are the fat-soluble vitamins.
- **On Old Olympus's Towering Tops, A Finn and a Swedish Girl Viewed Some Hops,** which stands for **Olfactory, Optic, Oculomotor, Trochlear, Trigeminal, Abducens, Facial, Sensorimotor** (vestibulocochlear), **Glossopharyngeal, Vagus, Spinal accessory,** and **Hypoglossal** nerves. These are the cranial nerves.

Mnemonics

A mnemonic is a variation of an acrostic. It is a phrase, motto, or verse that jogs the memory. It differs from an acrostic in that not every word is related to a specific piece of content. Mnemonics promote retention by connecting new or difficult information to known or less difficult information using mental associations or visual pictures.

- When studying apothecary and metric equivalents, remember this verse, "There are **15 grains** of sugar in **1 graham (gram)** cracker." This sentence should help you remember that **15 grains** are equivalent to **1 gram.**
- When trying to remember the difference between low-density lipoproteins (LDLs) and high-density lipoproteins (HDLs) refer to the following mnemonic: **LDH** is **L**ousy cholesterol and **HDL** is **H**appy cholesterol. This sentence should help you remember that increased LDH levels are associated with atherosclerosis and are undesirable (lousy cholesterol) and HDL promotes excretion of cholesterol from the body (happy cholesterol).

These techniques help increase the retention of information. The information is learned by rote without any in-depth understanding of the information learned. Information learned by repetition uses short-term memory and generally is quickly forgotten unless reinforced through additional study techniques or application in your nursing practice.

Comprehension Questions

Comprehension questions require you to **understand information.** To answer a comprehension question, you must commit facts to memory as well as translate, interpret, and determine the implications of that information. You demonstrate understanding when you translate or paraphrase information; interpret or summarize information; or determine the implications, consequences, corollaries, or effects of information. Comprehension questions expect you to know and understand the information being tested. After you understand basic information, you can identify the significance of data, which is an initial step in critical thinking.

SAMPLE ITEM 4-4

The nurse administers a cathartic to a patient. Which therapeutic outcome should the nurse expect when assessing the patient's response to this medication?

1. Increased urinary output
2. Decreased anxiety
3. Bowel movement
4. Pain relief

   To answer this question, you need to know not only that a cathartic is a potent laxative that stimulates the bowel (knowledge) but also that the increase in peristalsis will result in a bowel movement (comprehension).

SAMPLE ITEM 4-5

A nurse uses the interviewing technique of clarification when interviewing a patient. Which is the nurse doing when this communication technique is used?

1. Paraphrasing the patient's message
2. Restating what the patient has said
3. Reviewing the patient's communication
4. Verifying what is implied by the patient

   To answer this question, you need to know that clarifying is a therapeutic tool that promotes communication between the patient and nurse (knowledge) and you also must explain why or how this technique facilitates communication (comprehension).

SAMPLE ITEM 4-6

A nurse administers an intramuscular injection and then massages the insertion site after the needle is withdrawn. Which is the purpose of massaging the insertion site at the completion of the procedure?

1. Limit infection
2. Prevent bleeding
3. Reduce discomfort
4. Promote absorption

   To answer this question, you need to know that massage is one step of the procedure for an intramuscular injection (knowledge) and you also must understand the consequence of massaging the needle insertion site after the needle is withdrawn (comprehension).

STUDY TECHNIQUES TO INCREASE YOUR COMPREHENSION OF INFORMATION

Explore "Whys" and "Hows"

The difference between knowledge questions and comprehension questions is that you must know facts to answer knowledge questions, but you must understand the significance of the facts to answer comprehension questions. Facts can be understood and retained longer if they are relevant and meaningful to the learner. When studying information, ask yourself **why** or **how** the information is important. For example, when learning that immobility causes pressure ulcers, explore *why* they occur. Pressure compresses the capillary beds, which interferes with the transport of oxygen and nutrients to tissues, resulting in ischemia and necrosis. When studying a skill such as bathing, explore *how* soap cleans the skin. Soap reduces the surface tension of water and helps remove accumulated oils, perspiration, dead cells, and microorganisms. If you interpret information and identify *why* or *how* the information is relevant and useful, then the information has value. When information increases in value, it also increases in significance and is less readily forgotten.

Study in Small Groups

After you have studied by yourself, usually it is valuable to study the same information with another person or in a small group. The sharing process promotes your comprehension of information because you listen to the impressions and opinions of others, learn new information from a peer tutor, and reinforce your own learning by teaching others. In addition, the members of the group reinforce your interpretation of information and correct your misunderstanding of information. The value of group work is in the exchange process. Group members must listen, share, evaluate, help, support, reinforce, discuss, and debate to promote learning. There is truth in the saying "One hand washes the other." Not only do you help the other person when you study together, but you also help yourself.

Application Questions

The application of information demonstrates a higher level of understanding than just knowing or comprehending information because it requires the learner to **show, solve, modify, change, use, or manipulate information** in a real situation or presented scenario. To answer an application question, you must apply concepts you learned previously to a specific situation. The concepts may be theories, technical principles, rules of procedures, generalizations, or ideas that have to be applied in a presented scenario. Application questions test your ability to use information. The making of rational and reflective judgments, which are part of the critical-thinking process, results in a course of action.

SAMPLE ITEM 4-7

An older adult's skin looks dry, thin, and fragile. Which should the nurse do when providing back care to this patient?

1. Apply a moisturizing body lotion.
2. Massage using short, kneading strokes.
3. Use soap when washing the patient's back.
4. Leave excess lubricant on the patient's skin.

   To answer this question, you need to know that dry, thin, fragile skin is common in older adults (knowledge) and that moisturizing lotion helps the skin to retain water and become more supple (comprehension). When presented with this patient scenario, you have to apply your knowledge concerning developmental changes in older adults and the consequences of the use of moisturizing lotion (application).

SAMPLE ITEM 4-8

A nurse is caring for several patients on bladder-retraining programs and a variety of toileting time frames are employed. Which time frame for toileting is always included in a toileting schedule?

1. Every 2 hours when awake
2. When going to bed at night
3. At 8 a.m., 2 p.m., 8 p.m., and 2 a.m.
4. Every few hours and through the night

   To answer this question, you need to know the principle that nursing care should be individualized (knowledge). You also must understand the commonalities within the procedure of bladder retraining (comprehension). When presented with this concrete situation, you have to apply your knowledge about patient-centered care and the theoretical components of bladder-retraining programs (application).

SAMPLE ITEM 4-9

A nurse is to assist a heavy patient higher in bed. Which should the nurse do to prevent self-injury?

1. Keep the knees and ankles straight.
2. Straighten the knees while bending at the waist.
3. Place the feet together and keep the knees bent.
4. Position the feet apart with one foot placed forward.

　　To answer this question, you need to know (knowledge) and understand (comprehension) the principles of body mechanics. You also need to apply these principles in a particular patient-care situation, moving a heavy patient higher in bed (application).

STUDY TECHNIQUES TO INCREASE YOUR ABILITY TO APPLY INFORMATION

Relate New Information to Prior Learning

Learning is easier when the information to be learned is associated with what you already know. Therefore, relate new information to your foundation of knowledge, experience, attitudes, and feelings. For example, when studying the principles of body mechanics, review which principles are used when you carry a heavy package, move from a reclining to a standing position, or assist an older person to walk up a flight of stairs. When studying the principles of surgical asepsis, recall and review the various situations when you performed sterile technique and identify the principles that were the foundation of your actions. Applying concepts, such as principles and theories, in actual situations reinforces your ability to use them in future circumstances.

Identify Commonalities

A commonality exists when two different situations require the application of the same or similar principle. For example, when studying the principle of gravity, you must understand that it is the force that draws all mass in the earth's sphere toward the center of the earth. Now try to identify situations that employ this principle. As a nurse, you apply this principle when you place a urine collection bag below the level of the bladder, hang an intravenous bag higher than the intravenous insertion site, raise the head of the bed for a patient with dyspnea, and elevate the legs of a patient with edema of the feet. This study technique is particularly effective when working in small groups because it involves brainstorming. Others in the group may identify situations that you have not considered. Identifying commonalities reinforces information and maximizes the application of information in patient-care situations.

Analysis Questions

Analysis questions require you to **interpret a variety of data** and **recognize the commonalities, differences,** and **interrelationships among presented ideas.** To answer an analysis question, you must identify, examine, dissect, evaluate, or investigate the organization or structure of the information presented in the question. Analysis questions make the assumption that you know, understand, and can apply information. They then require an ability to examine information, which is a higher thought process than knowing, understanding, or applying information. For example, when studying blood pressure, you first memorize the parameters of a normal blood pressure (knowledge). Then you develop an understanding of what factors influence and produce a normal blood pressure (comprehension). Then you identify a particular patient situation that necessitates obtaining a blood pressure (application). Finally, you must differentiate among a variety of situations and determine which has the highest priority for assessing the blood pressure (analysis). Analysis questions are difficult because they demand scrutiny of a variety of complex data presented in the stem and options and require a higher-level critical-thinking process.

SAMPLE ITEM 4-10

A patient has dependent edema of the ankles and feet and is obese. Which diet should the nurse expect the primary health-care provider to order?

1. Low in sodium and high in fat
2. Low in sodium and low in calories
3. High in sodium and high in protein
4. High in sodium and low in carbohydrates

To answer this question, you need to know and understand the relationships between salt in the diet and fluid retention and between obesity and caloric intake (comprehension). You must also understand the impact of carbohydrates, proteins, and fats in a diet for a patient with edema and obesity (comprehension). When you answer this question, you must examine the information presented, identify the interrelationships among the elements, and arrive at a conclusion (analysis).

SAMPLE ITEM 4-11

A patient who is undergoing cancer chemotherapy says to the nurse, "This is no way to live." Which response uses reflective technique?

1. "Tell me more about what you are thinking."
2. "You sound discouraged today."
3. "Life is not worth living?"
4. "What are you saying?"

To answer this question, you need to know and understand the communication techniques of reflection, clarification, and paraphrasing (knowledge and comprehension). Also, you must analyze each statement and identify the communication technique being used. This question requires you to differentiate information presented in the four options to arrive at the correct answer.

SAMPLE ITEM 4-12

A nurse is assessing a patient who reports being incontinent. Which question should the nurse ask to elicit information related to urge incontinence?

1. "Does urination occur immediately after coughing?"
2. "Do you urinate small amounts of urine frequently?"
3. "Do you begin urinating immediately after feeling the need to urinate?
4. "Does urination occur at predictable intervals without feeling the need to urinate?"

To answer this question, you need to know and understand the characteristics associated with urge incontinence (knowledge and comprehension). Then you must analyze which question will obtain information that relates to urge incontinence. This question requires you to identify the various types of incontinence (e.g., stress, functional, urge, and continuous) and the question that will elicit information about each. You must differentiate among the statements in the four options to arrive at the correct answer (analysis).

STUDY TECHNIQUES TO INCREASE YOUR ABILITY TO ANALYZE INFORMATION

Identify Differences

To study for complex questions, you cannot just memorize and understand facts or identify the commonalities among facts; you must learn to discriminate. Analysis questions often require you to use differentiation to determine the significance of information. When studying the causes of an increased blood pressure, identify the different causes and why they may result in an increased blood pressure. For example, a blood pressure can increase for a variety of reasons: infection causes an increased metabolic rate; fluid retention causes hypervolemia; and anxiety causes an autonomic nervous system response that constricts blood vessels. In each situation the blood pressure increases, but for a different reason. Identifying differences is an effective study technique to broaden the interrelationship and significance of learned information.

Practice Test Taking

Taking practice tests is an excellent way to improve the effectiveness of your learning. Reviewing rationales for the right and wrong answers serves as an effective study technique. It reinforces learning, and it can help you identify areas that require additional study.

As you practice test taking, not only do you increase your knowledge but also you become more emotionally and physically comfortable in the testing situation. It is most effective if you gradually increase the time you spend taking practice tests to 2 to 3 hours. This will help build stamina, enabling you to concentrate more effectively during a shorter test. Marathon runners have long recognized the value of building stamina and the need for practice to achieve a "groove" that enhances performance. Marathon runners also manage their practice so that they "peak" on the day of the big event. The same principles can be applied to the nursing student preparing for an important test. You are at your peak and can achieve a groove when you feel physically, emotionally, and intellectually ready for the important test.

Practicing test taking should assist you to learn by:

- Acquiring new knowledge
- Comprehending information
- Understanding concepts
- Identifying rationales for nursing interventions
- Applying theories and principles
- Identifying commonalities and differences in situations
- Analyzing information
- Reinforcing previous learning
- Applying critical thinking

In addition, practicing test taking should assist you to:

- Use test-taking techniques
- Effectively manage time during a test
- Control your environment
- Control physical and emotional responses
- Feel empowered and in control
- Develop a positive mental attitude

4-1 1. Secondary prevention refers to strategies for people in whom disease is present. The goal is to halt or reverse the disease process.
2. There is no category called morbidity prevention. The word "morbidity" refers to illness; "mortality" refers to death.
3. Primary prevention refers to strategies used to prevent illness in people who are considered free from disease.
4. **Tertiary prevention uses strategies to assist people to adapt physically, psychologically, and socially to permanent disabilities.**

4-2 1. **Cleaning the hands removes microorganisms that can contaminate clean linen. Washing the hands or using a hand sanitizer is referred to as hand hygiene.**
2. Pulling the curtain is unnecessary when making an unoccupied bed; this is required to provide privacy when making an occupied bed.
3. Collecting clean linen is done after the hands are cleaned to prevent contamination of the linen.
4. Placing the bottom sheet is done after the hands are cleaned and the clean sheets are collected

4-3 1. 50 to 65 beats per minute is less than the expected range for the pulse of an adult.
2. **70 to 85 beats per minute is within the expected range of 60 to 100 beats per minute for the pulse of an adult.**
3. Although 90 beats per minute is within the high end of the expected range for the pulse of an adult, 105 beats per minute is above the expected range.
4. 110 to 125 beats per minute is above the expected range for the pulse of an adult.

4-4 1. Diuretics, not cathartics, produce an increase in urinary output.
2. Antianxiety agents (anxiolytics) reduce anxiety.
3. **Cathartics stimulate bowel evacuation; therefore, the patient should be assessed for a bowel movement.**
4. Analgesics, not cathartics, alter the perception and interpretation of pain.

4-5 1. Paraphrasing, also called "restating," is an interviewing skill that repeats the patient's basic message in similar words to encourage additional communication.
2. Restating, also called "paraphrasing," is a technique that repeats the patient's basic message in similar words to promote further communication.
3. Reviewing involves summarizing the main points in a discussion; this is useful at the end of an interview or teaching session.
4. **Clarification is a method of verifying that the patient's message is understood as intended; it is an attempt to obtain more information without interpreting the original statement.**

4-6 1. Using sterile equipment and sterile technique limits infection, not massaging the needle insertion site.
2. Removing the needle along the line of insertion limits trauma, which prevents bleeding.
3. Instilling the solution slowly and removing the needle along the line of insertion reduce discomfort.
4. **Massage disperses the medication in the tissues and facilitates its absorption.**

4-7 1. **Moisturizing lotion limits dryness and reduces the friction of the hands against the skin, which prevents skin trauma.**
2. Massaging with short, kneading strokes can cause injury to delicate, thin skin; light, long strokes should be used.
3. Soap should be avoided because it can further dry the skin.
4. Excess lubricant on the skin may promote skin maceration, and also it provides a warm, moist environment for the growth of microorganisms, which should be avoided.

4-8 1. Toileting a patient every 2 hours when awake may not be appropriate for all patients; some patients may need to be toileted every hour, and others may require toileting every 3 hours. The schedule should be individualized.
2. **All patients, regardless of the specifics of each individual bladder-retraining program, will be toileted before going to bed at night and after awakening in the morning.**

3. Toileting four times a day is too infrequent when implementing a bladder-retraining program.

4. Every few hours is a nonspecific time frame. It may not be necessary to awaken the patient every 4 hours during the night; this may interfere with the patient's sleep.

4-9 1. Keeping the knees and ankles straight places strain on the muscles of the back and should be avoided.

2. When moving patients, the nurse's knees should be flexed, not straight, and the knees and hips should be flexed, not the waist; these actions use the large muscles of the legs rather than the back.

3. Keeping the feet together produces a narrow base of support that can result in a fall.

4. **Both actions provide a wide base of support that promotes stability; placing one foot in front of the other facilitates bending at the knees, which permits the muscles of the legs, rather than the back, to bear the patient's weight.**

4-10 1. Although a low-sodium diet is appropriate to limit edema, a diet high in fat should be avoided by an obese individual because fats are high in calories.

2. **Sodium promotes fluid retention and increased calories add to body weight; therefore, both should be avoided by an obese patient with edema.**

3. Sodium promotes fluid retention and should be avoided by a patient with edema; protein may or may not be related to this patient's problem.

4. Although carbohydrates may be restricted in an obese individual to facilitate weight loss, a high-sodium diet promotes fluid retention and should be avoided.

4-11 1. This response is using the technique of clarification and asks the patient to expand on the message so that it becomes more understandable.

2. **This response is using reflective technique because it attempts to identify feelings in the patient's message.**

3. This response is using the technique of paraphrasing; it restates the patient's basic message in similar words.

4. This response uses the communication technique of clarification. The nurse is attempting to better understand what the patient is saying when this technique is used.

4-12 1. This option is related to stress incontinence. Stress incontinence occurs when intra-abdominal pressure increases (e.g., coughing, laughing).

2. This option is related to overflow incontinence. Overflow incontinence occurs when there is an involuntary passage of urine related to an over-distended bladder.

3. **Urge incontinence is associated with a sudden desire to void. Urge incontinence is related to a decreased bladder capacity and bladder irritation.**

4. This option is related to reflex incontinence. Reflex incontinence is the involuntary passage of urine in somewhat predictable intervals. It is associated with an inability to sense the urge to void or that the bladder is full.

The Multiple-Choice Question

In our society, success is generally measured in relation to levels of achievement. Before you entered a formal institution of learning, your achievement was subjectively appraised by your family and friends. Success was rewarded by smiles, positive statements, and perhaps favors or gifts. Lack of achievement or failure was acknowledged by omission of recognition, verbal corrections, and possibly punishment or scorn. When you entered school, your performance was directly measured against acceptable standards. In an effort to eliminate subjectivity, you were exposed to objective testing. These tests included true/false questions, matching columns, and multiple-choice questions. Achievement was reflected by numerical grades or letter grades. These grades indicated your level of achievement and by themselves provided rewards and punishments.

In nursing education, achievement can be assessed in a variety of ways: a patient's physiological response (Did the patient's condition improve?), a patient's verbal response (Did the patient verbalize improvement?), student nurses' clinical performance (Did the students do what they were supposed to do?), and student nurses' levels of cognitive competency (Did the students know what they were supposed to know?). You must pass the National Council Licensing Examination known as NCLEX-PN to work legally as a Licensed Practical Nurse or the NCLEX-RN to work legally as a Registered Nurse. These examinations consist of multiple-choice and alternate-format items. Consequently, both types of questions are frequently used in schools of nursing to evaluate student progress throughout the nursing curriculum. They also are used because they are objective, are time efficient, and can assess comprehensively the understanding of curriculum content that has depth and breadth. Therefore, it is important for you to understand the components and dynamics of multiple-choice and alternate-format items early in your nursing education.

In the spring of 2003, alternate-format items were introduced in nursing licensure examinations. **Alternate-format items** require the test taker to select multiple answers to a multiple-choice question, perform a calculation and fill in the blank, place options in priority order, or respond to a question in relation to an exhibit. For information about and examples of alternate-format items, review Chapter 8, Testing Formats Other Than Multiple-Choice Questions. Multiple-choice questions are addressed in this chapter.

COMPONENTS OF A MULTIPLE-CHOICE QUESTION

A multiple-choice question is an objective test item. It is objective because the perceptions or opinions of another person do not influence the grade. In a multiple-choice question, a question is asked, three or more potential answers are presented, and only one of the potential answers is correct. The student answers the question either correctly or incorrectly.

The entire multiple-choice question is called an **item.** Each item consists of two parts. The first part is known as the **stem.** The stem is the statement that asks the question. The second part contains the possible responses offered by the item, which are called **options.** One of the options answers the question posed in the stem and is the **correct answer.** The remaining options are the incorrect answers and are called **distractors.** They are referred to as "distractors" because they are designed to distract you from the correct answer.

The correct answers and the rationales for all the options of the sample items in this chapter are at the end of the chapter. Test yourself and see if you can correctly answer the sample items.

SAMPLE ITEM 5-1

Which should the nurse do immediately before performing any procedure?

1. Shut the door. (DISTRACTOR)

2. Wash the hands. (CORRECT ANSWER)

3. Close the curtain. (DISTRACTOR)

4. Drape the patient. (DISTRACTOR)

SAMPLE ITEM 5-2

A nurse is assessing placement of a nasogastric tube. Where should the distal end of the tube be within the body?

1. Stomach (CORRECT ANSWER)

2. Bronchi (DISTRACTOR)

3. Trachea (DISTRACTOR)

4. Duodenum (DISTRACTOR)

SAMPLE ITEM 5-3

A parent says to the nurse, "My kid is difficult to get along with and is only concerned about the opinions of friends." How old is the child?

1. 3 years old (DISTRACTOR)

2. 7 years old (DISTRACTOR)

3. 14 years old (CORRECT ANSWER)

4. 22 years old (DISTRACTOR)

THE STEM

The stem is the initial part of a multiple-choice item. The purpose of the stem is to present a problem in a clear and concise manner. The stem should contain all the details necessary to answer the question.

The stem of an item can be a complete sentence that asks a question. It also can be presented as an incomplete sentence that becomes a complete sentence when it is combined with one of the options of the item.

In addition to sentence structure, a characteristic of a stem that must be considered is its polarity. The polarity of the stem can be formulated in either a positive or negative context. A stem with a positive polarity asks the question in relation to what is true, whereas a stem with negative polarity asks the question in relation to what is false.

The Stem That Is a Complete Sentence

A complete sentence is a group of words that is capable of standing independently. When a stem is a complete sentence, it will ask a question and end with a question mark (?). It should clearly and concisely formulate a problem that can be answered before reading the options.

SAMPLE ITEM 5-4

Which should be the first action of the nurse when a fire alarm rings in a health-care facility?

1. Determine if it is a fire drill or a real fire.

2. Move patients laterally toward the stairs.

3. Take an extinguisher to the fire scene.

4. Close doors on the unit.

SAMPLE ITEM 5-5

Which is the most common reason why older adults become incontinent of urine?

1. They use incontinence to manipulate others.

2. The muscles that control urination become weak.

3. They tend to drink less fluid than younger patients.

4. Their increase in weight places pressure on the bladder.

SAMPLE ITEM 5-6

Which part of the body requires special hygiene when a patient has a nasogastric feeding tube?

1. Rectum

2. Abdomen

3. Oral cavity

4. Perineal area

The Stem That Is an Incomplete Sentence

When a stem is an incomplete sentence, it is a group of words that forms the beginning portion of a sentence. The sentence becomes complete when it is combined with one of the options in the item. Some tests will have a period at the completion of each option and others will not. Whether there is a period or not, each option should complete the sentence with grammatical accuracy. However, the answer is the only option that correctly completes the sentence in relation to the informational content. When reading a stem that is an incomplete sentence, usually it is necessary to read the options before the question can be answered.

SAMPLE ITEM 5-7

To **best** understand what a patient is saying, the nurse should:

1. Listen carefully.

2. Employ touch.

3. Show interest.

4. Remain silent.

SAMPLE ITEM 5-8

The **most** important reason why nurses should teach people not to smoke in bed is because it can:

1. Upset a family member.
2. Precipitate lung cancer.
3. Trigger a smoke alarm.
4. Result in a fire.

SAMPLE ITEM 5-9

When assisting a female patient with dementia to groom her hair, the nurse should:

1. Offer constant support and encouragement.
2. Set time aside for a long teaching session.
3. Alternate using a brush and a comb.
4. Teach her how to braid her hair.

The Stem With Positive Polarity

The stem with positive polarity is concerned with truth. It asks the question with a positive statement. The correct answer is accurately related to the statement. It is in accord with a fact or principle, or it is an action that should be implemented. A positively worded stem attempts to determine if you are able to understand, apply, or differentiate correct information.

SAMPLE ITEM 5-10

An older adult who is dying starts to cry and says, "I was always concerned about myself first, and I hurt many people during my life." Which is the underlying feeling being expressed by the patient?

1. Ambivalence
2. Sadness
3. Anger
4. Guilt

SAMPLE ITEM 5-11

Which nursing intervention most accurately supports the concept of informed consent for a surgical procedure?

1. Explaining what is being done and why
2. Involving the family in the teaching plan
3. Obtaining the patient's signature on the document
4. Teaching preoperative deep breathing and coughing

SAMPLE ITEM 5-12

Which should the nurse do when a patient appears to be asleep but does not react when called by name?

1. Loudly say, "Are you awake?"
2. Say to the patient, "Can you squeeze my hand?"
3. Inform the nurse manager in charge immediately.
4. Gently touch the patient's arm while saying the patient's name.

The Stem With Negative Polarity

The stem with negative polarity is concerned with what is false. It asks the question with a negative statement. The stem usually incorporates words such as "except," "not," or "never." These words are obvious. However, sometimes the words that are used are more obscure, for example, "contraindicated," "further," "unacceptable," "least," and "avoid." When a negative term is used, it may be emphasized by an underline (except), italics (*least*), boldface type (**not**), or capitals (NEVER). A negatively worded stem requires you to recognize exceptions, detect errors, or identify interventions that are unacceptable or contraindicated. Many nursing examinations do not have questions with negative polarity or do not emphasize the negative word when used in a stem. However, this information is included here in the event that you may be challenged by questions with negative polarity.

SAMPLE ITEM 5-13

On what part of the body should the nurse avoid using soap when bathing a patient?

1. Eyes
2. Back
3. Under the breasts
4. Glans of the penis

SAMPLE ITEM 5-14

The nurse determines that range-of-motion (ROM) exercises should NOT be done:

1. For comatose patients.
2. On limbs that are paralyzed.
3. Beyond the point of resistance.
4. For patients with chronic joint disease.

SAMPLE ITEM 5-15

Which suggestion by the nurse is the least therapeutic when teaching the patient about promoting personal energy?

1. Eat breakfast every day.
2. Exercise three times a week.
3. Get adequate sleep each night.
4. Drink a cup of coffee each morning.

SAMPLE ITEM 5-16

Which position is contraindicated for a patient who has dyspnea?

1. Fowler

2. Supine

3. Contour

4. Orthopneic

SAMPLE ITEM 5-17

Which action by the nurse is unacceptable during a bed bath?

1. Uncovering the area being washed

2. Using long, firm strokes toward the heart

3. Washing from the rectum toward the pubis

4. Replacing the top sheets with a cotton blanket

THE OPTIONS

All of the possible answers offered within an item are called "options." One of the options is the best response and is therefore the correct answer. The other options are incorrect and distract you from selecting the correct answer. These options are called "distractors." An item must have a minimum of three options to be considered a multiple-choice item, but the actual number varies among tests. The typical number of options is four or five responses, which reduces the probability of guessing the correct answer while limiting the amount of reading to a sensible level. Options usually are listed by number (1, 2, 3, and 4), lowercase letters (a, b, c, and d), or uppercase letters (A, B, C, and D). The grammatical presentation of options can appear in four different formats. An option can be a sentence, can complete the sentence begun in the stem, can be an incomplete sentence, or can be a single word.

The Option That Is a Sentence

A sentence is a unit of language that contains a stated or implied subject and verb. It is a statement that contains an entire thought and stands alone. Options can appear as complete sentences. Some tests have a period at the end of these options and others do not. Whether there is a period or not, each option should be grammatically correct. When the option is a verbal response, it should be grammatically correct and incorporate the appropriate punctuation, such as quotation marks (" "), comma (,) exclamation point (!), question mark (?), or period (.).

SAMPLE ITEM 5-18

Before performing a procedure, which should the nurse do first?

1. Collect the equipment for the procedure.

2. Position the patient for the procedure.

3. Explain the procedure to the patient.

4. Raise the bed to its highest position.

SAMPLE ITEM 5-19

A Catholic patient tells the nurse, "Before being hospitalized I went to mass and received Communion every morning." Which should the nurse do to meet this patient's spiritual needs?

1. Encourage the patient to say the rosary every day.

2. Make arrangements for the patient to receive communion.

3. Transfer the patient to a room with another Catholic patient.

4. Have a priest administer the Sacrament of Anointing of the Sick to the patient.

SAMPLE ITEM 5-20

A male patient is crying, and the only word the nurse understands is "wife." Which should the nurse say?

1. "I'm sure that your wife is fine."

2. "You are concerned about your wife?"

3. "What did your wife do to upset you?"

4. "Your wife will be visiting later today."

The Option That Completes the Sentence Begun in the Stem

When the option completes the sentence begun in the stem, the stem and the option together should form a sentence. Some tests have correct punctuation at the end of these options and others do not. Whether or not there is a period, each option should complete the stem in a manner that is grammatically accurate.

SAMPLE ITEM 5-21

A nurse understands that the primary etiology of obesity is a:

1. Lack of balance in the variety of nutrients

2. Glandular disorder that prevents weight loss

3. Caloric intake that exceeds metabolic needs

4. Psychological problem that causes overeating

SAMPLE ITEM 5-22

A nurse can best prevent the patient from getting a chill during a bed bath by:

1. Rubbing briskly to cause vasodilation.

2. Exposing only the area being washed.

3. Pulling the curtain around the bed.

4. Giving a hot drink before the bath.

SAMPLE ITEM 5-23

A nurse is to assist a patient with a bed bath. However, the patient has just returned from a diagnostic test, is in pain, and refuses the bath. The nurse should:

1. Encourage a shower instead.
2. Give a partial bath quickly.
3. Cancel the bath for today.
4. Delay the bath until later.

The Option That Is an Incomplete Sentence

When an option is an incomplete sentence, it does not contain all the parts of speech (e.g., subject and verb) necessary to construct a complete, autonomous statement. The option that is an incomplete sentence usually is a phrase or group of related words. Although not a complete sentence, it conveys a unit of thought, an idea, or a concept.

SAMPLE ITEM 5-24

Which nursing intervention is common when caring for all patients with infections?

1. Donning a mask
2. Wearing a gown
3. Washing the hands
4. Discouraging visitors

SAMPLE ITEM 5-25

When should the nurse administer mouth care to an unconscious patient?

1. Whenever necessary
2. Every four hours
3. Once a shift
4. Twice a day

SAMPLE ITEM 5-26

Which action by the nurse helps meet a patient's basic need for security and safety?

1. Addressing a patient by name
2. Accepting a patient's angry behavior
3. Ensuring a patient gets adequate nutrition
4. Explaining to a patient what is going to be done

The Option That Is a Word

A word is a series of letters that form a term. It is the most basic unit of language and is capable of communicating a message. The option that is a single word can be almost any part of speech (e.g., noun, pronoun, verb, or adverb) as long as it conveys information.

SAMPLE ITEM 5-27
Which is a primary source for obtaining information related to the independent functions of a nurse?

1. Chart
2. Patient
3. Nurse manager
4. Health-care provider

SAMPLE ITEM 5-28
A patient's spouse just died. Which approach should be used by the nurse when caring for this grieving patient?

1. Confronting
2. Supporting
3. Avoiding
4. Limiting

SAMPLE ITEM 5-29
What is the nurse doing when formulating a nursing diagnosis?

1. Planning
2. Assessing
3. Analyzing
4. Implementing

SAMPLE ITEM 5-30
Which word **best** describes feelings associated with a child in Erikson's stage of autonomy versus shame and doubt?

1. Hers
2. Mine
3. Theirs
4. Nobody's

5-1 1. Shutting the door should be done before washing the hands. The hands become contaminated when the door is touched.

2. **Before touching the patient, the nurse should wash his or her hands to remove microorganisms.**

3. Closing the curtain should be done before washing the hands. Curtains are considered contaminated. The hands should be washed after touching the curtains.

4. Draping the patient is done after washing the hands.

5-2 1. **The tube enters the nose, passes through the posterior nasopharynx and esophagus, and enters the stomach through the cardiac sphincter.**

2. The bronchi are passages between the trachea and bronchioles and are part of the respiratory system.

3. The trachea is a passage between the posterior nasopharynx and bronchi and is part of the respiratory system.

4. The duodenum is distal to the stomach and is the first portion of the small intestine; a nasogastric tube is designed to be advanced into the stomach, not the duodenum.

5-3 1. Toddlers are concerned about themselves and their autonomy, not others.

2. School-age children are easy to get along with and are concerned about performing and achieving.

3. **Adolescents are concerned about their identity, independence, and peer relationships; this causes tension between them and their parents.**

4. Young adults are developing intimate relationships and becoming socially responsible.

5-4 1. Whenever the fire alarm rings, it should always be considered an indication of a real fire.

2. Patients should be moved only if they are in danger.

3. The location of the fire must be identified before an extinguisher can be taken to the scene.

4. **Closing the doors on the unit should be the initial action of the options provided. A closed door provides for patient safety because it is a barrier that impedes the spread of the fire.**

5-5 1. This is untrue; most people want to be independent and in control of their bodily functions.

2. **Muscles, particularly the perineal muscles, tend to lose strength as people age.**

3. Incontinence is unrelated to fluid intake.

4. Older adults do not necessarily gain weight; many lose weight because of the loss of subcutaneous fat associated with aging. Body weight does not influence incontinence.

5-6 1. A nasogastric tube is unrelated to the rectum. Special care of this area of the body is unnecessary; care provided during a routine bed bath is adequate.

2. A nasogastric tube enters the body through the nose, not the abdomen. Cleansing of the abdomen during a routine bed bath is adequate.

3. **A nasogastric tube feeding generally negates the need to chew; with lack of chewing, salivation decreases, which causes the mucous membranes to become dry.**

4. The perineal area is unrelated to a nasogastric tube. Bathing of the perineal area during a routine bed bath is adequate.

5-7 1. **Attentive listening is important so that the nurse can pick up key words and identify emotional themes within the message.**

2. Touch is used to communicate a message of caring, not to receive, understand, or interpret a message from another person.

3. Although this may indicate acceptance and encourage ventilation of feelings, it does nothing to promote understanding by the nurse.

4. Although remaining silent may encourage further communication, it will not by itself promote understanding of the patient's message.

5-8 1. Although smoking can physically and emotionally disturb a family member, it is not the priority.

2. Although smoking may precipitate lung cancer, this is not the reason for not smoking in bed.

3. Smoke from a cigarette will not trigger a smoke alarm.

4. Confused, weak, or lethargic individuals may drop lighted cigarettes or ashes, which can ignite bed linens.

5-9 1. **People with dementia become confused easily and need support and encouragement to stay focused and motivated.**
2. People with dementia cannot concentrate long enough for a prolonged teaching session; learning occurs best with short, frequent teaching sessions.
3. Alternating a brush and a comb may promote confusion; patients with dementia need consistency.
4. Braiding the hair involves cognitive and psychomotor skills that the patient with dementia probably does not possess.

5-10 1. Ambivalence demonstrates two simultaneous conflicting feelings.
2. Although the patient may be unhappy about past behaviors, it is the underlying thoughts about hurting others that precipitated the patient's statement.
3. Anger is a feeling of displeasure caused by opposition or mistreatment and is demonstrated by the words or gestures used by the patient in an effort to fight back at the cause of the feeling.
4. **Guilt is a painful feeling of self-reproach resulting from the belief that one has done something wrong.**

5-11 1. **It is the surgeon's responsibility to explain what is going to be done and the potential negative and positive consequences (risks and benefits).**
2. Although the family may be involved, it is the patient who must sign the informed consent.
3. Legally a nurse may obtain a patient's signature on a consent form. The nurse's signature on the form only indicates that the patient was the person who signed the consent form. However, the nurse should identify the patient's understanding of the procedure to be performed and inform the surgeon if additional information is requested or necessary.
4. Preoperative teaching is necessary only if the patient consents to surgery.

5-12 1. Speaking loudly may frighten the patient; one of the patient's other senses should be stimulated because the patient

previously has not responded to a verbal intervention.
2. The nurse must get the patient's attention before giving a direction.
3. The nurse should assess the patient further before informing the nurse in charge.
4. **This action is the first step to assess this patient further. Touch and sound stimulate two senses, and using the patient's name is individualizing care.**

5-13 1. **Soaps usually contain sodium or potassium salts of fatty acids, which are irritating and can injure the sensitive tissues of the eyes.**
2. The back needs soap and water to remove perspiration that collects on the skin.
3. Body surface areas that touch are dark, warm, and moist and must be washed with soap and water to limit the growth of microorganisms.
4. The glans of the penis needs soap and water to remove perspiration, urine, and smegma.

5-14 1. Range of motion should be performed for unconscious patients because they usually are immobile and are at risk for developing contractures.
2. Paralyzed limbs must be moved through full range of motion by the nurse to prevent loss of range secondary to inactivity.
3. **Resistance indicates that there is strain on the muscles or joints; continuing range of motion beyond the point of resistance can cause injury and should be avoided.**
4. People with chronic joint disease usually need gentle range-of-motion exercises to keep the joints mobile.

5-15 1. Food contains nutrients and calories, which provide energy.
2. Exercise promotes muscle tone and energy.
3. Sleep is restful and restorative.
4. **Caffeine, although a stimulant, can be harmful to the body.**

5-16 1. When the patient is in a Fowler position, the diaphragm is not being compressed by the abdominal contents; this allows for maximal thoracic expansion.
2. **The abdominal contents press against the diaphragm when a person is in the supine position, which impedes**

expansion of the thoracic cavity and subsequently the lungs.

3. This position is desirable because the abdominal contents drop by gravity, permitting efficient contraction of the diaphragm and expansion of the thoracic cavity.

4. An upright position with the head higher than the hips (orthopneic position) allows the diaphragm to move toward the abdominal cavity during inspiration with minimal pressure of the abdominal organs against the diaphragm.

5-17 1. Only the area being washed should be exposed, to permit adequate bathing and inspection.

2. Using long, firm strokes toward the heart is desirable because it promotes venous return.

3. **This will contaminate the urinary meatus with microorganisms from the perianal area.**

4. Using a cotton blanket is desirable; it absorbs moisture, provides warmth, and promotes privacy.

5-18 1. Equipment should be gathered after the patient agrees to the procedure.

2. Positioning the patient is done immediately before the procedure is performed.

3. **Explaining the procedure meets the patient's right to know why and how care will be provided. It should be done before any step of the procedure is initiated.**

4. This may be frightening if the patient does not know why the action is being done; also, not every procedure needs the bed to be raised to its highest position.

5-19 1. This focuses on a different ritual and denies the patient's concerns about missing mass and not receiving communion.

2. **This helps to meet the patient's spiritual needs and is easily accomplished in a hospital setting.**

3. The nurse should assist the patient to meet spiritual needs. The nurse should not expect other Catholic patients to assume this role.

4. The sacrament of Anointing of the Sick is a different ritual than attending mass and receiving communion.

5-20 1. This statement offers false reassurance and draws a conclusion based on insufficient information.

2. **This response encourages further communication, which is necessary to obtain more information about what is upsetting the patient.**

3. This is a judgmental statement that is not based on fact.

4. This is not an open-ended question that allows the patient to express concerns; this is a statement that may or may not be true.

5-21 1. A lack of balance in nutrients can result in malnutrition, not necessarily obesity; it also can result in weight loss.

2. Although glandular disorders such as hypothyroidism may result in obesity, they are not the primary causes of obesity.

3. **If more calories are ingested than the body requires for energy, they will be converted to adipose tissue, which causes weight gain.**

4. A psychological problem is just one of many factors that influence overeating; it is not the primary cause of obesity.

5-22 1. Vasodilation promotes heat loss.

2. **Exposing only the area being washed limits the evaporation of fluids on the skin and radiation of heat from the body, which prevents the patient from getting a chill.**

3. Although this may prevent drafts, it will not prevent the patient's getting a chill from the environmental temperature, excessive exposure, or evaporation of water from the skin.

4. A hot drink will not prevent a chill.

5-23 1. A shower may be an unsafe activity when a patient is in pain. The patient has a right to refuse care.

2. This ignores the patient's right to refuse care and the fact that the patient is in pain.

3. The bath may eventually be cancelled, but it should be delayed first.

4. **Delaying the bath accepts the patient's present refusal to bathe; rest and pain reduction may make the patient more amenable to hygiene later in the day.**

5-24 1. Donning a mask is not necessary for Standard Precautions and is not required for all Transmission-Based Precautions.

2. Wearing a gown is not part of Standard Precautions and is not required for all Transmission-Based Precautions.

3. **Washing the hands before and after patient care and whenever contaminated**

is the most important action for preventing the spread of microorganisms.

4. After they have been taught how to use
   Standard and Transmission-Based
   Precautions, people are permitted to
   visit patients with infections.

5-25 1. **Unconscious patients usually have dry
   mucous membranes of the oral cavity
   because they frequently breathe
   through the mouth, are not drinking
   fluids, and may be receiving oxygen;
   oral hygiene is required whenever
   necessary, which usually is at least
   every 2 hours.**

2. Every 4 hours is too long a period of
   time between providing oral care for an
   unconscious patient; drying, sores, and
   lesions of the mucous membranes can
   occur.

3. Once a shift is too long a period of time
   to elapse before providing oral care for
   an unconscious patient.

4. Twice a day is too long a period of time
   between oral care for an unconscious
   patient.

5-26 1. Addressing a patient by name meets the
   patient's need for self-esteem.

2. Accepting a patient's expression of feelings, including feelings of anger, meets
   self-esteem needs. Limits may be set
   on feelings that escalate and place the
   patient and/or others in danger.

3. This action meets the patient's basic
   physiological need for adequate nutrients
   for body processes.

4. **Knowing what will happen and why
   provides for the patient's security
   needs; also, it is a patient's right. The
   unknown can be frightening.**

5-27 1. The chart is a secondary source; it also
   contains primary health-care providers'
   prescriptions and orders, which are dependent functions of the nurse.

2. **The primary and most important
   source for obtaining information referring to the patient is the patient.
   The independent functions of the
   nurse include interventions that relate
   to human responses, which are identified by direct contact with the patient.**

3. A nurse manager is a secondary source;
   independent functions of the nurse can be
   performed independently of others.

4. A primary health-care provider is a
   secondary source of information; when
   the nurse follows a primary health care
   provider's prescription or order, it is a
   dependent function of the nurse.

5-28 1. A confrontation may take away the
   patient's current coping mechanisms and
   leave the patient defenseless.

2. **A patient who is grieving is using
   defenses to cope with the crisis; these
   defenses should be supported.**

3. Avoiding the patient is a form of abandonment; the nurse should be present to
   provide support.

4. Setting limits may take away the patient's
   coping mechanisms and leave the patient
   defenseless.

5-29 1. Planning occurs after the assessment
   and analysis phases of the nursing
   process.

2. Assessing involves collecting data, which
   must be gathered before it can be analyzed and nursing diagnoses formulated.

3. **Data must be clustered and inter-
   preted to identify human responses
   that indicate potential or actual health
   problems that can be treated by the
   nurse; statements that indicate actual
   or potential health problems treatable
   by the nurse are nursing diagnoses.
   These actions require analysis.**

4. Implementation is putting the plan of
   care into action, which occurs after
   assessment, analysis, and planning.

5-30 1. The word "hers" is associated with others rather than the self or self-interests.

2. **Toddlers are developing a sense of
   autonomy and are discovering the
   difference between independence
   and dependence; they are concerned
   about themselves and their mastery
   over their environment.**

3. The word "theirs" is associated
   with others rather than the self or
   self-interests.

4. Toddlers are the center of their universe;
   they consider everything to be theirs.

The Nursing Process

Problem solving is a process that provides a framework for identifying solutions to complex problems. It is a step-by-step process that uses a systematic approach. One might say that problem solving is a "blueprint" that can be followed to identify and solve problems. The concept of problem solving is not used exclusively by nurses. It is used by other professionals to find solutions within the context of their own job responsibilities. Nurses use the problem-solving process to identify human responses and to plan, implement, and evaluate nursing care. When scientific problem solving is used within the context of nursing, it is known as the nursing process. The nursing process contains five steps:

1. **Assessment**
2. **Analysis**
3. **Planning**
4. **Implementation**
5. **Evaluation**

Because the nursing process incorporates critical thinking used by nurses to meet patients' needs, items on nursing examinations are designed to test the use of this process. Test items are not written haphazardly. They are carefully designed to test your knowledge of a specific concept, skill, theory, or fact from the perspective of one of the five steps of the nursing process. When reading an item, being able to recognize its place within the nursing process should contribute to your ability to identify what the test item is asking. To do this, you must focus on the critical words within the item.

   In this chapter the five steps of the nursing process are explored. Sample items are presented to demonstrate item construction as it relates to each step of this process. Critical words associated with each step of the nursing process are illustrated within the sample items. Attempt to identify variations of critical words within the sample items indicating activities associated with each step of the nursing process. Practice answering the questions. The better you understand the focus of the item you are reading, the better you will be at identifying what is being asked and the greater your chances of identifying the correct answer. The correct answers and the rationales for all the options of the sample items in this chapter are at the end of the chapter.

ASSESSMENT

During assessment, data must be accurately collected, verified, and document. Assessment items are designed to test your knowledge of information, theories, principles, and skills related to the assessment of the patient. This establishes the foundation on which nurses base the subsequent steps in the nursing process. Assessment questions ask you to:

- Obtain vital statistics
- Perform a physical assessment
- Collect specimens
- Identify clinical findings that are objective or subjective
- Identify patient communications that are verbal or nonverbal
- Identify clinical findings that are expected (normal) or unexpected (abnormal)
- Use various data collection methods
- Identify sources of data

- Verify critical findings
- Identify commonalities and differences in response to illness
- Document information about assessments

The critical words within a test item that indicate that the item is focused on assessment include the following: **inspect, identify, verify, observe, determine, notify, check, inform, question, verbal and nonverbal, signs and symptoms, stressors, adaptations, responses, stressors, clinical findings, clinical manifestations, sources, perceptions, and assess.** See whether you can identify variations of these critical words in the sample items in this chapter.

Most testing errors that occur on assessment items occur because options are selected that:

- Collect insufficient data
- Have data that are inaccurately collected
- Use unscientific methods of data collection
- Rely on a secondary source rather than the primary source—the patient
- Contain irrelevant data
- Fail to verify data
- Reflect bias or prejudice
- Fail to document data accurately

Collect Data

METHODS OF DATA COLLECTION

Collecting data is the first part of assessment. The nurse collects data through specific methods of data collection, such as performing a physical examination, interviewing, and reviewing records.

A **physical examination** includes the assessment techniques of inspection, palpation, auscultation, and percussion. Also, it includes obtaining the vital signs and recognizing acceptable and unacceptable parameters of obtained values.

Interviewing collects data using a formal approach (e.g., obtaining a health history) or an informal approach (e.g., exploring feelings while providing other nursing care).

Review of records includes consideration of reports such as the results of laboratory tests, diagnostic procedures, and assessments or consultations by other members of the health-care team.

SAMPLE ITEM 6-1

While making rounds, the nurse finds a patient on the floor in the hall. Which should be the nurse's initial response?

1. Inspect the patient for injury.

2. Transfer the patient back to bed.

3. Move the patient to the closest chair.

4. Report the patient's condition to the nurse manager.

This item tests your ability to recognize that, in an emergency situation, the nurse must first assess (inspect) the condition of the patient. This principle is basic to any emergency response by a nurse. Moving a patient before an assessment may worsen an injury. This item demonstrates how a basic concept related to assessment can be tested.

SAMPLE ITEM 6-2
Which should the nurse do to avoid patient accidents?
1. Provide a cane for walking if the patient is weak.
2. Determine the strength of a patient before walking.
3. Apply a vest restraint when a patient is using a wheelchair.
4. Keep the overbed table in front of a patient sitting in a chair.

  This item tests your ability to recognize the concept that the nurse must assess a patient before implementing care. The three distractors are all concerned with implementing care. This question also tests your ability to recognize physical examination as a method of collecting data about the status of a patient.

SAMPLE ITEM 6-3
Which assessment by the nurse most likely indicates that a patient is having difficulty breathing?
1. 18 breaths per minute and inhaled through the mouth
2. 20 breaths per minute and shallow in character
3. 16 breaths per minute and deep in character
4. 28 breaths per minute and noisy

  This item tests your ability to identify the option that reflects a respiratory rate and characteristic that is outside expected parameters. To answer this question successfully, you need to know the rate and characteristics of acceptable and unacceptable respirations.

SAMPLE ITEM 6-4
Which should a nurse always do when taking a rectal temperature?
1. Allow self-insertion of the thermometer.
2. Position the patient on the left side.
3. Use an electronic thermometer.
4. Lubricate the thermometer.

  Option 4 identifies what must be done (a critical element) to take a rectal temperature safely. The three distractors may or may not be done when obtaining a rectal temperature. Although this appears to be an implementation question because it involves an action, it is actually an assessment question because it is concerned with collecting data.

SAMPLE ITEM 6-5

A nurse is assessing a patient's ideal body weight. Which significant factor should be taken into consideration when performing this assessment?

1. Daily intake

2. Body height

3. Clothing size

4. Food preferences

This item tests the understanding that to calculate a patient's ideal body weight the nurse must also know the patient's height. The ideal body weight is the measurement that reflects the range of weight that is considered appropriate in relation to the patient's height. The ideal body weight is the measurement against which the patient's present weight is compared to determine if the patient is underweight or obese. Although the question does not address these concepts, the nurse also must know the patient's age and extent of bone structure.

SOURCES OF DATA

Data can be gathered not only by different methods but also from different sources. Sources of data available to the nurse include those that are primary, secondary, and tertiary. There is only one **primary source**—the patient. The patient is the most valuable source of information because the data collected are the most current and specific to the patient.

A **secondary source** produces information from someplace other than the patient. A family member is a secondary source who can contribute information about the patient's likes and dislikes, ethnic and cultural background, similarities and differences in behavior, and functioning before and during the health problem. The patient's medical record (chart) is another example of a secondary source. It is a legal document containing information that concerns the patient's physical, psychosocial, religious, and economic history and documents the patient's physical and emotional responses. Controversy surrounds the labeling of diagnostic test results in a chart as being from either primary or secondary sources. Although the chart itself is a secondary source, diagnostic test results are direct objective measurements of the patient's status and therefore are considered by some health-care professionals to be a primary source. The nurse must remember that the information in a chart is history and does not reflect the current status of the patient because the patient is dynamic and constantly changing. Secondary sources are valuable for gathering supplementary information about a patient.

A **tertiary source** provides information from outside the specific patient's frame of reference. Examples of tertiary sources include textbooks, the nurse's experience, and accepted commonalities among patients with similar physical and emotional responses. The nurse's or other health-care team members' responses to the patient are tertiary sources of patient data.

SAMPLE ITEM 6-6

A nurse asks a patient's wife specific questions about the patient's health status before admission. When collecting this information, the nurse is seeking information from a:

1. Primary source.

2. Tertiary source.

3. Subjective source.

4. Secondary source.

This item tests your ability to identify that a family member is a secondary source of information. Secondary sources provide information that is supplemental to the information collected from the patient.

TYPES OF DATA

The types of data collected when assessing a patient can be objective or subjective and verbal or nonverbal.

Objective data are measurable assessments collected when the nurse uses sight, touch, smell, or hearing to acquire information. Examples of objective data include an excoriated perineal area, diaphoresis, ammonia odor of urine, crackles, and vital signs. **Subjective data** can be collected only when the patient shares feelings, perceptions, thoughts, and sensations about a health problem or concern. Examples of subjective data include patient statements about pain, shortness of breath, or feeling depressed.

SAMPLE ITEM 6-7

A nurse is performing a physical assessment of a newly admitted patient. Which patient statement communicates subjective data?

1. "I have sores between my toes."

2. "I dye my hair but it is really gray."

3. "My joints hurt when I get up in the morning."

4. "My left leg drags on the floor when I am walking."

   This item tests your ability to differentiate between subjective and objective data. The nurse should know the types of data collected for the purposes of future clustering and determining their significance. Any information that the patient shares regarding feelings, thoughts, and concerns is subjective. Any information that the nurse verifies using the senses (e.g., vision, hearing, smell, and touch) or via some form of instrumentation (e.g., thermometer, pulse oximetry, laboratory data) is objective.

Communication can be verbal or nonverbal. **Verbal data** are collected via the spoken or written word. For example, statements made to the nurse by the patient are verbal data. **Nonverbal data** are collected via transmission of a message without words. Crying, a fearful facial expression, the appearance of the patient, and gestures are all examples of nonverbal data.

SAMPLE ITEM 6-8

Which is an example of nonverbal communication?

1. Letter

2. Holding hands

3. Noise in the room

4. Telephone message

   This item tests your ability to identify that holding hands is a form of nonverbal communication. Nonverbal communication does not use words. Touch, gestures, posture, and facial expressions are examples of nonverbal communication.

Verify Data

After data are collected, they must be verified. To verify data, information is confirmed by collecting additional data, questioning orders/prescriptions, obtaining judgments and/or conclusions from other team members when appropriate, and collecting data oneself rather than relying on technology. Verifying data ensures authenticity and accuracy. For example, when a vital statistic is outside the expected range, the nurse must substantiate the results first by collecting the data again and then collecting additional data to supplement the original information.

SAMPLE ITEM 6-9

A nurse takes a patient's blood pressure and records a diastolic pressure of 120 mm Hg. Which should the nurse do first?

1. Notify the primary health-care provider.

2. Retake the blood pressure.

3. Notify the nurse in charge.

4. Take the other vital signs.

This item tests your ability to identify that you must verify data when they are unexpectedly outside the acceptable range. Your first action should be to wait 2 minutes and then retake the blood pressure. An error may have been made when taking the person's blood pressure.

Document Information About Assessments

The last component of assessment includes the nurse's ability to document information obtained from assessment activities. Sharing vital information about a patient is essential if members of the health-care team are to be alerted to the most current status of the patient. Communication methods vary (e.g., progress notes, verbal notification, flow sheets); however, they all share the need to be accurate, concise, thorough, current, organized, and confidential.

SAMPLE ITEM 6-10

A patient returns to the surgical unit from the postanesthesia care unit after abdominal surgery. The primary health-care provider orders intravenous fluids, oxygen via nasal cannula at 2 L/min, I&O, and vital signs every 2 hours. Two hours after surgery the patient voids 400 mL of amber urine. What should the nurse do with this information?

1. Report this information to the primary health-care provider.

2. Record this amount on the patient's intake and output flow sheet.

3. Document this information on the patient's vital signs flow sheet.

4. Communicate this event verbally to the other members of the health-care team.

This item is testing your knowledge about the necessity of documenting a patient's status and on which part of the patient's clinical record the information should be placed.

ANALYSIS

Analysis, the second step of the nursing process, is the most difficult component. Analysis requires that data be validated and clustered and that their significance be determined. Analyzing data requires a strong foundation in scientific principles related to nursing theory, social sciences, and physical sciences. You need to know the commonalities and differences in patients' responses to various stresses. You must use reasoning to apply your knowledge and experience when answering analysis items. After the initial analysis of data, sometimes additional data need to be collected and analyzed. Only after all the data have been analyzed should a nursing diagnosis be made. Analysis questions ask you to:

- Validate interrelationship of data
- Cluster data
- Identify clustered data as meaningful
- Interpret validated and clustered data
- Identify when additional data are needed to further validate clustered data

- Identify nursing diagnoses
- Communicate nursing diagnoses to others

The critical words within a test item that indicate that the item is focused on analysis/nursing diagnosis include the following: **valid, organize, categorize, cluster, reexamine, pattern, formulate, nursing diagnosis, reflect, relate, problem, interpret, contribute, relevant, decision, significant, deduction, statement, and analysis.** See whether you can identify variations of these critical words in the sample items in this chapter.

Testing errors occur on analysis items when options are selected that:

- Omit data
- Cluster data prematurely
- Make a nursing diagnosis before all significant data have been clustered
- Force a nursing diagnosis to fit the signs and symptoms collected

Cluster Data

Clustering data groups related information together. Information is more meaningful when its relationship with other data is established. Clustering enables the nurse to organize data; eliminate that which is insignificant, irrelevant, or redundant; and reduce the data into manageable categories. First, data must be organized into general categories, such as physiological, sociocultural, psychological, and spiritual. Then data can be grouped into specific categories. For example, physiological data can be further grouped into categories such as nutrition, mobility, and elimination. Data can be obvious and easy to cluster or obscure and difficult to cluster. Some data are clustered easily because the information collected is clearly related to only one system of the body. For example, hard stool, a feeling of rectal fullness, and straining on defecation all relate to intestinal elimination. These clinical manifestations are easy to group and lead to the interpretation that the patient may be constipated. Other data are more difficult to cluster because the patient's clinical manifestations may involve a variety of systems of the body. A weak, thready pulse; weight loss; hypotension; and dry mucous membranes can be grouped together. At first, this information may not appear to be related because the clinical findings cross several body systems. However, with a thorough analysis the nurse should conclude that the data are interrelated and interpret that the patient may be dehydrated. Established frameworks such as Marjory Gordon's Functional Health Patterns (1994) and Abraham Maslow's Hierarchy of Human Needs (1970) (Fig. 6–1) provide structures for organizing and clustering data.

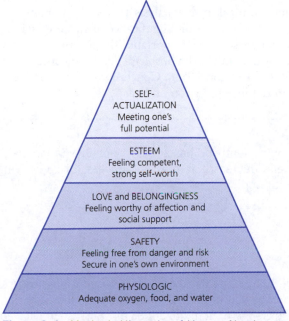

Figure 6–1. Maslow's Hierarchy of Human Needs

SAMPLE ITEM 6-11

A patient had a brain attack (i.e., stroke, cerebrovascular accident) that resulted in paralysis of the right side. When clustering data, the nurse grouped the following data together: drooling of saliva and slurred speech. Which information is most significant to include with this clustered data?

1. Receptive aphasia

2. Inability to ambulate

3. Difficulty swallowing

4. Incontinence of bowel movements

This item tests your ability to cluster clinical findings that indicate that a patient is at risk for aspiration. Oxygenation is a basic physiologic need. A patient who is drooling saliva and has slurred speech, right-sided paralysis, and difficulty swallowing is at serious risk for aspiration of material into the respiratory tract. Although the other options are all problems that must be addressed by the nurse, they are not data related to oxygenation and have no significance to this specific cluster.

SAMPLE ITEM 6-12

A nurse understands that pressure ulcers are most often associated with patients who:

1. Are immobilized.

2. Have psychiatric diagnoses.

3. Experience respiratory distress.

4. Need close supervision for safety.

This item tests your ability to identify the relationship between immobility and the formation of pressure ulcers. It is designed to test your knowledge of the fact that prolonged pressure on a site interferes with cellular oxygenation, which causes cell death, resulting in a pressure ulcer.

Interpret Data

Interpretation of data is critical in the analysis step of the nursing process. It is associated with the nurse's ability to determine the significance of clustered data. "Significance" in this context refers to some consequence, importance, implication, or gravity connected to the cluster as it relates to the patient's health problem. Finally, the interpretation of the significant clustered data should lead to a conclusion. Conclusions are the opinions, decisions, or inferences that result from the interpretation of data.

SAMPLE ITEM 6-13

A nurse is caring for a dying patient who has a loss of appetite (anorexia), difficulty falling asleep (insomnia), and decreased interest in activities of daily living. Which feeling reflects these clinical findings?

1. Anger

2. Denial

3. Depression

4. Acceptance

This item tests your ability to come to a conclusion based on a cluster of data. The word "reflect" in the stem cues you to the fact that this is an analysis question. You need to draw from your knowledge of commonalities of human behavior and theories of grieving to arrive at the conclusion that the patient probably is depressed.

SAMPLE ITEM 6-14

A patient who is debilitated and unsteady when standing insists on walking to the bathroom without calling for assistance. This behavior **best** reflects a need to be:

1. Alone.
2. Accepted.
3. Independent.
4. Manipulative.

This item tests your ability to come to a conclusion based on a cluster of data. To answer this question, you must analyze and interpret the information in the stem and come to a conclusion. Your knowledge of human behavior should enable you to select the correct answer.

Collect Additional Data

After arriving at an initial conclusion, additional data collection might be indicated to provide more information to support the suspected conclusion. This is done to ensure the relationship among the original data. The nurse continually reassesses the condition of the patient and the presence of needs, recognizing that the patient is dynamic and ever changing throughout all phases of the nursing process.

SAMPLE ITEM 6-15

A nurse assesses that a postoperative patient has a decreased blood pressure and weak, thready pulse and concludes that the patient may be hemorrhaging. For which additional signs of hemorrhage should the nurse assess the patient?

1. Pain
2. Jaundice
3. Tachycardia
4. Hyperthermia

This item is designed to test your understanding of the need to reassess a patient for additional data to reinforce the proposed conclusion that the patient is hemorrhaging. Hypotension, tachycardia, and a weak, thready pulse are related to a decreased blood volume that is associated with postoperative hemorrhage.

Identify and Communicate Nursing Diagnoses

Converting a conclusion into a diagnostic statement changes it from a general statement of a problem into a specific statement—or a nursing diagnosis. A nursing diagnosis is a statement of a specific health problem that a nurse is legally permitted to treat. The diagnostic statement should include the problem and the factors that contributed to the development of the problem.

It is necessary to include the contributing factors because, although two patients may have the same problem, it may have been caused by different stresses. This concept is important because the nature of the contributing factors generally drives the choice of interventions being planned. For example, two patients have impaired skin integrity. However, one patient's skin problem is related to incontinence and edema and the other patient's skin problem is related to immobility and pressure. The interventions may be very different because the factors contributing to the problem are different. This is discussed in more detail in the section in this chapter titled "Planning." Some nurses use the taxonomy of nursing diagnoses developed by the North American Nursing Diagnosis Association (NANDA) as a blueprint. This taxonomy provides for classifying nursing problems, standardizing language, facilitating communication, and focusing on an individualized approach to identifying and meeting a patient's nursing needs. The following are examples of nursing diagnoses:

- Risk for impaired skin integrity, related to incontinence
- Feeding self-care deficit, related to bilateral arm casts
- Ineffective airway clearance, related to excessive secretions

Nurses need to communicate nursing diagnoses to other nurses via a written plan of care. The plan should include the nursing diagnosis, expected outcomes, and planned interventions. The section of this chapter titled "Planning" discusses outcomes and planned nursing interventions in more detail.

SAMPLE ITEM 6-16

A patient who experienced a brain attack (i.e., stroke, cerebrovascular accident) has left-sided hemiparesis and is incontinent of urine. Which is an appropriately worded nursing diagnosis for this patient?

1. The patient has a need to maintain skin integrity.

2. The patient has a stroke evidenced by hemiparesis and incontinence.

3. The patient will be clean and dry and will receive range-of-motion exercises every four hours.

4. The patient is at risk for impaired skin integrity related to left-sided hemiparesis and incontinence.

This item tests your ability to identify language used by the NANDA taxonomy. To answer this item correctly, you must be able to identify the differences among a patient need, an expected outcome, a nursing intervention, and a properly stated nursing diagnosis associated with a cluster of data.

PLANNING

Planning is the third step of the nursing process. It involves identifying goals, projecting expected outcomes, setting priorities, identifying interventions, ensuring that the patient's health-care needs will be appropriately met, modifying the plan of care as needed, and collaborating with other health-care team members. To plan care, you must have a strong foundation of scientific theory, understand the commonalities and differences in response to nursing interventions, and know theories related to establishing priority of needs. You will need to use your knowledge and clinical experience when answering planning questions. Planning questions will ask you to:

- Involve the patient in the planning process
- Set goals
- Establish expected outcomes against which results of care can be compared for the purpose of evaluation
- Plan appropriate interventions based on their effects
- Establish priorities of nursing interventions
- Anticipate patient needs
- Collaborate with others
- Coordinate planned care with other disciplines
- Recognize that plans must be flexible and modified based on changing patient needs

The critical words within a test item that indicate that the item is focused on planning include the following: **achieve, desired, plan, effective, desired result, goal, priority, develop, formulate, establish, design, prevent, strategy, select, determine, anticipate, modify, collaborate, arrange, coordinate, expect, and outcome.** See whether you can identify variations of these critical words in the sample items in this chapter.

Testing errors occur during the planning phase when options are selected that:

- Do not include the patient in setting goals and priorities
- Are inappropriate goals
- Misidentify priorities
- Reflect goals that are unrealistic
- Reflect goals that are immeasurable
- Reflect planned interventions that are inappropriate or incomplete
- Fail to include family members and significant others when appropriate
- Fail to coordinate and collaborate with other health-care team members

Identify Goals

A **goal** is a broad, nonspecific statement concerning the desired result of nursing care. They are general statements that direct nursing interventions and stimulate motivation. Goals can be long term or short term. A **long-term goal** is one that will take time to achieve (months or years). A **short-term goal** is one that can be achieved relatively quickly (usually within days or weeks). Goals should be:

- Patient centered
- Specific (measurable)
- Realistic
- Achievable within a time frame

A short-term goal for a patient who has a respiratory tract infection might be, "The patient's sputum culture will be negative within in 1 week." "The patient" is the subject of the statement and therefore the goal is patient centered. "Sputum culture will be negative" is specific, realistic, and measurable. The phrase "within 1 week" establishes a time frame for the goal. A long-term goal for a patient who has a respiratory tract infection might be, "The patient will be free of infection within 1 month." "The patient" is the subject of the statement and therefore the goal is patient centered. Being "free of infection" is specific, realistic, and measurable. The phrase "within 1 month" indicates the time frame in which the goal should be achieved. Eventually a goal can be further developed to become an expected outcome. An outcome provides a standard of measure that can be used to determine whether the goal is reached. An expected outcome for the long-term goal listed above might be "The patient's sputum culture will be negative within 2 weeks." Outcomes are discussed in more detail next.

SAMPLE ITEM 6-17

A nurse is caring for a patient with a new temporary colostomy. Which is a realistic short-term goal for this patient?

1. The patient will have regular bowel elimination.

2. The patient's bowel will function within two days.

3. The patient is at risk for impaired skin integrity.

4. The patient's skin will remain intact around the stoma.

This item tests your ability to identify a short-term goal. To answer this question, you need to know commonalities related to caring for a patient with a new temporary colostomy and be able to identify the differences among short- and long-term goals and a nursing diagnosis.

Project Expected Outcomes

An **outcome** is any response (positive or negative) by an individual, family, or community to a nursing intervention. **Expected outcomes** are the predicted positive changes that should occur in response to care given. Expected outcomes are derived from goal statements, but they are more specific because they describe the behavior to be demonstrated or data to be collected. Expected outcomes are the benchmarks against which the patient's actual outcomes are compared to determine the effectiveness of the interventions provided. The Center for Nursing Classification and Clinical Effectiveness develops Nursing Outcome Classifications (NOC) which use standardized nursing terminology for outcomes across clinical settings and nursing care specialties. The NOC system identifies these outcomes as "indicators." Examples of NOC indicators are: "The patient will demonstrate meticulous hand washing technique", The patient will identify factors that increase the risk for injury", and "The patient will demonstrate the use of adaptive devices to increase mobility." Sometimes nurses may state goals and outcomes together. For example, "The patient will continuously maintain an effective airway clearance as evidenced by expectoration of sputum, clear lung fields, and noiseless breathing." The first part of the statement is the goal and what follows "as evidenced by" are the expected outcomes. The first part of the statement is general, and the second part is specific.

SAMPLE ITEM 6-18

A nurse is caring for a patient experiencing insomnia. The statement that is an expected · outcome is, "The patient:

1. has a sleep pattern disturbance."

2. can identify techniques to induce sleep."

3. will have privacy when attempting to sleep."

4. will report an optimal balance of sleep and activity."

    This item tests your ability to identify a statement that reflects an expected outcome. To answer this question, you should know commonalities of caring for a patient with insomnia. You also need to understand the differences among a goal, an expected outcome, a nursing diagnosis, and a nursing intervention.

Set Priorities

Setting priorities is an important step in the planning process. After patient needs and goals are identified, they must be ranked in order of importance. Maslow's Hierarchy of Needs (1970) is helpful in establishing priorities. Basic physiological needs are ranked first, with the need for safety and security, belonging and love, self-esteem, and self-actualization following in rank order. It is important, however, to understand that at one point in time any one of Maslow's needs may take priority depending on the needs of the individual patient. Obviously, if someone is choking on food, clearing the airway is the priority. However, there are times when the emergency or immediate need of the patient is in the psychological dimension. The nurse must identify the patient's perceptions and perspective when setting priorities because patients are the center of the health-care team. When possible, the patient should always be involved in setting priorities.

SAMPLE ITEM 6-19

A patient has just returned from surgery with an intravenous solution infusing and does not have a gag reflex. Which planned intervention takes priority?

1. Observe the dressing for drainage.

2. Ensure adequacy of air exchange.

3. Check for an infiltration.

4. Monitor vital signs.

    This item tests your ability to prioritize care. All of these planned interventions are important. However, oxygenation is essential to sustain life, and therefore maintaining a patent airway is the priority.

Identify Interventions

After priorities are established, a plan for nursing action must be formulated. To plan appropriately, the nurse must rely on scientific information, clinical judgment, and knowledge about the patient. By relying on this background, the nurse determines what nursing measures are most effective in assisting the patient to achieve a goal or outcome. Some nurses use the Nursing Interventions Classification (NIC) system, which is an evidenced-based, standardized classification of nursing interventions. The NIC system identifies nursing interventions as "any treatment, based upon clinical judgment and knowledge, that a nurse performs to enhance patient/client outcomes." Examples of NIC interventions include: Auscultate lung field every 8 hours; Set a relaxing routine to prepare for sleep; and Arrange for periodic respite care.

When using clinical judgment to identify appropriate nursing interventions a nurse must understand the rationale for the intervention. For example, when caring for a patient with a pressure ulcer, the nurse reasons, "If I turn and reposition the patient and massage around the area with lotion every 2 hours, then circulation will increase and healing will be promoted." When planning care, the nurse must know the scientific rationales for nursing interventions so that the interventions selected are the most appropriate for the patient-care situation. It is not enough to just know how; you also must know why.

When making decisions, the nurse must consider the concepts of "cause and effect," "risk and probability," and "value of the consequence to the patient." The action you plan is the "cause." The patient's response is the "effect." The likelihood of the occurrence of either a positive or negative effect is the "probability." The probability of the patient suffering harm from the action is the "risk." The value of the effect, in relation to its probability of occurring, influences the degree of risk one is willing to take to achieve the effect.

To facilitate this process of problem solving, an **information-processing model of decision making** should be used.

- First, identify all the possible nursing actions (cause) that may help the patient.
- Second, identify the all possible positive and negative consequences (effect) associated with each action.
- Third, determine the odds (probability) that each consequence will occur. This includes determining the probability of a negative effect occurring (risk).
- Fourth, arrive at a judgment based on the value of each effect to the patient.
- Fifth, choose the action that is "best" for the patient. The "best" action is one that has the lowest risk and the highest probability of helping the patient achieve the expected outcome (effect).

The concept of probability versus risk can be applied to buying a lottery ticket. If you buy one lottery ticket, your chances of winning are small (low probability). If you do not win, your risk will be small because you will lose only one dollar (low risk). On the other hand, if you spend your entire pay check on lottery tickets, you will not dramatically increase your chances of winning (low probability). However, if you do not win, you will lose your whole pay check and have no money to pay your bills (high risk). When making clinical decisions, you want to choose an action that has the highest probability of being successful with the lowest risk to the patient.

Also, the appropriateness of clinical decisions depends on the quality of the data collected and the accuracy of the inferences made in the earlier steps of the nursing process. Each step of the nursing process relies on the quality and accuracy of the preceding step.

SAMPLE ITEM 6-20

Which is the **most** effective way that nurses can prevent the spread of microorganisms in a hospital?

1. Washing the hands

2. Implementing contact precautions

Continued

Continued

3. Administering antibiotics to those who are sick

4. Using linen hampers with foot-operated covers

    This item tests your ability to identify that hand hygiene is the single most effective measure to prevent the spread of microorganisms. This is a question that focuses on a specific action that can contribute to the protection of all patients from the risk of infection.

SAMPLE ITEM 6-21

A patient on bedrest needs a complete change of linen. Which should the nurse plan to do?

1. Make an occupied bed.

2. Change the draw sheet and top sheet.

3. Use a mechanical lift to raise the patient.

4. Transfer the patient to a chair during the linen change.

    This item tests your ability to identify the needs of a patient on bedrest and, therefore, to plan to make an occupied bed. The word "plan" used in the stem is an obvious clue that this is a planning question.

SAMPLE ITEM 6-22

The nurse should make an occupied bed for a patient who is:

1. Obese.

2. In a cast.

3. Immobile.

4. On bedrest.

    This item is similar to sample item 6-21; however, the content of the stem and the correct option are reversed. This item is more difficult to identify as a planning item because the word "plan" is not in the stem.

Ensure That Health-Care Needs Will Be Appropriately Met

The nurse is obligated to take an action that will ensure that appropriate care will be provided. If adequate care cannot be administered because the nursing team member's expertise is unrelated to the patient's needs, the nursing team member is inexperienced for caring for a patient with a particular problem, or there is inadequate staffing, then a patient may be placed at risk. This might necessitate rearranging the assignment, or it might require intervention by the nurse supervisor. Once the nurse embarks on a "duty of care," the nurse is obligated to provide a standard of care defined by the Nurse Practice Act in the state in which the nurse works.

SAMPLE ITEM 6-23

The nurse manager arrives on duty and discovers that several staff members have just called in sick. Which is the nurse manager's most appropriate response?

1. Inform the supervisor and ask for additional staff.

2. Identify which patients need care and assign staff accordingly.

Continued

> 3. Explain to patients that when the unit is short staffed, only essential care can be provided.
>
> 4. Provide the best care possible, but refuse to accept responsibility for the standard of care delivered.
>
>   This item tests your ability to identify your responsibility to ensure that patients' needs are met appropriately. Once the nurse perceives a risk to patient safety, the nurse is obligated to take action that will ensure that appropriate care will be provided.

Modify the Plan of Care as Needed

Planning generally takes place before care is given. However, patient needs sometimes change while the nurse is in the process of implementing care, and a plan must be immediately modified. Modification of the plan of care also may take place after evaluation. The original plan may have been inadequate or inappropriate, or the patient's condition may have improved. It is important to recognize that plans of care are not set in stone but are modified in response to the changing needs of the patient. Because a patient's needs are dynamic, the nursing plan also is dynamic. It must continually be changed to be kept current, substituting new goals and planned interventions as indicated by the patient's changing needs.

> **SAMPLE ITEM 6-24**
>
> A patient is diaphoretic and is receiving oxygen by nasal cannula. During a bath, the patient experiences dyspnea and reports feeling tired. Which should the nurse plan to do?
>
> 1. Give a complete bath quickly.
>
> 2. Bathe only the body parts that need bathing.
>
> 3. Arrange for several rest periods during the bath.
>
> 4. Continue with the bath because dyspnea is unavoidable.
>
>   This item tests your ability to identify the need to modify a plan of care based on new data. The words "planning" in the stem and "arrange" in the correct answer are obvious clues that this is a planning question.

Collaborate With Other Health-Care Team Members

Another component of planning comprises consultation and collaboration with other health-care team members to brainstorm, seek additional input, and delegate and coordinate the delivery of health services. The nurse is responsible for coordinating the members of the nursing team as well as the entire health-care team. The nurse manages the members of the nursing team by appropriately delegating and supervising nursing interventions. The plan also identifies and coordinates the services of other health-care professionals. The nurse is responsible for ensuring that services such as laboratory tests, radiological studies, and physical therapy are performed within the context of the patient's physical and emotional abilities. For example, the nurse may arrange for a patient to go to physical therapy in the morning before the patient tires or the nurse may consult with the dietitian for help with designing a menu that incorporates a patient's preferences. Effective planning contributes to the delivery of patient care that has continuity and is patient centered, coordinated, and individualized.

SAMPLE ITEM 6-25

A nurse is caring for a patient with a large pressure ulcer that has not responded to common nursing interventions. With whom should the nurse consult first to **best** deal with this problem?

1. Plastic surgeon

2. Physical therapist

3. Clinical nurse specialist

4. Primary health-care provider

This item is designed to test your ability to identify that planning nursing care may require the nurse to seek the expertise of a nurse specialist. A clinical nurse specialist is educated and prepared to provide expert advice and lend problem-solving and educational skills to seek solutions to difficult clinical nursing problems. Although the nurse consults with health-care team members of other disciplines for various reasons, the nurse should consult with a clinical nurse specialist or other resources in nursing first for assistance with solving nursing problems.

IMPLEMENTATION

Implementation is the step of the nursing process in which planned actions are initiated and completed. It includes tasks such as organizing and managing planned care; providing total or partial assistance with activities of daily living (ADLs); counseling and teaching the patient and significant others; providing planned care; supervising, coordinating, and evaluating the process of the delivery of care by the nursing staff (this does not include the actual delegation of care that occurs in planning or the evaluation of the patient's response to care that occurs in evaluation); and recording and sharing data related to the care implemented.

To implement safe nursing care designed to achieve goals and expected outcomes, the nurse must understand and follow the implementation process. In addition, the nurse must have knowledge of scientific rationales for nursing procedures, psychomotor skills to implement procedures safely, and the ability to use different strategies to implement nursing care effectively. Implementation questions will ask you to:

- Identify steps in the implementation process
- Identify independent, dependent, and interdependent actions of the nurse
- Implement a procedure or treatment
- Respond to common or uncommon outcomes in response to interventions
- Respond to life-threatening or adverse events
- Prepare a patient for a procedure, treatment, or surgery
- Choose an approach that is most appropriate when implementing care
- Identify safe or unsafe practices
- Rationalize a step in a procedure
- Identify or apply concepts associated with teaching
- Identify or apply concepts associated with counseling
- Identify or apply principles associated with motivation
- Identify or apply techniques for therapeutic communication
- Identify when an intervention must be modified in response to a change in the patient's condition
- Identify when additional assistance is required to provide safe care
- Identify the nurse's responsibility associated with supervising and evaluating care delivered by those to whom interventions have been delegated
- Identify how and when to document or report care given along with the patient's response

The critical words within a test item that indicate that the item is focused on implementation include the following: **dependent, independent, interdependent, change, assist,** counsel, teach, give, supervise, perform, method, procedure, treatment, instruct, strategy, facilitate, provide, inform, refer, technique, motivate, delegate, and implement. See whether you can identify variations of these words indicating implementation activities in the sample items.

Testing errors occur on implementation items when options are selected that:

- Implement actions outside the definition of nursing practice
- Fail to respond to an adverse or life-threatening situation
- Fail to modify interventions in response to the changing needs of the patient
- Fail to identify when additional assistance is required for the delivery of safe care
- Reflect a lack of knowledge to safely implement interventions
- Do not accurately document the patient's response to the care given
- Fail to supervise and evaluate the delivery of delegated interventions

Legal Parameters of Nursing Interventions

Implementation occurs when the nurse uses an intervention to help a patient meet expected outcomes. Nursing interventions can be dependent, independent, or interdependent.

Dependent interventions are interventions that require an order/prescription by a health-care provider (e.g., physician, nurse practitioner, or physician's assistant). Administering a medication, providing IV fluids, and removing a nasogastric tube are examples of dependent interventions because they all require a legal order. When implementing a dependent intervention, the nurse does not blindly follow the order but determines whether the order is appropriate. A nurse who does not question and carries out an inappropriate order is contributing to the initial error and will be held accountable.

Independent interventions (nurse-prescribed) are those actions that a nurse is legally permitted to implement with no direction or supervision from others. Independent interventions do not require a health-care provider's order/prescription. Tasks related to collecting data and determining their significance, providing assistance with ADLs, teaching regarding health, and counseling are in the realm of independent legal nursing practice. Encouraging coughing and deep breathing, encouraging verbalization of fears, teaching principles related to nutrition, and providing a bed bath are examples of independent nursing interventions.

Interdependent interventions (collaborative) are actions implemented in partnership with other appropriate professionals. An example of an interdependent intervention is implementing actions identified in standing orders or a protocol. These situations delineate the parameters within which the nurse is permitted to administer to the patient. Protocols and standing orders are commonly found in emergency and critical care areas. Another example of an interdependent intervention is when a health-care provider orders, "Out of bed as tolerated." When assisting this patient to ambulate, the nurse must assess the patient's response to the activity. Based on the patient's response, the nurse can decide to terminate the activity or to increase the time and/or distance to be ambulated.

SAMPLE ITEM 6-26

A primary nurse assigns a staff nurse to insert an indwelling urinary (Foley) catheter. Which is the first thing the staff nurse should do?

1. Check the primary health-care provider's order.

2. Bring equipment to the patient's bedside.

3. Explain the procedure to the patient.

4. Wash hands thoroughly.

This question is designed to test your ability to identify that the insertion of a urinary catheter is a dependent nursing intervention that requires a primary health-care provider's order.

Types of Nursing Interventions

Examples of nursing actions associated with the implementation step of the nursing process include:

- **Assisting with Activities of Daily Living (ADLs):** Assisting with ADLs refers to activities associated with eating, dressing, hygiene, grooming, toileting, transfer, and locomotion. Situations associated with needs addressing ADLs can be acute, chronic, temporary, permanent, or related to maintaining or restoring function. ADLs are an integral part of daily life, and therefore their implementation is often tested.
- **Teaching:** To teach effectively in the cognitive (learning new information), psychomotor (learning new skills), and affective (developing new attitudes, values, and beliefs) domains, the nurse must apply teaching/learning principles to motivate patients to learn and grow. Health teaching activities are incorporated throughout the health-illness continuum, in a variety of health-care delivery settings, and across the life span. For these reasons, teaching principles are often incorporated into patient situations in test questions.
- **Responding to Life-Threatening Situations:** Responding to adverse or life-threatening situations requires the use of clinical judgment and decision making. Activities such as stopping the administration of an antibiotic in response to a patient's allergic reaction, initiating cardiopulmonary resuscitation, implementing the abdominal thrust procedure (Heimlich maneuver), and administering emergency medication are examples of measures that can be implemented in life-threatening situations. Most of these interventions address the basic physiological needs required for survival and are therefore frequently tested.
- **Implementing Preventive Actions:** Preventive actions are activities that help the patient to avoid a health problem. Administering immunizations, applying an allergy bracelet, employing medical and surgical asepsis, ensuring physical safety, and leading a group on weight reduction are examples of preventive measures. Because today's society emphasizes health, wellness, and illness prevention, these topics are often tested.
- **Performing Technical Skills:** The nurse must know how and when to implement a procedure and the expected outcomes of the procedure. Inserting a urinary catheter, providing a tube feeding, administering medication, performing an enema, and preparing a patient for a diagnostic test are examples of procedures implemented by the nurse. Steps, principles, rationales, and expected and potential adverse outcomes associated with procedures are concepts that are often tested in nursing questions.
- **Implementing Interpersonal Interventions:** Interpersonal activities help the nurse to assist a patient to adapt to changes that are caused by loss, illness, disability, or stress. Emotional care is provided by activities such as promoting a supportive environment, motivating a patient, providing for privacy, addressing spiritual needs, and accepting feelings. Counseling also is a component of interpersonal interventions. To counsel effectively, the nurse must apply therapeutic communication principles to explore patients' feelings and meet their emotional needs. Another aspect of interpersonal interventions is coordinating health-care activities. When the nurse collaborates with others and coordinates health-care activities, the nurse functions as the patient's advocate. People are complex human beings, and nursing care must address the mental, physical, emotional, spiritual, and legal/ethical realms. Because these realms are so important, associated nursing interventions are often tested in nursing questions.
- **Supervising and Evaluating the Effectiveness of Delegated Interventions:** Occasionally, the nurse who formulates the plan of care delegates all or part of the implementation of the plan to other members of the nursing team. Uncomplicated and basic interventions, particularly those associated with ADLs, are often delegated to a nursing assistant or licensed practical nurse. The nurse who delegates is responsible for the plan of care and is accountable for ensuring that the care is delivered according to standards of the profession. With the changing roles in health-care delivery, the importance of the nurse as manager is increasing and is therefore tested.
- **Reporting and Recording:** After care is given, it is recorded along with an assessment of the patient's response to care. Written communication establishes a permanent document

of the care patients receive and their responses. In addition to documenting, the nurse may verbally report to other health-care team members the care that was provided along with patients' responses. Also, verbal reports are given at the change of shifts, when responding to an emergency, or when transferring responsibility for a patient to another nurse. Because communication and documentation are essential to the provision of quality care, they are often tested.

SAMPLE ITEM 6-27

A patient has an order for a 2-gram sodium diet. Which should the nurse teach this patient to avoid?

1. Salt
2. Sugar
3. Liquids
4. Margarine

This item tests your ability to identify information that needs to be taught to a patient. Teaching is performed by the nurse to assist a patient to meet a health need. Mainly, this question tests your ability to identify that salt is sodium and thus it should be avoided when a patient is receiving a 2-gram sodium diet. The use of the word *avoid* indicates that the stem of this question has negative polarity.

SAMPLE ITEM 6-28

A patient vomits while in the supine position. Which should the nurse do?

1. Position the patient's head between the knees.
2. Raise the patient to a low-Fowler position.
3. Transfer the patient to the bathroom.
4. Turn the patient to the side.

This item is designed to test your ability to respond appropriately to an event. To answer this question, you must understand that it is important to assist the patient to expectorate the vomitus to avoid aspiration. In addition, you need to know that turning the patient on the side is putting the patient in the best position to facilitate drainage of matter from the mouth. Responding to an event by instituting an action is an implementation question.

SAMPLE ITEM 6-29

A patient reports feeling nauseated. Which should the nurse do to provide support for this patient?

1. Give mouth care every hour.
2. Delay meals until the nausea passes.
3. Position the emesis basin in easy reach.
4. Explain that the nausea will lessen with time.

Actions that anticipate an event is a type of implementation. The word "provide" in the stem gives you a clue that this is an implementation question. To answer this question correctly, you must understand that feeling nauseated is a precursor to vomiting and that providing an emesis basin will support the nauseated patient.

SAMPLE ITEM 6-30

Which is the underlying rationale for a nurse changing a patient's position every 2 hours?

1. Relieve pressure

2. Assess skin condition

3. Ensure that skin is dry

4. Provide massage to bony prominences

    This item tests your ability to identify the correct rationale for a nursing procedure. Relieving pressure is the rationale for regularly changing a patient's position. To implement safe and effective care, nurses must have a strong understanding of the scientific rationales for nursing actions.

SAMPLE ITEM 6-31

A nurse is administering medications to a group of patients. Which is the safest way for the nurse to identify a patient?

1. Ask the patient his or her name.

2. Check the identification bracelet.

3. Double-check the medication administration record.

4. Observe the response after stating the patient's name.

    This test item is designed to see if you can correctly identify a step in a procedure. Although more than one of the options might be an action implemented by the nurse, the question is asking you to choose the best answer from all the options offered. In this set of options, checking the identification bracelet is the most reliable and safest method to verify a patient's identity.

SAMPLE ITEM 6-32

To provide aseptically safe perineal care to all female patients, which should the nurse do?

1. Use a different part of the washcloth for each stroke.

2. Employ a circular motion when applying soap.

3. Apply deodorant spray to the perineal area.

4. Sprinkle talcum powder on the perineum.

    This item tests your ability to identify a step in a procedure based on a specific scientific principle (asepsis). To answer this question correctly, you need to know that medical asepsis is promoted when the spread of microorganisms is limited. Using one area of the washcloth for each stroke when washing the perineum contributes to aseptically safe perineal care. Identifying a step in a procedure is an implementation question.

SAMPLE ITEM 6-33

A Registered Nurse (RN) delegates the insertion of an indwelling urinary catheter (Foley) to a Licensed Practical Nurse (LPN). Which statement is accurate about the delegation of this procedure to the LPN?

1. The LPN will not be held accountable for the task because it was delegated by the RN.

2. The RN should have implemented the planned care and not have delegated it to the LPN.

Continued

3. The LPN should have respectfully refused to implement this task.

4. The RN will be held responsible for the delegated care.

This item tests your ability to understand that a nurse who delegates care to another nursing staff member is responsible for supervising and evaluating the delivery of that care. This is an important component of implementation and is a concept that may be tested.

SAMPLE ITEM 6-34

When a nurse signs a turning and positioning schedule form, it indicates that the patient:

1. Received a backrub with lotion.

2. Was turned at the time initialed.

3. Received range-of-motion exercises.

4. Was encouraged to turn to a different position.

This question tests your ability to understand the purpose of a turning and positioning flow sheet. Documenting the care given is a component of the step of implementation.

EVALUATION

Evaluation is the fifth and final step of the nursing process. Evaluation is a process that consists of four steps that must be implemented after care is delivered if the effectiveness of the nursing care is to be determined. The evaluation process includes identifying patient responses to care (actual outcomes), comparing a patient's actual outcomes to the expected outcomes, analyzing the factors that affected the outcomes for the purpose of drawing conclusions about the success or failure of specific nursing interventions, and modifying the plan when necessary. Evaluation questions will ask you to:

- Identify the steps in the evaluation process
- Identify whether an outcome is met or not met
- Identify progress or lack of progress toward a goal and/or expected outcome
- Identify the need to modify the plan of care in response to a change in the status of the patient or a plan that is ineffective
- Understand that the process of evaluation is continuous
- Understand that the nursing process is dynamic and cyclical

The critical words within a test item that indicate that the item is focused on evaluation include the following: **expected, met, desired, compared, succeeded, failed, achieved, modified, reassess, ineffective, effective, response, and evaluate.** See whether you can identify variations of these words indicating evaluation activities in the sample items. Most testing errors occur on evaluation items when options are selected that:

- Do not thoroughly and accurately reassess the patient after care is implemented
- Fail to cluster new data appropriately
- Fail to determine the significance of new data
- Come to inappropriate or inaccurate conclusions when comparing actual outcomes to expected outcomes
- Fail to modify the plan of care in response to the changing needs of the patient or in response to an ineffective plan

Identify Patient Responses (Actual Outcomes)

The process of evaluation begins with a reassessment that collects new information. After nursing care is implemented, the patient is reassessed and new clusters of data are identified and their significance determined. In the nursing literature the word "evaluation" has often been used interchangeably with the word "assessment," which causes confusion. It is important to remember that assessment is only one component in the process of evaluation. The nurse must first reassess to identify the patient's responses (actual outcomes). Actual outcomes are the patient's responses to nursing care.

SAMPLE ITEM 6-35

A patient on a bland diet reports a reduced appetite. Which is an initial way for the nurse to determine whether the patient's nutritional needs have been met?

1. Institute a three-day food intake study.

2. Weigh the patient at the end of the week.

3. Request an order for a dietary assessment.

4. Compare a current weight with the weight history.

This item is designed to test your ability to identify a common way to evaluate one aspect of a patient's nutritional status. In this situation, the results of nutritional care are determined by comparing a current weight assessment with a previous weight assessment in an effort to identify any gain or loss in the patient's weight. After a change in status is identified, a conclusion about the effectiveness of care can be determined from the data.

Compare Actual Outcomes With Expected Outcomes To Determine Goal Achievement

Expected outcomes and goals are the criteria that are established for the evaluation of nursing care. A comparison is made between the patient's actual outcomes and the expected outcomes to determine the effectiveness of nursing interventions. When reassessing the patient after care and comparing these new data with expected outcomes, it is possible to determine which expected outcomes have been achieved and which have not been achieved. The closer the patient's actual outcomes are to the expected outcomes, the more positive the evaluation. When expected outcomes are achieved, the goal is attained. Negative evaluations reflect situations in which the expected outcomes are not achieved. When expected outcomes are not achieved, the goal is not attained. Negative evaluations indicate that the nursing care was ineffective. For example: goal—"The patient will be free of a wound infection when discharged 5 days after abdominal surgery"; outcomes—"as evidenced by the presence of a normal white blood cell count, approximation of wound edges with granulated tissue, and vital signs within expected limits." If the patient's actual outcomes meet these expected outcomes, the goal is achieved. If the patient's actual outcomes indicate increased vital signs; an increased white blood cell count; and/or the presence of purulent exudate, erythema, or unapproximated wound edges at the incision site, the goal is not achieved.

SAMPLE ITEM 6-36

A nurse teaches a patient about the foods permitted on a 2-gram sodium diet. Which food selected by the patient indicates an understanding of the teaching?

1. Celery

2. Fresh fruit

3. Vegetables

4. Luncheon meat

This item is designed to test your ability to identify that of all the options presented, fruit has the least amount of sodium. In addition, the stem is worded in such a way that it requires the nurse to evaluate the correctness of the patient's response. The action described in the stem is an attempt to evaluate the patient's understanding of the teaching provided.

Analyze Factors That Affect Actual Outcomes of Care

After a determination is made of whether care is effective, the nurse must come to some conclusions about the potential factors that contributed to the success or failure of the plan of care. If a plan of care is ineffective, the nurse must examine what contributed to its failure. This requires the nurse to start at step 1 of the nursing process—assessment—and work through the entire process again in an attempt to identify why the plan was ineffective. Questions the nurse must ask include these: "Was the original assessment accurate?" "If a nursing diagnosis was made, was it accurate, and did it include all the *related-to* factors?" "Was the goal realistic?" "Were the outcomes measurable?" "Were the interventions consistently implemented?"

SAMPLE ITEM 6-37

A patient returns to the clinic after taking a 7-day course of antibiotic therapy and is still exhibiting signs of a urinary tract infection. Which should be the nurse's initial action?

1. Make an appointment for the patient to be seen by the primary health-care provider.

2. Arrange for the primary health-care provider to prescribe a different antibiotic.

3. Obtain another urine specimen for culture and sensitivity testing.

4. Determine if the patient took the medication as prescribed.

This item is designed to test your ability to identify that the nurse must analyze the factors that influence outcomes of care. Options 1, 2, and 3 can be eliminated because these actions immediately move to an intervention before collecting more information. They may be unnecessary, depending on the information gleaned from the patient. Option 4 is the correct answer because adherence with a medication administration schedule will influence the effectiveness of the medication.

Modify the Plan of Care

After it is determined that a plan of care is ineffective, the plan must be modified. The changes in the plan of care are based on new patient assessments, analysis of new data, goals, outcomes, and nursing strategies that are designed to address the new needs of the patient. The modified plan must then be implemented, and the whole evaluation process begins again. The process of evaluation is continuous.

SAMPLE ITEM 6-38

A newly admitted patient was provided with a regular diet consisting of three traditional meals a day. After several days it was identified that the patient was eating only approximately 50% of the meals and was losing weight. What should the nurse do?

1. Assist the patient until meals are completed.

2. Schedule several between-meal supplements.

3. Change the plan of care to provide five small meals daily.

4. Secure an order to increase the number of calories provided.

This item is designed to test your ability to identify that the nursing plan of care must be changed when care is ineffective. The new actions must be within the legal definition of nursing and address the specific needs of the patient.

Assessment

6-1 **1. An assessment must be made to determine if any intervention is necessary to stabilize an injured body part before moving the patient; moving an injured person can exacerbate an injury.**

2. Moving an injured patient before other nursing interventions can exacerbate an injury.

3. Moving an injured patient before other nursing interventions is unsafe because it can exacerbate an injury.

4. Reporting the incident should be done after the patient is safe.

6-2 1. This is unsafe because it is concerned with implementing care prematurely.

2. Nurses must always assess a patient before having the patient walk to ensure that the patient has the strength to ambulate safely.

3. Not all patients using a wheelchair need a vest restraint to maintain safety.

4. This is unsafe because an overbed table is a movable object.

6-3 1. 18 breaths per minute is within the expected range for an adult. Breaths can be inhaled through the mouth or nose.

2. 20 breaths per minute is within the expected range for an adult. The depth is not significant as long as the respirations appear effortless.

3. 16 breaths per minute is within the expected range for an adult. The depth is not significant as long as the respirations appear effortless.

4. 28 breaths per minute is outside the expected range for an adult; expected respirations should be between 14 and 20, effortless, and noiseless. This patient may be experiencing respiratory distress.

6-4 1. A nurse may permit an alert and capable patient to insert a rectal thermometer; however, if the patient has physical or cognitive deficits, this may not be possible. When a patient self-inserts an electronic thermometer, the handle of the probe must be decontaminated after its use.

2. When taking a rectal temperature, the patient can be safely positioned on either the right or left side.

3. The use of an electronic thermometer is not always practical. Electronic thermometers usually are not used in isolation because of the inconvenience related to the need to decontaminate equipment after use.

4. Lubricating a rectal thermometer is always done to facilitate entry into the rectum; a lubricant reduces resistance when the thermometer is inserted through the anal sphincters.

6-5 1. Daily intake reflects the amount of food the patient is ingesting; this information does not contribute to the calculation of ideal body weight.

2. To calculate ideal body weight, the nurse must know the patient's height, age, and extent of bone structure.

3. Clothing size is determined by weight and inches reflecting circumference of the chest and waist; this information does not contribute to the calculation of ideal body weight.

4. Determining food preferences supports the patient's right to make choices about care; this information does not contribute to the calculation of ideal body weight.

6-6 1. The primary source is the patient, not the wife.

2. A tertiary source provides information outside the patient's frame of reference.

3. The wife is not a subjective source. "Subjective" refers to a type of data; subjective data are collected when the patient shares feelings, perceptions, sensations, and thoughts.

4. Family members are secondary sources. Secondary sources provide supplemental information about the patient.

6-7 1. The nurse can examine between the patient's toes and visually verify the presence of sores. Because the sores can be visually verified, this information is objective.

2. The color of hair can be visually verified and, therefore, is considered objective information.

3. The experience of pain is subjective information because it can be verified only by the patient.

4. An altered gait can be visually verified and, therefore, is considered objective information.

6-8 1. A letter is considered verbal communication; words are written.
2. Holding hands is nonverbal communication; a message is transmitted without using words.
3. Sounds may or may not communicate meaning; however, a sound that communicates a meaning is considered verbal communication.
4. A telephone message is verbal communication; words generally are spoken in a telephone message.

6-9 1. Notifying the health-care provider may eventually be necessary, but it is not the priority.
2. The reading should be verified by retaking the blood pressure because the nurse may have made a mistake when originally taking the blood pressure.
3. Notifying the nurse in charge may be done after the blood pressure is verified and all the vital signs are taken.
4. Taking the other vital signs is done after the initial blood pressure is taken a second time; once one vital sign is identified as outside the expected range, all the vital signs should be assessed.

6-10 1. The primary health-care provider does not need to be notified at this time. The primary health-care provider should be notified if a patient does not void within 6 to 8 hours after surgery.
2. When a primary health-care provider writes an order for I&O, every fluid that goes into the patient (e.g., oral fluids, intravenous fluids, nasogastric instillations) is considered intake and every fluid that comes out of the patient (e.g., urine, vomitus, wound drainage) is considered output. The amount of urinary output must be documented in the patient's medical record.
3. The vital signs (e.g., temperature, pulse, respirations, blood pressure, and sometimes bowel movements) are recorded on the vital signs flow sheet.
4. Although this may be done, it does not provide a written record. Written documentation is necessary for a permanent record and to communicate the information to appropriate health-care team members other than those working on the surgical unit.

Analysis

6-11 1. Receptive aphasia is not associated with the data cluster presented in the stem. Receptive aphasia is an inability to understand either spoken or written language.
2. An inability to ambulate is not associated with the data cluster identified in the stem; this is associated with the inability to bear weight on the right leg because of hemiplegia.
3. Difficulty swallowing can contribute to a risk for aspiration; it is associated with the data identified in the stem (paralysis of the right side, drooling, slurred speech), and together they present a cluster of information that is significant.
4. Incontinence of stool is not associated with the data cluster identified in the stem; this is associated with hygiene needs and supports the fact that the patient is at risk for impaired skin integrity, not aspiration.

6-12 **1. Patients who are immobilized are subject to increased pressure over bony prominences with a subsequent decrease in circulation to tissues.**
2. A psychiatric diagnosis is unrelated to the development of pressure ulcers.
3. Respiratory distress is unrelated to the development of pressure ulcers.
4. A need for close supervision is unrelated to the development of pressure ulcers.

6-13 1. Acting-out behaviors commonly reflect anger.
2. Refusing to believe or accept a situation is reflective of denial.
3. Clinical manifestations commonly associated with depression include avoiding contact with others, withdrawal, loss of appetite (anorexia), and difficulty falling asleep (insomnia).
4. Acceptance is related to the final step of grieving; a patient reconciles and accepts the situation and is at peace.

6-14 1. The patient is not trying to be left alone. Avoiding others reflects this need.
2. A patient who wants to be accepted usually will follow directions.
3. The patient is attempting to perform self-care to demonstrate the ability to be self-sufficient and independent.

4. Manipulation is associated with intrigue, scheming, and conniving. This patient's behavior is clear and direct.

6-15 1. Pain generally is not associated with hemorrhage.
2. Jaundice is associated with a problem with the liver or biliary system.
3. Tachycardia, an increased heart rate, is a compensatory mechanism to increase oxygen to all body cells and is associated with hemorrhage.
4. Hyperthermia, increased body temperature, is unrelated to hemorrhage.

6-16 1. This statement is identifying a need, not a nursing diagnosis.
2. This statement is an incorrectly worded nursing diagnosis; a stroke is not something a nurse can diagnose or treat.
3. This statement is a combination of an expected outcome and an intervention, not a nursing diagnosis.
4. This statement is an appropriately worded nursing diagnosis that uses NANDA terminology; it contains a health problem appropriate for nursing interventions.

Planning

6-17 1. This is a long-term goal, not a short-term goal. Also, the statement does not contain a time frame.
2. This is correct wording for a goal, but it is unrealistic; it takes 3 to 5 days for a new colostomy to function.
3. This is the problem statement, the first part of a nursing diagnosis.
4. This is a short-term goal; it is patient centered and specific, and the word "remain" reflects the time frame.

6-18 1. This statement is the problem statement of a nursing diagnosis, not an expected outcome.
2. This statement is an expected outcome. It is specific knowledge the patient should demonstrate that may help the patient to attain the ultimate goal of relief from insomnia.
3. This statement is a planned nursing intervention, not an expected outcome.
4. This statement is a goal, not an expected outcome. It is a broad general statement about the status of the patient after the implementation of nursing care.

6-19 1. Observing the dressing for drainage is important, but it is not the priority.
2. Providing for a patient's oxygenation is essential to maintain life and is always the priority.
3. Checking for infiltration is important, but it is not the priority.
4. Monitoring vital signs is important, but it is not the priority.

6-20 **1. Washing the hands with soap and water mechanically removes microorganisms from the skin; hand hygiene is the most effective way to prevent cross-contamination.**
2. Usually this is necessary only when a patient has a virulent microorganism.
3. Antibiotics usually are given not to prevent infection but to treat it.
4. Although foot-operated linen hampers contain and limit the spread of microorganisms, they are not the most effective intervention to prevent cross-contamination.

6-21 **1. An occupied bed is made for a patient on complete bedrest; this patient is not permitted out of bed.**
2. All the linens should be changed regularly and whenever necessary.
3. An occupied bed can be made without a mechanical lift just by turning the patient.
4. A patient on bedrest is not allowed out of bed for any reason unless directed by a health-care provider's order.

6-22 1. An obese patient can be transferred out of bed while the linen is changed.
2. A patient in a cast can be transferred out of bed while the linen is changed.
3. An immobile patient can be transferred out of bed while the linen is changed.
4. Patients on bedrest must remain in bed when the linens are changed; this is called "making an occupied bed."

6-23 **1. The nurse manager has an obligation to ensure that all patients' needs will be appropriately met; this is the only option that addresses this concept.**
2. All patients must have their needs met.
3. Providing only essential care does not ensure that appropriate care will be provided; this action will increase anxiety and cause patients to doubt the quality of care being provided.
4. Once the nurse assumes a course of duty, the nurse is responsible for the care that is delivered.

6-24 1. Giving care as quickly as possible will increase the demand on the patient's cardiopulmonary system. This increases activity, which in turn increases oxygen needs; rushing may cause the patient to decompensate.
2. This does not address the patient's physical needs. The patient needs a full bath because of the diaphoresis.
3. **Providing rest periods conserves energy; this reduces the strain of activity by decreasing the demand for oxygen, which in turn decreases the rate and labor of respirations.**
4. The patient's dyspnea cannot be ignored. Continuing the bath will further jeopardize the patient's status.

6-25 1. When a patient does not respond to common nursing interventions for a large pressure ulcer there are other more appropriate resources available for consultation than a plastic surgeon.
2. The physical therapist is a specialist in the area of assisting a patient to achieve or maintain physical mobility and is not an expert in providing nursing care.
3. **The clinical nurse specialist is educated and prepared to provide expert assistance when other members of the health-care team seek solutions to difficult clinical nursing problems.**
4. A primary health-care provider is responsible for the patient's medical care and is not an expert in providing nursing care.

Implementation

6-26 1. **Inserting an indwelling urinary catheter is a dependent nursing intervention and requires an order that first must be verified by the nurse implementing the order.**
2. Bringing equipment to the patient's bedside is premature.
3. There are other things the nurse must do first.
4. Washing the hands is not the first step in this procedure.

6-27 1. **Salt used to season meals contains sodium; sodium must be avoided when a patient is receiving a 2-gram sodium diet.**
2. Sugar is avoided when a patient is receiving a reduced-calorie or diabetic diet, not a 2-gram sodium diet.

3. Fluids are avoided when the patient has fluid restrictions, not when receiving a 2-gram sodium diet; however, the patient must be alert to avoid fluids that are high in sodium such as diet sodas.
4. Margarine is to be avoided when a patient is receiving a low-fat diet, not a 2-gram sodium diet.

6-28 1. Positioning the head between the knees may exacerbate vomiting because the pressure of the abdomen against the chest and the force of gravity promote the flow of gastric content toward the mouth.
2. The high-Fowler, not low-Fowler, position may facilitate the exit of vomitus from the mouth.
3. Vomiting takes energy and can cause the patient to become weak during the transfer.
4. **Turning the patient on the side drains the mouth via gravity and reduces the risk of aspiration.**

6-29 1. Oral hygiene is sufficient every 8 hours and whenever necessary.
2. Delaying meals is inappropriate; nausea may be a long-standing problem.
3. **An emesis basin provides physical and emotional comfort; the emesis basin collects vomitus rather than soiling the bed linens and reduces the patient's concern regarding soiling.**
4. This action provides false reassurance; the nurse cannot predict when nausea will subside.

6-30 1. **Changing a patient's position relieves pressure from body weight and permits circulation to return to the area; prolonged pressure can cause cell death from lack of oxygen and nutrients needed to sustain cellular metabolism.**
2. Although skin condition should be assessed, it is not the primary reason for changing a patient's position every 2 hours.
3. The nurse should ensure the skin is clean and dry, but this is not the primary reason for changing a patient every 2 hours.
4. Massage should be performed around, not to, bony prominences.

6-31 1. Asking a patient his or her name is unsafe; the patient may be cognitively impaired.
2. **Checking the identification band is the safest method to identify a patient;**

it is the most reliable because each patient on admission receives an identification bracelet with his or her name and an identification number.

3. Checking the medication administration record will not verify the name of the person.

4. Calling the patient's name and observing the response are unsafe interventions because the patient may be cognitively impaired.

6-32 1. Using different parts of the washcloth with each stroke provides a clean surface for each stroke when washing; it avoids contaminating the meatus with soiled portions of the cloth.

2. Using a circular motion is unsafe because it may bring soiled matter into contact with the urinary meatus.

3. Applying deodorant spray to the perineal area can be irritating to some patients and can contribute to the risk of impaired skin integrity; also it does not remove bacteria.

4. Talcum powder is contraindicated because its application may aerosolize toxins that may be inhaled contributing to lung disease.

6-33 1. An LPN always is held responsible for care provided to patients and always works under the direction of an RN.

2. A nurse can delegate tasks to other qualified nursing staff members as long as delegated tasks are supervised and their delivery evaluated.

3. It is inappropriate to refuse to implement delegated tasks as long as the tasks are within the legal scope of LPN practice and the LPN can safely implement the task. This procedure is within the scope of practice of an LPN.

4. This is an accurate statement; the delegating nurse is responsible for supervising and evaluating the delivery of delegated tasks.

6-34 1. Although a backrub with lotion should be implemented when a patient is turned and positioned, it is not the purpose of a turning and positioning schedule form.

2. This indicates that turning and positioning were implemented as planned.

3. Although the patient should receive range-of-motion exercises, this is not the purpose of a turning and positioning schedule form.

4. A patient must actually be turned and positioned before the nurse signs the turning and positioning flow sheet; although a patient might be encouraged to turn, it does not mean that the patient was actually turned.

Evaluation

6-35 1. A food intake diary for 3 days might be done later if initial reassessments are inadequate.

2. It is unnecessary to wait until the end of the week; the patient's nutritional status can be assessed immediately.

3. It is not necessary to request a dietary assessment. The patient's nutritional status can be done easily and immediately by the nurse.

4. Measuring a patient's weight and comparing the weight with a previous weight is a quick and easy way to determine a patient's nutritional status.

6-36 1. Celery has more sodium than the nutrient in the correct option.

2. Fruit has the least amount of sodium compared with the other options.

3. Vegetables have more sodium than the nutrient in the correct option.

4. Luncheon meat is high in sodium because of the ingredients used to process the meat.

6-37 1. Making an appointment for the patient with the primary health-care provider is inappropriate before collecting additional data associated with the present plan of care.

2. Arranging for the primary health-care provider to prescribe a different antibiotic is inappropriate before collecting additional data associated with the present plan of care; this may be necessary later.

3. Obtaining another urine sample for a culture and sensitivity is inappropriate before collecting additional data about the present plan of care.

4. Determining adherence to the antibiotic regimen is the priority. Antibiotics must be taken routinely and consistently for the full course of treatment to maintain adequate blood levels of the drug.

6-38 1. Patients must not be forced to eat all their meals; the portions may be too large for an anorectic patient to ingest.
2. Adding between-meal supplements is a dependent intervention and requires a primary health-care provider's order.
3. **Arranging for five small meals daily is an interdependent nursing intervention. The primary health-care provider ordered a regular diet and** the nurse is providing this diet over five meals a day rather than the traditional three meals a day. Small, frequent feedings spread the meals throughout the day and provide a volume that is not as overwhelming as a full meal.
4. The problem is not the number of calories provided on the tray but the amount of food the patient is able to ingest at any one time.

Test-Taking Techniques

Performing well on nursing questions requires both roots and wings. The information in the previous chapters provided you with roots by giving you information about formulating a positive mental attitude, using critical thinking, employing time-management strategies, exploring a variety of study skills, and developing an understanding of the multiple-choice question and the nursing process. In this chapter an attempt is made to provide you with the wings necessary to "fly through" multiple-choice questions. Flying through multiple-choice questions has nothing to do with speed; it relates to being test wise and able to navigate through complex information with ease.

Tests in nursing involve complex information that has depth and breadth. In addition to having its own body of knowledge, nursing draws from a variety of disciplines, such as sociology, psychology, and anatomy and physiology. To perform well on a nursing examination, you must understand and integrate the subject matter. Nothing can replace effective study habits or knowledge about the subject being tested. However, being test wise can maximize the application of the information you possess. Being test wise entails specific techniques related to individual question analysis and general techniques related to conquering the challenge of an examination. One rationale for learning how to use these techniques is to provide you with skills that increase your command over the testing situation. If you are in control, you will maintain a positive attitude, which will affect your performance in a positive manner. When you have knowledge and are test wise, you should fly through a test by gliding and soaring, rather than by flapping and fluttering.

SPECIFIC TEST-TAKING TECHNIQUES

A specific test-taking technique is a strategy that uses skill and forethought to analyze a test item before selecting an answer. A technique is not a gimmick but a method of examining a question with consideration and thoughtfulness to help you select the correct answer. When an item has four options, the chance of selecting the correct answer is one out of four, or 25%. When you eliminate one distractor, the chance of selecting the correct answer is one out of three, or 33.3%. If you are able to eliminate two distractors, the chance of selecting the correct answer is one out of two, or 50%. Each time you successfully eliminate a distractor, you dramatically increase your chances of correctly answering the question.

Before you attempt to answer a question, break the question into its components. First, read the stem. What is it actually asking? It may be helpful to paraphrase the stem to focus on its content. Then, try to answer the question being asked in your own words before looking at the options. Often, one of the options will be similar to your answer. Then examine the other options and try to identify the correct answer.

If you know, understand, and can apply the information being tested, you can often identify the correct answer. However, do not be tempted to select an option too quickly, without careful thought. An option may contain accurate information, but it may not be correct because it does not answer the question asked in the stem. Be careful. Each option deserves equal consideration.

Use test-taking techniques for every question. However, the use of test-taking techniques becomes more important when you are unsure of the answer, because each distractor that you are able to eliminate will increase your chances of selecting the correct answer. Most nursing students are able to reduce the number of plausible answers to two. Contrary to popular belief, multiple-choice questions in nursing have only one correct answer. Use everything in your arsenal to conquer the multiple-choice question test: effective studying, a positive mental attitude, and, last but not least, test-taking techniques.

The correct answers for the sample items in this chapter and the rationales for all the options are at the end of the chapter.

Identify the Word in the Stem That Indicates Negative Polarity

Read the stem slowly and carefully. Look for key words such as **not, except, never, contraindicated, unacceptable, avoid, unrelated, violate,** and **least.** These words indicate negative polarity, and the question being asked is probably concerned with what is false. Some words that have negative polarity are not as obvious as others. A negatively worded stem asks you to identify an exception, detect an error, or recognize nursing interventions that are unacceptable or contraindicated. If you read a stem and several of the options appear correct, reread the stem because you may have missed a key negative word. These words are sometimes brought to your attention by an underline (not), italics (*except*), boldface (**never**), or capitals (VIOLATE). Many nursing examinations avoid questions with negative polarity. However, examples of these items are included for your information.

SAMPLE ITEM 7-1

Which action violates medical asepsis when the nurse makes an occupied bed?

1. Returning unused linen to a linen closet

2. Wearing gloves when changing the linen

3. Tucking clean linen against the frame of the bed

4. Using the old top sheet for the new bottom sheet

The key term in this stem is *violates.* The stem is asking you to identify the option that does <u>not</u> follow correct medical aseptic technique. If you missed the word *violates* and were looking for the answer that indicated correct medical aseptic technique, there will be more than one correct answer. When this happens, reread the stem for a word with negative polarity. In this item, you had to be particularly careful because the word *violates* is not emphasized for your attention.

SAMPLE ITEM 7-2

A patient is receiving a low-sodium diet. Which food should the nurse teach the patient to *avoid* because it is high in sodium?

1. Stewed fruit

2. Luncheon meats

3. Whole-grain cereal

4. Green, leafy vegetables

The key word in this stem is *avoid;* it is brought to your attention because it is italicized. The stem is asking you to select the food that a patient receiving a low-sodium diet should <u>not</u> eat. If you missed the word *avoid* and were looking for foods that are permitted on a low-sodium diet, then there will be more than one correct answer. When there appears to be more than one correct answer, reread the stem for a key negative word that you may have missed.

SAMPLE ITEM 7-3

Which should a nurse **never** do when rubbing a patient's back?

1. Apply pressure over vertebrae

2. Use continuous strokes

3. Wipe off excess lotion

4. Knead the skin

The key word in this stem is *never.* The stem is asking you to identify which option is <u>not</u> an acceptable practice associated with a back rub. If you missed the word *never* and were looking for what the nurse should do for a back rub, there will be more than one correct answer. This should alert you to the fact that you may have missed a key negative word.

Identify the Word in the Stem That Sets a Priority

Read the stem carefully while looking for key words such as **first, initially, best, priority, safest,** and **most.** These words modify what is being asked. This type of question requires you to put a value on each option and then place them in rank order. If the question asks what the nurse should do first, what the initial action by the nurse should be, or what the best response is, then rank the options in order of importance from 1 to 4, with the most desirable option as number 1 and the least desirable option as number 4. The correct answer is the option that you ranked number 1. If you are having difficulty ranking the options, eliminate the option that you believe is most wrong among all the options. Next, eliminate the option you believe is most wrong from among the remaining three options. At this point, you are down to two options, and your chance of selecting the correct answer is 50%. When key words such as "most important" are used, frequently all of the options may be appropriate nursing care for the situation. However, only one of the options is the *most* important. When all the options appear logical for the situation, reread the stem to identify a key word that asks you to place a priority on the options. These words occasionally are emphasized by an <u>underline</u>, *italics*, **boldface**, or CAPITALS.

Answering a test question that asks you to establish a priority (which is "most important," "best," "initial," and "first") requires you to make a decision using clinical judgment. It requires you to use perceptual, inferential, and/or diagnostic judgment to arrive at the correct answer based on the data in the question and options. To do this, you must draw on your knowledge of theory, concepts, principles, and nursing standards of practice. The student who has a strong foundation of knowledge and who is a critical thinker is best equipped to arrive at the correct answer. For additional information about making clinical decisions and types of clinical judgments, refer to Chapter 2, Critical Thinking, in the section titled Clinical Judgments.

A strategy you can draw on to help you answer priority questions is to refer to basic guiding theories that are part of the foundation of nursing. Maslow's Hierarchy of Needs, the Nursing Process, Kübler-Ross's Theory of Death and Dying, Man as a Unified Being, the theory that the patient is the center of the health team, teaching/learning theory, emotional support and communication theory, and the ABCs (Airway, Breathing, Circulation) of prioritizing physical care, to name a few, present clear parameters of practice that are the building blocks of the foundation of nursing practice. Choosing which theory or principle to draw on when answering a test question comes with practice. You first have to identify "what is happening" and "what should I do." You then have to identify which theory or principle applies best in the scenario presented in the question in light of the options offered.

Keeping these theories in mind when answering test questions, you should recognize that:

- Physiological needs generally need to be met first before higher-level needs.
- Disbelief and denial are generally a person's first response to news of a loss or anticipated loss.
- Meeting the needs of the patient comes first over other tasks.
- Patient readiness to learn must be assessed first before designing a teaching program.
- A patient's emotional status must be assessed as part of the first step in the nursing process.
- Nurses need to use interviewing techniques to effectively communicate in a nonthreatening way with patients.
- The nurse must deliver care in a nonjudgmental manner.
- Maintaining a patient's airway is always a priority.
- The patient's safety is always a priority.
- A thorough assessment must be completed before other steps in the nursing process.

Practice the questions in Chapter 11 that ask you to set a priority and study the rationales for the right and wrong answers. Priority questions are identified by the statement, "Identify key words in the stem that set a priority," which appears in the TEST-TAKING TIP after the question. This will help you build a body of knowledge associated with determining what the nurse should do first in different clinical situations presented in practice questions.

SAMPLE ITEM 7-4

Which should the nurse do <u>first</u> before administering an enema?

1. Collect the appropriate equipment.
2. Verify the order for the procedure.
3. Inform the patient about the procedure.
4. Ensure the patient's bathroom is empty.

The key word in this stem is *first*. Each of these options includes a step that is part of the procedure for administering an enema. You must decide which option is the *first* step among the four options presented. Before you can teach a patient, collect equipment, or actually administer the enema, you need to know the type of enema ordered. The type of enema will influence the other steps of the procedure. If option 2 were different, such as "Use medical asepsis to dispose of contaminated articles," the correct answer among these four options would be option 3. You can choose the first step of a procedure only from among the options presented.

SAMPLE ITEM 7-5

A patient has significant short-term memory loss and does not remember the primary nurse from day to day. When the patient asks, "Who are you?," which is the **most** appropriate response?

1. "You know me. I take care of you every day."
2. "Don't worry. I'm the same nurse you had yesterday."
3. Say nothing, because it probably will upset the patient.
4. State your name and say, "I am the nurse caring for you."

The key words in this stem are *most appropriate.* You are asked to select the <u>best</u> or <u>most suitable</u> response from among the four options presented. You may dislike all of the statements. You may even think of a response that you personally prefer to the offered options. YOU CANNOT REWRITE THE QUESTION. You must select your answer from the options presented in the item. The words *most appropriate* are not highlighted in this item, and therefore you must be diligent when reading the stem.

SAMPLE ITEM 7-6

A nurse is caring for a patient who just had a long leg cast applied for a compound fracture of the femur. Which is the **most** important nursing intervention when caring for this patient?

1. Turn and position every 4 hours.

2. Take pulses proximal to the casted area.

3. Cover rough edges of the cast with tape.

4. Inspect the cast for signs of drainage or bleeding.

   The word *most* in the stem sets a priority. Use the ABCs (Airway, Breathing, Circulation) to identify the *most* important option. No options are associated with airway or breathing. However, options 2 and 4 are associated with circulation. If you identify that assessing a distal, not proximal, pulse is important, then you can eliminate option 2. You have arrived at the correct answer.

Identify Key Words in the Stem That Direct Attention to Content

Generally, a stem of an item is short and contains only the information needed to make it clear and specific. Therefore, the use of a word or phrase in the stem has significance. A key word is the intentional or unintentional use of a word or phrase that provides information that leads you to the correct answer. Sometimes a key word is a word or phrase that modifies another word or phrase in the stem. It takes a broad concept and focuses the reader toward a more specific aspect of the concept (see Sample Item 7-7). Other times a word or phrase in the stem is significant because it is similar to or a paraphrase of a word or phrase in the correct answer (see Sample Item 7-8). Occasionally, a word or phrase in the stem is identical to a word or phrase in the correct answer and is called a **clang association** (see Sample Item 7-9). Every word in the stem is important, but some words are more significant than others. The identification of important words and the analysis of the significance of these words in relation to the stem and the options require critical thinking.

SAMPLE ITEM 7-7

To meet a patient's basic physiological needs according to Maslow's Hierarchy of Needs, which should the nurse do?

1. Maintain the patient's body in functional alignment.

2. Pull the curtain when the patient is on a bedpan.

3. Respond to a call light immediately.

4. Raise both side rails on the bed.

   An important word in the stem is *physiological.* It is an intentional use of a word to specifically limit consideration to one aspect of Maslow's theory.

SAMPLE ITEM 7-8

Which should the nurse do to help meet a patient's self-esteem needs?

1. Encourage the patient to perform self-care when able.

2. Ask family members to visit the patient more often.

Continued

Continued

3. Anticipate needs before the patient requests help.

4. Give the patient a complete bath.

An important word in the stem is *self-esteem*. The word "self-esteem" is similar to the word "self-care." Thoughtfully examine option 1. An option that incorporates words that are similar to words in the stem is often the correct answer. In addition, the word *self-esteem* in the stem is the intentional use of a word that focuses on one aspect of Maslow's theory. This question exemplifies the use of two clues in the stem when answering a question.

SAMPLE ITEM 7-9

Which should the nurse do to meet a patient's basic physical needs?

1. Pull the curtain when providing care.

2. Answer the call bell immediately.

3. Administer physical hygiene.

4. Obtain vital signs.

An important word in the stem is *physical*. It is a clue that should provide a hint that option 3 is the correct answer. The use of the word "physical" in both the stem and the option is called a *clang association*. It is the repetitious use of a word. Examine option 3 because when a clang association occurs, it is often the correct answer.

Identify the Central Person in the Question

Test questions usually require the nurse to respond to the needs of a patient. When a stem is limited to just the patient and the nurse, the patient is almost always the central person in the question. However, some questions focus on the needs of others, such as a child, parent, spouse, or roommate. To select the correct option, you have to identify the central (significant) person in the stem. The significant person is the person who is to receive the care. Sometimes, in addition to the patient, a variety of people are included in the stem. The inclusion of others may set the stage for the question or test your ability to discriminate. These people also may distract you from who is actually the significant person in the stem. Therefore, to answer the question accurately, you must determine WHO is the central person in the question.

SAMPLE ITEM 7-10

A nurse will be going on vacation. To involve the patient in the excitement, which is the **best** response by the nurse?

1. "Tell me about some of your favorite past vacations."

2. "Do you want to hear about the plans for my trip?"

3. "I'll bring the brochures for you to see."

4. "What do you think about vacations?"

Continued

There are two people in this stem, the patient and the nurse. There are two clues in the stem. The first clue is "involve the patient." To involve the patient, the patient must be active. Therefore, options 2 and 3 can be eliminated because they focus on the nurse, who is not the central person in the question. The second clue is the word *best*. The word "best" is asking you to set a priority. More than one option may include appropriate nursing care, but only one is the "best" action. Options 1 and 4 include appropriate nursing care. However, option 1 requires a more detailed response than option 4. Reminiscing involves more than just giving an opinion.

SAMPLE ITEM 7-11

A patient who has experienced the surgical removal of a breast (mastectomy) says to the nurse, "My husband can't look at my incision and hasn't suggested having sex since my surgery." Which should be the initial action of the nurse?

1. Arrange to speak with the husband about his concerns.

2. Plan to teach the husband that the wife needs his support.

3. Explore the patient's feelings about her husband's behavior.

4. Make an appointment with Reach for Recovery for the patient.

There are three people in this stem: the patient, the husband, and the nurse. There are two clues in the stem. The first clue is the quoted statement by the patient about her husband's behavior. The second clue is the word *initial*. The word "initial" is asking you to set a priority. The situation may require one or more of these responses, but only one of them should be done first. The patient's statement reflects the patient's concern. Addressing the patient's concern should come first. The patient is the central person in this question, not the husband. Options 1 and 2 focus on the husband, who is not the central person in this question and can be eliminated. In option 4, the nurse is using a referral to evade the issues involved and avoid professional responsibility.

SAMPLE ITEM 7-12

A patient is friendly, has many visitors, and appears happy. However, when the patient's daughter visits, the patient cries and reports the presence of pain. The daughter's eyes are filled with tears and she is visibly upset when she leaves her mother's room. Which should the nurse do?

1. Explore the situation with the daughter.

2. Encourage the patient to be more positive.

3. Tell the daughter that the patient usually does not cry.

4. Observe the interaction between them without intervening at this time.

There are many people in this situation: visitors, the patient, the daughter, and the nurse. The question expects the nurse to follow one course of action when the daughter becomes upset. The phrase "she is visibly upset" shifts the focus of the question to the daughter. Options 1 and 3 focus on the daughter. By eliminating two options (options 2 and 4) you have increased your chances of getting this question correct to 50%.

Identify Patient-Centered Options

Nursing is a profession that provides both physical and emotional care to patients. Therefore, the focus of the nurse's concern usually is the patient. Items that test your ability to be patient centered tend to explore patient feelings, identify patient preferences, empower the patient, afford the patient choices, or in some other way put emphasis on the patient. Because the patient is the center of the health-care team, the patient often is the priority.

SAMPLE ITEM 7-13

When assisting a patient who recently had an above-the-knee amputation to transfer into a chair, the patient starts to cry and says, "I am useless with only one leg." Which is a therapeutic response by the nurse?

1. "Losing a leg can be very difficult."

2. "You still have the use of one good leg."

3. "A prosthesis will make a big difference."

4. "You'll feel better when you can use crutches."

Option 1 is patient centered. It focuses on the patient's feelings by using the interviewing technique of reflection. Option 2 denies the patient's feelings, and options 3 and 4 provide false reassurance. When a patient's feelings are ignored or minimized, the nurse is not being patient centered. To be patient centered, the nurse should concentrate on the patient's feelings or concerns.

SAMPLE ITEM 7-14

An oriented patient states, "I always forget the questions I want to ask when my doctor visits me." Which is the nurse's **best** response?

1. Offer to stay when the doctor visits.

2. Remind the patient of the doctor's next visit.

3. Give the patient materials to write questions to ask the doctor.

4. Suggest that a family member be available to question the doctor.

Option 3 is patient centered. It focuses on the patient's ability, fosters independence, and empowers the patient. Option 2 does not address the patient's concern, and options 1 and 4 promote dependence, which can lower self-esteem. Avoiding patient concerns and promoting dependence are actions that are not patient centered. To be patient centered, the nurse should encourage self-care.

SAMPLE ITEM 7-15

Which should the nurse do first when combing a female patient's hair?

1. Use tap water to moisten the hair.

2. Apply a hair conditioner before combing.

3. Comb the patient's hair using long strokes.

4. Ask the patient how she prefers to wear her hair.

Option 4 is patient centered. It allows choices and supports the person as an individual. Options 1, 2, and 3 do not take into consideration patient preferences. A procedure that is begun before determining patient preferences is not patient centered. The Patient Care Partnership (formerly the Patient's Bill of Rights) mandates that the patient has a right to considerate and respectful care and to receive information before the start of any procedure and/or treatment.

SAMPLE ITEM 7-16

A patient enjoys television programs about animals. After one of these programs, the patient cries and sadly talks about a beloved cat that died. Which should be the nurse's initial response?

1. Tell the patient a story about a cat.
2. Hang a picture of a cat in the patient's room.
3. Ask the patient to share more about the cat she loved.
4. Obtain a book about cats for the patient from the library.

Option 3 is patient centered. It encourages the patient to communicate further. Options 1, 2, and 4 may eventually be done because they take into consideration the patient's interest in cats. However, they should not be the initial actions because they do not focus on the patient's feelings at this time. The nurse is being patient centered when encouraging additional communication and verbalization of feelings and concerns from the patient.

Identify Specific Determiners in Options

A specific determiner is a word or statement that conveys a thought or concept that has no exceptions. Words such as **just, always, never, all, every, none,** and **only** are absolute and easy to identify. They place limits on a statement that generally is considered correct. Statements that use all-inclusive terms frequently represent broad generalizations that usually are false. Frequently these options are incorrect and can be eliminated. However, some absolutes, such as "all patients should be treated with respect," are correct. Because there are few absolutes in this world, options that contain specific determiners should be examined carefully. Be discriminating.

SAMPLE ITEM 7-17

A nurse is giving a patient a bed bath. How can the nurse **best** improve the patient's circulation during the bath?

1. Use firm strokes.
2. Utilize only hot water.
3. Keep the patient covered.
4. Apply soap to the washcloth.

In option 2 the word *only* is a specific determiner. It allows for no exceptions. Hot water can burn the skin and also is contraindicated for patients with sensitive skin such as children, older adults, and people with dermatological problems. Because option 2 allows for no exceptions, it can be eliminated as a viable option.

SAMPLE ITEM 7-18

When providing perineal care for patients, by which action can nurses **most** appropriately protect themselves from microorganisms?

1. Washing their hands before giving care
2. Disposing contaminated water in the toilet
3. Wearing clean gloves when providing perineal care
4. Encouraging patients to provide all of their own care

In option 4 the word *all* is a specific determiner. It is a word that obviously includes everything. Expecting patients to provide all of their own care is unreasonable, is unrealistic, and may be unsafe. Option 4 can be eliminated. This increases your chances of choosing the correct answer because you have to choose from among three options rather than four.

SAMPLE ITEM 7-19

A patient states that the elastic straps of the oxygen face mask feel too tight. How should the nurse respond?

1. Explain the face mask must always stay firmly in place.

2. Replace the face mask with a nasal cannula.

3. Pad the straps with gauze.

4. Adjust the straps.

In option 1 the word *always* is a specific determiner. It is an absolute term that places limits on a statement that might otherwise be true. This option can be eliminated. By deleting option 1, the chances of your selecting the correct answer become 33.3% rather than 25%.

Identify Opposites in Options

Sometimes an item contains two options that are the opposite of each other. They can be single words that reflect extremes on a continuum, or they can be statements that convey converse messages. When opposites appear in the options, they must be given serious consideration. One of them will be the correct answer, or they both can be eliminated from consideration. When one of the opposites is the correct answer, you are being asked to differentiate between two responses that incorporate extremes of a concept or principle. When options are opposites, <u>more often than not, but not always,</u> one of them is the correct answer. When the opposites are distractors, they are attempting to divert your attention from the correct answer. This test-taking technique usually cannot be applied to options that reflect numerical values (e.g., heart rates, blood pressures, respiratory rates, laboratory values). If you correctly evaluate opposite options, you can increase your chances of selecting the correct answer to 50% because you have reduced the plausible options to two. The Sample Items that follow provide a variety of examples of how opposites appear in options.

SAMPLE ITEM 7-20

A nurse understands that the progress of growth and development in all older adults:

1. Slips backward.

2. Moves forward.

3. Becomes slower.

4. Remains stagnant.

Options 1 and 2 are opposites. They should be considered carefully in relation to each other and then in relation to the other options. These options are the reverse sides of a concept, movement in relation to growth and development. Options 3 and 4, although true for some individuals, are not true statements about *all* older adults as indicated in the stem. You now must select between options 1 and 2. Option 2 is the correct answer. By focusing on options 1 and 2 and then progressively examining and deleting options 3 and 4, you have systematically scrutinized this item.

SAMPLE ITEM 7-21

Anti-embolism stockings are ordered for a patient. When should the nurse apply the anti-embolism stockings?

1. While the patient is still in bed

2. Once the patient reports having leg pain

3. When the patient's feet become edematous

4. After the patient gets out of bed in the morning

Continued

Options 1 and 4 are opposites. Examine these options first. They are contrary to each other in relation to before or after an event, getting out of bed. Now assess options 2 and 3. These options expect the nurse to apply anti-embolism stockings after a problem exists. The purpose of these stockings is to foster venous return, thereby preventing edema and discomfort. Options 2 and 3 can be omitted from further consideration. The final selection is between options 1 and 4. You have increased your chances of correctly answering the question from 25% to 50%. Because edema can occur when the feet are dependent, anti-embolism stockings should be applied before, not after, the patient gets out of bed. You have arrived at the correct answer, option 1, using a methodical approach.

SAMPLE ITEM 7-22

A wrist restraint is ordered for a patient on bedrest. To which part of the patient's bed should the nurse tie the restraint?

1. Side rails
2. Footboard
3. Bed frame
4. Headboard

There are two sets of opposites in this question. Options 1 and 3 are opposites and options 2 and 4 are opposites. Examine each set of opposites in relation to each other. Options 2 and 4 are the opposite ends of a hospital bed. Neither option is more appropriate than the other. They are probably both distractors. Now examine options 1 and 3. Side rails are movable, and a restraint must be applied to something that is stationary. Now consider option 3. The bed frame is immovable. Options 1, 2, and 4 can be eliminated, and option 3 is the correct answer. In this question, two sets of opposites complicate analysis of these options. However, after examining each set of opposites, you should be able to use critical thinking to eliminate the incorrect options.

SAMPLE ITEM 7-23

Which type of intravenous solution is normal saline in relation to body fluids?

1. Hypertonic
2. Hypotonic
3. Acidotic
4. Isotonic

Options 1 and 2 are opposites. Appraise these words in relation to each other and their relationship to body fluids and normal saline. They are extremes in the concentration of solutes. Because normal saline is equal to body fluids in the concentration of solutes, these options are probably distractors. Now examine options 3 and 4. Acidotic refers to a low pH in body fluids and is not a type of intravenous solution. Option 3 can be deleted from consideration. In this question, the options that are opposites (1 and 2) are distractors and can be eliminated.

Identify Equally Plausible or Unique Options

Sometimes items contain two or more options that are similar. It is difficult to choose between two similar options because they are comparable. One option is no better or worse than the other option in relation to the statement presented in the stem. When analyzing options use the "If → Then" technique. Ask yourself, "If I perform this intervention in the option, then what will be the outcome?" In equally plausible options the outcomes frequently are the same or similar. Usually equally plausible options are distractors and can be eliminated from consideration. You have now improved your chances of selecting the correct answer to 50%. If you find three equally plausible options when initially examining the options, the fourth option probably will be different from the others and appear unique. Children's activity books present a game based on this concept. Four pictures are presented, and the child is asked to pick out the one that is different. "Which one of these is not like the others? Which one of these is not the same?" For example, the picture contains three types of fruit and one vegetable, and the child is asked to identify which one is different. The correct answer to a test item can sometimes be identified by using this concept of similarities and differences.

SAMPLE ITEM 7-24

Which should the nurse do to effectively help meet a patient's basic safety and security needs?

1. Serve adequate food.

2. Provide sufficient fluid.

3. Place the call bell near the patient.

4. Store the patient's valuables in the bedside table.

Options 1 and 2 are similar because they both provide nutrients. They are equally plausible when compared to each other and particularly when assessed in relation to the concepts of safety and security; neither relates to meeting a patient's safety and security needs. These options are distractors and can be eliminated from consideration. By just having to choose between options 3 and 4, you have raised your chances of correctly answering the question to 50%.

SAMPLE ITEM 7-25

How can the nurse promote circulation when providing a back rub?

1. Place the patient in the prone position.

2. Use moisturizing cream.

3. Apply Keri lotion.

4. Knead the skin.

Options 2 and 3 use substances when performing the back rub. Ask yourself, "If I use moisturizing cream, then what is the outcome?" Ask yourself, "If I use Keri lotion, then what is the outcome?" In both instances the outcome is the skin will become less dry and more supple. Because the outcomes are similar, the options are equally plausible. Equally plausible options usually are distractors; therefore, you can delete these options. Now evaluate the remaining options. One of them is the correct answer.

SAMPLE ITEM 7-26

Which is the reason why passive range-of-motion (PROM) exercises are performed?

1. Increase endurance

2. Prevent loss of mobility

3. Strengthen muscle tone

4. Maximize muscle atrophy

Continued

> Options 1, 3, and 4 all include words (increase, strengthen, and maximize) that address improvement of something (endurance, muscle tone, and atrophy). They are alike. Option 2 is different. It prevents something from happening, loss of mobility. Option 2 is unique when compared with the presentation of the other options, and it should be given careful consideration. Even if you do not know the definition of "atrophy" and do not understand that the loss of muscle mass should not be maximized, you can still use the test-taking technique of identifying similar and unique options. "Which one of these is not like the others? Which one of these is not the same?"

SAMPLE ITEM 7-27

Which should the nurse plan to do immediately before performing any patient procedure?

1. Shut the door.

2. Wash the hands.

3. Close the curtain.

4. Drape the patient.

> Options 1, 3, and 4 are similar in that they all somehow enclose the patient. Ask yourself about the outcome of each intervention (If → Then). Options 1, 3, and 4 all provide for patient privacy. They are all plausible interventions when providing patient care. It is difficult to choose the most correct answer from among these three options. Option 2 is different. It relates to microbiological safety rather than emotional safety. Because this option is unique when compared with the other options, it should be thoroughly examined in relation to the stem because it is likely to be the correct answer.

Identify the Global Option

A global option is more comprehensive and general than the other options. Although unspoken, the global option may include under its mantle a specific concept identified in one or more of the other options. Identifying global options is similar to identifying unique options. The global option usually is a broad general statement, whereas the three distractors generally are specific. You must pick out the option that is different. "Which one of these is not like the others? Which one of these is not the same?"

SAMPLE ITEM 7-28

The most effective way for the nurse to prevent the spread of infection in a nursing home is by:

1. Administering antibiotics to sick patients.

2. Limiting the spread of microorganisms.

3. Isolating residents who are sick.

4. Keeping all unit doors closed.

> Options 1, 3, and 4 are all incorrect as indicated in the rationales. However, if you did not know that they were incorrect and you just examined the four options, you should have noticed that options 1, 3, and 4 all identify specific actions while option 2 is broad and general and is different from the other options.

SAMPLE ITEM 7-29

When the nurse is repositioning a patient, which is the **most** important principle of body mechanics?

1. Elevating the arms on pillows
2. Maintaining functional alignment
3. Preventing external rotation of the hips
4. Placing a small pillow under the lumbar curvature

Options 1, 3, and 4 are something you might do to support a patient in a specific position. However, option 2 is comprehensive and broad and identifies something the nurse should do when positioning all patients regardless of the specific position.

Identify Duplicate Facts Among Options

Sometimes items are designed so that each option contains two or more facts. Usually identical or similar facts appear in at least two of the four options. If you identify a fact as incorrect, you can eliminate all the options that contain this fact. By deleting distractors, you increase your chances of selecting the correct answer.

SAMPLE ITEM 7-30

A patient has a vest restraint. While making this patient's occupied bed, which must the nurse do to promote patient safety?

1. Keep the vest restraint tied, and lower both side rails.
2. Keep the vest restraint tied, and lower one side rail.
3. Untie the vest restraint, and lower both side rails.
4. Untie the vest restraint, and lower one side rail.

This item is testing two concepts: whether a vest restraint should be tied or untied when providing direct care and whether one or both side rails should be lowered when providing direct care. If you only know the fact that the side rail should be lowered just on the side on which you are working, you can eliminate options 1 and 3. If you only know the fact that a vest restraint can be untied when the nurse is at the bedside providing direct care, you can eliminate options 1 and 2. In either case, you can eliminate two options as distractors, and you have increased your chances of selecting the correct answer from 25% to 50%.

SAMPLE ITEM 7-31

A 2-gram sodium diet is ordered for a patient. Which group of nutrients is **most** appropriate for this diet?

1. Fruit, vegetables, and bread
2. Hot dogs, mustard, and pickles
3. Hamburger, onions, and ketchup
4. Luncheon meats, rolls, and vegetables

This item is testing your knowledge about the sodium content of foods. If you know that hot dogs and luncheon meats are both processed foods that are high in sodium, you can eliminate options 2 and 4. If you understand that ketchup and mustard are both condiments that are high in sodium, you can delete options 2 and 3. By knowing either fact, you can reduce the final selection to between two options. The similarities between these options are less clear than if the parts were identical, but the technique of identifying duplicate facts in options can still be used.

SAMPLE ITEM 7-32

A nurse is monitoring a patient who is at risk for hemorrhage. For which clinical manifestations should the nurse assess the patient?

1. Warm, dry skin; hypotension; bounding pulse

2. Hypertension; bounding pulse; cold, clammy skin

3. Weak, thready pulse; hypertension; warm, dry skin

4. Hypotension; cold, clammy skin; weak, thready pulse

This item is testing your knowledge about patient responses associated with hemorrhage. Three patient responses are presented: the condition of the skin, the blood pressure, and the characteristic of the pulse. Even if you know only one of these facts about hemorrhage, you can reduce your final selection to between two options. If you know that hypotension is associated with hemorrhage, you can eliminate options 2 and 3. If you know that cold, clammy skin is related to hemorrhage, you can delete options 1 and 3. If you know that a weak, thready pulse is associated with hemorrhage, you can eliminate options 1 and 2. If you know only one or two of the facts presented, you can maximize your chance of correctly answering this type of item. Options that have two or three parts work to your advantage if you use the technique of identifying duplicate facts in options.

Identify Options That Deny Patient Feelings, Concerns, or Needs

Because nurses are human and caring, and primarily want their patients to get well, they often assume the role of champion, protector, or savior. However, by inappropriately adopting these roles, nurses often diminish patient concerns, provide false reassurance, and/or cut off further patient communication. To be a patient advocate, the nurse cannot always be a Pollyanna. Pollyanna, the heroine of stories by Eleanor Hodgman Porter, was a person of irrepressible optimism who found good in everything. Sometimes nurses must focus on the negative rather than the positive, acknowledge that everything may not have the desired outcome, and concentrate on patients' feelings as a priority. Options that imply everything will be all right deny patients' feelings, change the subject raised by the patient, encourage the patient to be cheerful, or transfer nursing responsibility to other members of the health-care team usually are distractors and can be eliminated from consideration.

SAMPLE ITEM 7-33

The day before surgery for a hysterectomy, a patient says to the nurse, "I am worried that I might die tomorrow." Which response by the nurse is therapeutic?

1. "It is really routine surgery."

2. "The thought of dying can be frightening."

3. "You need to tell your surgeon about this."

4. "Most people who have this surgery survive."

Options 1 and 4 minimize the patient's concern because these messages imply that there is nothing to worry about; the surgery is routine and most patients survive. In option 3 the nurse avoids the opportunity to encourage further discussion of the patient's feelings and surrenders this responsibility to the surgeon. After collecting more information, the nurse should inform the surgeon of the patient's concern about death. Options 1, 3, and 4 deny the patient's feelings and can be eliminated because they are distractors. Option 2 is the correct answer because it encourages the patient to focus on the expressed feelings about death.

SAMPLE ITEM 7-34

After surgery, a patient reports mild incisional pain while performing deep-breathing and coughing exercises. Which is the nurse's **best** response?

1. "Each day it will hurt less and less."
2. "This is an expected response after surgery."
3. "With a pillow, apply pressure against the incision."
4. "I will get the pain medication that was prescribed."

Option 1 is a Pollyanna-like response that may provide false reassurance. The nurse does not know that the pain will get less and less for this patient. Option 1 can be deleted from consideration. Although option 2 is a true statement, it cuts off communication because it diminishes the patient's concern and does not explore a solution for minimizing the pain. Option 2 can be eliminated as a distractor. You now must choose between options 3 and 4. The stem indicates that the patient has pain when coughing; the pain is not continuous. Option 4 can be deleted because it is inappropriate to administer an analgesic at this time. Mild pain should subside after the activity is completed. The correct answer is option 3 because it recognizes the mild pain and offers an intervention to help relieve the temporary discomfort. Each time you eliminate an option that denies a patient's feelings, you increase your chances of selecting the correct answer.

SAMPLE ITEM 7-35

An older woman with a right-sided hemiplegia and tears in her eyes sadly states, "I used to brush my hair 100 strokes a day and now I have to rely on others to do it." Which should be the initial response by the nurse?

1. "It's hard not being able to do things for yourself."
2. "With physical therapy you will be able to brush your own hair someday."
3. "Let me brush your hair 100 strokes, and then I'll help you with breakfast."
4. "That's true, but there are lots of other things you are capable of doing for yourself."

Option 2 is a Pollyanna-like response because it implies that everything will be all right eventually. Option 3 changes the subject and cuts off communication. Option 4 initially accepts the patient's statement but then attempts to refocus the patient on the positive. Options 2, 3, and 4 in one way or another deny the patient's feelings, concerns, and/or needs. The correct answer is option 1 because it is an open-ended statement that focuses on the patient's feelings.

Use Multiple Test-Taking Techniques

You have just been introduced to a variety of test-taking techniques. As you practice applying each of these techniques to test items, you will become more skillful at being test wise. As you become better at applying test-taking techniques, you can further maximize success in choosing the correct option if you use more than one test-taking technique within an item.

SAMPLE ITEM 7-36

A patient's plan of care indicates that active range-of-motion (AROM) exercises of the right leg are to be done every 4 hours while the patient is awake. Which should the nurse do?

1. Explain that all patients do AROM exercises by themselves.
2. Take the patient to physical therapy for the AROM exercises.
3. Move the patient's leg through AROM exercises as ordered.
4. Demonstrate for the patient how to perform AROM exercises.

Continued

Option 1 includes the specific determiner *all* and should be carefully evaluated. Some patients are able to perform AROM exercises themselves and others require assistance. Because some patients cannot totally perform AROM exercises independently, there are exceptions to the statement in option 1. This option can be deleted from consideration by using the technique *Identify Specific Determiners in Options.* Option 2 transfers the responsibility for care that the nurse is educated and licensed to provide. This option can be eliminated from consideration by using the technique *Identify Options That Deny Patient Feelings, Concerns, or Needs.* By using two test-taking techniques, you have eliminated options 1 and 2, reduced the number of options to two, and increased your chances of selecting the correct answer to 50%.

SAMPLE ITEM 7-37

Which patient responses are unexpected in response to the general adaptation syndrome?

1. Dilated pupils and bradycardia

2. Mental alertness and tachycardia

3. Increased blood glucose level and tachycardia

4. Decreased blood glucose level and bradycardia

By carefully reading the stem, you should identify that the word *unexpected* is a significant word in this item. You have just used the test-taking technique *Identify the Word in the Stem That Indicates Negative Polarity.* If you know that tachycardia is associated with the general adaptation syndrome, you can eliminate options 2 and 3. This reasoning uses the test-taking technique *Identify Duplicate Facts Among Options.* If you identify that options 3 and 4 are opposites, you should give these options particular consideration. By seriously considering these options, you are using the test-taking technique *Identify Opposites in Options.* A variety of test-taking techniques can be applied to analyze and answer this item.

SAMPLE ITEM 7-38

Which patient need is being met when the nurse administers a back rub to reduce the physical discomfort of a backache?

1. Safety

2. Security

3. Self-esteem

4. Physiological

By thoughtfully reading the stem, you should identify that the important words are "reduce the physical discomfort of a backache." When reviewing the options, you should recognize that the word "physiological" in option 4 is closely related to the word "physical" in the stem. Option 4 should be given serious consideration. This reasoning uses the test-taking technique *Identify Key Words in the Stem That Direct Attention to Content.* Options 1 and 2 present the words "safety" and "security." They are comparable, and choosing between them is difficult. They are distractors. This reasoning uses the test-taking technique *Identify Equally Plausible Options.* Options 1, 2, and 3 all begin with the letter "S" whereas option 4 begins with the letter "P." Option 4 is different from the others and should be considered carefully because it may be the correct answer. You have just used the test-taking technique *Identify the Unique Option.* The use of multiple test-taking techniques in considering an item can facilitate the deletion of distractors and the selection of the correct answer.

GENERAL TEST-TAKING TECHNIQUES

A general test-taking technique is a strategy that is used to conquer the challenge of an examination. To be in command of the situation, you must be able to manage your internal and external domains. The test taker who approaches a test with physical, mental, and emotional authority is in a position to regulate the testing situation, rather than to have the testing situation dominate.

Follow Your Regular Routine the Night Before a Test

Follow your usual routine the night before a test. This is not the time to make changes that may disrupt your balance. If you do not normally eat pepperoni pizza, exercise, or study until 2 a.m., do not start now. Go to bed at your usual time. Avoid the temptation to have an all-night cram session. Studies have demonstrated that sleep deprivation decreases reaction times and cognitive skills. An adequate night's sleep is necessary to produce a rested mind and body that provide the physical and emotional energy required to maximize performance on an examination.

Arrive Early for the Examination

Plan your schedule so that you arrive at the testing site 15 to 30 minutes early. Arrange extra time for unexpected events associated with traveling. There may be a traffic jam, a road may have a detour, the car may not start, the train may be late, the bus may break down, or you may have to park in the farthest lot from the testing site. If the location of the testing site or classroom is unfamiliar to you, it is wise to take a practice run at the same time of day of the scheduled test and locate the room. On the day of the examination, this should help you avoid getting lost or being late.

By arriving early, you have an opportunity to visit the rest room, survey the environment, and collect your thoughts. Because anxiety is associated with an autonomic nervous system response, you may have urgency, frequency, or increased intestinal peristalsis. Visit the rest room before the test to avoid using testing time to meet physical needs. The test may or may not be administered in the room in which the content is taught. Arriving early allows you to become more comfortable in the testing environment. Decide where you want to sit if seats are not assigned. Students have preferences such as sitting by a window, being in the back of the room, or surrounding themselves with friends. Selecting your own seat allows you to manipulate one aspect of your environment. In addition, this time before the test provides you with an opportunity to collect your thoughts. You may desire to review content on a flash card, perform relaxation exercises, or reinforce your positive mental attitude. However, avoid comparing notes with other students. They may have inaccurate information or be anxious. Remember, anxiety is contagious. If you are the type who is affected by the anxiety of other people, avoid these people until after the test.

Bring the Appropriate Tools

To perform a task, you need adequate tools. A pen may be required to complete the identifying information on a form or answer sheet. A pencil usually is necessary to record your answers on the answer sheet if it is a paper and pencil test that uses a computer answer form. Use number 2 pencils because they have soft lead that facilitates the computer scoring of the answer sheet. Bring at least two pens and two or more pencils. Backup equipment is advisable because ink can run out and points can break. Have at least one eraser. You may decide to change an answer or need to erase extraneous marks that you make on the question book or the answer sheet. A watch also is a necessary tool if permitted when a clock is not available in the room. Depending on your individual needs, other tools might include eyeglasses or a hearing aid. If you are taking the test using a computer students often are not permitted to bring anything into the testing environment. All electronic devices including watches and calculators must be left outside the room. A clock and calculator may be accessed on the computer when desired. Assemble all your equipment the night before the test, and be sure to take them with you to the testing site.

Understand All the Directions for the Test Before Starting

It is essential to understand the instructions before beginning the test. On some tests you are responsible for independently reading the instructions, whereas on others the proctor verbally announces the instructions. However, more often than not you will have a written copy of the instructions while the proctor reads them aloud. In this instance, do not read ahead of the proctor. The proctor may elaborate on the written instructions, and you do not want to miss any additional directions. If you do not understand a particular part of the instructions, immediately request that the proctor explain them again. You must completely understand the instructions before beginning the examination.

Manage the Allotted Time to Your Advantage

All tests have a time limit. Some tests have severe time restrictions in which most test takers do not complete all the questions on the examination. These are known as "speed tests." Other tests have a generous time frame in which the majority of test takers have ample time to answer every question on the examination. These are known as "power tests." The purpose of tests in nursing is to identify how much information the test taker possesses about the nursing care of people. Most nursing examinations are power tests. Regardless of the type of test, you must use your time well.

To manage your time on an examination, you must determine how much time you have to answer each item, leaving some time for review at the end of the testing period if permitted. To figure out how much time you should allot for each item, divide the total time you have for the test by the number of items on the test. For example, if you have 90 minutes to take a test that has 50 items, divide 90 by 50. This allots 1 minute and 48 seconds for each item. If you actually allot 1½ minutes per item, you will leave 15 minutes for a final review. Be aware of the time as you progress through a test. If you determine that you have approximately 1½ minutes for each question, by the time you have completed 10 items, 15 minutes should have passed. Pace yourself so that you do not spend more than 1½ minutes on an item if possible. If you answer an item in less than 1½ minutes, you can use the extra time for another item that may take slightly longer than 1½ minutes or add this time to the end for review. The allocation of time for test completion depends on the complexity of the content, the difficulty of the reading level, and the number of options presented in the items.

Read each item slowly and carefully including all the options presented. It may be necessary to read the question twice. If you process items too quickly, you may overlook important words, become careless, or arrive at impulsive conclusions. If you find that you are spending too much time, you may want to immediately eliminate obvious distractors and not belabor them. Then only work with the remaining viable options. In addition, you want to avoid getting bogged down on a difficult question because you can lose valuable time, become flustered, and lose focus and concentration when upset. Clearly indicate the question so that you can return to it later if permitted. Move on; this puts you back in control! Some computerized tests do not allow you to review past items. In this situation a question must be answered before the next question is presented. Answer the question to the best of you ability and then move on. Work at your own pace. Do not be influenced by the actions of other test takers. If other test takers complete the examination early, ignore them and do not become concerned. Just because they finish early does not indicate that they will score well on the test. They may be imprudent speed demons. A cautious, discriminating, and judicious approach is to your advantage. Be your own person and remember that time can be your friend rather than your enemy.

Time allocation varies for tests taken on a computer. See Chapter 9, Computer Applications in Education and Evaluation, for more information.

Concentrate on the Simple Before the Complex

Answer the easy questions before the difficult questions. This uses the basic teaching/learning principle of moving from the simple to the complex. By doing this, you can maximize your use of time and maintain a positive mental attitude. Begin answering questions. When you are confronted with a difficult item, have already used your allotted time to answer it, and still do not know the answer, then skip over this item and move on to the next one. Make a notation on scrap paper, next to the item in the question booklet, next to the number of the skipped item on the answer sheet or in the appropriate location on a computer administered examination so that you can return to this item later in the test if permitted. When you reach the end of the test, return to those items that you saved for the end. You should have time to spend on these items, and you may have accessed information from other items that can assist you in answering these questions. Concentrating on the simple before the complex permits you to answer the maximum number of items in the time allocated for the examination.

On computer-administered examinations this strategy may not be applicable. You may be required to enter an answer before the next item will appear on the screen.

Avoid Reading Into the Question

A nursing question has two parts. The first part is known as the stem. The stem is the statement that asks a question. The second part contains the possible responses, which are called options. The stem of a question also has two parts. One part presents information about a clinical event, topic, concept, or theory. The other part asks you to respond in some way. The response part asks you to choose the best option that answers the question based on the information presented in the stem. The information presented in the stem needs to be separated in your mind from the response part of the stem. In some questions the information and response parts of the question are very clear. Other questions are presented in a manner that is less clear about which is the information part and which is the response part.

The following questions illustrate the difference between the information and the response parts of the stem. In each example, the information part of the stem is boldfaced and the response part is italicized.

While walking, a patient becomes weak and the patient's knees begin to buckle. *What should the nurse do?*

Which is an example of **a patient goal?**

Before administering medication for pain, *what should the nurse do first?*

Questions generally are designed to test common principles and concepts. Therefore it is important that you avoid overanalyzing the facts in the question. In an attempt to achieve this goal, consider the following suggestions.

When reading the stem:

- Identify the important words.
- Do not add information from your own mind.
- Do not make assumptions (read between the lines) about the information presented in the stem.

When reading the options:

- Read all the options before choosing the correct answer.
- Refer back only to the words that you identified as being important in the stem.
- Do not add information to an option.

- Relate an option to just what is being asked in the response part of the stem.
- Focus on commonalities, principles, and concepts associated with your level of learning that is being tested.
- Do not focus only on your experiences, which may be too narrow for a point of reference.
- Recognize that an option can contain correct information but it may or may not have anything to do with the information and response parts of the stem.

When reading options, it is important that you read all the options before selecting the correct answer. This may sound like a ridiculous suggestion; however, we found that students often selected options 1, 2, or 3 over option 4. We tested this theory by placing the correct answer as option 1 and then placing it as option 4 on a different examination. When the correct answer was 4 instead of 1, fewer students selected the correct option. When we asked students who got the question wrong when the correct answer was option 4, did they examine option 4, the students admitted that they did not read all the options.

Most students find it helpful when they can separate the information part of the question from the response part of the question. By incorporating these suggestions, you should have a better ability to identify what information is in the scenario and what you are being asked to do. As a result, your chances of answering the question correctly, without reading into the question, should increase.

Make Educated Guesses

An educated guess is the selection of an option based on partial knowledge, without knowing for certain that it is the correct answer. When you have reduced the final selection to two options, usually it is to your advantage to reassess these options in the context of the knowledge you do possess and make an educated guess. Making a wild guess by flipping a coin or choosing your favorite number should depend on whether the test has a penalty for guessing.

Some examinations assign credit when you answer a question correctly and do not assign credit when you answer a question incorrectly. The directions for these examinations may state that only correct answers will receive credit, that you should answer every question, that you should not leave any blanks, or that there are no penalties for guessing. In these tests it is to your advantage to answer every question. First, select answers based on knowledge. If you are unsure of the correct answer, reduce the number of options and then make an educated guess. If you have absolutely no idea what the answer can be, then make a wild guess because you will not be penalized for a wrong answer.

Some tests assign credit when you answer a question correctly and subtract credit when you answer a question incorrectly. The instructions for these examinations may inform you not to guess, that credit will be subtracted for incorrect answers, or that there is a penalty for guessing. In these tests a statistical manipulation is performed to mathematically limit the advantage of guessing. When taking these tests, it is still to your advantage to make an educated guess if through knowledge you can reduce your final selection to two options. However, wild guessing is not to your advantage because your chance of selecting the correct answer is only 25%.

Maintain a Positive Mental Attitude

It is important that you foster a positive mental attitude and a sense of relaxation. A little apprehension can be motivating, but too much can interfere with your attention, concentration, and problem-solving ability. Use the positive techniques you have practiced and that work for you to enhance relaxation and a positive mental attitude. For example, feel in control by skipping the difficult questions; enhance relaxation by employing diaphragmatic breathing for several deep breaths, rotating your shoulders, or flexing and extending your head; foster a positive mental attitude by telling yourself, "I am prepared to do this well!" or "I know I have studied hard and I will be successful!"

Check Your Answers and Answer Sheet

It is important to record your answers accurately, particularly when using a computer scoring sheet. Paper and pencil computer-scored tests usually use separate answer sheets in which each item has numbers or letters that represent the corresponding responses to each item in the test. You do not want to lose points because you placed your answer in the wrong row. You need to verify the number of the question with the number on the answer sheet at least two times when recording your answer. You should conscientiously do this every time you record an answer.

At the end of the examination, again review your answer sheet for accuracy. Make sure that every mark is within the lines, heavy and full, and in the appropriate space. Erase any extraneous marks on the answer sheet. Additional pencil marks, inadequately erased answers, and marks outside the lines will confuse the computer and alter your score. Also, make sure that you have answered every question, especially on tests that do not penalize for guessing. An effective and thorough review should leave you with a feeling of control and a sense of closure at the end of the examination.

If you take an examination on a computer you may be able to select or change an answer before submitting your final choice. Double-check your selected response before hitting the key that finalizes your answer.

7-1 1. **Linens cannot be returned to a linen storage area once they are removed because they are exposed to microorganisms in the hallways and/or patient rooms.**
2. Used linens may be contaminated with body secretions; wearing gloves is part of standard precautions.
3. Tucking clean linen against the frame of the bed is an acceptable practice; the entire bed is washed with a disinfectant between patients.
4. Reusing a top sheet for the bottom sheet is an acceptable practice if the sheet is not wet or soiled.

7-2 1. Stewed fruit is low in sodium.
2. **Luncheon meats generally are processed with large amounts of sodium.**
3. Whole-grain cereal is low in sodium.
4. Green, leafy vegetables are low in sodium.

7-3 1. **Applying pressure over the vertebrae should be avoided because it can cause unnecessary pressure over bony prominences; back rub strokes should massage muscle groups, not vertebrae.**
2. Using continuous, firm strokes is soothing and relieves muscle tension; this action is based on the gate-control theory of pain relief.
3. Excess lotion can be an irritant to the skin and should be removed.
4. Kneading the skin increases circulation and should be part of a back rub unless contraindicated.

7-4 1. Collecting equipment is not done first because each type of enema has different equipment requirements.
2. **The order should be verified first. It is essential that the specific type of enema ordered be given; enemas have different solutions, volumes, and purposes.**
3. Informing the patient about the procedure is not done first because the nurse's explanation depends on the type of enema being administered.
4. Arranging for an empty bathroom should be done after the equipment and patient are prepared and ready.

7-5 1. This statement is a demeaning response and does not answer the patient's question.
2. This statement denies the patient's concern and does not answer the question.
3. Not responding may make the patient more upset; the patient has a right to know who is providing care.
4. **This statement answers the question, which meets the patient's right to know; also, it is a respectful response.**

7-6 1. The patient should be turned and positioned every 1 to 2 hours to help expose the cast to air, which facilitates even drying of the cast. Also, frequent changes of position will help minimize venous stasis, which may contribute to deep vein thrombosis, as well as relieve pressure, which can contribute to skin breakdown.
2. Distal, not proximal, pulses should be taken to ensure that circulation is not compromised by the pressure of the cast.
3. Although it is important to cover rough edges of the cast with tape, these interventions are not the priority.
4. **Bleeding may occur with a compound fracture. Drawing a ring around the drainage on the cast and adding the date, time, and initials helps to establish the degree of bleeding or discharge over time.**

7-7 1. **Maintaining functional alignment supports a basic physiological need; this reduces physical strain and potential injury to joints, muscles, ligaments, and tendons and can prevent the formation of contractures.**
2. Pulling the curtain supports the patient's need for self-esteem; it provides privacy.
3. Responding to the call light immediately supports the patient's need for security and safety; patients should know that help is available immediately when needed.
4. Raising both side rails on the bed supports the patient's need for safety and security; bed rails prevent a patient from falling out of bed.

7-8 1. **Self-care encourages a patient's independence, which increases self-esteem.**

2. Family member visits generally meet the patient's need for love and belonging, not self-esteem.
3. When a person is dependent on another, such dependency often lowers self-esteem.
4. Providing a complete bath promotes dependency; the patient should be as independent as possible.

7-9 1. Pulling a curtain when providing care supports the patient's self-esteem needs.
2. Answering a call bell immediately meets the patient's safety needs.
3. **Administering hygiene meets a patient's basic physiological need to be clean.**
4. Vital signs are not a physiological need of the patient. They are an assessment done by the nurse to determine the patient's needs.

7-10 1. **This response directly involves the patient and invites the patient to relive a past vacation.**
2. This response focuses on the nurse rather than the patient.
3. This response focuses on the nurse's vacation rather than focusing on the patient.
4. This question by the nurse asks for an opinion, which can be answered with a short response.

7-11 1. Speaking with the husband might be done later. It is not the initial action.
2. Eventually the husband also will need support after the patient's needs are met first. This intervention avoids the husband's needs.
3. **The fact that the patient raised the issues about her husband indicates that she is concerned about his behavior. Her feelings need to be explored and her self-esteem supported.**
4. Making an appointment with Reach to Recovery is not the initial intervention. This may be done eventually after the patient's initial needs are met.

7-12 1. **Exploring the situation provides the daughter with an opportunity to verbalize her feelings with regard to her mother's behavior. All behavior has meaning, and talking about the situation may provide insight. Eventually, the situation should be explored with the patient and the daughter together.**

2. Encouraging the patient to be more positive denies the patient's feelings and ignores the daughter's feelings; both cut off communication.
3. This information may further upset the daughter and may precipitate feelings such as guilt or anger.
4. The nurse has a responsibility to intervene.

7-13 1. **This statement focuses on the patient's feelings by the use of reflection.**
2. This statement denies the patient's feelings.
3. This statement is an assumption and offers false reassurance.
4. The nurse cannot predict that the patient will feel better. This response offers false reassurance.

7-14 1. Although this may eventually be done, it does not promote independence; also, it may violate the patient's privacy if the patient's questions are personal.
2. Reminding the patient of the primary health-care provider's next visit does not address the patient's concern; the patient forgets the questions to be asked, not when the primary health-care provider will visit.
3. **Providing a paper and pen to write down questions promotes independence, self-esteem, and privacy.**
4. This may foster feelings of dependence and may violate the patient's privacy if the questions to be asked are personal.

7-15 1. Moistening the hair may be done after obtaining the patient's permission.
2. Applying a hair conditioner may be done if desired by the patient. A procedure should be explained and the patient's consent obtained before beginning a procedure.
3. Initially short strokes, beginning at the ends and progressively moving toward the roots as tangles are removed, should be used to comb/brush the hair.
4. **Seeking preferences promotes individualized care by allowing personal choices.**

7-16 1. This intervention is not patient centered. This intervention focuses on the nurse's perspective, not the patient's perspective.
2. Although this may eventually be done if desired by the patient, it is not the primary intervention.
3. **This intervention is patient centered. Asking the patient to share more encourages verbalization of feelings.**

4. The nurse may eventually do this if the patient expresses an interest in reading a book about cats.

7-17 1. **Pressure and friction produce local heat, which dilates blood vessels, improving circulation.**
2. Hot water can damage delicate tissue and should be avoided; bath water should be between 110°F and 115°F.
3. Keeping the patient covered prevents chilling.
4. Soap lowers the surface tension of water, which promotes cleaning.

7-18 1. Hand hygiene before care protects the patient from the nurse.
2. The nurse is still exposed to body secretions if not wearing gloves when discarding contaminated water.
3. **Gloves are a barrier against body secretions and are used with standard precautions.**
4. Expecting patients to provide all of their own care is unreasonable and inappropriate; some patients require assistance with meeting their needs.

7-19 1. Straps and a mask that are firm against the skin can cause tissue trauma.
2. Changing the method of oxygen delivery requires a primary health-care provider's order.
3. Padding the straps with gauze without adjusting the straps will make the mask tighter against the face.
4. **Loosening the elastic straps will reduce the pressure of the mask against the face; the elastic straps can be adjusted for comfort while keeping the edges of the mask gently against the skin.**

7-20 1. Aging is progressive and does not move backward.
2. **Aging, from conception to death, advances and moves onward.**
3. Although this may be true for some older adults, it is not true for all.
4. Although this may be true for some older adults, it should not be generalized to the entire population of older adults.

7-21 1. **Dependent edema is minimal while the feet are still elevated; anti-embolism stockings should be applied before the legs are moved to a dependent position.**
2. The purpose of anti-embolism stockings is to promote venous return, not reduce pain.
3. This will cause tissue trauma because of the presence of fluid in the interstitial compartment; anti-embolism stockings are applied to prevent, not treat, edema.
4. Fluid will accumulate in an extremity when dependent in patients with peripheral vascular disease or congestive heart failure. The application of anti-embolism stockings when there is fluid in the interstitial compartment will cause tissue trauma.

7-22 1. Side rails do not provide a stable base of support. Injury can occur if the rails are lowered before the straps are removed.
2. Tying a restraint to the footboard requires an excessively long strap in which the patient's legs may get entangled.
3. **The bed frame is a stable base of support and is beyond the patient's reach.**
4. Tying a restraint to the headboard may result in an uncomfortable line of pull with the arm above the head.

7-23 1. A solution is hypertonic when the electrolyte content is more than the electrolyte content of body fluid.
2. A solution is hypotonic when the electrolyte content is less than the electrolyte content of body fluid.
3. Acidotic refers to excessive levels of hydrogen ions in the blood affecting pH values. This term is not related to intravenous fluids.
4. **A solution is isotonic when the electrolyte content is approximately equal to the electrolyte content of body fluids. Normal saline (0.9% sodium chloride) is isotonic.**

7-24 1. Serving adequate food meets basic physiological needs, not safety and security needs.
2. Providing sufficient fluid meets basic physiological needs, not safety and security needs.
3. **Being able to summon help when needed provides a sense of security and physical safety for the patient.**
4. The bedside table is not a secure place to store valuables.

7-25 1. Placing the patient in the prone position exposes the entire area to permit a thorough back rub; it does not promote circulation.

2. Moisturizing creams hold moisture within the skin, making it more supple; they do not promote circulation.

3. Keri lotion is a moisturizing lotion that helps make skin more supple. Keri lotion does not promote circulation,

4. Kneading causes friction and pressure against the skin that promotes localized heat, which precipitates vessel dilation, improving circulation.

7-26 1. Active range-of-motion (AROM), not passive range-of-motion (PROM), exercises can increase endurance.

2. PROM exercises prevent shortening of muscles, ligaments, and tendons, which causes joints to become fixed in one position, limiting mobility.

3. Active, not passive, range-of-motion exercises can strengthen muscle tone.

4. Maximizing muscle atrophy will never be a patient goal. Atrophy is the loss of muscle mass because of lack of muscle contraction. AROM exercises will minimize, not maximize, muscle atrophy.

7-27 1. Shutting the door provides privacy and prevents drafts, but it may contaminate the nurse's hands.

2. Between patients and before and after providing care the nurse must wash the hands to remove dirt and microorganisms; otherwise, equipment and the patient will be affected by cross-contamination. Medical asepsis is a priority. Hand washing is also known as hand hygiene.

3. Closing the curtain should occur before washing the hands; curtains are considered contaminated.

4. Draping the patient provides for privacy and prevents chilling, but if the nurse's hands are not clean they will contaminate the linen and the patient.

7-28 1. Antibiotics are administered to treat patients with infections, not all sick patients.

2. This is a broad statement that incorporates under its mantle many different actions that may be implemented to prevent the spread of microorganisms.

3. Isolating a resident is not necessary unless the resident has a communicable disease; implementing standard precautions is sufficient.

4. Keeping all unit doors closed is unnecessary; this action is not part of standard precautions. Closing the door is part of airborne precautions.

7-29 1. This is not required for all positions. The arms are supported when a patient is placed in a lateral or a Sims position.

2. Functional alignment refers to maintaining the body in an anatomical position that supports physical functioning, minimizes strain and stress on muscles, tendons, ligaments, and joints, and prevents contractures.

3. This is not required for all positions. External rotation of the hips is prevented when a patient is in the supine (dorsal recumbent) position.

4. This is not required for all positions. A pillow is placed under the lumbar curvature when a patient is in the low-Fowler or supine (dorsal recumbent) positions.

7-30 1. Both actions may injure the patient. The patient may fall out of bed on the side opposite the nurse, and moving a restrained patient exerts stress on the patient's musculoskeletal system.

2. Although one side rail can be lowered, moving a restrained patient may injure the patient.

3. Although the vest restraint can be untied while the nurse is at the bedside, lowering the rail on the side opposite to which the nurse is working may result in the patient falling out of bed.

4. Untying a restraint permits free movement, which limits stress on the patient's musculoskeletal system. Lowering one side rail allows the nurse to provide direct care. Keeping the side rail raised on the side opposite to which the nurse is working provides a barrier to prevent the patient from falling out of bed.

7-31 **1. These foods—fruits, vegetables, and bread—contain the least amount of sodium compared with the foods listed in the other options.**

2. Hot dogs, mustard, and pickles all contain a high level of sodium and should be avoided.

3. Ketchup is high in sodium and should be avoided.

4. Luncheon meats are processed foods that contain a high level of sodium and should be avoided.

7-32 1. With hemorrhage, the patient's skin will be cold and clammy, not warm and dry, and the pulse will be weak and thready, not bounding. Hypotension is associated with hemorrhage because of hypovolemia.

2. Because of the reduced blood volume associated with hemorrhage, the patient's blood pressure will decrease, not increase, and the pulse will be weak and thready, not bounding. Cold, clammy skin is associated with hemorrhage because of peripheral vasoconstriction.

3. With hemorrhage, the patient's blood pressure will decrease, not increase, and the skin will be cold and clammy, not warm and dry. A weak, thready pulse is associated with hemorrhage because of hypovolemia.

4. Because of the decreased blood volume associated with hemorrhage, the blood pressure will be reduced and the pulse will be weak and thready; because of the autonomic nervous system response and the constriction of peripheral blood vessels, the patient's skin will be cold and clammy.

7-33 1. This statement denies the patient's feelings about death and cuts off further communication.

2. This statement uses reflective technique because it focuses on the underlying feeling expressed in the patient's statement.

3. This statement abdicates the responsibility of the nurse (to explore the patient's feelings) to the surgeon; it cuts off communication and does not meet the patient's immediate need to discuss fears of death; eventually the surgeon should be notified of the patient's feelings.

4. This statement minimizes the patient's concern about dying; it cuts off communication.

7-34 1. Although this is true for most patients, it may not be true for this patient. This is a Pollyanna-like response that may provide false reassurance.

2. Although this is a true statement, it cuts off communication and does not present an intervention to help limit the patient's present discomfort.

3. This response recognizes the mild pain and offers the patient an intervention to help limit the temporary discomfort.

4. This response is inappropriate at this time. If more than mild pain is expected, analgesics should be administered before pain-inducing activities.

7-35 **1. This response identifies the patient's concern and offers an opportunity to further discuss the topic.**

2. This is a Pollyanna-like response that provides false reassurance; the patient may never be able to brush her own hair.

3. This response offers a solution before allowing the patient to discuss concerns, thereby cutting off communication.

4. After the patient's present feelings are explored, then pointing out the patient's abilities is appropriate.

7-36 1. Some patients are not capable of performing AROM exercises, depending on the strength of the affected and unaffected extremities and their physical, mental, and/or emotional status.

2. Taking the patient to physical therapy every 4 hours is unrealistic and transfers the nurse's responsibility to another member of the health team.

3. AROM exercises should be performed by the patient. Passive range-of-motion exercises should be performed by a nurse.

4. Assisting patients with mobility issues is within the scope of nursing practice.

7-37 1. Tachycardia, not bradycardia, is associated with the general adaptation syndrome; dilated pupils are expected.

2. Both mental alertness and tachycardia are expected autonomic nervous system responses that occur during the alarm stage of the general adaptation syndrome. These are part of the "fight or flight" mechanism.

3. Both increased blood glucose level and tachycardia are expected autonomic nervous system responses that occur during the alarm stage of the general adaptation syndrome. These are part of the "fight or flight" mechanism.

4. During the alarm stage of the general adaptation syndrome, both the blood glucose level and heart rate of the patient increase not decrease.

7-38 1. Safety and security needs, the second level of needs according to Maslow, are met when the patient is protected from harm.
2. Security needs are related to safety needs, the second level of needs according to Maslow. A patient will feel protected and safe when safety and security needs are met.

3. Self-esteem needs, a third-level need, are met when the patient is treated with dignity and respect.
4. **Being free from pain or discomfort is a basic physiological need; a back rub improves local circulation, reduces muscle tension, and limits pain.**

Testing Formats Other Than Multiple-Choice Questions

Teachers make many decisions that influence students. Some are instructional decisions. What teaching strategies should be used to teach certain content? Some decisions are curricular decisions. What information should be included in a unit of instruction? The decisions teachers make that produce the most anxiety for most students are the measurement and evaluation decisions. What does the student know? What can the student do? To make these decisions, teachers use tests to appraise progress toward curricular goals, assess mastery of a skill, and evaluate knowledge of what was learned in a course. Three factors are involved in making measurement and evaluation decisions.

1. **What knowledge or ability is to be measured?**
   Generally, that which is most important or relevant is measured. Examples include the expected range of vital signs in an adult, the principles of patient teaching, legal and ethical implications of health-care delivery, and patient safety. You usually can identify what is most significant by the emphasis placed on the material. Content in a textbook that is highlighted, boldfaced, capitalized, or repeated several times usually is important. Information that appears in the textbook and is incorporated into the teacher's classroom instruction also is significant. Concepts that are introduced in the classroom setting and then applied in a classroom laboratory or clinical setting are critical concepts. You often can predict the content that will be on a test and therefore use your study time more efficiently.

2. **How can the identified knowledge or ability be measured?**
   A set of operations must be devised to isolate and display the knowledge or ability that is to be measured. Examples include multiple-choice questions, true-false questions, completion items, matching columns, extended essay questions, and the performance of a procedure. To feel in control when taking tests, you should be familiar with the various testing formats. Dealing with a particular test format is a skill, and to develop a skill you must practice. Student workbooks that accompany required textbooks, questions at the end of chapters, and books devoted to testing usually contain numerous questions. Practice answering these questions. Experience promotes learning and practice makes perfect!

3. **How can the results of the devised operations be measured or expressed in quantitative terms?**
   In other words, the unit of measure that indicates a passing grade or an acceptable performance must be identified by the instructor. Examples of acceptable results include a grade within 10% of the average grade in the class, a grade of 80%, or the correct performance of previously identified steps (critical elements) of a procedure. When taking tests, you should be aware of the criteria for scoring the test. You should ask the following questions: What is the passing grade? How many points are allocated to each question? Can partial credit be received for an answer? Is there a penalty for guessing? What are the critical steps that must be performed for each skill to pass the test? Answers to these and other questions can help you make decisions such as how much time to devote to certain questions or whether to guess at an answer.

In previous chapters, the multiple-choice question was discussed in detail. In this chapter, testing formats other than multiple-choice questions are presented. Test questions can be classified as structured-response questions, restricted-response questions, extended essay questions, or performance appraisals.

A **structured-response question** requires you to select the correct answer from among available alternatives. Multiple-choice, multiple-response, true-false, and matching items are examples of structured-response questions.

A **restricted-response question** requires you to write a short answer. The response is expected to be a word, phrase, sentence, or product of a mathematical calculation. Short-answer, completion, and fill-in-the-blank items are examples of restricted-response questions.

An **extended essay question** requires you to generate the answer, via a free-response format, in reply to a question or problem that is presented.

A **performance appraisal** presents a structured situation and requires you to demonstrate part or all of a skill.

The answers and rationales for all the sample items in this chapter are at the end of the chapter. Test-taking tips do not always apply to alternate-item questions. When applicable, test-taking tips will be presented and discussed.

STRUCTURED-RESPONSE QUESTIONS

A structured-response item is one that asks a question and requires you to select an answer from among the options presented. These items include multiple-choice, multiple-response, true-false, and matching questions. These formats usually are efficient, dependable, and objective. Because multiple-choice questions are discussed in Chapter 5, only multiple-response, true-false, and matching questions are presented here.

Multiple-Response Questions

A multiple-response question is a variation of a regular multiple-choice question. A regular multiple-choice question asks a question and then provides three or four potential answers. The test taker must select the one correct answer from among the presented potential answers. A multiple-response question is similar in that it presents a question and potential answers. However, it varies in that it requires the test taker to identify two or more correct answers from among numerous potential answers (usually five or six).

TEST-TAKING TIPS: See Multiple Response Items under Alternate Question Formats Reflective of NCLEX on page 143 for Test-Taking Tips.

SAMPLE ITEM 8-1
When assessing a stage III pressure ulcer, the nurse identifies the extent of tissue damage. **Select all that apply.**

1. _____ Undermining of adjoining tissue

2. _____ Limited to partial-thickness loss

3. _____ Damage to subcutaneous tissue

4. _____ Extension through the fascia

5. _____ Damage to muscle

SAMPLE ITEM 8-2
Which actions must be implemented to meet the criteria of Transmission-Based Precautions to reduce the spread of infection when the nurse is caring for a patient with primary pulmonary tuberculosis? **Select all that apply.**

1. _____ Donning a gown when entering the room

2. _____ Putting on gloves when delivering a food tray

3. _____ Placing a mask on the patient during transport

Continued

> 4. _____ Admitting the patient to a private room that has negative air pressure
> 5. _____ Wearing a respiratory device when entering the room (N95 respirator)
> 6. _____ Keeping the door to the room closed except when entering or leaving

True-False Questions

In a true-false question a statement is presented, and only two options are given from which to select an answer. True-false questions frequently are used to test knowledge of facts because the response must be absolutely true or false. It can be a demanding format because no frame of reference is provided. The question usually is constructed out of context, and the truth or falsity of the statement can be difficult to evaluate. However, true-false questions can work to your benefit because you have a 50% chance of getting the answer right. If you do not know the answer and there is no penalty for guessing, make an educated guess. Never leave a blank answer if there is no penalty for guessing. Follow the instructions for selecting the correct answer; for example, you may be told to circle your answer or instructed to place an X on a line next to your answer.

> **SAMPLE ITEM 8-3**
> When providing a bed bath, the nurse understands that soap helps in cleaning because it decreases the surface tension of water. Place an X on the line that indicates your answer.
>
> True _____   False _____

> **SAMPLE ITEM 8-4**
> A nurse should assume a broad stance when transferring a patient from the bed to a wheelchair. Circle your answer.
>
> True   False

> **SAMPLE ITEM 8-5**
> The nurse should teach a patient experiencing insomnia that exercising just before going to bed promotes sleep. Place an X on the line that indicates your answer.
>
> True _____   False _____

> **SAMPLE ITEM 8-6**
> When obtaining a patient's vital signs the nurse understands that pulse pressure is the difference between the apical and radial pulse rates. Circle your answer.
>
> True   False

Variations of true-false items have been developed to simplify and clarify what is being asked. These questions may also obtain more information about what you know and limit guessing. **Highlighting a word or phrase in the question** (by CAPITALIZING it or by using **bold type**, *italics*, or <u>underlining</u>) is a simple variation that helps to reduce ambiguity and increase precision. You can also use this technique when answering true-false questions in which certain words are not highlighted. Underline key words, as well as words that modify key words, to focus your attention on the most important part of the statement.

SAMPLE ITEM 8-7
Palpation is the examination of the body using the sense of **touch.** Place an X on the line that indicates your answer.

True _____   False _____

SAMPLE ITEM 8-8
The process in which solid, particulate matter in a fluid moves from an area of increased concentration to an area of decreased concentration is known as <u>osmosis</u>. Circle your answer.

True   False

Grouping short true-false items under a common question, another variation of the true-false question, attempts to arrange affiliated information together. It is an effective approach to assess knowledge about related categories, classifications, or characteristics. Each statement that is being evaluated must be considered in relation to the original question. This variation reduces the amount of reading and provides a greater frame of reference for evaluating each statement. This type of question increases specificity and clarity.

SAMPLE ITEM 8-9
Indicate if the following choices are true or false in relation to the introductory statement. Place an X on the lines that indicate your answers.
   Surgical asepsis is maintained when the nurse:
1. Removes the drape from a sterile package by touching the outer 1 inch with ungloved hands.

   True _____ False _____
2. Dons the first sterile glove by touching just the inside of the glove.

   True _____ False _____
3. Keeps hands below the elbows during a surgical hand scrub.

   True _____ False _____
4. Holds a sterile object below waist level.

   True _____ False _____

SAMPLE ITEM 8-10
Signify whether or not each procedure employs the principle of positive pressure. Circle your answers.
1. Mechanical ventilation

   True   False
2. Continuous bladder irrigation

   True   False
3. Chest tubes (chest drainage system)

   True   False
4. Instillation of fluid into a nasogastric tube with a piston syringe

   True   False

Requiring the test taker to correct false statements is another variation of the true-false question. With this type of question, you are instructed to rewrite the question whenever you determine that the statement is false. This approach guarantees that you understand the information underlying a false statement. It also decreases guessing because you will receive credit only if able to revise the question to make it a correct statement. This variation is sometimes combined with the true-false variation that highlights a word or phrase in the original question.

SAMPLE ITEM 8-11

Mark your answer with an X in the space provided. If you identify the statement as false, revise the statement so that it is accurate.

The expected range of the heart rate for an adult is 70 to 110 beats per minute.

True _____ False _____

Correction _____

SAMPLE ITEM 8-12

Indicate with an X if the statement is true or false. Correct the underlined words if the statement is false.

According to Erikson's developmental theory, the central task of <u>young adulthood</u> is identity versus role confusion.

True _____ False _____

Correction _____

True-false items can be asked in relation to specific stimulus material included with the question. This variation of the true-false question provides a frame of reference for the specific questions being asked within the item. Examples of stimulus material include a graph, map, chart, table, or picture. Memorization of information generally is not sufficient for answering these types of questions because they test more than the recall or regurgitation of facts. These questions test comprehension, interpretation, application, and reasoning, which are higher levels of cognitive ability.

SAMPLE ITEM 8-13

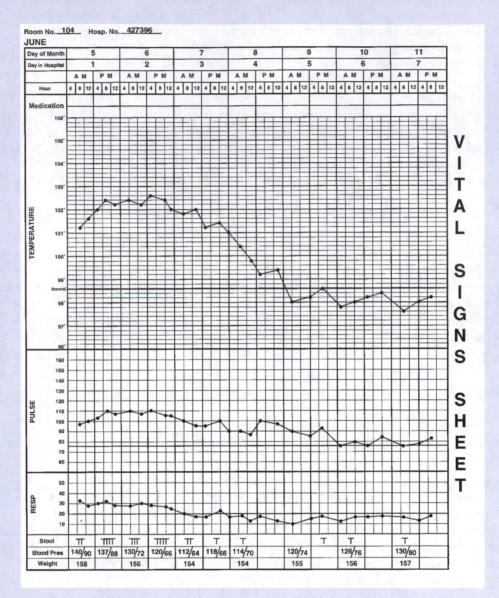

The vital signs sheet reflects an adult patient's 7-day hospitalization.

Determine if each statement is true or false in relation to the information plotted on the vital signs sheet. Circle your answers.

1. On June 7 at 10 p.m., the patient's temperature was 101.2°F.

   True   False

2. During the last 3 days of the patient's hospitalization, the patient's temperature reflected a normal circadian rhythm.

   True   False

3. During the first 4 days of the patient's hospitalization, the patient's blood pressure was consistent with a developing fluid volume deficit.

   True   False

4. During hospitalization, the patient's pulse rate ranged from 76 to 110 beats per minute.

   True   False

Continued

5. The patient's baseline pulse rate on admission to the hospital was within expected limits.

   True False

6. When the patient's temperature increased during the acute phase of the illness, the patient's respirations decreased.

   True False

SAMPLE ITEM 8-14

DAILY INTAKE AND OUTPUT RECORD

DATE JUNE 5

INTAKE								OUTPUT			
I.V. FLUIDS							ORAL	URINE	EMESIS	N.G. TUBE	HEMOVAC
Time	Bottle	Amount	Solution	Medication and Dosage	* ABS.	∓ LIB					
8	1	1000	NS	20 mEq KCl	↓			650			
8:30							360				
10:00							120				
11:30							240	150			
12:00									160		
1:40									90		60
2.15								250			
3:00					525	475					45
7-3 TOTAL		8-HR TOTAL			525	475	720	1050	250		105
3-11 TOTAL		8-HR TOTAL									
11-7 TOTAL		8-HR TOTAL									
24 HOUR TOTAL											

INTAKE GRAND TOTAL ____ OUTPUT GRAND TOTAL ____

* ABS. = amount absorbed ∓ LIB = Left in bag

A patient's daily intake and output (I&O) record for the 7 a.m. to 3 p.m. shift is illustrated above. Identify whether the following statements correctly or incorrectly reflect the information presented in the I&O record. Place an X on the line to indicate your answer.

1. If the intravenous solution infused at an equal volume per hour, the hourly rate was 75 mL per hour.

   True __________ False __________

2. If the patient had 4 oz. of orange juice with breakfast at 8:30 a.m., the patient also drank another 10 oz. of fluid with breakfast.

   True __________ False __________

Continued

Continued

3. The patient's intake and output was equal at the completion of the 7 a.m. to 3 p.m. shift.

   True _____ False _____

4. The additive to the patient's intravenous solution was 20 mg of vitamin K.

   True _____ False _____

Matching Questions

A matching question begins by establishing a frame of reference for the question. It explains the topic of the question and the basis on which matches should be made. The item then divides into a double-column format. It presents a statement in Column I and then requires you to select a corresponding, related, or companion statement from among a list of possible options in Column II. Usually the question assesses information about related categories, classifications, or characteristics. Sometimes the items in the two columns are equal in number, and sometimes Column I will have fewer statements than Column II. When the columns are equal in length, the format can work either for you or against you. If the columns have seven items each and you know six of the answers, you will automatically get the last answer correct. On the other hand, if you make an incorrect choice, you will automatically get two answers wrong. These problems are minimized if the response column (Column II) has more options than the question column (Column I). The matching question is a relatively superficial testing format that lends itself to factual information that usually is memorized.

TEST-TAKING TIP:
- **Read the directions for matching questions carefully because they specify the basis for the matching. In addition, they will tell you where to place the correct answer and the number of times an option can be selected.**
- **Cover Column II and for each item in Column I attempt to recall the memorized information without being cued by the content in Column II. Hopefully the information you memorized will appear as an option in Column II. By doing this you may become less confused or distracted by the list of options.**
- **Match items you are absolutely certain are correct matches. This leaves a reduced list on which to focus. Now consider the remaining options moving from the simple to the complex as determined by your frame of reference.**
- **Make an educated decision if you do not know an answer.**

SAMPLE ITEM 8-15
Column I contains terminology used to describe types of breathing exhibited by patients. Match each term to its correct description in Column II. Place the number you select from Column II on the line at the left of the term in Column I. Use each number only once.

Column I	Column II
_____ a. Bradypnea	1. Respirations that are increased in depth and rate
_____ b. Apnea	2. Difficulty breathing
_____ c. Hyperpnea	3. Respiratory rate less than 10 breaths per minute
_____ d. Tachypnea	4. Absence of breathing
_____ e. Eupnea	5. Respiratory rate greater than 20 breaths per minute
_____ f. Dyspnea	6. Normal breathing
	7. Shallow breathing interrupted by irregular periods of apnea

SAMPLE ITEM 8-16
Column I lists types of exercises. Match a type of exercise with its most therapeutic value or outcome. Indicate, in the space provided, the number from Column I that matches the letter in Column II. Options from Column I can be used more than once.

Column I—Exercises

1. Passive range of motion
2. Aerobic
3. Isometric
4. Kegel

Column II—Outcomes

a. Promote urinary continence (_____)
b. Improve strength of pelvic floor muscles (_____)
c. Promote pulmonary functioning (_____)
d. Improve cardiovascular conditioning (_____)
e. Increase muscle mass, tone, and strength of an extremity in a cast (_____)
f. Maintain joint mobility (_____)

RESTRICTED-RESPONSE QUESTIONS

Restricted-response questions are also known as free-response questions. Completion and short-answer questions are examples of restricted-response questions. These questions pose a simple question and expect you to furnish the answer. The response can be a word, phrase, sentence, or product of a mathematical calculation. Because these types of questions usually have an uncomplicated, direct format, they are most effective for assessing the understanding of simple concepts, the definition of terms, the knowledge of facts, or the ability to solve mathematical problems.

Completion Questions

A completion question generally is a short statement with one or more blanks. You are required to furnish the word, words, or phrase that accurately completes the sentence. In a completion question, the key word or words are the ones that are omitted. This forces you to focus on the important information reflected in the question rather than trivia. This type of question does not permit flexibility or creativity in your response. The question anticipates a particular word or phrase that will produce an accurate statement.

SAMPLE ITEM 8-17
Flexion and fixation of a joint is called a _____.

SAMPLE ITEM 8-18
Postural drainage uses gravity to drain secretions from the _____.

SAMPLE ITEM 8-19
The expected respiratory rate for an adult is _____ to _____ breaths per minute.

The inclusion of two possible answers to fill in the blank is a simple variation of a completion question. This format resembles an alternate-response question because you are asked a question and two choices are presented from which to pick an answer. This type of question gives you an advantage because the words presented are clues. These words nudge your memory and the recall of information necessary to answer the question. When faced with a question that has only two possible options, the chance of selecting the correct answer is 50%.

SAMPLE ITEM 8-20
When describing "radiating pain," the nurse is referring to its (intensity/location).

SAMPLE ITEM 8-21
The feeling that a person needs to void immediately is called (frequency/urgency).

Short-Answer Questions

A short-answer question is a free-response item because it asks a question and expects you to compose an answer. It provides some flexibility and creativity because the response does not have to complete a sentence or fill in a blank. You usually can use anywhere from one word to several sentences to answer the question. A short-answer question that needs only a word or a phrase to answer the question is similar to a completion question, but the original question is a complete sentence rather than an incomplete sentence. A short-answer question that requires several sentences to answer the question goes beyond the standards or criteria of a completion question, but it still focuses on the knowledge of facts, terminology, simple concepts, or the ability to perform mathematical computations.

Short-answer and completion questions can be used interchangeably to address the same content. For example, compare Sample Items 8-17 through 8-19 with Sample Items 8-22 through 8-24, respectively.

TEST-TAKING TIP:
- **Write as much relevant information as the format permits in the hope that what you include answers the question and contains the specific information expected. The more relevant information you include in the response, the better you can demonstrate comprehension of the information being tested.**

SAMPLE ITEM 8-22
What is the definition of the word *contracture?*

_____

SAMPLE ITEM 8-23
What is the purpose of postural drainage?

_____

SAMPLE ITEM 8-24
What is the normal range of respirations per minute in an adult?

_____

SAMPLE ITEM 8-25

An intravenous solution of 1000 mL of D_5W to be administered at 100 mL/hr is prescribed for a patient. The drop factor of the intravenous administration set is 15 drops/mL. How many drops per minute should the patient receive?

_____ drops/min

EXTENDED ESSAY QUESTIONS

An extended essay is a free-response question because the answer is drafted by you in reply to a question. It requires higher cognitive skills than just recall and comprehension. You must be able to write to answer an extended essay question. Essay questions expect you to select, arrange, organize, integrate, synthesize, and compare or contrast information. You must be able to use language constructively, be creative when solving problems, and use critical thinking to manipulate complicated information. The extended essay is most suitable for evaluating mastery of complex material.

Generally, instructors examine your writing from the viewpoint of **writing for evaluation.** Instructors measure your knowledge by evaluating an end product such as a written assignment or essay question on an examination. To answer an essay question, you must be able to put your thoughts on paper in a logical manner using correct spelling, grammar, and punctuation. There is no easy way to develop effective writing skills without practice. Most learning institutions today have writing centers that provide specialized faculty to assist you with writing activities. To maximize your success in formulating written assignments, you must view writing from the perspectives of **learning to write** and **writing to learn.**

Learning to Write

When learning to write, you are not looking at an end product that will be evaluated by the instructor but rather focusing on the process of writing. Writing requires a basic understanding of the English language. For example, you need to have an adequate vocabulary, understand the rules of grammar and punctuation, and be able to spell. When learning to write, you also must focus on the organizational and analytical skills that help you to assess, advise, teach, argue a point of view, and challenge new and old theories. Critical thinking is an essential skill needed to process the information that is to be written. Techniques that can be used to promote learning to write include brainstorming, setting priorities, and editing and revising previously written material.

Brainstorming is a method of exploring a topic by spontaneously listing thoughts or ideas. Making lists of words or phrases that relate to a topic allows you to explore a topic and your perspectives on the topic. For example, when students were asked to make a list of everything and anything relevant to patient progress notes, interesting insights developed. Some students were content oriented, in that they listed everything a health-care provider should include in progress notes, such as vital signs, specific care provided, and patients' responses to care. Other students were process oriented, in that they stated that notes should be specific, legible, and comprehensive. Brainstorming helps you not only to learn to write but also to explore topics through writing. If you take the time to examine what you have written, it also may tell you a lot about yourself.

Setting priorities is an analytical skill that requires you to compare and contrast information and identify that which is most important or significant. Use a systematic method or theoretical base to make priority setting easier. Maslow's Hierarchy of Needs is an excellent framework because it also helps to organize information. Data can be clustered in each of the five levels or categories of needs. These needs are ranked according to how critical they are to survival. The physiological needs are the most basic and carry the highest priority; safety and security, love and belonging, self-esteem, and self-actualization follow. You can practice setting priorities each day just by ranking your activities for the day in order of importance.

Analyzing, editing, and revising previously written material are other ways to learn to write. Consider writing directly on a computer. On a computer, it is easy to move around words, phrases, and sentences as you edit and revise your writing. Seeing your words in print helps to separate you from your own handwriting, making it easier to examine the content of your writing. When you have the luxury of time, it is always to your advantage to write an assignment one day and then several days later review this first draft. Your analytical skills may improve; you may acquire new information since you first wrote the material; or your perspective may be different or clearer. Also, you probably will be more open to constructive criticism when it comes from within. Analyzing, editing, and revising your own written work are excellent ways to improve your writing abilities.

The hardest thing to overcome when engaging in learning-to-write activities is the feeling that, because you may not have completed a project, you have not learned. Remember, learning takes place in the learner and is a lifelong process.

Writing to Learn

When writing to learn, you are focusing on what you will eventually understand or remember, not on the process of writing. You learn content by the very act of writing because at least two cognitive domains are being integrated: cognitive (thinking) and psychomotor (writing). You learn the course content you are writing about and discover what you know, what you need to know, and what you think about certain topics. When you are writing to learn, you are writing for yourself, and what you learn is the end product. Techniques that can be used to promote writing to learn include writing lists, writing journals, posing and answering questions, and note taking.

Writing a list can be a simple or complex task. A simple list is repetitiously writing a phrase or fact in an effort to reinforce learning. This requires a low-level thinking process that involves the recall of information—for example, writing common equivalents (30 cc × 30 mL = 1 ounce). A complex list might require the writer to discriminate between the commonalities and differences of content material. This requires higher levels of the thinking process and includes comprehension, application, and analysis. An example would be making a list of nursing interventions that use the concept of gravity (intravenous infusion, urinary catheter, elevation of an extremity to promote venous return). To compile this list, you must comprehend a concept and be able to identify the commonalities among the applications of this concept.

Writing a journal focuses on the use of words, the expression of ideas and feelings, and the documentation of activities; no consideration should be given to format, grammar, or punctuation. For 5 to 10 minutes each day, write a diary. It will improve your thinking and learning as well as document where you have been, where you are, and where you are going.

Posing and answering questions can lead to a better understanding of the content you are learning as well as improve your critical-thinking skills. Many textbooks have a companion study guide or workbook. Answering questions from these books and questions that you make up for yourself are excellent ways to reinforce the understanding of information. Putting your thoughts into concrete words and using the psychomotor skill of writing help you to learn.

Note taking can be a simple or complex task. A simple note-taking strategy is the rewriting of class notes. When you rewrite notes, you revise information so that it is more organized and clear. A complex note-taking strategy is to add relevant information from the textbook to your class notes. You can even add to your notes your own thoughts and reactions.

TEST-TAKING TIP
- Learn to write.
- Write to learn.
- Follow a three part format when answering an extended essay question.

    Write an introduction. An introduction should, in a general way, indicate what will be discussed. It introduces the topic and serves as a preface for what will follow.

Write the central part of the answer. The central part of the answer should explore all the information that is being presented to answer the question. Organize this part of the answer by writing a topical outline. This blueprint promotes an orderly flow of information, prevents departure from your script, and ensures that significant material is included.

Write a summary. The summary should recap what was discussed and come to several conclusions. It serves as a finale and brings closure to your answer.

SAMPLE ITEM 8-26

Compare and contrast critical thinking and clinical judgment and include at least three characteristics of each.

PERFORMANCE APPRAISAL

Nursing care is an art and a science. Nurses must not only comprehend information but also be able to perform skills safely. Therefore, testing the ability to identify and implement steps in a procedure accurately is essential in evaluating the achievement of skills. It is impossible to physically demonstrate an entire psychomotor skill on paper-and-pencil or computer-administered examinations. However, skills can be tested in a variety of ways. Questions that require you to identify a step in a procedure can be asked in the typical multiple-choice format. An example is "What should the nurse do first when preparing to give a bed bath to a patient?" This question requires you to select one correct answer out of four presented options. (See SAMPLE ITEM 5-1 in Chapter 5.) Questions that require you to select related steps in a procedure also can be presented in the multiple-response format. An example is "Identify all the actions that should be implemented when maintaining Airborne Transmission-Based Precautions." This question requires you to select two or more options to answer the question. (See SAMPLE ITEM 8-2 in this chapter.)

Questions that ask you to demonstrate knowledge about a skill in relation to a realistic image such as an illustration or a photograph expect you to respond in some way. An example is "Place an X over the area where the nurse should insert the needle of the syringe when accessing the *vastus lateralis* muscle." This question requires you to implement just one step of a procedure in relation to a visual cue. (See SAMPLE ITEM 8-30 in this chapter.) Another question format that can test knowledge about the steps of a procedure are drag and drop/ordered response questions. When a drag and drop question is evaluating your knowledge about a skill it will ask you to place the options presented in the question into the order in which they should be performed. For example, "A nurse identifies that a patient is unresponsive. List the following steps in order of priority." (See SAMPLE ITEM 8-34 in this chapter.)

The ability to demonstrate a procedure safely can also be evaluated when you actually implement the skill on a patient simulator manikin.

This type of performance appraisal evaluates your ability to complete all the steps of a psychomotor skill. Obtaining a blood pressure, changing a sterile dressing, administering a tube feeding, performing tracheal suctioning, and obtaining a patient's temperature are examples of psychomotor skills. When evaluating these skills, the criteria (critical elements) for passing should be identified before you attempt the procedure.

A **critical element** is any step that must be performed accurately to receive a passing score. Critical elements may be general or list very specific criteria. For example, general critical elements for obtaining a temperature reading may include maintain medical asepsis, provide for physical safety, and ensure privacy. These are less specific because there are numerous ways to meet each of these critical elements. Specific critical elements may include use a probe cover on the thermometer before placing it in the patient's mouth, hold the thermometer while it is in place, or pull the curtain around the patient before obtaining a rectal temperature.

TEST-TAKING TIPS
- Use clinical techniques/skills textbooks when practicing procedures and preparing for performance appraisals. A clinical checklist of step-by-step critical elements can be used by another student to assess your performance of a psychomotor skill in a laboratory setting. This supports reciprocal study relationships.
- Practice psychomotor skills using a patient simulator manikin. Practicing on a manikin provides a hands-on experience that is a nonthreatening way to practice a skill. It also provides an opportunity to simulate a testing situation and helps with desensitization, which may give you a feeling of control.

ALTERNATE QUESTION FORMATS REFLECTIVE OF NCLEX

Before April 2003, all of the questions on NCLEX examinations were presented in the typical multiple-choice format. This type of question requires you to select one correct answer of four presented options. In April 2003, The National Council of State Boards of Nursing (NCSBN) incorporated item formats other than the typical multiple-choice question. These items are called alternate-format items. **Alternate-format items** use the benefits of computer technology to assess knowledge via questions that require you to identify multiple answers, perform a calculation, prioritize information, or respond to a question in relation to a graphic image, picture, audio recording, video, or exhibit. The NCSBN believes that test takers can demonstrate their entry-level nursing competence in ways that are different from the typical multiple-choice format and that some nursing content will be more readily and authentically evaluated.

Alternate-format items include fill-in-the-blank calculation items, hot spot items, multiple-response items, graphic and illustration items, drag and drop/ordered response items, and exhibit items. The following sample questions are examples of these types of alternate-format items.

Fill-in-the-Blank Calculation Items

A fill-in-the-blank calculation item asks a question that requires you to perform a mathematical computation and type in your answer. You will be directed to include a whole number or the number of decimal places that should be used. Only numbers and decimal points can be entered. If the test is taken on a computer, usually you can access a calculator on the computer to assist you with your computation.

TEST-TAKING TIPS
- Memorize important formulas when studying for a test.
- Read the question carefully to identify the unit of measure required and if the answer is to be a whole number or have 1 or more decimal places.
- Write several important formulas or equivalent conversions on provided scrap paper or an erasable noteboard immediately after beginning a test.

OR
- When confronted with a calculation question, visualize the formula required to answer the question and write it down before answering the question.
- Insert the information presented in the scenario into the formula and perform the computation using a calculator. Do not perform calculation problems in your head.

- Review your answer to ensure that it is in the unit of measure requested in the question and that the answer is realistic.
- Ensure that the numerical answer is presented accurately:
  If the answer is less than a whole number place a 0 before the decimal point (e.g., 0.25). Some computer programs automatically insert the 0.
  If instructed to use 1 or 2 decimal places ensure that only 1 or 2 numbers follow the decimal point (e.g., 0.2, 0.25).
  If the question asks that the answer be a whole number and the mathematical calculation results in an answer that is less than a whole number you must round up or down to the next whole number. To round up a tenth of a number it has to be 0.5 to 0.9. For example, 21.75 should be rounded up to 22. To round down to a whole number it has to be 0.1 to 0.4. For example, 21.3 should be rounded down to 21.

SAMPLE ITEM 8-27

A primary health-care provider orders 1500 mL to be administered every 24 hours. At what hourly rate should the nurse set the infusion pump? **Record your answer using a whole number.**

Answer: _____ mL/hr

SAMPLE ITEM 8-28

A primary health-care provider prescribes 500 mg of an antibiotic to be administered IVPB every 6 hours. One gram of the medication is supplied in a vial that states: "add 2.5 mL of sterile water to yield 3 mL of solution." How much solution should the nurse administer?
Record your answer using one decimal place.

Answer: _____ mL

Hot Spot Items

A hot spot item asks a question in relation to a presented illustration. When a test is taken on the computer, you need to place the cursor on the area you want to select and left-click on the mouse.

TEST-TAKING TIPS

- Read the question twice to ensure that you understand what the question is asking. Briefly look at the visual cue (e.g., illustration, photograph).
- Visualize the anatomy and consider its associated physiology in relation to the question being asked.
- In your mind identify the location of your answer. Then examine the visual cue provided in the question and insert your answer.

SAMPLE ITEM 8-29

A patient is on complete bedrest in the semi-Fowler position because of excessive fluid volume and difficulty breathing. Place an X over the area of the body that is at the greatest risk for dependent edema.

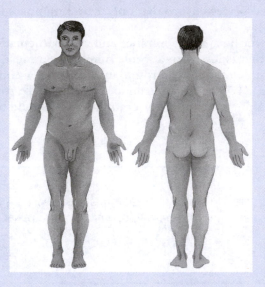

SAMPLE ITEM 8-30

The nurse must administer an intramuscular injection. Place an X over the area where the nurse should insert the needle of the syringe when utilizing the *vastus lateralis* muscle.

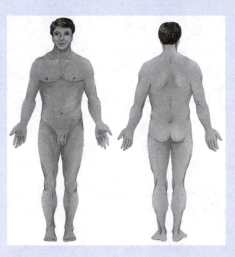

Graphic and Illustration Items

A graphic item presents a question with several options as potential answers. Each option contains a graphic image rather than textual material. You must analyze the images and select the correct answer from among the presented options. In a graphic item the illustrations appear in the options.

An illustration item is a variation of a graphic item. It presents a question accompanied by a chart, table, or visual image. You must analyze the options in relation to the illustration before selecting the option you believe is the correct answer. Illustrations can appear in a variety of formats such as multiple choice, multiple response, and fill-in-the-blank calculation items but the illustration will always be part of the stem of the question.

TEST-TAKING TIPS

- **When reading your textbook or other resources, graphic material such as illustrations often are presented to support written content. Concentrate on these images and commit them to memory when studying because they reinforce the content you are learning. Examples include illustrations of range-of-motion exercises, the chain of infection, or a person with Parkinson's disease. Remember, "A picture is worth a thousand words."**
- **When confronted with a question with graphic material, recall similar visual images you have studied and draw on your knowledge related to those visual images to attempt to answer the question.**

SAMPLE ITEM 8-31

Identify positions used by the nurse that reflect correct body mechanics to help prevent stress and strain on back muscles. **Select all that apply.**

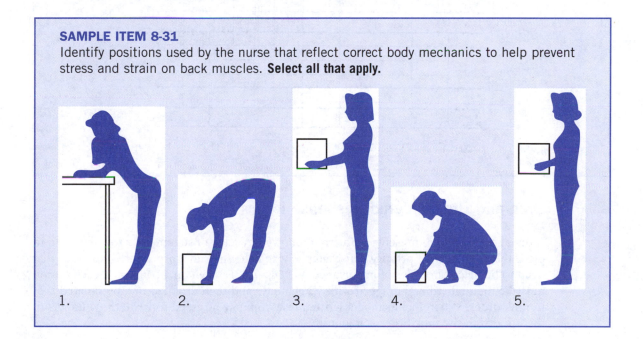

1.   2.   3.   4.   5.

SAMPLE ITEM 8-32

Referring to the I&O flow sheet on page 142 for a patient admitted at 8 a.m. what was the patient's total fluid intake for the 7 hours between 8 a.m. and 3 p.m.? **Record your answer using a whole number.**

Answer: _____ mL

Continued

Continued

DAILY INTAKE AND OUTPUT RECORD

DATE   JUNE 5

Time	Bottle	Amount	Solution	Medication and Dosage	* ABS.	∓ LIB	ORAL	URINE	EMESIS	N.G. TUBE	HEMOVAC
8	1	1000	NS	20 mEq KCl				650			
8:30							360				
10:00							120				
11:30							240	150			
12:00									160		
1:40									90		60
2:15								250			
3:00						525	475				45
7-3 TOTAL		8-HR TOTAL			525	475	720	1050	250		105
3-11 TOTAL		8-HR TOTAL									
11-7 TOTAL		8-HR TOTAL									
24 HOUR TOTAL											

INTAKE GRAND TOTAL [   ]   OUTPUT GRAND TOTAL [   ]

* ABS. = amount absorbed   ∓ LIB = Left in bag

Drag and Drop/Ordered Response Items

A drag and drop item presents a situation followed by a list of statements. You are asked to place them in order of priority. For example, it may be steps in a procedure or actions that need to be placed in order of importance. When a test is taken on a computer, each option must be highlighted and dragged with your mouse and then dropped in a designated area in rank order. When included on a written test, you may be asked to write the numbers of the options in the rank order you identify.

TEST-TAKING TIPS
- **Explore priorities related to nursing care when studying. For example, washing your hands before a procedure, maintaining a patent airway, and assessing a patient before planning or implementing care. Also, explore a variety of care that may be performed last. For example, leaving a bed in the lowest position, washing your hands after removing gloves, documenting all care provided, and positioning a call bell near the patient before leaving the room.**
- **Use theories or scientific processes to help prioritize options. For example, the ABCs (Airway, Breathing, and Circulation), Maslow's Hierarchy of Needs, and the steps of the Nursing Process.**
- **If the question is about a procedure, visualize yourself performing the procedure and then analyze the options.**
- **Place options in order of priority or importance by beginning with your first selected option and progressing to the last option from among the options presented. If you have difficulty progressing from 1 through 5/6 options then select the option you believe should be first and then select the option you think should be last. Alternate selecting the first and last options from the remaining options until one option is left or all the options have been selected.**

SAMPLE ITEM 8-33

A nurse discovers a fire in the dayroom where a patient is watching television. Rank the following actions from 1 to 5 in the order in which they should be performed in accordance with the RACE acronym associated with fire safety.

1. Pull the fire alarm.

2. Shut the doors on the unit.

3. Move all patients off the unit.

4. Take the patient out of the dayroom.

5. Move patients in adjacent rooms to an area down the hall.

Answer: _____.

SAMPLE ITEM 8-34

A nurse in a hospital identifies that an adult patient is unresponsive. Place the following steps in the order in which they should be performed.

1. Direct another nurse to activate the emergency response system.

2. Deliver 30 fast, 2 inches in depth chest compressions.

3. Check for the presence of a carotid pulse.

4. Check for breathing.

5. Deliver 2 breaths.

Answer: _____

Multiple Response Items

A multiple response item requires you to identify one or more correct options from among a list of presented options. It is similar to a multiple choice question except that it has more than four options and there are two or more correct options. All the correct options must be identified to receive credit for the question.

TEST-TAKING TIPS

- Use test-taking techniques that apply to traditional multiple-choice questions such as identify specific determiners in options, identify opposites in options, and identify options that deny patient feelings, concerns, or needs.
- Identify each option you know is a correct answer. Then identify each option you know is an incorrect answer. Finally, examine any remaining options and make an educated decision as to whether they are correct or incorrect.

OR

- Identify one option you know is a correct answer. Then identify one option you know is an incorrect answer. Continue to alternate the identification of correct and incorrect options until all options have been determined to be correct or incorrect or if there are remaining options that you cannot classify as correct or incorrect. Then examine these final options and make an educated determination as to whether they are correct or incorrect.

SAMPLE ITEM 8-35

A nurse assesses a patient and concludes that the patient has a fluid volume deficit. Which assessments support this conclusion? **Select all that apply.**

1. _____ Tenting of skin

2. _____ Decreased pulse

Continued

Continued

3. _____ Sudden weight loss
4. _____ Increased blood pressure
5. _____ Longitudinal furrows in the tongue

SAMPLE ITEM 8-36

A nurse manager of a medical/surgical unit is making the assignments for the day for the nursing members of the health-care team. Which activities can be delegated to a nursing assistant? **Select all that apply.**

1. _____ Changing the linen of a patient in traction
2. _____ Massaging the back of a patient who is on complete bedrest
3. _____ Transferring a patient from the bed to a chair by using a mechanical lift
4. _____ Teaching a patient who is receiving an opioid how to prevent constipation
5. _____ Reinforcing a postoperative dressing that is saturated with a bloody discharge
6. _____ Obtaining vital signs of a patient who is returning from the postanesthesia care unit

Exhibit Items

An exhibit item presents a situation and asks a question. It provides information that can be accessed via a variety of tabs. Each tab must be reviewed to collect information within the tab. When taken on a computer you must click on one tab to collect the information within the tab before moving to the next tab. When included on a written test you probably will be able to view the information within all the tabs at the same time. You must identify significant information within each tab and integrate the information from among the tabs. From this analysis you can make inferences, deductions, and/or conclusions that eliminate options and support the correct answer.

TEST-TAKING TIPS

* **Read the stem of the question carefully to determine what the question is asking. Identify important words that focus your attention on significant information in the tabs that follow.**
* **Read all the information presented in the tabs of the exhibit item. They may include information such as laboratory results, vital signs, prescriptions for medications, primary health-care provider orders, patient assessment, patient statements, or progress notes. Identify data that are significant such as abnormal laboratory values, vital signs that are outside expected values, medications that may have drug-to-drug interactions, inappropriate orders, and patient concerns.**
* **Reread the stem of the question and compare and contrast the information in the stem with the information in the tabs.**
* **Compare and contrast your conclusions about significant information in the stem and the tabs with the information in each option.**
* **Ensure that the option you selected has a relationship with the main topic of the question in the stem and information presented in one or more tabs.**

SAMPLE ITEM 8-37

A 90-year-old man is admitted to the hospital with a diagnosis of change in mental status. A family member states that the patient has not eaten much for the last week and seemed very confused this morning. The nurse completes a physical assessment and reviews the patient's medical record. Which human response does the nurse determine the patient is exhibiting?

1. Dehydration

2. Hypervolemia

Continued

3. Urinary tract infection

4. Increased blood glucose level

Laboratory Results
Sodium: 155 mEq/L
WBC: 8000 µL
Hct: 60%
Fasting blood sugar (FBS): 114 mg/dL

Vital Signs at 2:00 p.m.
Temperature: 100°F
Pulse: 88 beats/min, regular
Respirations: 24 breaths/min

Nursing Progress Note
Patient is oriented to place and person but is easily distracted, is unable to follow directions, and voided a small amount of clear amber urine; the tongue has furrows and there is tenting of the skin.

SAMPLE ITEM 8-38
A patient comes to the emergency department with concerns about extreme fatigue and prolonged episodes of menstruation. The primary health-care provider performs a battery of tests. When reviewing the patient's record, the nurse identifies that the patient's oxygen problem is related to an impairment of which mechanism?

1. Osmosis

2. Diffusion

3. Transport

4. Ventilation

Laboratory Tests
RBC: 2.9 (10^6 cells/mm^3)
WBC: 7000 mm^3
Hb: 8.5 g/dL
Hct: 34%

Radiology Report
Chest radiograph: normal findings; all bones aligned and symmetrical; normal positioned soft tissues, mediastinum, lungs, pleura, heart, and aortic arc.

Vital Signs Sheet
Temperature: 98.8°F (oral)
Pulse: 92 beats/min, regular rhythm
Respirations: 24 breaths/min, regular rhythm, unlabored

SUMMARY

To promote success when challenged by an examination with a variety of testing formats, it is wise to be familiar with the various formats. Structured-response, restricted-response, extended-essay, and performance-appraisal formats are commonly used in schools of nursing in addition to the alternate-formats items found on the NCLEX, such as fill-in-the-blank calculation, multiple-response, hot spot, drag and drop/ordered response, graphic and illustration, and exhibit items. These questions have some commonalities, but each is unique. Understanding the commonalities and differences in these formats and using a variety of test-taking techniques facilitate a feeling of control, which contributes to a positive mental attitude.

8-1   **Answer: 1 and 3.**

1. <u>X</u> Undermining of adjoining tissue can occur with a stage III pressure ulcer. Undermining is a wider area of tissue damage that extends under and beyond the opening of the wound (under the surface of adjoining tissue). The wound with undermining is more extensive than that which is visible from the surface.

2. _____ A stage III pressure ulcer is not limited to partial-thickness loss. Partial-thickness loss (e.g., blister, abrasion, shallow crater) is associated with a stage II pressure ulcer.

3. <u>X</u> A stage III pressure ulcer involves full-thickness skin loss (through the dermis and epidermis) with damage or necrosis extending to subcutaneous tissue.

4. _____ A stage III pressure ulcer does not involve damage through the fascia. A stage IV pressure ulcer involves damage to muscle, bone, or supporting tissue (e.g., tendon or capsule of a joint). Undermining and sinus tracts are relatively common with a stage IV pressure ulcer.

5. _____ A stage III pressure ulcer does not involve muscle damage. A stage IV pressure ulcer involves damage to muscle, bone, or supporting tissue (e.g., tendon or capsule of a joint). Undermining and sinus tracts (tunneling) are relatively common with a stage IV pressure ulcer.

8-2   **Answer: 3, 4, 5, and 6.**

1. _____ Donning a gown when entering a room where Airborne Transmission-Based Precautions are required is unnecessary unless there is a likelihood of splashing of blood, body fluids, body secretions, or excretions.

2. _____ Putting on gloves when delivering a food tray where Airborne Transmission-Based Precautions is required is unnecessary unless there is a likelihood of splashing of blood, body fluids, body secretions, or excretions.

3. <u>X</u> A patient requiring Airborne Transmission-Based Precautions must wear a surgical mask when transported outside the room to protect others from the patient's respiratory microorganisms.

4. <u>X</u> A patient requiring Airborne Transmission-Based Precautions must be cared for in a monitored negative air pressure room that maintains 6 to 12 air changes per hour. A negative air pressure room prevents room air from flowing through the door to the nursing unit; it expels room air to the outside environment unless a high-efficiency particulate air (HEPA) filtration system is used.

5. <u>X</u> An N95 respirator mask must be worn when entering a room where Airborne Transmission-Based Precautions are required. An N95 respirator mask protects the wearer from the transfer of oral and nasopharyngeal organisms from the patient. N95 respirators demonstrate a filtration efficiency of the most penetrating particle size (0.1 to 0.3 micrometers) at 99.5% to 99.75%.

6. <u>X</u> The door to a room with monitored negative air pressure must be kept closed at all times except when entering or exiting the room. This prevents air in the room from flowing through the door to the nursing unit and expels the room air to the outside environment unless a high-efficiency particulate air (HEPA) filtration system is used.

8-3 **TRUE**

Soap decreases the surface tension of water. Surface tension is the tendency of a liquid to minimize the area of its surface by contracting. Decreasing the surface tension increases the ability of water to wet another surface.

8-4 **TRUE**

A broad stance widens the nurse's base of support, which promotes stability.

8-5 **FALSE**

Exercise is a stimulating activity that should be avoided before bedtime. Adequate exercise during the day promotes sleep later in the day.

8-6 **FALSE**

Pulse pressure is the difference between the systolic and diastolic blood pressures. Pulse deficit is the difference between the apical and radial pulse rates.

8-7 TRUE
Palpation is a technique in which the examiner applies the fingers or hands to the body to assess the texture, size, consistency, and location of body parts.

8-8 FALSE
The process in which solid, particulate matter in a fluid moves from an area of higher concentration to an area of decreased concentration is known as *diffusion*. The process in which a pure solvent, such as water, moves through a semipermeable membrane from an area that has a decreased solute concentration to one that has an increased solute concentration is known as *osmosis*.

8-9 1. TRUE
The outer border of a drape is considered contaminated. After sterile gloves are donned, the nurse can touch only inside this border to maintain sterility of the field.
2. TRUE
Because the hands are not sterile, the nurse avoids contaminating the sterile glove by touching only the inside of the glove. The second sterile glove is donned by touching just the outside of the glove with the hand that is already covered by the first sterile glove.
3. FALSE
During a surgical hand scrub, the hands are held above the elbows; this allows water to flow downward by gravity without contaminating the nurse's hands. Hand hygiene associated with medical asepsis requires the hands to be held below the elbows.
4. FALSE
Sterile objects held below the waist are not within the nurse's direct visual field and inadvertently may become contaminated.

8-10 1. TRUE
Mechanical ventilation uses positive pressure to push air and/or oxygen into the lungs during the inspiratory phase of the respiratory cycle. Positive pressure is pressure greater than that of the atmosphere.
2. FALSE
A continuous bladder irrigation uses the principle of gravity to instill fluid into the bladder as well as to promote the flow of fluid out of the bladder through the triple-lumen indwelling urinary catheter.

Gravity is the force that draws all masses in the earth's sphere toward the center of the earth.
3. FALSE
Chest tubes (chest drainage system) exert negative pressure to remove air and fluids from the pleural space. Negative pressure is pressure less than that of the atmosphere, and it is the opposite of positive pressure.
4. TRUE
Positive pressure is exerted when the plunger of a piston syringe is pushed toward its cone tip.

8-11 FALSE
This statement can be revised in the following way: The expected range of the heart rate for an adult is *60 to 100* beats per minute.

8-12 FALSE
To revise this question as directed, the words *young adulthood* must be changed to *adolescence*. You will not receive credit for this question if you changed *identity versus role confusion* to *intimacy versus isolation*. Although this statement is accurate, the instructions for revising the statement have not been followed.

8-13 1. FALSE
The patient's temperature was 101.4°F. Each line above 101 is 0.2 of a degree.
2. TRUE
Body temperature varies throughout the day with the lowest temperature in the early morning and the highest temperature between 8 p.m. and midnight. A circadian rhythm (diurnal variation) is a pattern based on a 24-hour cycle.
3. TRUE
With fluid volume deficit, the volume in the intravascular compartment decreases (hypovolemia), resulting in a decreased blood pressure (hypotension).
4. TRUE
This patient's pulse rate per minute ranged from 76 (on June 10th and 11th) to 110 (on June 5th and 6th).
5. TRUE
A pulse rate of 98 is within the expected range of 60 to 100 beats per minute.
6. FALSE
During the acute phase of the illness, the patient's temperature, pulse, and respirations were all increased.

8-14 1. TRUE

The intravenous solution was hung at 8 a.m. and infused 525 mL over the next 7 hours. The total volume (525) divided by the number of hours (7) equals 75 mL/hr.

2. FALSE

If each ounce is equal to 30 mL, 4 ounces is equal to 120 mL. If you subtract 120 from the total volume of fluid taken at 8:30 a.m. (360), the amount of additional fluid consumed was 240 mL. If you divide 240 mL by 30 mL, it equals 8 ounces, not 10.

3. FALSE

The intake was 525 + 720 = 1245 mL. The output was 1050 + 250 + 105 = 1405 mL. The output exceeded the intake by 160 mL.

4. FALSE

The additive to the patient's intravenous solution was 20 mEq of potassium chloride.

8-15 a. 3

Bradypnea is abnormally slow breathing with a regular rhythm (respiratory rate less than 10 breaths/min).

b. 4

Apnea is the temporary cessation of breathing (absence of breathing).

c. 1

Hyperpnea is deep, rapid, labored respirations, usually associated with strenuous exercise.

d. 5

Tachypnea is abnormally rapid breathing with a regular rhythm (respirations that are increased in depth and rate).

e. 6

Eupnea is breathing that is expected at a rate of 12 to 20 breaths per minute and depth with a tidal volume of approximately 500 mL (normal breathing).

f. 2

Dyspnea is difficulty breathing characterized by an increased effort and use of accessory muscles (difficulty breathing). "Shallow breathing interrupted by irregular periods of apnea" (option 7) was an extra option included in Column II that did not have a matching term in Column I.

8-16 a. 4

Kegel exercises consist of repetitive contractions of the muscles of the pelvic floor. These muscles facilitate voluntary control of urination.

b. 4

Kegel exercises, which are performed by voluntarily starting and stopping the urinary stream, tone the perineal muscles of the pelvic floor.

c. 2

Aerobic exercises involve activity that demands that oxygen be taken into the body at a rate greater than the amount the body usually requires, promoting respiratory functioning.

d. 2

Aerobic exercises involve sustained muscle movements that increase blood flow, heart rate, and metabolic demand for oxygen over time, promoting cardiovascular functioning.

e. 3

Isometric exercises cause a change in muscle tension but no change in muscle length; no muscle or joint movement occurs.

f. 1

Passive range-of-motion exercises occur when another person moves each of the patient's joints through their full range of movement, maximally stretching all muscle groups within each plane over each joint.

8-17   *Contracture* is the only acceptable answer to this question.

Contractures are permanent flexion deformities of joints caused by disuse, atrophy, and shortening of muscles.

8-18   *Respiratory passages* or *lung* are both acceptable answers to this question.

With postural drainage, the patient is placed in various positions to promote the movement of secretions from smaller to larger pulmonary airways, where they can be removed by coughing or suctioning.

8-19   The correct answer for this question is *12* to *20*.

8-20   The correct answer is *location*.

Radiating pain is a description that relates to where the pain is experienced in the body. It includes the initial site of the pain and its extension to other parts of the body. Intensity refers to the perceived severity of the pain; intensity can be measured on a scale of 0 (no pain) to 10 (severe pain).

8-21   The correct answer is *urgency*.
Urgency is the feeling that the person must void immediately whether or not there is much urine in the bladder. It is precipitated by psychological stress and/or irritation of the vesical trigone and/or urethra. Frequency is the increased incidence of voiding.

8-22   Acceptable answers include permanent flexion and fixation of a joint or an abnormal shortening of a muscle that results in limited range of motion of a joint and eventually ankylosis.
Compare this item with Sample Item 8-17.

8-23   Acceptable answers include mobilize respiratory secretions; loosen pulmonary secretions to facilitate their expectoration; or promote a clear airway by draining respiratory secretions toward the oral cavity.
Compare this item with Sample Item 8-18.

8-24   Acceptable answers may include just stating the numbers 12 to 20.
A more complex answer might state: The expected (normal) number of breaths per minute for an adult ranges from 12 to 20 with an average of 16. Compare this item with Sample Item 8-19.

8-25   Answer: 25 drops/min.
To arrive at the correct answer, you have to perform the following calculation:

$$\frac{\text{Volume to be infused}}{\text{Number of hours}} \times \frac{\text{drop factor}}{60 \text{ minutes}}$$

$$\frac{100 \times 15}{1 \times 60}$$

$$\frac{1500}{60} = 25 \text{ drops/min}$$

8-26   To answer this question, use the three-part format:

INTRODUCTION: The introduction functions as a preface, preamble, or prologue for what information will follow.

Although there are many detailed definitions of the practice of nursing, in the simplest terms nursing consists of helping people meet needs. To do this, nurses must employ cognitive skills such as critical thinking and problem solving. The commonalities and differences of critical thinking and problem solving will be discussed.

CENTRAL PART: The central part of the answer presents and explores the information necessary to answer the question. Make a topical outline of the facts to be included, and then write a narrative that incorporates and elaborates on the information in the outline.

Definition of critical thinking
Definition of clinical judgment
Commonalities of critical thinking and
   clinical judgment
  Strong knowledge base
  Attitude of inquiry and intellectual
    humility
  Purposeful process
  Employs reasoning
Differences of critical thinking
  Proactive
  Uses thinking processes to clarify and
    improve understanding
  Open ended
Differences of clinical judgment
Reactive
Uses the mental operation of critical thinking to explore possibilities
Starts with a problem and ends with an enlightened conclusion

SUMMARY: The summary should briefly recap or review the general theme of the discussion and come to one or more conclusions. It serves to close the response to the essay question.

The nurse of today and especially of the future must be able to integrate critical thinking and clinical judgment to maximize human potential. Although they have a common foundation, each mode of thinking is unique. Nurses should blend them into a repertoire of cognitive strategies.

ALTERNATE-FORMAT ITEMS REFLECTIVE OF NCLEX

Fill-in-the-Blank Calculation Items

8-27   **Answer: 63 mL/hr.**
The question directed you to use a whole number for your answer.
1500 ÷ 24 = 62.5 mL. When a portion of a mL is 0.5 or greater, round up to the next full number.

8-28   **Answer: 1.5 mL.**
The question directed you to use one decimal place in your answer.
1 gram is equal to 1000 mg. Solve the problem using ratio and proportion.

$$\frac{\text{Desired}}{\text{Have}} \quad \frac{500 \text{ mg}}{1000 \text{ mg}} = \frac{x \text{ mL}}{3 \text{ mL}}$$

$$1000x = 1500$$
$$x = 1500 \div 1000$$
$$x = 1.5 \text{ mL}$$

Hot Spot Items

8-29   **The sacral area (shaded) is at greatest risk for dependent edema for this patient. Fluid volume excess increases capillary pressures causing fluid to move from the intravascular compartment into interstitial tissue. Because fluid flows by gravity, edema is observed in dependent tissues. A patient who has difficulty breathing is generally positioned in a semi- or high-Fowler position. In the Fowler position the sacrum is the most dependent area and is therefore at greatest risk for interstitial edema.**

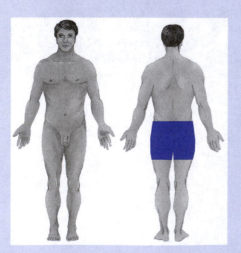

8-30   **The *vastus lateralis* site (shaded) is located on the middle third and anterior lateral aspect of the thigh, one handbreadth above the knee (from the lateral femoral condyle) and one handbreadth below the greater trochanter.**

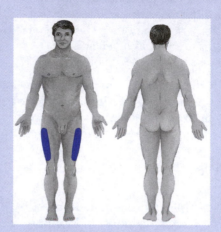

Graphic and Illustration Items

8-31 1. Bending over without bending the knees places undue stress and strain on lower back muscles and should be avoided. The illustration below demonstrates correct body mechanics.

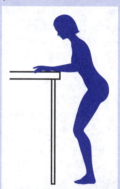

2. Lifting an object without bending the knees and standing close to the object should be avoided. It requires upper body muscles to lift the object causing undue stress and strain on upper body structures. In addition, the center of gravity is outside the base of support. The illustration below demonstrates correct body mechanics.

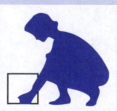

3. Holding objects in front of and away from the body places the center of gravity outside the base of support, which places undue stress and strain on muscles of the upper body and should be avoided. In addition, balance is less stable when the line of gravity falls outside the base of support. The illustration below demonstrates correct body mechanics.

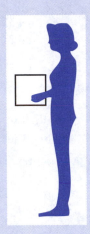

4. Standing close to an object to be lifted, flexing the back and knees, and then straightening the knees and unflexing the back cause the large muscles of the legs to bear most of the burden. Doing so places less stress and strain on the muscles of the upper body.

5. Holding objects close to the body places the line of gravity closer to the base of support, facilitating balance and reducing stress and strain on the muscles of the upper body.

8-32   **Answer: 1245 mL.**
To arrive at the total intake for the 7 hours between 8 a.m. and 3 p.m., the nurse has to add the 525 mL of IV fluid absorbed (indicated in the box at the bottom of the "Abs" column in the row labeled "7-3 total" and the 720 mL of oral intake (indicated in the box at the bottom of the "ORAL" column in the row labeled "7-3 total." 525 mL of IV fluids plus 720 mL of oral intake equals 1245 mL of total fluid intake for the 7 hours between 8 a.m. and 3 p.m. The LIB column indicates the volume of fluid that remains in the intravenous bag at the end of the time frame.
Urine, emesis, and Hemovac output.

DAILY INTAKE AND OUTPUT RECORD

DATE   JUNE 5

Time	Bottle	Amount	Solution	Medication and Dosage	ABS	LIB	ORAL	URINE	EMESIS	N.G. TUBE	HEMOVAC
8	1	1000	NS	20 mEq KCl			650				
8:30							300				
10:00							120				
11:30							240	150			
12:00									160		
1:40									90		60
2:15								250			
3:00						525	475					45
7-3 TOTAL		8-HR TOTAL			525	475	720	1050	250		105
8-11 TOTAL		8-HR TOTAL									
11-7 TOTAL		8-HR TOTAL									
24 HOUR TOTAL											

INTAKE GRAND TOTAL [   ]   OUTPUT GRAND TOTAL [   ]

* ABS. = amount absorbed   ∓ LIB = left in bag

Drag and Drop/Ordered Response Items

8-33   Answer: 4, 1, 2, 5, 3

4. Take the patient out of the dayroom—Remove: The priority is to remove the patient, who is in the immediate vicinity of the fire and is at risk for injury.
1. Pull the fire alarm—Activate: Once the patient is protected from harm, the fire alarm can be activated.
2. Shut the doors on the unit—Contain: After the patient is protected from harm and the alarm is sounded, measures can be implemented to contain the fire by actions such as closing doors.
5. Move patients in adjacent rooms to an area down the hall. Evacuate: This is necessary only after the previous three steps are implemented and if it is determined that patients are at risk.
3. Move all patients off the unit—Evacuate: This is necessary if the fire escalates and the patients are at risk.

8-34   Answer: 4, 1, 3, 2, 5

4. Feeling or hearing air movement determines if there is gas exchange in and out of the lung.
1. Members of the emergency response team will bring equipment (e.g., defibrillator, medications) and assist with the administration of CPR and other medical interventions.
3. The absence of a pulse indicates that the patient has experienced a cardiac arrest.
2. Chest compressions push blood and the oxygen it contains out of the heart to body cells. Thirty compressions within 18 seconds should be performed (a rate of 100 per minute) to a depth of 2 inches with complete chest recoil after each compression. Research demonstrates that compressions are the critical elements in adult resuscitation.
5. Opening the airway and giving 2 breaths is performed after the first 30 compressions and each subsequent cycle of 30 compressions if performing one person CPR. The compression to ventilation ratio is 15 to 2 when CPR is performed by 2 health care providers.

Multiple Response Items

8-35 1. X___ Tenting of skin occurs because of the decrease in interstitial and intracellular fluid.
2. ____ The pulse increases to compensate for hypovolemia.
3. X___ One liter of fluid weighs 2.2 pounds. The patient will lose weight as fluid is excreted.
4. ____ The blood pressure decreases because of the decreased intravascular fluid volume.
5. X___ Interstitial and intracellular fluid shifts to the intravascular compartment to maintain cardiovascular function. As a result, the tongue becomes furrowed and dry.

8-36 1. X___ Assisting patients with the activities of daily living, which includes maintaining clean linen for a patient in traction, is within the scope of practice of a nursing assistant.
2. X___ Providing a backrub is considered an activity of daily living, which is within the scope of practice of a nursing assistant.
3. X___ Assisting patients with the activities of daily living, which includes transferring patients from the bed to a chair, is within the scope of practice of a nursing assistant.
4. ____ Patient teaching is an independent role of a nurse, not a nursing assistant. Teaching requires the knowledge of anatomy, physiology, pharmacology, teaching/learning principles, and rationales for appropriate nursing interventions.
5. ____ Caring for surgical dressings, which requires the use of sterile technique, is not within the scope of practice of a nursing assistant.
6. ____ Although nursing assistants can take routine vital signs of patients who are physiologically stable, immediate postoperative patients and patients who are physiologically unstable should have their vital signs assessed by a nurse.

Exhibit Items

8-37
Laboratory Results
Sodium: 155 mEq/L
WBC: 8000 µL
Hct: 60%
FBS: 114 mg/dL

Vital Signs at 2:00 p.m.
Temperature: 100°F
Pulse: 88 beats/min, regular
Respirations: 24 breaths/min

Nursing Progress Note
Patient is oriented to place and person but is easily distracted, is unable to follow directions, and voided a small amount of clear amber urine; the tongue has furrows and there is tenting of the skin.

ANSWER AND RATIONALES
1. The physical assessment and laboratory results indicate that the patient is dehydrated. Oliguria, furrows of the tongue, tenting of the skin, and increased vital signs are all signs of dehydration. The serum sodium level that is higher than the expected range of 135 to 145 mEq/L and the hematocrit that is higher than the expected range of 40% to 54% indicate hemoconcentration associated with dehydration.
2. With hypervolemia, the patient's hematocrit will be decreased, indicating hemodilution.
3. With a urinary tract infection there is not just an increase in the temperature; the WBCs also will be increased and the urine will be cloudy.
4. The physical assessment data do not support the inference that the patient has hyperglycemia. The FBS is within the expected limits of 70 to 120 mg/dL in the older adult, and there is an absence of polyuria, polyphagia, polydipsia, fatigue, weakness, and vision changes.

8-38
Laboratory Tests
RBC: 2.9 (10^6 cells/mm^3)
WBC: 7000 mm^3
Hb: 8.5 g/dL
Hct: 34%

Radiology Report
Chest radiograph: normal findings; all bones aligned and symmetrical; normal positioned soft tissues, mediastinum, lungs, pleura, heart, and aortic arc.

Vital Signs Sheet
Temperature: 98.8°F (oral)
Pulse: 92 beats/min, regular rhythm
Respirations: 24 breaths/min, regular rhythm, unlabored

ANSWER AND RATIONALES
1. Osmosis is unrelated to this patient situation. Osmosis is related to fluid balance. It is the movement of water through a semipermeable membrane from an area of decreased concentration of constituents to an area of increased concentration of constituents.

Continued

Continued

2. The patient's respiratory status—an unlabored respiratory rate of 24 breaths/min with a regular rhythm—does not reflect a problem with diffusion. The slight increase in respiratory rate is a compensatory response to the decreased number of red blood cells that carry oxygen to all body cells. The chest radiograph rules out primary lung disease, indicating that problems with diffusion do not exist.

3. **The patient has a problem with oxygen transport because of an inadequate number of red blood cells; the hemoglobin component of red blood cells carries oxygen to body cells. When comparing the patient's laboratory results to the expected values below, the results indicate that the patient's RBC, Hb, and Hct are all decreased, reflecting a reduced ability to transport oxygen on the hemoglobin molecule of the RBCs. The expected ranges for these laboratory tests for women are:**
    RBC: 3.6 to 5.0 (10^6 cells/mm^3)
    WBC: 5000 to 7000 mm^3
    Hb: 12.0 to 16.0 g/dL
    Hct: 36% to 48%

4. Although increased pulse and respirations may indicate a problem with ventilation, the fact that the respirations are unlabored and the chest radiograph results are within expected limits shows that there is not a problem with ventilation.

Computer Applications in Education and Evaluation

We are members of an informational society in which information is created, stored, retrieved, manipulated, and communicated. Exploding knowledge and technology, the emerging health-care reform initiatives, and the intensified and diversified role of the nurse all add to the complexity of functioning within this informational society. To process information efficiently, effectively, and economically, computers are essential. They have become a reality in every aspect of our world and are used in private homes, educational settings, industry, and health-care facilities. To prepare for a career in nursing, you must have the basic skills to use computers in a comfortable manner and be a willing learner to keep pace with rapidly advancing computer technology. Although computers are used in the practice of nursing, this chapter will focus on the use of computers only in relation to education and evaluation.

Computing across the curriculum is not new in the educational setting. Educators immediately identified the potential of interactive participation to facilitate learning. Programmed-instruction textbooks were the predecessors of computer programs. These textbooks presented information within blocked narrative material. Each grouping of material was called a frame. Each frame required a response from the learner before moving on to the next narrative frame. These textbooks required active involvement by the learner. Computers make this programmed approach more interactive by increasing the potential, richness, and variety of frame styles, which improves the effectiveness of the lesson. Computers also use graphics, color, and sound to facilitate learning in a way that programmed-instruction textbooks were unable to do because of the limitations of the written format.

Students generally enjoy using the computer to facilitate learning because programs hold their attention, provide immediate feedback, and never become impatient. Also, they are accessible, challenging, and fun. Computer-based instruction is not designed to replace the more traditional forms of teaching in most settings but to augment them. Computers allow you to review difficult material at your own rate, increase critical thinking, experience simulated clinical situations, and assess your knowledge and judgment. The greatest advantage of computer-based instruction is that you become an active participant, not just a passive spectator.

To be an active participant, you should have a simple understanding of a few essential keyboard keys. Most programs are "user friendly" and include on-screen instructions, help menus, and/or tutorials. Generally, students do not have difficulty manipulating the keyboard or mouse. However, some students have "computer anxiety." Only exposure to computers in a secure and positive learning environment can lessen computer anxiety and promote computer literacy.

The computer can enhance student learning by accessing professional resources, managing information, teaching, simulating clinical situations, and evaluating knowledge. The following are examples of how computers can be used in education and evaluation.

THE COMPUTER AS A RESOURCE TOOL

The computer is a resource tool that can be used to obtain information for academic assignments. A computerized literature search that uses national databases or networks can provide rapid access to current literature in nursing and its related fields. A modem (a device that allows transmission of data between computers over a telephone or cable line) connects you to the information retrieval system, and specific protocols may be required to gain entry to a database. These searches usually can be conducted in most libraries with the assistance of the research librarian. However, cost may be a factor because lines must be maintained to transmit and receive information. Most systems also have online connect charges for accessing the database as well as for the length of time the database is being used, and a fee may be charged for online or off-line printing. Online printing provides an immediate hard copy of the desired information, whereas off-line printing provides a hard copy that is sent by mail at a later date. Sometimes the fees incurred are beyond the financial means of the average student. Literature searches on the computer save time and energy. Therefore, you must decide whether these activities are cost effective for you by measuring the time saved against the money spent.

THE COMPUTER AS AN INFORMATION MANAGER

The computer has revolutionized the way in which information is managed, not only outside the home but inside the home. Many people now compose written material immediately on the computer. This is possible because you no longer need to have strong keyboard skills or expend extensive time and energy to learn how to use software programs. Today, user-friendly software programs have on-screen commands and effective help menus. Touch, a stylus, or a mouse also help facilitate computer use. The personal computer can be used for word processing, spreadsheets, data processing, creating graphs of data, and so on. You can now manipulate data, words, and images to complete your academic assignments with ease.

THE COMPUTER AS AN INSTRUCTOR

Computer-assisted instruction (CAI) is an excellent addition to the repertoire of strategies available to educators and nursing students to facilitate the learning process. In CAI, information is communicated from the computer to the learner without direct interaction with the teacher. These instructional delivery systems can present principles and theory, enhance comprehension, promote creative problem solving, and provide immediate feedback to enrich independent learning.

Some computer programs display information in a textual format that has limited interaction between you and the computer. These programs really function as an automated textbook. Other tutorial approaches present new information in small steps or frames and then require you to make responses to demonstrate your comprehension of the material just delivered. Such programs function as an automated, programmed-instruction textbook. These types of programs generally use a linear format that proceeds from the beginning of the program to the end of the program without deviation. They present information in a straight line, with one beginning and one end, and every student is exposed to the same information. Although valuable, these programs do not recognize the learner as an individual with specific needs, interests, and abilities.

With the advent of CD-ROM (Compact Disk-Read-Only Memory) technology and sophisticated software programs, the computer learning experience has become more individualized. Programs that use a branching format allow you to select a path that focuses on information relevant to your ability and interest. When programs meet individualized needs, learning is more effective, use of time is more efficient, and student motivation increases.

THE COMPUTER AS A TOOL FOR DISTANCE EDUCATION

Computers and the technology that affects their use are revolutionizing the existing parameters about what is a teaching/learning environment. The age of the Internet has enabled a shift from the typical classroom setting to distance learning/education via the Internet/World Wide Web.

Distance education has created communities of learning that maximize communication between and among students and faculty. Many colleges and universities offer distance education courses in response to the needs of students who have part-time or full-time jobs, family responsibilities, or study-time constraints or who are geographically isolated. Originally, distance education involved print materials; instruction via audio or video cassettes; and communication via telephone, voice mail, and faxing. Today, technological advances, including fixed computer media (e.g., CD-ROM), room-based video conferencing (e.g., interactive television), desktop video conferencing, the World Wide Web (e.g., Internet-based programming), and so on, provide multimedia methods of instruction that many students find more challenging and interesting than the traditional text-based materials. These new methods of delivery promote learning in the cognitive (thinking), affective (feeling), and psychomotor (skills) learning domains inherent in nursing practice, which is an intellectually challenging and social, behavioral, and practice-oriented profession.

Distance education has both advantages and disadvantages and requires a special type of learner.

Advantages of distance education include:

- Accessibility to education for those who are geographically isolated
- Opportunities for learning within a flexible time frame
- Individualized pace of learning
- Active participation
- Self-motivation
- Development of computer literacy

Disadvantages of distance education include:

- Lack of face-to-face communication
- Sense of isolation
- Difficulty with course content in the affective (feelings) and psychomotor (skills) learning domains
- Adjustment to innovative teaching/evaluation strategies
- Pressure to master the technology

Characteristics of students who participate successfully in distance education are:

- Risk takers
- Assertive
- Self-directed
- Responsible

Distance education, particularly in nursing education, is still in its infancy. Important questions exist regarding student financial aid, confidentiality, source of finances for infrastructure, availability of qualified nursing faculty, transferability of credit, delivery of academic support services, appropriate/effective clinical experiences, and valid and reliable methods of evaluation. These concerns have legal and ethical implications that must be addressed for distance education to be a viable alternative for students who want to become nurses. The computer as a tool for distance education has unlimited potential and has already revolutionized higher education. Only the future will tell if computers in relation to distance education will increase the number of graduate nurses and help reverse the nursing shortage.

THE COMPUTER AS A SIMULATOR

The role of the nursing educator is to assist you to move beyond the mere memorization of facts to the application of information in clinical situations. To do this, you must use critical thinking to integrate information into a meaningful frame of reference. Computer simulations are designed to enhance your ability to use critical thinking and safely make sound clinical judgments in a fabricated situation. These simulation programs provide a supportive environment because they usually produce less anxiety and are obviously safe for the "patient." Although computer simulation has long been used in aeronautics and flight training, it is in its childhood in simulating experiences within the health-care professions.

Nursing simulations may present a patient database that requires you to input, sort, and retrieve data. Simulations may focus on the application of information processing skills, which assist you to select sources of data that are most appropriate, classify data, cluster and sequence data, and even evaluate data. Simulations may focus on components of critical thinking. A program addressing critical thinking may require you to identify relationships, recognize commonalities and differences, and use deductive and inductive reasoning to support inferences. Simulations may also be designed to improve decision making by requiring you to identify the nature of the problem, choose a course of action from multiple options, establish priorities, and evaluate the outcome of the final decision. These simulations are maximized by the use of patient simulator manikins that can be programed to reflect human responses. The use of manikins is a fairly recent innovation in nursing education. Historically manikins have been used in nursing education since 1911 when a simple manikin called Mrs. Chase was introduced. Mrs. Chase manikins are still used today to practice the performance of basic fundamental nursing skills. In 1960 Resusci Anne was developed to teach, practice, and evaluate the performance of cardiopulmonary resuscitation (CPR). Numerous forms now available include adult, child, and infant manikins. Resuscitation manikins are more advanced than the Mrs. Chase manikin but not as advanced as high fidelity integrated manikins (e.g., SimMan). These computerized manikins were not routinely used in nursing education until approximately 2009. At that time they became more affordable, and the National Council of State Boards of Nursing issued a position paper that advocated the inclusion of innovative teaching strategies in nursing education. The computers within the manikin are preprogrammed and/or allow faculty to program the manikin to produce human responses such as palpable pulses; normal and abnormal heart, lung, and bowel sounds; the chest rising and falling; blinking the eyes; changing pupillary accommodation; as well as speaking. Preprogrammed scenarios are available that allow students to practice simulated experiences in preparation for clinical experiences or evaluations on the simulator.

Lastly, simulations can present clinical situations that are difficult to present in a classroom setting or events that a student may not have had the opportunity to experience in the clinical setting. Curricula cannot guarantee that every student will have an opportunity to experience each and every situation that may be important to learning. However, computer simulations help to fill this void.

The disadvantage of simulation programs in nursing is that they cannot include all the unpredictable variables that occur in real-life situations. However, interactive videodisc instruction (IVD, IVI), a sophisticated form of computer-assisted instruction, uses the newest computer technology to enrich the clinical situations presented and encourage the highest degree of interaction between a student and the computer. Studies have demonstrated that there is a highly significant degree of student satisfaction with interactive videodisc instruction and that a positive mental attitude is significant to the learning process because of its influence on student motivation, learning rate, and retention and application of information.

THE COMPUTER AS AN EVALUATOR

Evaluation (test-taking) programs are designed to measure your knowledge, skills, and abilities in relation to the practice of nursing. They can be self-administered or administered by a person in authority. Programs devised to be self-administered generally contain both a learning mode and a self-evaluation mode.

In the learning mode, you are presented with a question and are asked to select the correct answer. After you select an option, the program provides immediate feedback regarding the correctness of the choice. Rationales for the correct and wrong answers may be provided, depending on how the program is designed. The learning mode that provides rationales for all the choices has the potential to promote new learning or reinforce previous learning. These types of programs are a form of CAI.

The evaluation mode enables you to conduct an assessment of your test-taking abilities regarding a specific body of knowledge addressed in the program. The evaluation mode also allows you to experience a testing situation. Some programs provide rationales for all the options at the completion of the program. Other, more detailed programs may allow you to design self-tests according to specific parameters (e.g., number of questions, clinical content, steps in the nursing process, difficulty level of the questions, parameters reflective of the NCLEX test plan). Also, it may supply an individualized analysis of your performance after you take a test. This analysis may include information such as the questions you got wrong with rationales, the content areas that you need to study further, your performance in relation to other nursing students, or predictions for passing future examinations. Self-administered evaluation programs are particularly successful because they focus on competency and provide immediate feedback.

An evaluation program conducted by a person in authority may be administered to assess your ability to pass a course of study or to demonstrate your competency for certification or licensure. These programs use computer technology and replace paper-and-pencil tests. Some programs use question and answer testing formats and others use patient simulator manikins. Computer programs that present questions that require the test-taker to select an answer are used to evaluate the competence of a nursing student. Some programs may use a format in which you and every other test taker are confronted by the exact same questions. Other programs may use **computerized-adaptive testing** (CAT), a unique format in which your examination is assembled interactively as you answer each question. In a typical CAT format, all the questions in the test bank have a calculated level of difficulty. You are presented with a question. If you answer the question correctly, you are presented with a slightly more difficult question. If you answer the question incorrectly, you are presented with a slightly easier question. This process is repeated for each question until a pass-or-fail decision is made. Passing is determined by your demonstration of knowledge, skills, and abilities in relation to a standard of acceptable performance. The advantages of the CAT format are that it individualizes each test, provides for self-paced testing, reduces the amount of time needed to complete the test, and produces greater measurement precision. The disadvantages of the CAT format are that you cannot review the entire test before starting, you cannot skip difficult questions and return to them at a later time, and you cannot go back and change an answer once it is selected and entered.

Patient simulator manikins are often used by faculty to evaluate a nursing student's ability to perform specific skills, assess a patient, and/or use clinical judgment in a simulated scenario. Evaluations on a patient simulator manikin can be a stressful experience. Therefore, students should utilize every opportunity to use these patient simulator manikins to advance their knowledge, "clinical experience," and ability to think critically when making clinical judgments.

In 1994 the NCLEX-RN and the NCLEX-PN, the licensure examinations for registered nurses and practical nurses, respectively, changed from standard paper-and-pencil tests to examinations using CAT. Although no previous computer experience is necessary to take a test using CAT, it is always better to be familiar with the particular testing format used. There are many commercial products available that use the CAT format. Practice can only improve your performance on future CAT examinations.

SUMMARY

Computers are causing major changes in the traditional ways things are done in health-care education and evaluation. In our information-savvy society, some certainties exist: we are on information overload; the manipulation of information has become more sophisticated than ever before; and computers will be used more extensively in education, evaluation, and practice in the future. You must become computer literate and be willing to learn about new computer technology as it emerges, such as high-fidelity integrated manikins (Sim Man) used in practice and evaluation of nursing skills and clinical judgment. The most important implication of computer applications in learning, practice, and evaluation is that you can use the computer and simulator manikins to increase the efficiency of your work and study, thereby leaving more time to interact with instructors, peers, and patients.

Analyze Your Test Performance

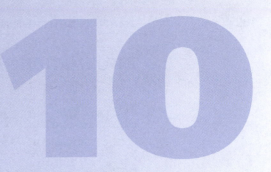

Students work hard at studying course content and learning and using test-taking strategies. However, they seldom progress to the important step of analyzing their test performance to determine their knowledge and information-processing strengths and needs. When reviewing a wrong answer, usually you are able to identify when you did not know the theory or principles being tested. However, without a performance analysis, you may not identify the trends in the gaps in your knowledge because you are lacking the "big picture." In addition, errors often occur because of inept information processing rather than because of lack of knowledge. When reviewing an examination, you might say, "What a silly mistake. I knew that content." This suggests that you probably made an information-processing error. Unless you identify your knowledge gaps and information-processing errors and take corrective action, you probably will continue to make the same mistakes over and over.

Students frequently do not review their test performance because they believe it is time consuming or they do it in a haphazard, rather than a systematic, manner. A methodical analysis of your test performance is well worth the time and effort. It does take time because you have to stop and think critically about each item you answered incorrectly. However, you must spend time to save time. When you focus your study, you will study "better," not longer or harder. Also, the results of an analysis of your test performance should identify your information-processing errors. When you are aware of these errors, you can correct them, which should improve your test-taking abilities and ultimately your test grades.

You may find it threatening to analyze your test performance because it requires you to admit that you may be doing something wrong or that you are unprepared in some manner. You need to *get a grip!* Get over this kind of negative thinking! Finding fault is not the focus of a performance review. We all make mistakes. If we were perfect, we would not be human. The important point is that you must learn from your mistakes. If you are having difficulty with controlling negative thoughts, review Chapter 1, Empowerment. Your goal is to improve your test performance. Identifying your knowledge deficits and information-processing errors should provide a focus for corrective action. This places you in a position of control, which is essential if you are to be successful.

Two tools are presented in this chapter to analyze questions that you answer incorrectly. The first tool, **Information-Processing Analysis,** focuses on the "process" of test taking. This tool has two parts: Processing Errors and Personal Performance Trends. It discloses processing errors in relation to the stem of a question and the options in a question. It also addresses trends in your personal performance in relation to time management, concentration, empowerment, decisiveness/indecisiveness, and clusters of errors. It includes a section for comments for you to make notes about your reactions or questions you may want to explore with your instructor. The second tool, **Knowledge Analysis,** focuses on the "content" aspect of a test. It may identify clusters of errors in specific knowledge categories as well as errors in the steps of the nursing process.

This chapter also contains corrective action guides that address each tool. These guides discuss how to correct your identified errors in the "Analysis" tools and direct you to sections in this text that will help you avoid your errors in the future.

INFORMATION-PROCESSING ANALYSIS TOOL

Information-Processing Analysis Tool

Processing Errors	Question Number																Total
STEM																	
Missed word indicating negative polarity																	
Missed word setting a priority																	
Missed key words that direct attention to content																	
Misinterpreted information presented																	
Missed the central point/theme																	
Missed the central person																	
Read into the question																	
Missed the step in the nursing process (NP)																	
Incompletely analyzed the stem; read it too quickly																	
Did not understand what the question was asking																	
Did not know or did not remember the content associated with the question																	
OPTIONS																	
Answered quickly without reading all the options																	
Failed to respond to negative polarity in stem																	
Misidentified the priority																	
Misinterpreted information																	
Read into option																	
Did not know or did not remember the content																	
Knew content but inaccurately applied concepts and principles																	
Knew the right answer but recorded it inaccurately																	

Personal Performance Trends	Comments
1. I finished the exam with time to review YES { } NO { }	
2. I was able to focus with little distraction YES { } NO { }	
3. I felt calm and in control YES { } NO { }	
4. When I changed answers, I got more questions right rather than wrong YES { } NO { }	

5. Identify error clusters:
   a. First third of exam   { }
   b. Middle third of exam   { }
   c. Last third of exam   { }
   d. "Runs" of errors   { }
   e. No clusters identified { }	

Complete the Processing Errors portion of the Information-Processing Analysis Tool in the following way:

- Review a question you got wrong and determine which processing error caused you to answer the question incorrectly.
- Place the number of the question in the first box to the right of the identified processing error on the tool.
- If you cannot decide between two processing errors or more than one error was involved, put the number of the question next to more than one processing error.
- When another question you got wrong has the same processing error, place the number of the subsequent question in the box to the right of the number of the previous question.
- Insert the number of every question you got wrong on the test into the Processing Errors portion of the Information-Processing Tool.
- Tally the total number of answers you got wrong for each processing error in the last column on the right. Students often will notice a clustering of errors in one area or another.

You can individualize this tool to reflect your specific processing error. For example, if you find that you frequently got questions wrong because you "Read into the question," you could subdivide this area into "Added information from my own mind" and/or "Made assumptions."

Complete the Personal Performance Trends portion of the Information-Processing Analysis Tool in the following way:

- Answer questions 1, 2, 3, and 4. Identify your answer as either YES or NO by placing a mark in the brackets accompanying the question.
- Divide the number of the questions in the test by 3 to determine how many questions are in the first, middle, and last third of the test.
- Count the number of questions you got wrong in the first third of the test and enter that number in the brackets next to 5.a. Do the same for 5.b. and 5.c.
- Look at the questions you got wrong and identify if 2 or more occur in a row or if 3 or more occur close proximity. Enter the number of "runs" you identify in the brackets next to 5.d.
- Place a mark in the brackets next to 5.e. if no error clusters are identified.

CORRECTIVE ACTION GUIDE FOR THE INFORMATION-PROCESSING ANALYSIS TOOL

This Guide has two parts: one that addresses Processing Errors and the other that addresses Personal Performance Trends. Both of these are included in the Information-Processing Analysis Tool. After you have completed the Processing Errors portion of the Information-Processing Analysis Tool, investigate your results with the *Corrective Action Guide for Information-Processing Analysis: Processing Errors*. This section of the guide has three columns:

- Column 1 lists Processing Errors, which are identical to the Processing Errors in column 1 of the Information-Processing Analysis Tool.
- Column 2 refers you to the chapters and sections in this textbook that address information related to the Processing Errors listed in column 1.
- Column 3 indicates the pages where you can find the information listed in column 2.

This portion of the Guide directs you to information that you can review to correct your information-processing problems. For example, if you have multiple "Xs" in the row related to "Missed the word setting a priority," you should review the information about "Identify the Word in the Stem That Sets a Priority" that is included in Chapter 7, Test-Taking Techniques. Review the sections in the book included in column 2 for every processing error that you identify that relates to your performance.

The Processing Errors section of the Guide directs you to information that you can review to enhance your ability to examine the stem of a question and explore the options presented to arrive at the correct answer.

Corrective Action Guide for Processing Errors in the Information-Processing Analysis Tool—cont'd

Processing Errors	Review the Following Sections in this Textbook	Page Number
STEM Missed word indicating negative polarity	**Chapter 7,** Test-Taking Techniques (Identify the Word in the Stem That Indicates Negative Polarity)	98
Missed word setting a priority	**Chapter 7,** Test-Taking Techniques (Identify the Word in the Stem That Sets a Priority)	99
Missed key words that direct attention to content	**Chapter 7,** Test-Taking Techniques (Identify Key Words in the Stem That Direct Attention to Content)	101
Misinterpreted information presented	**Chapter 2,** Critical Thinking (Practice Critical Thinking and Apply Critical Thinking to Multiple-Choice Questions)	12 14
Missed the central point/theme	**Chapter 2,** Critical Thinking (Practice Critical Thinking and Apply Critical Thinking to Multiple-Choice Questions)	12 14
Missed the central person	**Chapter 7,** Test-Taking Techniques (Identify the Central Person in the Question)	102
Read into the question	**Chapter 7,** Test-Taking Techniques (Avoid Reading Into the Question) **Chapter 2,** Critical Thinking (Avoid Reading Into the Question)	116 15
Missed the step in the nursing process (NP)	**Chapter 6,** The Nursing Process (Focus on the step of the nursing process that you misidentified in the knowledge analysis tool)	67–89
Incompletely analyzed the stem	**Chapter 7,** Test-Taking Techniques (Avoid Reading into the Question and Identify Key Words in the Stem That Direct Attention to Content) **Chapter 2,** Critical Thinking (Apply Critical Thinking to Multiple-Choice Questions)	116 101 14
Did not understand what the question was asking	**Chapter 7,** Test-Taking Techniques (Identify Key Words in the Stem That Direct Attention to Content and Avoid Reading Into the Question) **Chapter 2,** Critical Thinking (Practice Critical Thinking and Apply Critical Thinking to Multiple-Choice Questions) **Chapter 11,** Practice Questions with Answers and Rationales (Study answers and rationales of practice questions)	101 116 12 14 173–411
Did not know or did not remember the content associated with the question	**Chapter 4,** Study Techniques (Specific Study Techniques Related to Cognitive Levels of Nursing Questions) **Chapter 11,** Practice Questions with Answers and Rationales (Study answers and rationales of practice questions)	41 173–411

Continued

Corrective Action Guide for Processing Errors in the Information-Processing Analysis Tool—cont'd

Processing Errors	Review the Following Sections in this Textbook	Page Number
OPTIONS Answered quickly without reading all the options	**Chapter 7,** Test-Taking Techniques (Avoid Reading Into the Question)	116
Failed to respond to negative polarity in the stem	**Chapter 7,** Test-Taking Techniques (Identify the Word in the Stem That Indicates Negative Polarity)	98
Misidentified the priority	**Chapter 7,** Test-Taking Techniques (Identify the Word in the Stem That Sets a Priority)	99
	Chapter 11, Practice Questions With Answers and Rationales (Study answers and rationales of practice questions)	173–411
Misinterpreted information	**Chapter 2,** Critical Thinking (Practice Critical Thinking and Apply Critical Thinking to Multiple-Choice Questions)	12 14
Read into options	**Chapter 7,** Test-Taking Techniques (Avoid Reading Into the Question) **Chapter 2,** Critical Thinking (Avoid Reading Into the Question)	116 15
Did not know or did not remember the content	**Chapter 4,** Study Techniques (Specific Study Techniques Related to Cognitive Levels of Nursing Questions) **Chapter 11,** Practice Questions With Answers and Rationales (Study answers and rationales for practice questions)	41 173–411
Knew content but inaccurately applied concepts and principles	**Chapter 2,** Critical Thinking (Apply Critical Thinking to Multiple-Choice Questions) **Chapter 11,** Practice Questions With Answers and Rationales (Study answers and rationales for practice questions)	14 173–411

Personal Performance Trends	Comments
1. I finished the exam with time to review YES { } NO { }	
2. I was able to focus with little distraction YES { } NO { }	
3. I felt calm and in control YES { } NO { }	
4. When I changed answers, I got more questions right rather than wrong YES { } NO { }	

5. Identify error clusters:
    a. First third of exam   { }
    b. Middle third of exam   { }
    c. Last third of exam   { }
    d. "Runs" of errors   { }
    e. No clusters identified { }	

Corrective Action Guide for Personal Performance Trends in the Information-Processing Analysis Tool

The Personal Performance Trends section of the Guide provides a global perspective of your functioning throughout the examination rather than your performance on specific test items. After you have completed the Personal Performance Trends portion of the Information-Processing Analysis Tool, investigate your results with the corrective actions suggested below. This section of the Guide includes issues such as:

Time management (I finished the exam with time to review)

Concentration (I was able to focus with little distraction.)

Empowerment (I felt calm and in control.)

Decisiveness/indecisiveness (When I changed answers, I got the questions right.)

Error clusters (I had no cluster errors; I had error clusters in the first, middle, or last third of an exam or "runs" of error clusters.)

This portion of the Guide focuses on issues that can promote or hinder your performance on an examination. Each personal performance trend statement is accompanied by:

- Comments that specifically relate to the trend being discussed.
- Questions you must ask yourself if you answer NO to statements 1 through 4 or if you identify error clusters in statement 5.
- A Review that refers you to content in the book that explores information related to the personal performance trend being discussed.

1. I FINISHED THE EXAM WITH TIME TO REVIEW

If your answer was YES, you have managed your time well. If your answer was NO, you are not managing your time effectively and you need to identify why you are taking too long to proceed through the test. You must answer the following questions:

- Am I taking too much time to answer each question?
- Am I getting bogged down and spending too much time on a few difficult questions that prevent me from finishing or reviewing the test?
- (Other) Identify your own questions.

Review

Chapter 7, Test-Taking Techniques: Manage the Allotted Time to Your Advantage, page 115.

Chapter 7, Test-Taking Techniques: Concentrate on the Simple Before the Complex, page 116.

2. I WAS ABLE TO FOCUS WITH LITTLE DISTRACTION

If your answer was YES, you have sufficient concentration and the ability to block out distractions. If your answer was NO, you must answer the following questions:

- Am I fatigued before and/or during the test?
- Do distractions in the environment cause me to lose focus?
- Was I physically uncomfortable during the test?
- (Other) Identify your own questions.

Review

Chapter 1, Empowerment: Establish Control Before and During the Test, page 6.

3. I FELT CALM AND IN CONTROL

If your answer was YES, you have anxiety under control and are able to focus on the test rather than having to cope with anxious responses. If your answer was NO, you must answer the following questions:

- Do I experience uncomfortable, fearful responses during exams?
- Do I experience internal mental stressors (negative self-talk) that block my confidence?

- Do I get flustered when confronted with a question that I am unable to answer?
- (Other) Identify your own questions.

Review

Chapter 1, Empowerment: Develop a Positive Mental Attitude, page 1.
Chapter 7, Test-Taking Techniques: Maintain a Positive Mental Attitude, page 117.

4. WHEN I CHANGED ANSWERS I GOT MORE QUESTIONS RIGHT RATHER THAN WRONG

Some examinations, especially those taken on a computer, do not permit a review of previously answered questions. However, others allocate time for a short review at the end of the examination. During review of your answers at the end of an examination you may be tempted to change your original answer to another option that you now believe is the correct answer. It is critical for you to know if you are changing correct answers to wrong answers or wrong answers to correct answers when reviewing questions. If you answered YES to the question, "When I changed answers, I got more questions right rather than wrong" you are able to change answers based on careful review of the stem and options. If you answered NO to the question you must ask yourself the following questions:

- What causes me to change my answers?
- Do I lack confidence when I answer a question?
- Why do I keep changing answers when I know I always change correct answers to wrong answers?
- (Other) Identify your own questions.

Analyze whether changing answers works to your advantage. Every time you review a test, evaluate your accuracy in changing answers. Keep score of how many answers you changed from wrong to right and how many you changed from right to wrong.

If the number of items you changed from wrong to right is greater than the number of items you changed from right to wrong, it probably is to your advantage to change answers you ultimately believe you answered incorrectly. Subsequent questions may have contained content that was helpful in answering a previous question, you may have accessed information you did not remember originally, or you may be better able to assess the question with more objectivity at the end of the test when you personally feel less pressure to finish.

If the number of items you changed from right to wrong is greater than the number of items you changed from wrong to right, you should avoid changing your answers unless you are absolutely positive that your second choice is the correct answer. As the end of an examination approaches, some people tend to experience more anxiety, not less, which interferes with perception and the processing of information. If you tend to change answers to the wrong answer, leave your eraser home or sit on your hands so that you do not change the answer!

When considering changing an answer to a previously answered question, use test-taking techniques to increase your ability to focus on what the question is asking and eliminate distractors. A careful review may dissect the question into its component parts, thereby revealing a key word or clue that assists you to reconsider your previous answer.

Review

Chapter 7, Test-Taking Techniques, page 97.

Chapter 8, Testing formats Other Than Multiple-Choice Questions, page 125.

Chapter 11, Practice Questions With Answers and Rationales (Most questions contain test-taking tips), pages 173–411.

5. IDENTIFY ERROR CLUSTERS

The purpose of identifying error clusters is to determine if anxiety or fatigue is affecting your performance. If you identify a group of errors at the beginning, middle, or end of an examination or you identify "runs" of incorrect answers (two or more incorrect answers in a row or three or more in close proximity) you need to analyze what is happening. You must ask yourself the following questions:

- Do I get anxious before or during the exam?
- Do I get tired?
- Do I get flustered when confronted with a difficult question?
- Do I lose my ability to concentrate?
- (Other) Identify your own questions.

Review

Errors that occur in the first third of an exam: If your errors occur in the beginning of an exam, you may want to use techniques that allow you to control the testing environment or use anxiety reduction techniques just before the exam begins to feel more in control and therefore less anxious.

> Chapter 1, Empowerment: Establish Control Before and During the Test, page 6.
> Chapter 1, Empowerment: Develop a Positive Mental Attitude, page 1.

Errors that occur in the middle third of an exam or in clusters throughout an exam: If you find that errors occur in the middle third of the exam or runs of error clusters occur after every 20 or 30 questions, you may need to reduce tension and anxiety. We counselled a graduate nurse who did not pass the National Council Licensure Examination for Registered Nurses (NCLEX-RN) after two attempts. When assessing her performance on a practice examination, we identified the fact that every 30 minutes she made four or five errors in a row. We encouraged her to take a break every 25 minutes until she completed the examination. On her next attempt, she passed the NCLEX-RN. A break every 25 minutes was the key change in her approach to the NCLEX-RN. In the classroom setting, this may be impossible; therefore, you should engage in a relaxation technique that works for you for 2 or 3 minutes. In addition you can visualize a person who supports you emotionally standing beside you and giving you encouragement during the examination or use positive self-talk by saying, "I can do this," or "I studied hard for this exam." Remember, relaxation techniques must be practiced to be effective and should be conducted in a simulated testing situation before a real testing situation. Recognize that if you implement relaxation techniques during a test, you must adjust the time you allot for each question and your review.

> Chapter 1, Empowerment: Challenge Negative Thoughts, page 2.
>
> Chapter 1, Empowerment: Use Controlled Breathing (Diaphragmatic Breathing), page 2.
>
> Chapter 1, Empowerment: Perform Muscle Relaxation, page 4.
>
> Chapter 1, Empowerment: Use Imagery, page 5.

Errors that occur in the last third of an exam: If you find that the majority of your errors occur during the last third of an exam, you may need to practice increasing your test-taking stamina by practicing test taking for longer periods of time. Stamina also can be increased by practicing test taking in a simulated testing environment.

> Chapter 1, Empowerment: Exercise Regularly, page 6.
>
> Chapter 4, Study Techniques: Simulate a Testing Environment, page 38.
>
> Chapter 4, Study Techniques: Practice Test Taking, page 49.

KNOWLEDGE ANALYSIS TOOL

The Knowledge Analysis Tool has two parts: Knowledge Categories and Nursing Process. Knowledge categories include the range of basic information that is the foundation of nursing practice. The Nursing Process section of the tool includes the steps of the nursing process: assessment, analysis, planning, implementation and evaluation. The nursing process provides a systematic approach to the delivery of nursing care.

Knowledge Analysis Tool

Knowledge Categories	Question Number
Legal/ethical issues	
Health-care delivery systems	
Basic human needs	
Growth and development	
Communication	
Emotional needs	
Physical assessment	
Physical safety	
Mobility	
Hygiene	
Pain and comfort	
Rest and sleep	
Nutrition	
Fluid and electrolytes	
Urinary elimination	
Bowel elimination	
Oxygen	
Microbiological safety	
Administration of medications	
Pharmacology	
Perioperative	
Community setting	
Pathophysiology	
Anatomy and physiology	
Computations	
Nursing Process	
Assessment	
Analysis	
Planning	
Implementation	
Evaluation	

Complete the Knowledge Categories portion of the Knowledge Analysis Tool in the following way:

- Review a question you got wrong and determine which knowledge category best represents the content being tested in the question.
- Place the number of the question in the first box to the right of the identified knowledge category on the tool.
- If you cannot decide between two knowledge categories, put the number of the question next to more than one knowledge category.
- When another question you got wrong has the same knowledge category, place the number of the subsequent question in the box to the right of the previous question.
- Insert the number of every question you got wrong on the test into the Knowledge Categories portion of the Knowledge Analysis Tool.
- Tally the total number of answers you got wrong for each knowledge category in the last column on the right. Students often will notice a clustering of errors in one or more category.

If you find that you got many questions wrong in one of the categories, you may identify subdivisions to the category. For example, if you got many questions wrong in the area of perioperative nursing, you could subdivide this area into "Preoperative," "Intraoperative," and "Postoperative."

Complete the Nursing Process portion of the Knowledge Analysis Tool in the following way:

- Review a question you got wrong and determine which step of the nursing process best represents the content being tested in the question. Identify just one step of the nursing process for each question you got wrong.
- Place the number of the question in the first box to the right of the step in the nursing process you identified.
- When another question you got wrong reflects the same step of the nursing process, place the number of the subsequent question in the box to the right of the previous question.
- Insert the number of every question you got wrong on the test into the Nursing Process portion of the Knowledge Analysis Tool.
- Tally the total number of answers you got wrong for each step of the nursing process in the last column on the right. Students often will notice a clustering of errors in one or two steps of the nursing process.

CORRECTIVE ACTION GUIDE FOR THE KNOWLEDGE ANALYSIS TOOL

This Guide has two parts: Knowledge Categories and Nursing Process. Knowledge Categories include the broad areas of information that form the basics of nursing practice. Evaluating your performance using this section of the tool will help identify your gaps in knowledge. The Nursing Process portion of the tool reflects the steps of the nursing process: assessment, analysis, planning, implementation, and evaluation. Exploring your performance using this section of the tool will help identify your difficulties in performing critical thinking and problem-solving behaviors within the practice of nursing. Remember, the nursing process is a systematic approach that uses critical thinking to provide nursing care.

Corrective Action Guide for the Knowledge Categories in the Knowledge Analysis Tool

First, complete the Knowledge Categories portion of the Knowledge Analysis Tool. Then, identify the knowledge categories that have question numbers indicating answers that are incorrect. The more wrong answers within a category, the less knowledge you have of the content within the category. The more categories in which you have wrong answers the broader your lack of nursing knowledge. The related nursing content for each wrong answer should be explored. However, when time is limited, focus on those knowledge areas with the most wrong answers.

Studying is essential to learning, which is a complex activity. Most people study before a test. However, it is essential also to study after a test. When you identify a practice question that you answered incorrectly, reread your class notes and textbook regarding that topic. Discuss it with your instructor if you still do not understand the content. When you have a thorough understanding of the content being tested you will be better able to identify the correct answer. In addition, you will have more confidence in the option you select and be less likely to change your answer later during the examination.

One of the best ways to achieve a higher grade on a test is to be overprepared. Compare and contrast class notes with information within your textbook. Study in a small group with your peers to obtain different perspectives on material in a specific knowledge category or when analyzing a test item. Practice the questions in Chapter 11 and review the rationales for the correct and incorrect answers. Understanding complex concepts usually requires a variety of study approaches and repetition.

Review

Chapter 4, General Study Techniques, page 37.

Chapter 4, Specific Study Techniques Related to Cognitive Levels of Nursing Questions, page 41.

Chapter 1, Empowerment: Overprepare for a Test, page 5.

Chapter 11, Practice Questions with Answers and Rationales, pages 173–411.

Corrective Action Guide for the Nursing Process in the Knowledge Analysis Tool

First, complete the Nursing Process portion of the Knowledge Analysis Tool. Then, identify the steps of the nursing process that have question numbers indicating answers that are incorrect. The more wrong answers within a particular step of the nursing process, the more significant your difficulties will be in answering questions that require the typical thinking behaviors associated with that step. For example, assessment questions may require you to collect or analyze data, whereas planning questions may require you to set goals or identify priorities.

Read the stem and each option carefully when taking a simulated practice examination. Determine which step of the nursing process is reflected by the question before even attempting to answer the question. When you are able to identify the question's placement within the nursing process it will provide a focus for a more in-depth review of the stem and options. It should facilitate your identification of what the test item is asking.

Review

Chapter 2, Critical Thinking, page 9.

Chapter 6, The Nursing Process, page 67.

SUMMARY

You should use these test-analysis tools to assess your test performance after taking a practice examination. Then you should use these tools when reviewing every examination you take in class. Do not be shy in asking your instructor for help with your analysis. Nursing instructors who are student centered will help you with this analysis during class or office hours because instructors have a vested interest in your success. Analysis of your test performance is essential if you are to identify your own individual learning needs. After your learning needs are identified using the presented tools, the Corrective Action Guides should direct you to information that can improve your abilities. Engaging in activities that analyze your test performance is time well spent!

Practice Questions With Answers and Rationales

Chapter 11 contains 500 questions divided into 14 categories of basic nursing practice. Each category contains between 25 and 40 test items. These items provide an opportunity for you to apply the test-taking techniques that were presented in Chapter 7. A test-taking technique is a strategy that uses skill and forethought to analyze a test item before selecting an answer. Every test item should be examined to determine if any of the test-taking techniques apply. When it is appropriate to use a test-taking technique, a **Test-Taking Tip** follows the item. Some items do not have a Test-Taking Tip because test-taking techniques do not pertain to every item.

The Test-Taking Tip cues you to one or more of the strategies that can assist you in arriving at the correct answer. These strategies were discussed in Chapter 7 under Specific Test-Taking Techniques. Use the Test-Taking Tip to examine the question with consideration and thoughtfulness. The rationales for items are given at the end of each category and address the following:

- Application of the Test-Taking Tip
- Identification of the correct answer
- Rationale for why the correct answer is correct
- Rationale for why each distractor is incorrect

THE WORLD OF THE PATIENT AND NURSE

This section includes factors that influence the role of the nurse and the delivery of health care. Questions address ethics, legal aspects of nursing practice, the nursing process, the responsibilities associated with the management of nursing practice (including delegation to and supervision of members of the nursing team), meeting the spiritual needs of patients, patients' rights, the difference between dependent and independent roles of the nurse, standards of nursing practice, and agencies that provide structure for the delivery of health care.

QUESTIONS

1. A patient tells the nurse, "My new bathrobe is missing." Which is the **most** appropriate response by the nurse?
   1. Determine if the patient is angry.
   2. Initiate a search for the patient's bathrobe.
   3. Provide an isolation gown that can be used as a robe.
   4. State that it must have gone down with the soiled linen.

   TEST-TAKING TIP Identify the word in the stem that sets a priority. Identify the clang association. Identify the patient-centered option. Identify the option that denies the patient's feelings, concerns, or needs.

2. Which is the **most** important reason why it is necessary that the nurse understand the scientific rationale for the actions that constitute a procedure?
   1. Document the nursing care given.
   2. Explain the required nursing care.
   3. Implement the nursing care safely.
   4. Formulate the nursing plan of care.

   TEST-TAKING TIP Identify the word in the stem that sets a priority.

3. A nurse observes a patient going into another patient's room without permission, which upsets the other patient. Which should the nurse do **first** when responding to the wandering patient?
   1. Help the patient to the correct room.
   2. Place the patient in restraints temporarily.
   3. Determine the motivation for the patient's behavior.
   4. Share the observation about the patient with the health-care team.

   TEST-TAKING TIP Identify the word in the stem that sets a priority. Identify the central person in the question. Identify patient-centered options.

4. Which information **best** describes a voluntary agency?
   1. Supported by unpaid helpers and contributors
   2. Privately owned and operated for profit
   3. Health maintenance organization
   4. Nonprofit organization

   TEST-TAKING TIP Identify the word in the stem that sets a priority. Identify the key word in the stem that directs attention to content. Identify opposites in options.

5. A nurse in charge directs another nurse to do something that is outside the legal role of the nurse. Which should the nurse do in response to this direction?
   1. Decline the assigned task.
   2. Complete the delegated task.
   3. Inform the union representative.
   4. Notify the supervisor immediately.

   TEST-TAKING TIP Identify opposites in options.

6. A patient is legally determined to have died. When should the nurse begin postmortem care?
   1. As soon as death is pronounced
   2. After significant others have left
   3. Once the nursing supervisor is informed
   4. Only after the primary health-care provider is notified

   TEST-TAKING TIP Identify the option with a specific determiner. Identify the unique option.

7. An example of a goal identified by a nurse when planning a patient's plan of care is, "The patient will:
   1. Maintain a weight of 140 pounds."
   2. Need small, frequent feedings."
   3. Be at risk for weight loss."
   4. Be assisted with meals."

   TEST-TAKING TIP Identify the unique option.

8. Which is the **first** task to be completed by the nurse when arriving on the unit for work?
   1. Count controlled drugs with the nurse going off shift.
   2. Make rounds to check on the safety of patients.
   3. Prioritize care to be completed during the shift.
   4. Receive a report on the status of patients.

   TEST-TAKING TIP Identify the word in the stem that sets a priority. Identify the key word in the stem that directs attention to content.

9. A nurse breaks a patient's dentures because of carelessness. Which specific legal term applies to this action?
   1. Battery
   2. Assault
   3. Negligence
   4. Malpractice

10. A nurse is caring for a patient who is often argumentative and demanding. Which is the **best** intervention when planning care for this patient?
    1. Bring another nurse as a witness.
    2. Involve the patient in decision making.
    3. Accept the behavior as probably a lifelong pattern.
    4. Explain that the staff would appreciate the patient's cooperation.

    TEST-TAKING TIP Identify the word in the stem that sets a priority. Identify key words in the stem that direct attention to content. Identify opposites in options. Identify the patient-centered option. Identify the option that denies the patient's feelings, concerns, or needs.

11. Which statement describes the purpose of the American Nurses' Association (ANA) Standards of Nursing Practice?
    1. Legal statutes that guide nursing actions
    2. Progressive actions for a nursing procedure
    3. Requirements for registered nurse licensure
    4. Policy statements defining the obligations of nurses

    TEST-TAKING TIP Identify the key word in the stem that directs attention to content.

12. A patient with dementia needs assistance with hygiene, grooming, eating, and toileting. Which agency **best** meets this patient's needs after discharge from the hospital?
    1. Nursing home
    2. Psychiatric institution
    3. Outpatient care facility
    4. Adult day-care program

    TEST-TAKING TIP Identify the word in the stem that sets a priority. Identify key words in the stem that direct attention to content.

13. A nurse observes a multiple-vehicle collision in which several people are seriously injured and stops to offer assistance. Which legal principle is in operation in this situation?
    1. A legal trust that accompanies a nursing license applies to this situation.
    2. The nurse can be held legally responsible for care provided.
    3. Immunity is afforded because a contract does not exist.
    4. Immunity is provided by the Good Samaritan Law.

    TEST-TAKING TIP Identify clang associations. Identify opposites in options.

14. A nurse says to a patient, "You should get a second opinion because your primary health-care provider is not the best." For which can the nurse be sued?
    1. Libel
    2. Assault
    3. Slander
    4. Negligence

15. A nurse obtains an informed consent from a patient who is to have an invasive procedure. Which does the nurse's signature on the informed consent form indicate?
    1. Surgeon described the procedure and its potential risks
    2. Patient knows and understands expected outcomes
    3. Patient actually signed the consent form
    4. Surgeon is protected from being sued

    TEST-TAKING TIP Identify the clang association. Identify equally plausible options.

16. A nurse observes another nurse treating a patient in an abusive manner. Which should the nurse do **first?**
    1. Tell the nurse in charge and write a report.
    2. Become a role model for the other nurse.
    3. Talk with the nurse about the incident.
    4. Reassure and calm the patient.

    TEST-TAKING TIP Identify the word in the stem that sets a priority. Identify the central person in the question. Identify the unique option. Identify the patient-centered option.

17. Which is the purpose of the National Council Licensure Examination for Registered Nurses (NCLEX-RN)?
    1. Identify minimal safe practice
    2. Accredit schools of nursing
    3. Control nursing education
    4. Verify graduation

    TEST-TAKING TIP Identify equally plausible options. Identify the unique option.

18. When obtaining a health history, the nurse identifies that a patient has gained 10 pounds in the past week. Which step of the nursing process is performed when the nurse documents this information in the patient's clinical record?
    1. Analysis
    2. Planning
    3. Evaluation
    4. Assessment

19. A nurse assigns a Nursing Assistant to a patient who transfers to a chair with a mechanical lift. It has been a long time since the Nursing Assistant has used the lift. Which should the nurse do to ensure the safety of the patient?
    1. Request that another Nursing Assistant assist with the patient's care.
    2. Ask the Nursing Assistant to demonstrate how to use the lift.
    3. Explain to the Nursing Assistant how to use the lift.
    4. Assign the patient to another Nursing Assistant.

    TEST-TAKING TIP Identify equally plausible options. Identify clang associations.

20. A male patient has dementia. He is verbally and physically abusive and paranoid. Which should the nurse always do when providing care?
    1. Compliment him on how nice he looks.
    2. Administer care as quickly as possible.
    3. Explain what care is to be done.
    4. Tell him what he wants to hear.

    TEST-TAKING TIP Identify the word in the stem that sets a priority. Identify the key word in the stem that directs attention to content. Identify equally plausible options.

21. A patient says, "I don't like anyone to go into my closet or drawers." Which should the nurse do when returning hygiene equipment to the patient's bedside cabinet?
    1. Store the materials on the overbed table.
    2. Allow the patient to put the equipment away.
    3. Provide reassurance that personal things will not be taken.
    4. Explain the hazard of not putting equipment away as it is being done.

    TEST-TAKING TIP Identify the clang association. Identify opposites in options. Identify the patient-centered option. Identify options that deny patient feelings, concerns, or needs.

22. A primary nurse, responsible for a group of patients, is delegating responsibilities to the other members of the nursing team. Which tasks should the nurse include when formulating an assignment for the nursing assistant? **Select all that apply.**
    1. _____ Monitoring patients' tube feedings
    2. _____ Assisting patients with eating meals
    3. _____ Ambulating patients outside their rooms
    4. _____ Regulating patients' intravenous solutions
    5. _____ Supervising patients when they are taking medications

    TEST-TAKING TIP Identify key words in the stem that direct attention to content.

23. The nurse is involved in a patient situation that presents an ethical dilemma. The nurse refers to an ethical decision-making algorithm to assist in arriving at a solution. Place the steps presented in the order in which they should occur?
    1. State the dilemma.
    2. List potential solutions.
    3. Collect, analyze, and interpret data.
    4. Determine if the dilemma can be resolved by a nurse.
    5. Implement nursing actions that have acceptable consequences.

    Answer: _____

24. Which situation is an example of an intentional tort? **Select all that apply.**
    1. _____ Forgetting to administer a STAT medication
    2. _____ Performing a procedure without informed consent
    3. _____ Carelessly administering a medication to the wrong patient
    4. _____ Threatening to withhold pain medication if a patient does not behave
    5. _____ Applying a restraint without an order when a patient is at risk for self-harm

    TEST-TAKING TIP Identify key words in the stem that direct attention to content.

25. Which actions by a nurse violate patient confidentiality and privacy? **Select all that apply.**
    1. _____ Interviewing a patient in the presence of others
    2. _____ Writing patient statements in the progress notes
    3. _____ Disclosing patient information to family members
    4. _____ Presenting the patient's problems at a team conference
    5. _____ Sharing data about a patient at the change of shift report

    TEST-TAKING TIP Identify the word in the stem that indicates negative polarity. Identify key words in the stem that direct attention to content.

26. Nurses must respect the expectations and responsibilities of patients and inform them of the Patient Care Partnership (formerly Patient Bill of Rights). Which patient expectations are included in the Patient Care Partnership? **Select all that apply.**
    1. _____ Being able to smoke in their rooms
    2. _____ Requesting to know the identity of caregivers
    3. _____ Demanding that they be moved to private rooms
    4. _____ Receiving accurate information about their diagnosis
    5. _____ Refusing a treatment ordered by their primary health-care provider

27. A nurse is completing an Unusual Occurrence Report because of an event that occurred in the hospital. The nurse entered a description of the event in the section titled, "Provide a Brief Description of the Event." Place a check in the box in front of the **most** appropriate contributing factor in the "What are the Contributing Factors" section of the report that relates to this event.

Unusual Occurrence Report

Date of Event: _____ Time of Event: _____ Department: _____

Patient Last Name:	First Name:	MI:
Patient #:	Attending Physician:	
Visitor Last Name:	First Name:	Phone #:
Employee Name:	Dept:	
Physician Name:	Specialty:	

Occurrence Category (Check most appropriate)

☐ Agency nurse-related	☐ AMA	☐ Delay in treatment
☐ Diet-related	☐ HIPAA compliance	☐ Loss of personal property
☐ Medication-related	☐ Narcotics-related	☐ Order not executed
☐ Patient injury	☐ Peer-review related	☐ Restraint-related
☐ Staff injury	☐ Supplies/Equipment	☐ Visitor injury

☐ Other (please explain):

Description of Occurrence:

A patient overheard a nurse sharing information about the patient's diagnosis and treatment to a visitor in the hall. The patient reported this event to the nurse in charge and stated, "I am very upset".

Contributing Factors (Check all that apply)

☐ Individual:	☐ System:
Knowledge, skills, and/or experience: ☐ Unclear ☐ Incomplete	Policies/procedures not in place: ☐ Unclear ☐ Outdated
☐ Non-adherence to standard of care or practice	Environmental: ☐ Staffing ☐ Patient acuity ☐ Congestion
☐ Documentation incomplete or inadequate	Communications and work flow: ☐ Intradepartmental ☐Interdepartmental
	☐ Equipment failure

Other (please explain):

Submitted by:	Dept:	Date:

TEST-TAKING TIP Identify the word in the stem that sets a priority.

28. A registered nurse is the leader of a team consisting of 1 licensed practical nurse and 2 nursing assistants. Which assignments should the registered nurse delegate to the licensed practical nurse? **Select all that apply.**
1. _____ Administer a medication via the direct intravenous push technique
2. _____ Develop a nursing plan of care for a newly admitted patient
3. _____ Perform a venipuncture to obtain a blood specimen
4. _____ Change a dressing on a pressure ulcer
5. _____ Collect clinical data about patients

29. Which activities are dependent functions of the nurse? **Select all that apply.**
1. _____ Ambulating a patient down the hall
2. _____ Documenting perioperative nursing care
3. _____ Changing a sterile dressing that is soiled
4. _____ Providing oxygen for acute shortness of breath
5. _____ Assisting with selection of choices on the menu

TEST-TAKING TIP Identify the key word in the stem that directs attention to content.

30. Ethics is specifically concerned with which of the following? **Select all that apply.**
1. _____ Preventing a crime
2. _____ Protecting civil law
3. _____ Making value judgments
4. _____ Identifying negligent acts
5. _____ Determining right or wrong

31. A nurse is formulating a Nursing Assistant assignment. Which activities should the nurse delegate to the Nursing Assistant? **Select all that apply.**
1. _____ Reporting unusual clinical manifestations to the nurse
2. _____ Ensuring that patients swallow their medication
3. _____ Orienting a new employee to the unit
4. _____ Teaching patients personal hygiene
5. _____ Distributing meal trays to patients

TEST-TAKING TIP Identify key words in the stem that direct attention to content.

32. Place the following nursing activities in the order in which they should be performed when progressing through the *nursing process*, beginning with assessment and ending with evaluation.
1. Changing a sterile dressing
2. Formulating a short-term goal
3. Obtaining a patient's vital signs
4. Concluding a patient is dehydrated
5. Identifying a need to modify the plan of care

Answer: _____

TEST-TAKING TIP Identify key words in the stem that direct attention to content.

33. A nurse who is a member of a quality improvement committee reviews a chart detailing trends of 4 problem categories identified in Incident Reports over a 4-month period of time. Corrective action plans were implemented to address each problem category. After analyzing the chart documenting trends over the successive months of March, April, and May, which problem category should cause the **most** concern?

1. Falls
2. Medication errors
3. Violations of confidentiality
4. Failures to maintain standards of practice

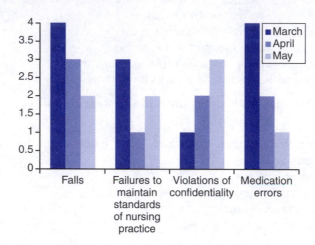

TEST-TAKING TIP Identify the word in the stem that sets a priority.

34. Which statement indicates that the nurse is using deductive reasoning? **Select all that apply.**

1. _____ A patient is admitted with a diagnosis of dehydration and the nurse assesses the patient's skin for tenting.
2. _____ A nurse observes a patient fall out of bed on the right hip and immediately assesses the patient for pain in the right hip.
3. _____ A patient has an elevated white blood cell count and a fever. The nurse concludes that the patient may have an infection.
4. _____ A patient is scheduled for surgery and is crying, trembling, and has a rapid pulse. The nurse makes the inference that the patient is anxious.
5. _____ A nurse in the emergency department reports to a nurse on a medical unit that a patient with hypoglycemia is being admitted. The nurse assesses the patient for pale, cool, clammy skin and a low blood glucose level.

TEST-TAKING TIP Identify key words in the stem that direct attention to content.

35. Which action or inaction by a nurse is an example of an unintentional tort? **Select all that that apply.**

1. _____ Failure to stop at an automobile collision to render first aid
2. _____ Failure to recognize a cluster of data that indicated a safety problem causing injury to a patient
3. _____ Failure to identify the signs and symptoms of hyperglycemia causing a life-threatening event
4. _____ Fracturing a patient's rib while implementing cardiopulmonary resuscitation that followed appropriate standards of care
5. _____ Refusal to be transferred to a unit for which the nurse does not feel adequately prepared to provide an acceptable level of care

TEST-TAKING TIP Identify key words in the stem that direct attention to content.

36. A registered nurse is the leader of a team consisting of two nursing assistants. Which assignments should the registered nurse keep rather than assign to one of the nursing assistants? **Select all that apply.**
    1. ____ Evaluating a patient's response to the administration of an analgesic
    2. ____ Emptying the collection bag of a urinary retention catheter
    3. ____ Obtaining a specimen of exudate from a draining wound
    4. ____ Taking routine vital signs of patients who are stable
    5. ____ Assisting patients with range-of-motion exercises

37. An older adult is to be discharged from the hospital after being treated with intravenous antibiotics for pneumonia. A nursing case manager is assessing the patient's physical, emotional, and socioeconomic needs. The nurse reviews the primary health-care provider's summary and interviews the patient and the patient's son. Which setting should the nurse explore with the patient and son because it is the **most** appropriate setting for the patient when discharged from the hospital?
    1. Independent living facility
    2. Assisted living facility
    3. Day-care program
    4. Nursing home

PATIENT INFORMATION

Primary Health-Care Provider's Summary
The patient is an 86-year-old woman who has emphysema and arthritis of the hands and knees. She is capable of performing the activities of daily living but should use a wheelchair when walking long distances. Her vital signs are within acceptable limits of an individual her age. She should continue medical supervision every 3 months.

Interview of Patient
Patient looking forward to discharge. She stated, "I like my privacy. I prefer to take care of myself." Patient indicated difficulty getting to the store now that she no longer drives. She also stated, "I am a little lonely living by myself and I am so sick of making the same old meals all the time."

Interview of Patient's Son
Patient's son works full time and has an active social life on the weekends. He stated, "I would like her to live with me but it really is impossible. I am never home." The son indicated that his mother has ample financial resources for whatever she decides to do.

TEST-TAKING TIP Identify the word in the stem that sets a priority.

38. An emergency department nurse is caring for a patient with a history of chronic pulmonary disease who presented with shortness of breath, a dry oral cavity, and furrows of the tongue. In addition, the patient is using accessory muscles to breathe. Which actions can be implemented independently by the nurse? **Select all that apply.**
    1. ____ Take the vital signs
    2. ____ Encourage fluid intake
    3. ____ Monitor oxygen saturation
    4. ____ Place the patient in the high-Fowler position
    5. ____ Assess the lungs for adventitious breath sounds

    TEST-TAKING TIP Identify key words in the stem that direct attention to content.

39. A nurse is caring for a patient who has a small statue on the bedside table similar to the illustration. Which should the nurse recognize that this rendition of a revered figure represents?

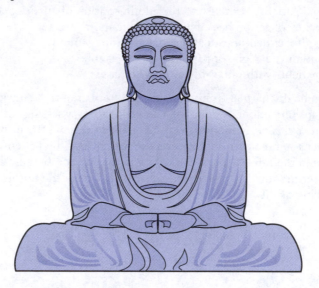

1. A model of the right way of life
2. Allah and the six articles of faith
3. The mediator between God and humankind
4. Belief that the Old Testament shows them how to worship

40. A nurse is planning to delegate patient care to a Nursing Assistant. Which are appropriate activities for a Nursing Assistant? **Select all that apply.**
1. _____ Evaluating vital signs
2. _____ Making occupied beds
3. _____ Monitoring tube feedings
4. _____ Providing patients with physical hygiene
5. _____ Assisting postoperative patients with their first ambulation

TEST-TAKING TIP Identify key words in the stem that direct attention to content.

1. **TEST-TAKING TIP** The word "most" in the stem sets a priority. The word "bathrobe" in the stem and in option 2 is a clang association. Option 2 is patient centered. Option 4 denies the patient's feelings, concerns, or needs.
   1. Determining if the patient is angry does not address the problem of the missing bathrobe.
   2. **Patients have a right to expect that efforts will be implemented to ensure security for their belongings.**
   3. Although this may be done, it does not address the problem of the missing bathrobe.
   4. Explaining what may have happened does not address the feeling of loss or the need to find the bathrobe.

2. **TEST-TAKING TIP** The word "most" in the stem sets a priority.
   1. Knowledge of the scientific rationale for care given is not necessary for the act of documentation.
   2. Although it is important to explain all care to the patient, it is not the priority.
   3. **The safety of the patient always takes priority; the nurse must perform only those skills that are understood and have been practiced.**
   4. Although nurses need to understand scientific rationales to appropriately plan care, it is not the priority.

3. **TEST-TAKING TIP** The word "first" in the stem sets a priority. The patient in the room was the patient who was violated and is the central person in the question. Options 1 and 2 are patient centered. Controlling the wandering patient's behavior protects the violated patient. Options 2 and 3 focus on the wandering patient, not on the patient who was violated. Because restraints are inappropriate unless less restrictive measures are tried first to control the wandering patient's behavior, option 2 can be eliminated.
   1. **Patients have a right to privacy and security for themselves and their belongings; helping the patient to the correct room protects the other patient.**
   2. Restraining patients for any reason other than their own physical safety or the safety of others is illegal; it is false imprisonment.
   3. This is not the priority. The nurse can explore the motivation for the behavior later.
   4. Sharing the observation with the health-care team does not address the immediate need. After the behavior is addressed, it can be communicated.

4. **TEST-TAKING TIP** The word "best" in the stem sets a priority. The word "voluntary" is the key word in the stem that directs attention to content. Options 2 and 4 are opposites.
   1. Although volunteers serve as helpers and contributors provide financial support to voluntary agencies, these are not the reason for the classification; voluntary agencies are nonprofit organizations.
   2. A privately owned and operated agency for profit is a proprietary agency.
   3. A health maintenance organization (HMO) is a form of health-care delivery and does not reflect how the organization is funded. An HMO can be voluntary (nonprofit) or proprietary (for profit) and, with emerging health-care reform, some may be official agencies (supported by government funds).
   4. **Voluntary agencies may not make a profit; any money made must be applied to operating expenses and provision of services.**

5. **TEST-TAKING TIP** Options 3 and 4 are opposites.
   1. **Performing a task that is outside the legal definition of the nurse is illegal; a nurse has the responsibility to refuse to follow an order that is illegal.**
   2. Nurses should perform only those tasks that they are licensed to perform.
   3. Eventually the union representative may be notified if the nurse is threatened with repercussions for not following the order. Not all agencies are unionized.
   4. The nurse should notify the supervisor only if the nurse in charge continues to insist that the task be performed.

6. **TEST-TAKING TIP** Option 4 contains the word "only," which is a specific determiner. In options 1, 3, and 4 the final word in the statements end in "ed." Option 2 is unique.
   1. This does not recognize the right of the family to see the deceased one last time before postmortem care.

2. **This allows the family members time to make a last visit before the body is prepared for transfer to a mortuary.**

3. Postmortem care at this time is premature.

4. Postmortem care should not begin until after death is pronounced and the family has an opportunity to make a last visit.

7. **TEST-TAKING TIP** Option 1 is unique because it is the only option with a number.

1. **This is a goal statement that is specific and measurable and contains a time frame; "maintain" implies continuously.**

2. This statement identifies a need or an intervention in response to an identified problem, not a goal.

3. This is an inference about the patient's status, not a goal.

4. This is an intervention, not a goal.

8. **TEST-TAKING TIP** The word "first" in the stem sets a priority. The word "arriving" is the key word in the stem that directs attention to content. It establishes a time frame.

1. Controlled drugs can be counted at any time during the change of shift.

2. Rounds are implemented after report. The nurse first needs to know the status of the patients; a report provides baseline data about patients before additional assessments can be conducted. Some institutions have walking rounds in which report and assessment of patients are conducted simultaneously.

3. Before the nurse can prioritize care, the nurse must first know about each patient's status.

4. **Before care can be planned and implemented, the nurse needs to know the condition and immediate needs of patients.**

9. 1. *Battery* is the purposeful, angry, or negligent touching of a patient without consent.

2. *Assault* is an act intended to provoke fear in a patient.

3. ***Negligence*** **occurs when the nurse's actions do not meet appropriate standards and result in injury to another or one's belongings; negligence can occur with acts of omission or commission.**

4. *Malpractice* is misconduct performed in professional practice that results in harm to another.

10. **TEST-TAKING TIP** The word "best" in the stem sets a priority. The words "argumentative" and "demanding" are key words in the stem that direct attention to content. Options 2 and 4 are opposites. Option 2 offers the patient choices, and option 4 implies that the patient is to comply with what the patient is told to do. Option 2 is patient centered. Option 4 denies the patient's feelings, concerns, or needs.

1. This is a defensive response. All behavior has meaning; the nurse should initially identify the reason for the behavior.

2. **The patient is the center of the health-care team and has a right to be involved in the decision making concerning care; this individualizes care and promotes self-esteem, which often prevents argumentative and demanding behavior.**

3. This is an assumption. The patient's behavior may not be a lifelong pattern. Many people cope with anxiety by this behavior. This behavior may be an attempt to gain control in a situation in which the individual feels out of control and should be addressed.

4. This response is judgmental and takes away the patient's coping mechanism.

11. **TEST-TAKING TIP** The word "purpose" is the key word in the stem that directs attention to content.

1. Legal statutes are laws created by elected legislative bodies; they are not nursing standards.

2. Step-by-step actions in a procedure or protocol are the critical elements for completing an intervention.

3. Requirements for licensure and the ANA Standards of Nursing Practice are unrelated. All state licensing acts require a specified level of education and the passing of a special examination.

4. **The ANA has general resolutions that recommend the responsibilities and obligations of nurses; these standards help determine if a nurse has acted as any prudent, reasonable nurse would given a similar education, experiential background, and environment.**

12. **TEST-TAKING TIP** The word "best" in the stem sets a priority. The words "needs assistance with hygiene, grooming, eating,

and toileting" are key words in the stem that direct attention to content because they indicate the significant amount of assistance needed.

1. **This patient needs long-term nursing care as well as 24-hour supervision.**
2. A psychiatric institution is inappropriate for this patient. Patients with dementia need supportive care for the rest of their lives. Psychiatric settings today generally provide acute care services for mentally ill patients.
3. Outpatient care facilities usually provide acute care services, not long-term nursing care or 24-hour supervision.
4. Many day-care programs function 5 days a week from 8 a.m. until 6 p.m. to assist working family members. There are no data given that indicate the support of the family to meet the patient's needs or the ability of the patient to provide self-care when not at the day-care program.

13. **TEST-TAKING TIP** The word "legal" in the stem and the word "legally" in option 2 and "legal" in option 1 are clang associations. Option 2 is opposite to both options 3 and 4. However, options 3 and 4 are distractors because they are incorrect.

1. Assistance at the scene of an accident is an ethical, not a legal, duty.
2. **Nurses are responsible for their own actions, and the care provided must be what any reasonably prudent nurse would do under similar circumstances.**
3. A contract does not have to exist for a nurse to commit negligence.
4. The Good Samaritan Law does not provide legal immunity; the nurse can still be held accountable for gross departure from acceptable standards of practice or willful wrongdoing.

14. 1. *Libel* is defamation of character via print, writing, or pictures, not spoken words.
2. *Assault* is an attempt or threat to touch another person unjustifiably.
3. ***Slander* is defamation of character by spoken words.**
4. *Negligence* is the failure to do something a reasonably prudent nurse would do under similar circumstances or the commission of an act that a reasonably prudent nurse would not do under similar circumstances.

15. **TEST-TAKING TIP** The term "consent form" in the stem and option 3 is a clang association. Options 1 and 2 are equally plausible.

1. The nurse's signature does not document that the surgeon described the procedure and its risks; the patient's signature documents that the procedure and its risks are understood.
2. The nurse's signature does not document that the patient was properly informed about expected outcomes.
3. **The nurse only witnesses the patient's signature and examines the document for the correct date.**
4. The nurse's signature on an informed consent form does not protect the surgeon from being sued. Reasonably prudent practice protects the surgeon from being sued.

16. **TEST-TAKING TIP** The word "first" in the stem sets a priority. The patient is the central person in the question, not the abusive nurse. Option 4 is unique because it is the only option that addresses the needs of the patient. Option 4 is patient-centered.

1. Telling the nurse in charge about the behavior should be done later; another action is the priority.
2. Becoming a role model will be done later; another action is the priority.
3. This may be done later; it is not the priority at this time.
4. **The patient is the priority at this point in time; after the patient is protected and safe, the actions of the abusive nurse must be addressed.**

17. **TEST-TAKING TIP** Options 2, 3, and 4 are equally plausible because they all address aspects associated with nursing education. Option 1 is unique because it addresses safe practice.

1. **The NCLEX-RN® examination is designed to identify whether a candidate has met a minimum level of performance to safely practice as a licensed registered nurse.**
2. State boards of nursing, Accreditation Commission for Education in Nursing (ACEN), and the American Association of Colleges of Nursing accredit schools of nursing.

3. Controlling nursing education is not the purpose of NCLEX-RN®.
4. A degree or diploma, not NCLEX-RN®, verifies that the student has met the criteria for graduation from the granting institution.

18. 1. Analysis involves interpretation of data, collection of additional data, and identification and communication of nursing diagnoses. Analysis does not include the communication of data collected during the assessment phase of the nursing process.
2. Planning involves setting goals, establishing priorities, identifying expected outcomes, identifying interventions designed to achieve goals and outcomes, ensuring that the patient's health-care needs are met appropriately, modifying the plan as necessary, and collaborating with other health-care team members to ensure that care is coordinated. Planning does not include the communication of data collected during assessment.
3. Evaluation involves identifying a patient's response to care, comparing a patient's actual responses with the expected outcomes, analyzing factors that affected the actual outcomes for the purpose of drawing conclusions about the success or failure of specific nursing activities, and modifying the plan of care when necessary; evaluation does not include the communication of data collected during the assessment phase.
4. **Communicating important assessment data to other health-care team members is a component of the assessment phase of the nursing process.**

19. **TEST-TAKING TIP Options 1 and 4 are equally plausible. The words "used the lift" in the stem and "use the lift" in options 2 and 3 are clang associations.**
1. Another Nursing Assistant should not be held accountable for the care assigned another staff member. The nurse is directly responsible for ensuring that delegated care is safely delivered to patients.
2. **Demonstration is the safest way to assess whether the Nursing Assistant has the knowledge and skill to safely transfer a patient using a mechanical lift.**
3. This teaching method does not take into consideration the need for the Nursing

Assistant to practice the psychomotor skills associated with this task. Explaining is not sufficient.
4. This does not address the Nursing Assistant's need to know how to move a patient safely with a mechanical lift.

20. **TEST-TAKING TIP The word "always" in the stem sets a priority. The word "abusive" is the key word in the stem that directs attention to content. Options 1 and 4 are equally plausible because neither option is better than the other.**
1. This may not be true; trust is based on honesty.
2. This does not address the patient's needs. Rushing may increase the patient's anxiety.
3. **This supports every patient's right to know what care is being given and why.**
4. Telling a patient what he wants to hear is patronizing; when patients feel they are being humored, trust deteriorates.

21. **TEST-TAKING TIP The word "equipment" in the stem and in option 2 is a clang association. Options 2 and 4 are opposites. Option 2 gives the patient control and therefore is the most patient-centered option. Options 3 and 4 deny patient feelings, concerns, or needs.**
1. This does not support the patient's need to be in control of the immediate environment; equipment should be stored appropriately to protect it from pathogens in the environment.
2. **This supports the patient's right to control personal space.**
3. This still results in a violation of the patient's personal space.
4. Logic generally does not reduce a patient's concern; the patient needs to feel in control, and this action does not support this need.

22. **TEST-TAKING TIP The words "nursing assistant" are key words in the stem that direct attention to content.**
1. ____ Monitoring patients' tube feedings is the legal responsibility of the nurse, not the nursing assistant.
2. **X Most interventions that relate to activities of daily living can be delegated to a nursing assistant.**
3. **X Nursing assistants are responsible for meeting patients' basic activities of daily living under the supervision of the nurse.**

4. ____ Regulating patients' intravenous solutions is the legal responsibility of the nurse, not the nursing assistant.

5. ____ Assisting patients with taking medication is the legal responsibility of the nurse, not the nursing assistant.

23. **Answer: 3, 1, 4, 2, 5**

Refer to the Ethical Decision-Making Algorithm indicated below that highlights the steps in the question as they appear in the algorithm.

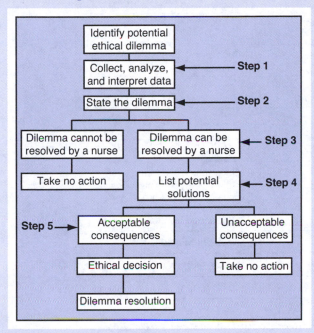

24. **TEST-TAKING TIP** The words "intentional tort" are key words in the stem that direct attention to content.

1. ____ This is an unintentional tort. The nurse did not intentionally forget to administer the STAT medication.

2. **X This action is an intentional tort. Intentionally touching a patient's body or clothing or anything held by or attached to a patient in an angry, willful, negligent, or violent manner without consent or providing treatment without informed consent is battery.**

3. ____ This is an unintentional tort. The medication was carelessly, not intentionally, administered to the wrong patient.

4. **X This action is an intentional tort. Intentionally threatening to harm or touch a patient in an insulting, unjustifiable, or offensive manner is assault.**

5. ____ This action is not an intentional tort. This is appropriate nursing care. A nurse may apply a restraint without an order by a primary health-care provider in an emergency when a patient is at risk of hurting others or oneself. The nurse is obligated to seek an order from a primary health-care provider as soon as possible.

25. **TEST-TAKING TIP** The word "violate" in the stem indicates negative polarity. The question is asking, "Which actions *do not* support a patient's right to confidentiality and privacy?" The words "confidentiality" and "privacy" are key words in the stem that direct attention to content.

1. **X Interviewing a patient in the presence of others violates confidentiality; others may overhear information that should be kept confidential.**

2. ____ Documenting statements in the patient's medical record is an acceptable practice.

3. **X The nurse legally is not permitted to divulge patient information to anyone without the patient's consent.**

4. ____ A team conference enables professionals to share important information about patients and is an acceptable practice.

5. ____ Sharing information at a change of shift report notifies nursing team members of the patient's changing status and is an appropriate practice.

26. 1. ____ Patients are not permitted to smoke in their rooms. The Joint Commission, the agency responsible for accrediting hospitals, requires that accredited facilities be "smoke-free." However, some facilities still provide limited, designated smoking areas.

2. **X Patients have a right to know the names of caregivers and their roles.**

3. ____ A private room is generally a privilege, not a right, that is provided at extra expense; it is not automatically provided on demand. However, a patient requiring isolation may be transferred to a private room at no additional expense to the patient.

4. **X Patients have a right to accurate information about their diagnosis, treatment, and prognosis in terms they can understand.**

5. **X Patients have a right to refuse care against medical advice; the primary health-care provider must explain to the patient the risks involved in lack of treatment.**

27. **TEST-TAKING TIP** The word "most" in the stem sets a priority.

A breach of duty occurred when the nurse's actions failed to meet the standard of care established by authoritative entities such as legislation, professional organizations, job descriptions, and agency policies and procedures regarding maintaining confidentiality. In this situation, the nurse's breach of duty caused emotional harm to the patient and is considered malpractice.

Unusual Occurrence Report

Date of Event: _____   Time of Event: _____   Department: _____

Patient Last Name:	First Name:	MI:
Patient #:	Attending Physician:	
Visitor Last Name:	First Name:	Phone #:
Employee Name:	Dept:	
Physician Name:	Specialty:	

Occurrence Category (Check most appropriate)

☐ Agency nurse-related	☐ AMA	☐ Delay in treatment
☐ Diet-related	☐ HIPAA compliance	☐ Loss of personal property
☐ Medication-related	☐ Narcotics-related	☐ Order not executed
☐ Patient injury	☐ Peer-review related	☐ Restraint-related
☐ Staff injury	☐ Supplies/Equipment	☐ Visitor injury
☐ Other (please explain):		

Description of Occurrence:

A patient overheard a nurse sharing information about the patient's diagnosis and treatment to a visitor in the hall. The patient reported this event to the nurse in charge and stated, "I am very upset".

Contributing Factors (Check all that apply)

☐ Individual:	☐ System:
Knowledge, skills, and/or experience: ☐ Unclear ☐ Incomplete	Policies/procedures not in place: ☐ Unclear ☐ Outdated
☑ Non-adherence to standard of care or practice	Environmental: ☐ Staffing ☐ Patient acuity ☐ Congestion
☐ Documentation incomplete or inadequate	Communications and work flow: ☐ Intradepartmental ☐ Interdepartmental
	☐ Equipment failure

Other (please explain):

Submitted by:	Dept:	Date:

28. 1. ____ Licensed practical nurses cannot administer medication via the direct intravenous push technique. Also, they cannot administer intravenous antineoplastic medications or the initial bag of an intravenous solution. These situations have a risk of untoward patient effects that a licensed practical nurse is not prepared to address.

2. ____ Licensed practical nurses do not have the educational depth and breadth necessary to develop nursing plans of care. Nursing plans of care should be developed by registered nurses.

3. **X Licensed practical nurses can perform a venipuncture to obtain a blood specimen. Licensed practical nurses learn anatomy and physiology, sterile technique, and how to perform simple nursing procedures.**

4. **X Licensed practical nurses can change dressings on wounds. Licensed practical nurse educational programs include the principles of sterile technique and uncomplicated sterile nursing procedures. The clinical data obtained during a dressing change must be reported to a registered nurse for evaluation and intervention if necessary.**

5. **X Licensed practical nurses can assess patients to collect clinical data but they cannot interpret the information or determine which clinical action is required.**

29. **TEST-TAKING TIP** The word "dependent" is the key word in the stem that directs attention to content.

1. **X Ambulation of a patient requires a primary health-care provider's order. Patient activity (e.g., bedrest, out of bed to chair, out of bed) is a dependent function of a nurse.**

2. ____ Documenting nursing care is an independent function of the nurse and does not require a primary health-care provider's order.

3. **X Dependent activities of the nurse are those activities that require a primary health-care provider's order; changing a sterile dressing requires a primary health-care provider's order.**

4. ____ In an emergency, a nurse may administer oxygen to a patient experiencing acute shortness of breath until a primary health-care provider's order is obtained.

5. ____ Selecting among choices of foods offered within a diet is an interdependent function; however, the type of diet is a dependent function.

30. 1. ____ Criminal law is concerned with crimes.

2. ____ Civil law is concerned with wrongs committed by one person against another.

3. **X Ethics is concerned with value judgments and behavior that is acceptable or unacceptable.**

4. ____ Negligence is concerned with a careless act of commission or omission that results in injury to another.

5. **X Ethics is concerned with value judgments such as behaviors that are considered acceptable or unacceptable.**

31. **TEST-TAKING TIP** The words "Nursing Assistant" are key words in the stem that direct attention to content.

1. **X The Nursing Assistant is trained to identify major abnormal or unexpected signs and symptoms and to notify the nurse when they are changed from the patient's baseline; the nurse then completes a professional assessment of the patient's condition.**

2. ____ It is illegal for the Nursing Assistant to administer drugs, even if under the supervision of the nurse.

3. ____ A Nursing Assistant should not be responsible for the supervision of other employees.

4. ____ The Nursing Assistant is not prepared for this responsibility. Teaching requires a strong scientific knowledge base and an ability to use scientific teaching/learning principles when planning and implementing an educational plan.

5. **X Nursing Assistants are permitted to distribute meal trays to patients. They just have to verify the patient's name to the name on the menu on the tray.**

32. **TEST-TAKING TIP** The words "nursing process" are key words in the stem that direct attention to content.

Answer: 3, 4, 2, 1, 5

3. **Assessment, the first step of the nursing process, involves collecting, verifying, and documenting patient information/data; this includes information such as vital signs and physical assessments.**

4. Analysis, the second step of the nursing process, involves clustering and analyzing data and arriving at conclusions about the significance of the data. It also involves the identification of nursing diagnoses.

2. Planning, the third step of the nursing process, involves setting goals, objectives, and expected outcomes. In addition, priorities of care are identified and interventions are planned to meet the goals, objectives, and expected outcomes.

1. Implementation, the fourth step of the nursing process, involves the actual delivery of nursing care. It includes activities such as executing the proposed plan of care, performing dependent and independent interventions, reacting to life-threatening/adverse responses, and communicating with or teaching patients.

5. Evaluation, the fifth step of the nursing process, involves identifying patient responses to care, comparing actual patient outcomes with expected outcomes, determining factors that affected outcomes, and modifying the plan of care if necessary.

33. **TEST-TAKING TIP** The word "most" in the stem sets a priority.

1. The *Falls* category demonstrates a downward trend in the number of events indicating improvement. This indicates a positive trend and is not a cause for concern.

2. The *Medication errors* category demonstrates a downward trend in the number of events indicating improvement. This indicates a positive trend and is not a cause for concern.

3. The *Violations of confidentiality* category results should cause the most concern. The chart indicates that the number of events increased rather than decreased each month in spite of the implementation of a corrective action plan.

4. The *Failures to maintain standards of nursing practice* category initially demonstrates improvement in April; however, it indicates an increase in events in May when compared with April. Although this is a concern, it is not as alarming as a progressively negative trend demonstrated in another problem category.

34. **TEST-TAKING TIP** The words "deductive reasoning" are key words in the stem that direct attention to content.

1. X This statement reflects the nurse using deductive reasoning. It moves from a general premise (the patient is dehydrated) to a specific deduction (the patient will probably have tenting of the skin, which is a sign of dehydration).

2. X This statement reflects the nurse using deductive reasoning. It moves from a general premise (the patient may have fractured the head of the femur in the fall) to a specific deduction (the patient will probably have pain in the hip if it is fractured).

3. ____ This statement reflects the nurse using inductive reasoning. It moves from the specific to the general. A pattern of information (an elevated white blood cell count and fever) leads to a generalization (the patient may have an infection).

4. ____ This statement reflects the nurse using inductive reasoning. It moves from the specific to the general. A pattern of information (crying, trembling, and a rapid pulse) leads to a generalization (the patient may be anxious).

5. X This statement reflects the nurse using deductive reasoning. It moves from a general premise (the patient is experiencing hypoglycemia) to a specific deduction (the patient will probably have pale, cool, clammy skin and a low blood glucose level).

35. **TEST-TAKING TIP** The words "unintentional tort" are key words in the stem that direct attention to content.

1. ____ A nurse is not obligated to stop at the scene of an accident to render first aid.

2. X This is an example of an unintentional tort. The nurse's lack of action failed to meet standards of care established by a job description, agency policy or procedures, the state nurse practice act, or standards established by professional organizations that caused the patient to experience a life-threatening situation.

3. X This is an example of an unintentional tort. The nurse's lack of action failed to meet standards of care established by a job description,

agency policy or procedures, the state nurse practice act, standards established by professional organizations that caused the patient to sustain an injury.

4. ____ While an unintentional injury occurred there are no grounds for a tort because appropriate standards of care were followed.

5. ____ This is not an unintentional tort. A patient is not involved. This is associated with management. State nurse practice acts protect a nurse from suspension, termination, disciplinary action, and/or discrimination if the nurse refuses to do or not do something because he or she believes that it is inappropriate and could be harmful.

36. 1. **X Evaluating patient responses to medications is the responsibility of a licensed nurse. Nursing assistants do not have the educational background related to the expected, nontherapeutic effects of medications.**

2. ____ Nursing assistants are taught to follow medical aseptic principles when performing basic skills such as emptying the collection bag of a urinary retention catheter.

3. **X Obtaining a specimen of exudate from a draining wound involves the use of sterile technique. The use of sterile technique is beyond the scope of practice of a nursing assistant.**

4. ____ Nursing assistants are capable of taking the vital signs of patients who are stable. Obtained vital signs are then reported to the registered nurse who evaluates the values obtained by the nursing assistant.

5. ____ Nursing assistants are capable of assisting patients with range-of-motion exercises. It is a repetitive activity that nursing assistants are taught to perform.

37. **TEST-TAKING TIP The word "most" in the stem sets a priority.**

1. **Each patient in an independent living facility has his or her own apartment. It can be as small as one room with a kitchenette, living room, and sleeping area or as large as a 1-, 2-, or 3-room apartment. These facilities usually provide 2 or 3 meals a day and social activities. This patient has difficulty getting to the stores, is bored with meal preparation, is lonely, and has**
ample financial resources. An independent living facility can best meet the patient's needs after discharge from the hospital.

2. An assisted living facility is unnecessary for this patient at this time. This patient is capable of performing her own activities of daily living (e.g., bathing, toileting, and dressing) and she prefers privacy. This type of facility may be appropriate in the future if her emphysema or arthritis get progressively debilitating.

3. Most day-care programs function only 5 days a week and may require patients to supply their own transportation to and from the program. Also, many day-care programs are designed for cognitively impaired individuals. There are no data that indicate that this patient is cognitively impaired and the patient no longer drives.

4. This patient does not require the services of a nursing home. The patient is able to perform the activities of daily living and has no health problems that require either skilled nursing care or custodial nursing care.

38. **TEST-TAKING TIP The words "implemented independently" are key words in the stem that direct attention to content.**

1. **X Taking the vital signs provides important information about the overall status of the patient and is an independent function of a nurse.**

2. ____ The intake of fluid and food requires an order by the primary health-care provider and is a dependent function of the nurse.

3. **X Pulse oximetry is a noninvasive procedure that measures the oxygen saturation level in the blood. It is commonly used to assess the oxygen status of a patient, the effect of medications on the respiratory system, and a patient's tolerance to a change in activity level. Pulse oximetry does not require an order by a primary health-care provider and is within the scope of independent nursing practice.**

4. **X The high-Fowler position facilitates ventilation by using gravity to lower abdominal organs away from the diaphragm, thereby promoting better expansion of the thoracic cavity on inspiration. The greater expansion of**

the thoracic cavity facilitates gas exchange, promoting oxygenation of body cells. Positioning patients appropriately is an independent function of the nurse and does not require an order by a primary health-care provider.

5. X Assessing a patient's lung sounds is an independent function of the nurse. Identifying various breath sounds such as rales, rhonchi, stridor, or wheezing can assist the primary health-care provider in planning medical intervention. In addition, nurses can evaluate the outcomes of interventions such as position changes; encouragement of coughing; increased fluid intake; and nembulizer treatments and other medications, such as bronchodilators, based on the improvement or lack of improvement in breath sounds.

39. 1. Those who follow the Buddhist religion revere Buddha (reflected in the illustration) not as a god but as a model of the right way of life. According to Buddhism, humankind will develop when evil is avoided and morality, purity, and good works prevail.

2. This is a statue of Buddha and is unrelated to those who believe in Allah and the six articles of faith, which are associated with Islam.

3. This is a statue of Buddha and is not the figure that is considered the mediator between God and humankind. Those who follow Christian religions believe that Jesus is the mediator between God and humankind.

4. This is a statue of Buddha and is unrelated to those who believe in the Old Testament. Followers of Judaism believe that the laws in the Old Testament teach them how to show devotion to God and how to act toward others.

40. **TEST-TAKING TIP** The words "Nursing Assistant" are key words in the stem that direct attention to content.

1. ____ Evaluating vital signs requires professional nursing judgment. The nurse is educationally prepared to determine the significance of vital sign measurements, not the Nursing Assistant.

2. X Making occupied and unoccupied beds is within the role of Nursing Assistants. Nursing Assistants are taught to perform this activity safely.

3. ____ It is not legal for a Nursing Assistant to monitor tube feedings; this action is within the legal practice of a licensed nurse.

4. X Nursing Assistants are trained to provide basic hygiene measures under the direction of a nurse.

5. ____ Nurses should ambulate postoperative patients for the first time after surgery; nurses have the knowledge to analyze a patient's response to ambulating postoperatively. Nursing Assistants can ambulate patients who have simple, noncomplex needs.

COMMON THEORIES RELATED TO MEETING PATIENTS' BASIC HUMAN NEEDS

This section includes questions related to the work of theorists such as Kübler-Ross, Maslow, Selye, Dunn, Engel, Kohlberg, and Erikson. It also includes questions related to principles of teaching, growth and development, stress and adaptation, and the definition of health.

QUESTIONS

1. Which developmental task according to Erikson should the nurse assist older adult patients to achieve?
   1. Establishing trust
   2. Becoming dependent
   3. Reconciling one's life
   4. Assisting grown children

   TEST-TAKING TIP Identify key words in the stem that direct attention to content.

2. A nurse is teaching a patient with diabetes how to self-monitor blood glucose levels. What is the **most** important factor when predicting the success of a teaching program regarding the learning of this skill?
   1. Interest of the learner
   2. Extent of family support
   3. Amount of reinforcement
   4. Level of learner's cognitive ability

   TEST-TAKING TIP Identify the word in the stem that sets a priority. Identify clang associations.

3. Which describes the pattern of the process of growth and development?
   1. Uncertain
   2. Nonpredictable
   3. Based on motivation
   4. Influenced by the previous steps

   TEST-TAKING TIP Identify equally plausible options.

4. A nurse is assessing a patient with a severe sunburn. In which classification of stress should the nurse place the sun that caused the sunburn?
   1. Physical
   2. Chemical
   3. Physiological
   4. Microbiological

5. A nurse is interviewing an adolescent during a yearly physical examination. Which patient activity identified by the nurse supports the developmental task of adolescence?
   1. Reading a book
   2. Learning how to use a computer
   3. Helping parents with household chores
   4. Attending a high school basketball game

   TEST-TAKING TIP Identify the key word in the stem that directs attention to content.

6. Which word **best** describes the feelings associated with an infant in Erikson's stage of trust versus mistrust?
   1. Me
   2. We
   3. You
   4. They

   TEST-TAKING TIP Identify the word in the stem that sets a priority. Identify key words in the stem that direct attention to content. Identify opposites in options.

7. A nurse is obtaining the psychosocial history of a patient. Which event generally precipitates the highest degree of stress when considering theories about stress?
   1. Marriage
   2. Pregnancy
   3. Relocation
   4. Retirement

   TEST-TAKING TIP Identify the word in the stem that sets a priority. Identify the key word in the stem that directs attention to content.

8. A nurse is collecting information to prepare a teaching plan for a patient with type 1 diabetes. Which question asked by the nurse is associated with collecting information in the cognitive domain of learning?
   1. "How do you inspect your feet each day?"
   2. "Can you measure a serum glucose level?"
   3. "What do you know about diabetes mellitus?"
   4. "Are you able to perform a subcutaneous injection?"

   TEST-TAKING TIP Identify the key word in the stem that directs attention to content. Identify the unique option. Identify the clang association.

9. A nurse is teaching a patient about self-injection with insulin. Which is the **most** effective approach to use in this situation?
   1. Book
   2. Video
   3. Discussion
   4. Demonstration

   TEST-TAKING TIP Identify the word in the stem that sets a priority.

10. A nurse identifies that a patient has been exposed to the stress of air pollution caused by a wood-burning fireplace in the home. Which classification of stress is air pollution?
    1. Physical
    2. Chemical
    3. Physiological
    4. Microbiological

11. A nurse is interviewing a patient who is terminally ill. Which is an unexpected behavior associated with the usual process of grieving?
    1. Talking about the illness
    2. Seeking alternative therapies
    3. Becoming angry with people
    4. Attempting to commit suicide

    TEST-TAKING TIP Identify the word in the stem that indicates negative polarity. Identify key words in the stem that direct attention to content.

12. A nurse is assessing a patient coping with multiple stresses and knows that one body system has a major impact on how a patient responds to stress. Which body system should the nurse assess **first** because it primarily controls the general adaptation syndrome?
    1. Endocrine
    2. Respiratory
    3. Integumentary
    4. Cardiovascular

    TEST-TAKING TIP Identify the word in the stem that sets a priority. Identify key words in the stem that direct attention to content.

13. A patient asks a nurse, "What is health?" Which concept basic to **most** definitions of health should the nurse consider when answering the patient's question?
    1. A progressive state
    2. The absence of disease
    3. Relative to one's value system
    4. An extreme of the wellness–illness continuum

    TEST-TAKING TIP Identify key words in the stem that direct attention to content. Identify the word in the stem that sets a priority. Identify the patient-centered option. Identify the unique option. Identify equally plausible options.

14. A nurse is planning to provide personal health care information to several patients. Which patient should the nurse anticipate will be **most** motivated to learn?
    1. A 55-year-old woman who had a mastectomy and is very anxious about her body image
    2. A 56-year-old man who had a heart attack last week and is requesting information about exercise
    3. An 18-year-old man who smokes two packs of cigarettes and is in denial about the dangers of smoking
    4. A 47-year-old woman who has a long-leg cast after sustaining a broken leg and is still experiencing severe pain

    TEST-TAKING TIP Identify the word in the stem that sets a priority.

15. A patient is readmitted to the hospital because of complications resulting from non-adherence to the prescribed health-care regimen. Which should the nurse do **first**?
    1. Encourage healthy behaviors.
    2. Develop a trusting relationship.
    3. Use educational aids to reinforce teaching.
    4. Establish why the therapeutic plan is not being followed.

    TEST-TAKING TIP Identify the word in the stem that sets a priority.

16. A patient with type 2 diabetes mellitus and restrictive airway disease comes to the emergency department of the hospital because of a productive cough and fever. The patient is diagnosed with pneumonia and is admitted for treatment. During the admission health history the patient tells the nurse, "I work full time as a high school English teacher and I am very healthy." Which is the **most** important intervention by the nurse during the patient's hospitalization?
    1. Explain why the patient is really not well.
    2. Identify the patient's perception of the sick role.
    3. Foster patient independence concerning self-care.
    4. Give the patient written materials about the identified illness.

    TEST-TAKING TIP Identify the word in the stem that sets a priority. Identify the option that denies patient feelings, concerns, or needs. Identify the patient-centered option.

17. A nurse is interviewing the wife of a patient who died 2 weeks ago. The wife states, "I go to the cemetery every day and say several prayers." Which stage of grieving according to Engel's model of grieving is the patient exhibiting?
    1. Developing awareness
    2. Resolving the loss
    3. Idealization
    4. Restitution

    TEST-TAKING TIP Identify key words in the stem that direct attention to content.

18. A nurse is assessing a patient's readiness to learn about smoking cessation. Which patient factor does the nurse consider is **most** important when determining if a teaching program is needed by the patient?
    1. Previous experience
    2. Perceived need
    3. Expectations
    4. Flexibility

    TEST-TAKING TIP Identify the word in the stem that sets a priority.

19. What should the nurse do to meet a patient's basic physiological needs? **Select all that apply.**
    1. ____ Raise the side rails
    2. ____ Provide a bed bath
    3. ____ Converse with the patient
    4. ____ Explain procedures to the patient
    5. ____ Ambulate the patient to the bathroom

    TEST-TAKING TIP Identify the key word in the stem that directs attention to content.

20. A nurse educator is teaching a class on the concepts of stress and adaptation and reinforced the content using the following illustration. Which is the **most** important reason why the nurse educator presented this illustration?

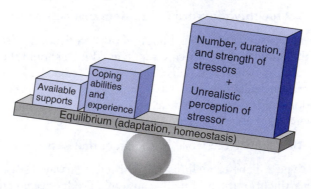

    1. It appeals to participants of the class.
    2. It employs the concept of positive reinforcement.
    3. It stimulates learning in those with an internal locus of control.
    4. It improves students' conceptual understanding of presented content.

    TEST-TAKING TIP Identify the word in the stem that sets a priority.

21. A mentally disadvantaged adult patient is learning self-care. What should the nurse do to help the patient increase learning? **Select all that apply.**

1. _____ Verbally recognize when goals are met.
2. _____ Use demonstration as a teaching strategy.
3. _____ Offer candy as a reward when learning occurs.
4. _____ Disregard the behavior when goals are not met.
5. _____ Set a variety of short-term objectives to be met.
6. _____ Conduct several short teaching sessions for each skill.

22. The nurse refers to Maslow's Hierarchy of Human Needs to organize a patient's basic human needs. Place the following patient statements that reflect basic needs in order from the most to the least basic.

1. "How soon are visiting hours so that my family can visit me?"
2. "Promise me that someone will answer my call bell when I ring."
3. "I would like you to help me with the arrangements for my funeral."
4. "Can you please close the door when you help me to the bathroom?"
5. "I am sitting here a long time and I am very thirsty. Can I have a glass of water?"

Answer: _____

23. Lawrence Kohlberg's theory of stages of moral development is based on the ability to think at progressively higher levels as one matures. Place the following motivations for thinking in the order as one advances from a basic to a higher level of moral development.

1. Adhering to societal standards while individualizing values and beliefs
2. Using abstract reasoning based on universal ethical principles
3. Pleasing others based on what they expect
4. Performing actions based on rules
5. Fearing negative consequences
6. Wanting positive consequences

Answer: _____

TEST-TAKING TIP Identify key words in the stem that direct attention to content.

24. Which of the following patients' level of wellness does the nurse determine best represents the placement of the X on Dunn's Health Grid?

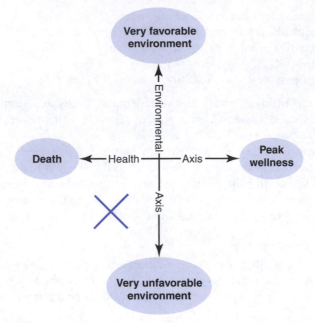

1. A person with emphysema and a history of a brain attack with left-sided weakness who lives in a nursing home while receiving respiratory rehabilitation
2. A relatively healthy person who is recovering from the birth of a stillborn and who shares a small apartment with several other unrelated individuals
3. A teenager who recently recovered from a fractured femur who lives with caring parents in a middle-class family home
4. A person who is receiving treatment at the local clinic for cirrhosis of the liver and who lives in an abandoned van

25. A nurse is caring for an eleven-year-old child who was recently diagnosed with type 1 diabetes. In addition to encouraging the child to practice with the equipment associated with diabetes, which additional interventions should the nurse implement to support this patient? **Select all that apply.**
1. ____ Gently identify non–age-appropriate behavior and suggest corrective actions.
2. ____ Explain that expressing feelings of sadness and anger is acceptable.
3. ____ Provide honest, concrete, and detailed answers to questions.
4. ____ Assign the patient to a private room if available.
5. ____ Encourage visits from peers and siblings.

TEST-TAKING TIP Identify patient-centered options. Identify options that deny patient feelings, concerns, or needs.

26. Place the following statements made by a patient with a terminal illness in order according to Kübler-Ross's five stages of Grief in Death and Dying.
1. "I will never see my grandchildren grown up and married."
2. "I will give up my cigars to see my grandchild born this summer."
3. "I'm working on a tape recording that I'm making for my grandchildren."
4. "I'm getting another opinion because I was told 3 months ago everything was fine."
5. "I cannot believe the doctor missed the tumor 3 months ago when I was last examined."

Answer: _____

TEST-TAKING TIP Identify key words in the stem that direct attention to content.

27. According to Maslow's Hierarchy of Needs, which **most** clearly reflect(s) physiological needs? **Select all that apply.**
  1. _____ Fever
  2. _____ Trauma
  3. _____ Puberty
  4. _____ Restraints
  5. _____ Menopause

   TEST-TAKING TIP Identify the word in the stem that sets a priority. Identify key words in the stem that direct attention to content.

28. A nurse is considering the principles of stress and adaptation. Which words describe the concept of adaptive capacity? **Select all that apply.**
  1. _____ Safety
  2. _____ Health
  3. _____ Restore
  4. _____ Imbalance
  5. _____ Reestablish

   TEST-TAKING TIP Identify key words in the stem that direct attention to content.

29. A nurse is preparing a teaching plan for a patient who was just diagnosed with type 1 diabetes. Which are the most effective teaching strategies that can be used in the cognitive domain? **Select all that apply.**
  1. _____ Explanation
  2. _____ Demonstration
  3. _____ Group discussion
  4. _____ Written materials
  5. _____ Individual practice

   TEST-TAKING TIP Identify the word in the stem that sets a priority. Identify the key word in the stem that directs attention to content.

30. A nurse is caring for a variety of patients on a medical unit in the hospital. In which order should the nurse perform the following actions using Maslow's Hierarchy of Needs as a basis for prioritizing care?
  1. Administering two liters of oxygen via a nasal cannula
  2. Encouraging a family member to visit as often as desired
  3. Arranging for a minister to visit when requested by a patient
  4. Asking a patient about personal preferences before beginning care
  5. Placing the call bell within easy reach after a patient is transferred to a chair

   Answer: _____

   TEST-TAKING TIP Identify key words in the stem that direct attention to content.

31. Which statements are associated with the task of generativity versus stagnation according to Erikson's developmental theory? **Select all that apply.**
  1. _____ "I want to do it myself."
  2. _____ "I will be getting married next week."
  3. _____ "I enjoy mentoring the new employees."
  4. _____ "I am pleased with the decisions I have made."
  5. _____ "I am teaching my children how to manage their money."

   TEST-TAKING TIP Identify key words in the stem that direct attention to content.

32. A nurse is completing a health history for a 90-year-old woman being admitted to a home health-care program. The patient has Parkinson disease and stage 3 lung cancer that currently is in remission. The patient said that she is able to get around all right as long as she stops frequently to catch her breath. She further explained that, other than knowing that she has cancer, she felt that "healthwise I'm in pretty good shape." She said her children insisted that she get help with bathing several mornings a week but said, "I don't feel that I need any help." The primary health-care provider's history and physical stated that the patient's activities of daily living are significantly impaired as a result of the Parkinson disease and she may have less than 6 months to live. Where should the nurse place an X on the Health-Illness Continuum to reflect the patient's perception of her health?

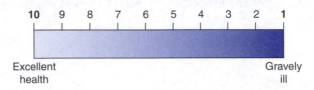

33. A nurse provides preoperative teaching for a patient scheduled for surgery. What should the nurse do to ensure that the patient understands the content of the teaching session? **Select all that apply.**
1. ____ Use simple vocabulary.
2. ____ Obtain a return demonstration.
3. ____ Ask the patient what was learned.
4. ____ Speak distinctly when giving directions.
5. ____ Talk slowly when speaking with the patient.

TEST-TAKING TIP Identify the clang association. Identify patient-centered options.

34. A nurse is admitting the child in this photograph to the hospital for testing and treatment. Which should the nurse implement when caring for this child? **Select all that apply.**

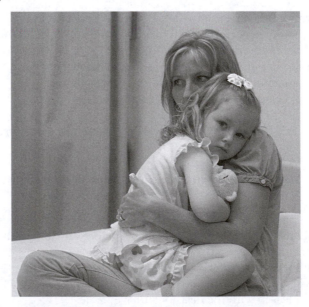

1. ____ Explain to the child that an intervention may "hurt" but that medicine can be given to make the "hurt" go away.
2. ____ Use a doll to explain what is going to be done and why in terms that the child can understand.
3. ____ Encourage the parent to stay with the child as much as possible.
4. ____ Examine the child while she is sitting on her mother's lap.
5. ____ Remind the child that she is a big girl.

TEST-TAKING TIP Identify the option that denies patient feelings, concerns, or needs. Identify patient-centered options.

35. A nurse is caring for a female patient who is dying and the patient's family members. The nurse has verbal interactions, listed below, with the patient and several family members, who tend to hover around the patient. Which is the **best** nursing action based on patient and family member statements?
   1. Reinforce with the patient the son's desire for his mother to keep on fighting.
   2. Explain to the granddaughter that she should focus on her grandmother.
   3. Help family members to understand the patient's need to withdraw.
   4. Tell the husband about bereavement counseling that is available.

Patient

"I know my time is up. Everyone is hanging around and talking to me. I am so tired. I just want to rest."

Patient's Husband

"We are so in love and we have been a great team. I don't know what I am going to do when this is over."

Patient's Son

"My mother was a strong independent woman all her life. I keep telling her to fight."

Patient's Granddaughter

"My grandmother has been a fabulous grandmother. I am getting married in 3 weeks and I want her at the ceremony."

TEST-TAKING TIP Identify the word in the stem that sets a priority. Identify the unique option. Identify the central person in the question. Identify the patient-centered option. Identify options with clang associations.

COMMON THEORIES RELATED TO MEETING PATIENTS' BASIC HUMAN NEEDS ANSWERS AND RATIONALES

1. **TEST-TAKING TIP** The words "older adult" are key words in the stem that direct attention to content.
   1. Establishing trust is the major task of infants.
   2. Dependency is not a task for which one strives; dependency results if an 8- to 12-year-old is unable to resolve the conflict of industry versus inferiority.
   3. **Older adults need to come to terms with the fact that the end of life is near; reviewing one's life is a step in this process.**
   4. Middle-aged adults may help grown children; this is usually a task of this age group.

2. **TEST-TAKING TIP** The word "most" in the stem sets a priority. The word "learning" in the stem and the words "learner" in option 1 and "learner's" in option 4 are clang associations.
   1. **The motivation of the learner to acquire new attitudes, information, or skills is the most important component for successful learning; motivation exists when the learner recognizes the future benefits of learning.**
   2. Although family support is important, the patient's interest and readiness to learn are the priorities for successful learning of a skill; some patients do not have a family support system.
   3. Although reinforcement is important, it is not the most significant factor in learning.
   4. Although a teaching program must be designed within the patient's developmental and cognitive abilities, it is useless unless the patient recognizes the value of what is to be learned.

3. **TEST-TAKING TIP** Options 1 and 2 are equally plausible.
   1. Although growth and development progress through some stages faster than others, they still follow a certain predictable pattern.
   2. Stages of growth and development do follow a predictable pattern.
   3. Motivation may influence the achievement of tasks in some stages of growth and development; however, growth and development do not rely on motivation.
   4. **Success or failure of task achievement in one stage of development influences succeeding stages; failure to resolve a crisis at one stage damages the ego, which makes the resolution of the following stages more difficult.**

4. 1. **Physical stresses are stresses from outside the body and include light, environmental temperature, sound, pressure, motion, gravity, and electricity.**
   2. Chemical stresses relate to toxic substances such as acids, alkalines, drugs, and exogenous hormones.
   3. Physiological stresses are disturbances in structure or function of any tissue, organ, or system within the body.
   4. Microbiological stresses are organisms such as bacteria, viruses, molds, or parasites that can cause disease.

5. **TEST-TAKING TIP** The word "adolescent" is the key word in the stem that directs attention to content.
   1. Middle childhood (6 to 12 years), not adolescence, is concerned with developing fundamental skills in reading and writing; the school-age child is very industrious.
   2. Middle childhood (6 to 12 years), not adolescence, is concerned with developing fundamental skills such as using a computer; the school-age child is very industrious.
   3. The childhood years, not adolescence, are related to helping behaviors; 3- to 5-year-olds like to imitate parents and 6- to 12-year-olds are developing appropriate social roles.
   4. **Adolescents are concerned with developing new and more mature relationships with their peers; adolescents tend to associate with their peers rather than with their parents.**

6. **TEST-TAKING TIP** The word "best" in the stem sets a priority. The words "trust versus mistrust" are key words in the stem that direct attention to content. Options 1 and 3 are opposites, and options 2 and 4 are opposites. In this instance, identifying opposites is not helpful in focusing on the correct answer.
   1. **The infant is egocentric and unaware of boundaries between the self and others; the infant is concerned with needs being met immediately.**

2. The infant has not identified the difference between self and others.

3. The infant has not identified the difference between self and others.

4. The infant has not identified the difference between self and others.

7. **TEST-TAKING TIP** The word "highest" in the stem sets a priority. The word "stress" is the key word in the stem that directs attention to content.

   1. **Holmes and Rahe (1967) determined stress units for life events based on the readjustment required by individuals to adapt to particular situations or events. The mean stress unit for marriage is 50, which is more than the other options presented.**
   2. The mean stress unit for pregnancy is 40, which is less than the correct answer.
   3. The mean stress unit for a change in residence is 20, which is less than the correct answer.
   4. The mean stress unit for retirement is 45, which is less than the correct answer.

8. **TEST-TAKING TIP** The word "cognitive" is the key word in the stem that directs attention to content. Option 3 is unique because it is the only option that is concerned with "what is" rather than "how to." Options 1, 2, and 4 all relate to the performance of a skill. The word "diabetes" in the stem and in option 3 is a clang association.

   1. This statement focuses on the performance of a skill that relates to the psychomotor, not cognitive, domain.
   2. This statement focuses on the performance of a skill that relates to the psychomotor, not cognitive, domain.
   3. **This is the cognitive domain because it deals with the comprehension of information.**
   4. This statement focuses on the performance of a skill that relates to the psychomotor, not cognitive, domain.

9. **TEST-TAKING TIP** The word "most" in the stem sets a priority.

   1. Although a book can be used for learning a skill (psychomotor domain), it is not as effective as other methods; it is more appropriate for learning and comprehending information (cognitive domain).
   2. Although a video can be used for learning a skill (psychomotor domain), it is not as effective as other methods.
   3. Learning via discussion is appropriate for the cognitive (knowing) and affective (feeling) domains.
   4. **Demonstration uses a variety of senses, such as sight, hearing, and touch. The opportunity to observe and manipulate equipment promotes learning a skill.**

10. 1. Air pollution is not a physical stress; physical stresses include temperature, sound, pressure, light, motion, gravity, and electricity.
    2. **Burning wood releases toxic substances and gases into the air; these are considered chemical stresses. Acids, alkalines, drugs, and exogenous hormones are also considered chemical stresses.**
    3. Air pollution is not a physiological stress; disturbances in the structure or function of any tissue, organ, or system of the body are considered physiological stresses.
    4. Air pollution is not a microbiological stress; bacteria, viruses, molds, and parasites are considered microbiological stresses.

11. **TEST-TAKING TIP** The word "unexpected" in the stem indicates negative polarity. You must identify the behavior that is *not* usually associated with the grieving process. The words "behavior" and "grieving" are key words in the stem that direct attention to content.

    1. Although talking about the illness occurs throughout the grieving response, it is most expected during the early stage of disbelief (No, not me).
    2. Seeking alternative therapies occurs most often during the stage of bargaining (Yes me, but . . .).
    3. Anger is expected and occurs when there is a developing awareness of the impending loss (Why me?).
    4. **Although some people who are terminally ill attempt suicide, it is not an expected response to loss.**

12. **TEST-TAKING TIP** The word "first" in the stem sets a priority. The words "controls" and "general adaptation syndrome" are key words in the stem that direct attention to content.

    1. **The general adaptation syndrome (GAS) primarily involves the endocrine system and autonomic nervous system; antidiuretic hormone, adrenocorticotropic hormone, cortisol, aldosterone, epinephrine, and norepinephrine**

are all involved with the fight-or-flight response.

2. The respiratory system does not control the GAS. It is stimulated by a component of the syndrome.

3. The integumentary system does not control the GAS. It is stimulated by a component of the syndrome.

4. The cardiovascular system does not control the GAS. It is stimulated by a component of the syndrome.

13. **TEST-TAKING TIP The words "basic to most" are key words in the stem that direct attention to content. The word "most" in the stem sets a priority. Option 3 is patient centered. Option 3 is unique because it relates to the patient. Options 1, 2, and 4 relate to the disease process. Options 2 and 4 are equally plausible.**

1. Health fluctuates on a continuum that has extremes of wellness to illness; movement can occur up or down the continuum, not only in one direction.

2. The World Health Organization's definition of health is "A state of complete physical, mental, and social well-being, and not merely the absence of disease or infirmity." Some people who have a chronic illness consider themselves healthy because they are able to function independently.

3. **A definition of health is highly individualized; it is based on each person's own experiences, values, and perceptions. Health can mean different things to each individual; people tend to define health based on the presence or absence of symptoms, their perceptions of how they feel, and their capacity to function on a daily basis.**

4. Although high-level wellness is one extreme of the wellness–illness continuum and severe illness the other, where one plots a position on the continuum is based on the individual's value system.

14. **TEST-TAKING TIP The word "most" in the stem sets a priority.**

1. When a nurse is caring for a person who is coping with the diagnosis of cancer and a change in body image, the nurse should encourage the expression of feelings, not engage in teaching.

2. **A patient who is requesting information is indicating a readiness to learn.**

3. People in denial are not ready to learn because they do not admit they have a problem. In addition, adolescents believe that they are invincible.

4. A person who is in pain is attempting to cope with a physiological need. This patient is not a candidate for teaching until the pain can be lessened; pain can preoccupy the patient and prevent focusing on the information being presented.

15. **TEST-TAKING TIP The word "first" in the stem sets a priority.**

1. Several other important factors that support adherence to a health-care regimen come before encouraging healthy behaviors.

2. **A trusting relationship between the patient and the nurse is essential. Patients have to be confident that the nurse will maintain confidentiality, has credibility, is nonjudgmental, and is genuinely interested in their success.**

3. Although using educational aids to reinforce teaching supports adherence to a health-care regimen, an action in another option has priority.

4. This is not the first thing the nurse should do to facilitate adherence to a health-care regimen. After the action in another option is completed, then the nurse can assess the factors contributing to the cause for nonadherence to the prescribed health-care regimen.

16. **TEST-TAKING TIP The word "most" in the stem sets a priority. Option 1 denies patient feelings, concerns, or needs. The nurse is explaining that the patient is "not well" while the patient stated, "I am very healthy." Option 3 is patient centered because it focuses on supporting the patient's perception of being healthy, which is associated with independence.**

1. This intervention is judgmental and argumentative and may cut off communication between the patient and nurse.

2. Although identifying the patient's perception of the sick role may be done eventually by assessing the patient's verbal and nonverbal interactions, it is not the priority.

3. **The nurse should ensure that the patient is as independent as possible to help the patient avoid the sick role and maintain the patient's self-concept. According to the Role Performance**

Model of Health, individuals who are able to fulfill their roles in life consider themselves healthy even though they may have an illness or disability.

4. Although giving the patient written materials about the identified illness may be done, it is not the priority.

17. **TEST-TAKING TIP The words "Engel's model of grieving" are key words in the stem that direct attention to content.**

1. During the *developing awareness stage* of Engel's model of grieving, people begin to internalize the loss and psychological pain is experienced.

2. During the *resolving the loss stage* of Engel's model of grieving, people center their energy on thoughts and beliefs about the deceased.

3. During the *idealization stage* of Engel's model of grieving, people initially repress negative thoughts and feelings about the deceased. Later in this stage people tend to incorporate some unique characteristics of the deceased into their own personalities.

4. **According to Engel's model of grieving, the wife is in the restitution stage of grieving. During the *restitution stage*, grieving people are involved with religious practices and rituals.**

18. **TEST-TAKING TIP The word "most" in the stem sets a priority.**

1. Although previous experience is important to know when designing a teaching program, it is not as important as another option when determining whether a teaching program is needed.

2. **Readiness to learn and motivation, which are closely tied together, are the two most important factors contributing to the success of any learning program. The learner must recognize that the learning need exists and that the material to be learned is valuable.**

3. Although expectations are important to know so the teacher can incorporate them into the teaching plan, particularly when setting goals, it is not as important as another option when determining whether a teaching program is needed.

4. Although it is important to know how flexible a patient is when designing a teaching plan, particularly when setting goals, it is not as important as another

option when determining whether a teaching program is needed.

19. **TEST-TAKING TIP The word "physiological" is the key word in the stem that directs attention to content.**

1. ____ Raising side rails relates to the patient's need for safety and security, the second level in Maslow's Hierarchy of Needs.

2. **X A bed bath supports the patient's physiological need to be clean and is related to the first level, physiological needs, in Maslow's Hierarchy of Needs.**

3. ____ Conversing with a patient relates to the need for love and belonging, the third level in Maslow's Hierarchy of Needs.

4. ____ Explaining procedures relates to the patient's need for safety and security; patients have a right to know what is happening to them and why.

5. **X Elimination is a basic physiological need according to Maslow's Hierarchy of Needs. Basic needs relate to food, air, water, elimination, rest, sex, physical activity, temperature regulation, and cleanliness.**

20. **TEST-TAKING TIP The word "most" in the stem sets a priority.**

1. Although a graphic may appeal to visual learners, graphics may not appeal to all learners.

2. The concept of positive reinforcement is not associated with presenting an illustration to reinforce learning. Positive reinforcement is associated with using praise and encouragement to enhance motivation. Research by Ivan Pavlov and B. F. Skinner presented the theory of positive reinforcement.

3. An internal or external locus of control is associated with motivational theory and is unrelated to the rationale for using illustrations to explain complex information.

4. **Research demonstrates that when illustrations are used in conjunction with reading content learners outperform students who just read the content. Illustrations attract attention, facilitate retention of information, and improve understanding of complex content by creating a context.**

21. 1. **X Recognizing goal achievement supports feelings of self-esteem and**

independence; it provides external reinforcement and promotes internal reinforcement.

2. **X Self-care requires performing skills; a demonstration and return demonstration use a variety of senses (e.g., sight, touch) that reinforce learning a psychomotor skill.**

3. ____ The routine ingestion of candy is not healthy; praise is a more acceptable reward.

4. ____ A patient's behavior should never be disregarded; all behavior should be addressed in a nonjudgmental and supportive manner.

5. ____ A mentally disadvantaged person generally can focus on only one objective at a time; several may be overwhelming.

6. **X Short sessions with a limited amount of information/practice may prevent a cognitively impaired person from becoming overwhelmed.**

22. Answer: 5, 2, 1, 4, 3

5. **This statement reflects the most basic level in Maslow's Hierarchy of Human Needs, which is Physiological. This level is associated with concerns such as elimination, nutrition, rest and sleep, and oxygenation.**

2. **This statement is associated with Safety and Security, a second-level need according to Maslow. Second-level needs are related to feeling safe from danger or risk and the need to feel secure in one's own environment.**

1. **This statement is associated with Love and Belonging, a third-level need according to Maslow. Third-level needs relate to the need to feel worthy of affection and support and identification with a group.**

4. **This statement indicates a need for privacy, which supports self-esteem, a fourth-level need according to Maslow. This level also includes the need to feel competent and respected.**

3. **This statement indicates Self-Actualization, the highest level need according to Maslow. Planning one's own funeral reflects reaching a stage of acceptance in the dying process. Acceptance is the highest level of achievement in the dying process according to Kübler-Ross. This demonstrates fulfillment of potential.**

23. **TEST-TAKING TIP The words "Lawrence Kohlberg's theory of stages of moral development" are key words in the stem that direct attention to content.**

Answer: 5, 6, 3, 4, 1, 2

5. **Fearing negative consequences is the motivation for behavior that reflects the first stage of moral development – Obedience and punishment.**

6. **Wanting positive consequences reflects the second stage of moral development—Individualism and exchange.**

3. **Pleasing others based on what they expect reflects the third stage of moral development—Interpersonal relationships.**

4. **Performing actions based on rules reflects the fourth stage of moral development—Maintaining social order.**

1. **Adhering to societal standards while individualizing values and beliefs reflects the fifth stage of moral development—Societal contracts and individual rights.**

2. **Using abstract reasoning based on universal ethical principles reflects the sixth stage of moral development – Universal principles.**

24.

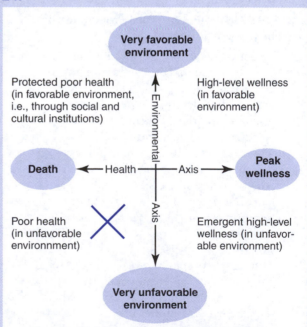

1. **This patient is in protected poor health and lives in a favorable environment. This person should be plotted on the upper left side of Dunn's Health Grid.**

2. This person reflects emergent high-level wellness and lives in an unfavorable environment. This person should be plotted on the lower right side of Dunn's Health Grid.
3. This person reflects high-level wellness living in a favorable environment. This person should be plotted on the upper right side of Dunn's Health Grid.
4. **This person is in poor health and lives in an unfavorable environment. This person should be plotted on the lower left side of Dunn's Health Grid.**

25. **TEST-TAKING TIP Options 2 and 5 are patient-centered options. Options 1, 3 and 4 deny patient feelings, concerns, or needs.**

1. ____ The nurse should accept non–age-appropriate behaviors such as regression, resistance, or crying as long as they does not place the patient or others in danger. These are features of illness in a child and should be accepted as normal reactions to hospitalization. The child needs to feel supported and accepted, not criticized.
2. **X Explaining that expressing feelings of sadness and anger are acceptable gives the patient permission to express these feelings in a nonjudgmental environment. These are expected reactions to grieving.**
3. ____ Although honest and concrete answers to questions expressed by a school-aged child are appropriate, too much detail can be overwhelming and should be avoided. A nurse should always ask the patient if the patient has any questions, and if so, more detail can be provided based on the questions asked.
4. ____ A school-aged child should be assigned to a room with an age- and gender-appropriate roommate when possible because socialization with peers is an important aspect of social development in a school-aged child. Also, roommates can engage in diversional activities such as crafts and board or electronic games.
5. **X Encouraging visits from peers and siblings supports the patient's need to maintain significant interpersonal relationships. These relationships support love and belonging needs.**

26. **TEST-TAKING TIP The words "Kübler-Ross's five stages of Grief in Death and Dying" are key words in the stem that direct attention to content.**

Answer: 4, 5, 2, 1, 3
4. **This statement indicates Stage I—denial. The patient is not ready to believe that something is wrong. During the denial stage the patient may be artificially cheerful, prolonging denial, or unable to deal with practical problems associated with the diagnosis or prognosis.**
5. **This statement indicates Stage II—anger. During the anger stage the patient may displace angry feelings on the primary health-care provider, other caregivers, and/or loved ones. Also, patients may overreact to situations that generally would not anger them prior to the loss.**
2. **This statement indicates Stage III—bargaining. During the bargaining stage the patient may promise to change negative behaviors if just given more time.**
1. **This statement indicates Stage IV—depression. During the depression stage the patient may withdraw and become isolated, or the patient may grieve over past behavior or what will not happen.**
3. **This statement indicates Stage V—acceptance. During the acceptance stage the patient has come to terms with the loss. However, that is not to say that the patient is happy about the impending loss. Behaviors such as having a decreased interest in support people or surroundings, making plans such as saying goodbye to significant others, getting financial affairs in order, or making funeral arrangement are associated with the acceptance stage.**

27. **TEST-TAKING TIP The word "most" in the stem sets a priority. The words "Maslow's Hierarchy of Needs" and "physiological" are key words in the stem that direct attention to the content.**

1. **X An increase in body temperature (fever) is either the body's attempt to regain homeostasis or is a response to an invading microorganism. It is a basic physiological response.**
2. **X Trauma can be life threatening and interfere with basic physiological functioning.**

3. ____ Although physiological changes are associated with the growth spurt and development of secondary sexual characteristics during puberty, self-identity and self-esteem often take priority at this time.

4. ____ Restraints meet safety and security needs because they protect the patient from harm.

5. ____ Although physiological changes are associated with menopause, love, self-esteem, and self-actualization are often the priorities at this time.

28. **TEST-TAKING TIP The words "adaptive capacity" are key words in the stem that direct attention to content.**

1. ____ Safety refers to a basic human need, not adaptive capacity.

2. ____ Health refers to a relative state of a person at a particular moment in time in the physical, emotional, spiritual, and mental dimensions, not adaptive capacity.

3. **X Adaptive capacity refers to the physical, emotional, mental, and spiritual resources one can draw on to reestablish or restore one's previous state or original condition.**

4. ____ Imbalance occurs when a person is threatened by a stressor. Adaptive capacity refers to the physical, emotional, mental, and spiritual resources one can draw on to seek to correct the imbalance and return to a state of homeostasis.

5. **X Adaptive capacity refers to the physical, emotional, mental, and spiritual resources one can draw on to return to one's previous state or original condition.**

29. **TEST-TAKING TIP The word "most" in the stem sets a priority. The word "cognitive" is the key word in the stem that directs attention to content.**

1. **X An *explanation* is within the cognitive domain. An explanation defines, describes, and interprets information so that it is understood.**

2. ____ A *demonstration* is most effective when teaching skills, which are part of the psychomotor domain.

3.. ____ A *group discussion* is most effective when coping with feelings, which are part of the affective domain.

4. **X Factual information can be presented in written materials (e.g., book, pamphlet). It provides reinforcement after**

a verbal explanation from the primary health-care provider or nurse.

5. ____ *Practice* is most effective when learning skills, which are part of the psychomotor domain.

30. **TEST-TAKING TIP The words "in which order" and "Maslow's Hierarchy of Needs" are key words in the stem that direct attention to content.**

Answer: 1, 5, 2, 4, 3

1. **Administering 2 liters of oxygen via a nasal cannula—Meeting basic physiological needs (e.g., patent airway, nutrition, elimination) are first-level needs according to Maslow.**

5. **Arranging the call bell within easy reach after a patient is transferred to a chair—Promoting a feeling of safety and security addresses second-level needs according to Maslow.**

2. **Encouraging a family member to visit as often as desired—Maintaining support systems provides for love and belonging needs, third-level needs according to Maslow.**

4. **Asking a patient about personal preferences before beginning care—Promoting self-control supports self-esteem needs, fourth-level needs according to Maslow.**

3. **Arranging for a minister to visit when requested by a patient—Meeting spiritual need relates to self-actualization, the highest-level need according to Maslow.**

31. **TEST-TAKING TIP The words "generativity versus stagnation" are key words in the stem that direct attention to content.**

1. ____ This statement relates to the conflict of autonomy versus shame and doubt. The 2- to 4-year-old seeks a balance between independence and dependence and attempts to achieve autonomy.

2. ____ This statement relates to the conflict of intimacy versus isolation. The young adult aged 20 to 30 years seeks to select a partner for a life relationship.

3. **X This statement relates to the conflict of generativity versus stagnation. The person aged 30 to 60 years is interested in guiding younger individuals.**

4. ____ This statement relates to the conflict of integrity versus despair. The person aged 60 years or older struggles to feel

a sense of worth about past experience and goals achieved and seeks a sense of integrity.

5. X **This statement relates to the conflict of generativity versus stagnation. A parent is guiding children to be independent.**

32.

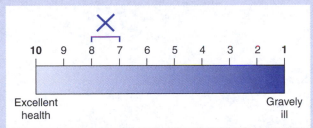

10　9　8　7　6　5　4　3　2　1

Excellent health　　　　　　　　　　　　Gravely ill

A patient's nursing admission history and physical examination should reflect the physical and emotional status of the patient and include the patient's perception of one's level of wellness. An X next to either number 7 or number 8 reflects the *patient's perception of her level of wellness*. The patient said that *she is able to get around all right as long as she stops frequently to catch her breath*. She went on to explain that other than knowing that she has cancer she felt that *"healthwise I'm in pretty good shape."* She said that the only reason she accepted home-health care was because her children insisted that she get help with bathing several mornings a week but went on to say, *"I don't feel that I need any help."* The nurse may place the patient lower on the Health-Illness Continuum; however, that would reflect the nurse's perception, not the patient's perception.

33. **TEST-TAKING TIP** The word "understands" in the stem and the word "learned" in option 3 illustrate a covert clang association. Although they are different words, both have a similar meaning. Options 2 and 3 are patient centered because they are the only options that seek feedback from the patient.

　1. ____ Using simple vocabulary helps to send a clearer message, but it does not inform the sender whether the receiver understood the message.

　2. X **When a patient performs a return demonstration the nurse can observe the patient's technique. Incorrect actions can be corrected, and correct actions can be reinforced.**

3. X **Seeking feedback enables the caregiver to know whether the message was understood as intended.**

4. ____ Speaking distinctly when giving directions helps to send a clearer message, but it does not inform the sender whether the receiver understood the message.

5. ____ Speaking slowly helps to send a clearer message, but it does not inform the sender whether the receiver understood the message.

34. **TEST-TAKING TIP:** Option 5 denies patient feelings, concerns, or needs because it is judgmental and intimidating. Option 5 denies the patient's need to be a "little girl" supported by her mother. Options 1, 2, 3, and 4 are patient-centered options.

　1. X **Explaining that an intervention may "hurt" but that medicine can be given to make the "hurt" go away supports a trusting patient-nurse rapport and reassures the child that care will be provided to support comfort.**

　2. X **Using a doll to explain what is going to be done and why in terms that the child can understand helps to reduce fear of the unknown.**

　3. X **Encouraging a parent to stay with the child as much as possible supports a child's need to feel safe, secure, and protected.**

　4. X **Examining the child while she is sitting on her mother's lap supports the child's need to feel safe, secure, and protected.**

　5. ____ Reminding the child that she is a big girl denies the child's potential need to regress to protect the ego.

35. **TEST-TAKING TIP** The word "best" in the stem sets a priority. Option 3 is unique because it includes all members of the family. Option 3 focuses on the needs of the patient who is the central person in the question and is a patient-centered option. All options contain clang associations; therefore, this technique is not helpful in selecting the correct answer: option 1—son, option 2—granddaughter, option 3—family members, option 4—husband.

　1. This is an inappropriate intervention. The nurse is meeting the son's needs rather than the patient's needs.

2. Explaining to the granddaughter that she should focus on her grandmother is a judgmental response and may cut off further communication between the granddaughter and the nurse. The granddaughter is in the bargaining stage of grieving.

3. **Although the nurse is caring for family members as well as the patient, the patient must be the nurse's priority.**

The patient is entering the acceptance stage of grieving and has decreased interest in environmental activities and people. The patient needs a quiet, peaceful environment.

4. Tell the husband about the availability of bereavement counseling at this time is premature. The nurse should first listen to the husband's feelings and concerns.

COMMUNICATION AND MEETING PATIENTS' EMOTIONAL NEEDS

This section includes questions related to assessing and meeting patients' sociocultural, psychological, and spiritual needs. It also includes questions that focus on the principles of communication, communication skills, interventions that support emotional needs, and communicating with the confused or disoriented patient. Additional questions focus on patterns of behavior in response to illness, nursing interventions that assist patients to adapt to illness, caring for the dying patient's emotional needs, defense mechanisms, and responding to the crying patient.

QUESTIONS

1. A nurse is conducting an intake interview with a patient. Which should the nurse do **first** to facilitate therapeutic communication with this patient?
   1. Use probing questions.
   2. Teach about hygiene.
   3. Ask direct questions.
   4. Listen attentively.

   TEST-TAKING TIP Identify the word in the stem that sets a priority. Identify the unique option. Identify equally plausible options.

2. A patient's son has just died. The patient states, "I can't believe that I have lost my son. Can you believe it?" Which is the nurse's **best** response?
   1. Touch the patient's hand and say, "I am very sorry."
   2. Encourage a family member to stay and provide support.
   3. Leave the room and allow the patient to grieve privately.
   4. Assume a serious facial expression and say, "I can't believe it either."

   TEST-TAKING TIP Identify the word in the stem that sets a priority. Identify patient-centered options. Identify the option that denies the patient's feelings, concerns, or needs. Identify equally plausible options.

3. A patient is admitted to the hospital with multiple health problems. Which nursing intervention is **least** effective in meeting the patient's psychosocial needs?
   1. Addressing the patient by name
   2. Assisting the patient with meals
   3. Identifying achievement of patient goals
   4. Explaining care before it is to be given to the patient

   TEST-TAKING TIP Identify the word in the stem that indicates negative polarity. Identify the key word in the stem that directs attention to content. Identify the unique option.

4. A dying patient says to the nurse, "I was much more religious when I was young." How should the nurse respond to the patient's statement?
   1. "Do you still believe in God?"
   2. "Do you want us to pray for you?"
   3. "Would you like me to call a chaplain?"
   4. "Are you concerned about life after death?"

5. A nurse identifies that a usually talkative patient is withdrawn. Which is the nurse's **best** response?
   1. "What is bothering you?"
   2. "You are very quiet today."
   3. "Tell me what you're upset about."
   4. "Why are you so withdrawn today?"

   TEST-TAKING TIP Identify the word in the stem that sets a priority. Identify the unique option.

6. A patient's spouse died 1 week ago. When reminiscing about their life together, the patient begins to cry. Which is the nurse's **best** response?
   1. Leave the patient alone to provide privacy.
   2. Say, "Things will get better as time passes."
   3. Encourage the patient to get grief counseling.
   4. Say, "This must be a very difficult time for you."

   TEST-TAKING TIP Identify the word in the stem that sets a priority. Identify options that deny patient feelings, concerns, or needs. Identify patient-centered options.

7. A patient has a history of verbally aggressive behavior. One afternoon the patient starts to shout at another patient in the lounge. Which is the **most** appropriate statement by the nurse?
   1. "Stop what you are doing."
   2. "Let's go talk in your room."
   3. "Please sit down until you are calm."
   4. "Do not raise your voice in a hospital."

   TEST-TAKING TIP Identify the word in the stem that sets a priority. Identify key words in the stem that direct attention to content. Identify options that deny patient feelings, concerns, or needs. Identify the patient-centered option. Identify the unique option.

8. A patient is being discharged to a nursing home. While preparing the discharge summary, the patient says, "I feel that nobody cares about me." Which is the nurse's **best** response?
   1. "You feel as if nobody cares."
   2. "We all are concerned about you."
   3. "It's hard to be angry at your family."
   4. "Your family doesn't have the skills to care for you."

   TEST-TAKING TIP Identify the word in the stem that sets a priority. Identify the clang association. Identify opposites in options. Identify the option that denies patient feelings, concerns, or needs. Identify the patient-centered option.

9. A female patient talks about her children when they were young and states, "I was a very strict mother." Which response by the nurse exhibits the technique of paraphrasing?
   1. "It must have been difficult to be a disciplinarian."
   2. "Sometimes we are sorry for our past behaviors."
   3. "You don't seem like a very strict person."
   4. "You believe you were a firm parent."

   TEST-TAKING TIP Identify the key word in the stem that directs attention to content. Identify the option that denies patient feelings, concerns, or needs. Identify the patient-centered option.

10. A patient who is withdrawn says, "When I have the opportunity, I am going to commit suicide." Which is the **best** response by the nurse?
    1. "You have a lovely family. They need you."
    2. "Let's explore the reasons you have for living."
    3. "You must feel overwhelmed to want to kill yourself."
    4. "Suicide does not solve problems. Tell me what is wrong."

    TEST-TAKING TIP Identify the word in the stem that sets a priority. Identify the key word in the stem that directs attention to content. Identify options that deny patient feelings, concerns, or needs. Identify the unique option. Identify the patient-centered option.

11. A patient asks for advice regarding a personal problem. Which is the **most** appropriate response by the nurse?
    1. Explain that nurses are not permitted to give advice to a patient.
    2. Encourage the patient to speak with a family member.
    3. Ask the patient what would be the best thing to do.
    4. Offer an opinion after listening to the patient.

    TEST-TAKING TIP Identify the word in the stem that sets a priority. Identify the option that denies patient feelings, concerns, or needs. Identify opposites in options. Identify the patient-centered option.

12. A newly admitted patient appears upset and agitated. Which should the nurse do to **best** assist this patient?
    1. Arrange for the patient to remain on bedrest.
    2. Encourage the patient to share feelings.
    3. Keep the patient as active as possible.
    4. Point out the behavior to the patient.

    TEST-TAKING TIP Identify key words in the stem that direct attention to content. Identify the option that denies patient feelings, concerns, or needs. Identify the patient-centered option. Identify opposites in options.

13. An older adult reminisces extensively and attempts to keep the nurse from leaving the room. Which nursing action is a therapeutic response?
    1. Encouraging the patient to focus on the present
    2. Limiting the amount of time the patient talks about the past
    3. Setting aside time to listen to the stories about the patient's past
    4. Suggesting that the patient reminisce with other patients of the same age

    TEST-TAKING TIP Identify key words in the stem that direct attention to content. Identify options that deny patient feelings, concerns, or needs. Identify opposites in options.

14. Several times a day, every day, a patient who is experiencing short-term memory loss asks when medication is to be given. The patient receives medication at the same time every day. Which is the **most** therapeutic nursing intervention?
    1. Inform the patient when the time for medication has arrived.
    2. Tell the patient to go to the nurse when it is time for medication.
    3. Encourage the patient to remember when it is time for medication.
    4. Make the patient a sign to hang on a wall indicating the time for medication.

    TEST-TAKING TIP Identify the word in the stem that sets a priority. Identify key words in the stem that direct attention to content. Identify equally plausible options.

15. A patient is upset and rambles about an incident that occurred earlier in the week. Which should the nurse do **first**?
    1. Ask the patient what is wrong.
    2. Identify the patient's concerns.
    3. Recognize the patient is confused.
    4. Encourage the patient to focus on the present.

    TEST-TAKING TIP Identify the option that denies patient feelings, concerns, or needs.

16. A nurse is assessing patients who are coping with multiple stresses to identify the use of defense mechanisms as coping behaviors. Which type of behavior is related to defense mechanisms?
1. Relief
2. Conscious
3. Somatizing
4. Manipulative

TEST-TAKING TIP Identify key words in the stem that direct attention to content.

17. A dying patient says, "All my life I was fairly religious, but I am still worried about what happens after death." Which is the nurse's **best** response?
1. "The unknown is often frightening."
2. "Devout people know that God is forgiving."
3. "You must feel good about being faithful all your life."
4. "People with near-death experiences say it is peaceful."

TEST-TAKING TIP Identify the word in the stem that sets a priority. Identify options that deny patient feelings, concerns, or needs. Identify opposites in options. Identify the patient-centered option.

18. A patient becomes upset whenever anyone mentions an upcoming birthday and does not want to talk about age. Which does this behavior reflect?
1. Denial
2. Sorrow
3. Loneliness
4. Suppression

19. A patient is confused and disoriented. Which route of communication used by the nurse is **most** effective in this situation?
1. Touch
2. Talking
3. Writing
4. Pictures

TEST-TAKING TIP Identify the word in the stem that sets a priority. Identify the unique option.

20. A patient tells the nurse, "The doctor just told me I have cancer" and then begins to cry. Which is the **best** response by the nurse?
1. "Things will seem better tomorrow."
2. "Sometimes it helps to talk about it."
3. "Deep breathing may help you regain control."
4. "Tears are good because it gets it out of your system."

TEST-TAKING TIP Identify the word in stem that sets a priority. Identify the unique option. Identify options that deny patient feelings, concerns, or needs. Identify equally plausible options. Identify the patient-centered option.

21. A nurse is performing a self-appraisal concerning the use of statements that do not support a patient's needs. Which statements by the nurse are nontherapeutic? **Select all that apply.**
1. _____ "This is minor surgery."
2. _____ "You're smiling this morning."
3. _____ "A lot of people hate injections."
4. _____ "It is difficult to cope with pain."
5. _____ "You'll walk better after you have physical therapy."

TEST-TAKING TIP Identify the word in the stem that indicates negative polarity.

22. A nurse is caring for the toddler in the photograph. Which nursing actions support the emotional needs of this child? **Select all that apply.**
    1. ____ Demonstrating to the child how the pen light works before using it
    2. ____ Maintaining a smiling expression when talking with the child
    3. ____ Placing oneself within several inches of the child
    4. ____ Encouraging the child to hold a soft, cuddly toy
    5. ____ Allowing the child to sit on the mother's lap

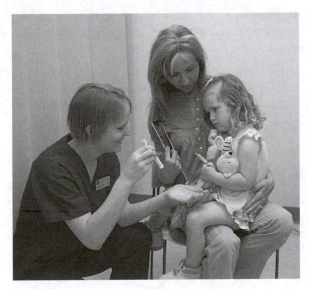

    TEST-TAKING TIP Identify patient-centered options. Identify the option that denies patient feelings, concerns, or needs.

23. A patient who is hearing impaired tells the nurse, "I have difficulty hearing what people say to me." Which should the nurse do? **Select all that apply.**
    1. ____ Face the patient directly when talking.
    2. ____ Provide pencil and paper for communication.
    3. ____ Enunciate clearly when speaking with the patient.
    4. ____ Shout with a loud voice in the patient's better ear.
    5. ____ Ask the patient questions that require a yes or no answer.
    6. ____ Encourage the patient to use gestures and facial expressions when talking.

24. Which concepts are important for the nurse to consider when interacting with others? **Select all that apply.**
    1. ____ Personal appearance can be a source of information about a person.
    2. ____ Progress notes are a form of nonverbal communication.
    3. ____ Patients with expressive aphasia cannot communicate.
    4. ____ Touch has various meanings to different people.
    5. ____ Words have the same meaning for all people.

    TEST-TAKING TIP Identify specific determiners in options.

25. A nurse obtains a health history from a patient with a chronic illness. Which behaviors support the nurse's conclusion that the patient may be depressed? **Select all that apply.**
    1. ____ Wishing to attend a nephew's wedding
    2. ____ Seeking multiple medical opinions
    3. ____ Evading activities of daily living
    4. ____ Lacking interest in appearance
    5. ____ Being sarcastic to caregivers

    TEST-TAKING TIP Identify the key word in the stem that directs attention to the content.

26. A dying patient is withdrawn and depressed. Which are the **most** therapeutic actions by the nurse? **Select all that apply.**
1. _____ Explaining the fact that patient goals still can be accomplished
2. _____ Assisting the patient to focus on positive thoughts
3. _____ Offering the patient advice when appropriate
4. _____ Accepting the patient's behavioral response
5. _____ Telling the patient you are available to talk

TEST-TAKING TIP Identify the word in the stem that sets a priority. Identify key words in the stem that direct attention to content. Identify options that deny patient feelings, concerns, or needs.

27. Alprazolam 0.5 mg PO three times a day is prescribed for a patient with generalized anxiety disorder. It is supplied in an oral solution of 1 mg/mL. How much solution should the nurse administer? **Record your answer using one decimal place.**

Answer: _____ mL

28. A nurse in the emergency department is caring for several patients who are anxious. Place the following patients in the order that reflects the levels of anxiety progressing from mild, to moderate, to severe, and finally to panic levels of anxiety.
1. Patient who has vocal pitch changes, is focusing on one topic, and is exhibiting slight muscle tremors
2. Patient who has normal vital signs, is asking numerous questions, and is exhibiting slight muscle tension
3. Patient who has distorted perception, is hyperventilating, and is exhibiting erratic behavior
4. Patient who has increased motor activity, is irritable, and is exhibiting dilated pupils

Answer: _____

29. A patient who is incontinent of urine becomes upset. Which are the **best** responses by the nurse while changing the patient's gown and linens? **Select all that apply.**
1. _____ "This must be difficult for you."
2. _____ "I am a nurse. This is part of my job."
3. _____ "This doesn't bother me. It often happens."
4. _____ "This occurs all the time. Try not to feel bad."
5. _____ "I am your nurse. I will change your gown and linens."

TEST-TAKING TIP Identify the word in the stem that sets a priority. Identify the clang association. Identify options that deny patient feelings, concerns, or needs. Identify patient-centered options.

30. A patient has difficulty communicating verbally (expressive aphasia) because of a brain attack (stroke). Which should the nurse do when caring for this patient? **Select all that apply.**
1. _____ Anticipate needs to reduce frustration.
2. _____ Teach the patient how to use a picture board.
3. _____ Encourage the patient to elaborate with gestures.
4. _____ Be patient when the patient is attempting to speak.
5. _____ Ask the patient questions that require a yes or no response.

31. A patient who usually is verbal appears sad and withdrawn. Which should the nurse do? **Select all that apply.**
    1. ____ Use open-ended questions.
    2. ____ Describe the behavior to the patient.
    3. ____ Continue to observe the patient's behavior.
    4. ____ Ensure that the patient has time to be alone.
    5. ____ Attempt to engage the patient in cheerful conversation.

    TEST-TAKING TIP Identify key words in the stem that direct attention to content. Identify opposites in options. Identify patient-centered options. Identify options that deny patient feelings, concerns, or needs.

32. A patient verbally communicates with the nurse while exhibiting nonverbal behavior. How should the nurse confirm the meaning of the nonverbal behavior? **Select all that apply.**
    1. ____ Look for similarity in meaning between the patient's verbal and nonverbal behavior.
    2. ____ Ask family members to help interpret the patient's behavior.
    3. ____ Validate inferences by asking the patient direct questions.
    4. ____ Recognize that what a patient says is most important.
    5. ____ Point out the behavior to the patient.

    TEST-TAKING TIP Identify clang associations.

33. A primary health care provider prescribes alprazolam 0.5 mg PO tid for a patient experiencing panic attacks. What should the nurse do when caring for this patient? **Select all that apply.**
    1. ____ Assess for signs of alprazolam abuse.
    2. ____ Ensure that naloxone is readily available.
    3. ____ Teach the patient to provide for personal safety.
    4. ____ Encourage the intake of grapefruit juice during therapy.
    5. ____ Advise the patient not to abruptly discontinue the medication.
    6. ____ Encourage the patient to take an additional prn dose when experiencing high-anxiety situations.

    TEST-TAKING TIP Identify clang associations.

34. A hospice nurse is working with several dying patients. Place the following patients' statements in the order that reflect the stages of Kübler-Ross's grieving theory progressing from diagnosis to impending death.
    1. "I am going to fight this disease with every ounce of energy I've got."
    2. "I don't trust my doctor's diagnosis that I have inoperable cancer."
    3. "I always wore a condom. How could I have gotten AIDS?"
    4. "I can't fight anymore. Please tell my family to let me go."
    5. "I am not going to grow old with my wife."

    Answer: _____

35. Which level anxiety is the patient currently experiencing based on the information in the patient's clinical record?
1. Mild
2. Moderate
3. Severe
4. Panic

PATIENT'S CLINICAL RECORD

Progress Note

Admitted to the coronary care unit (CCU) from the emergency department for observation because of chest pain and palpitations. On admission to the unit, patient reports the presence of a headache, dizziness, and nausea but no longer feels chest pain or palpitations. Asking numerous questions about the chest pain previously experienced; continually focusing on the potential for pain.

Vital Signs on Admission to the CCU

Temp: 99°F, oral route
Pulse: 120 beats/min, regular rhythm
Respirations: 32 breaths/min, deep and rapid
Pulse oximetry: 98%

Physical Assessment

Patient has increased motor activity and a fearful facial expression.
Demonstrates a decreased ability to focus or concentrate when asked questions and is easily distracted. Is still experiencing tachycardia and is hyperventilating.

1. **TEST-TAKING TIP** The word "first" in the stem sets a priority. Option 4 is unique because it is a receptive, nonverbal action, whereas the other options are all active verbal interventions. Options 1 and 3 are equally plausible because both involve direct questioning.

   1. Direct, not probing, questions might be asked later; probing questions violate a patient's right to privacy.
   2. Teaching self-care might be done later; it is not the priority.
   3. Asking direct questions may be done later; it is not the priority.
   4. **Reception of a message must occur before the nurse can intervene; by listening, the nurse collects information that influences future care.**

2. **TEST-TAKING TIP** The word "best" in the stem sets a priority. Options 1 and 4 are patient-centered. Option 3 abandons the patient and denies the patient's feelings, concerns, or needs. Options 2 and 3 abdicate nursing responsibility and are equally plausible.

   1. **Touch denotes caring; this statement is direct and supportive but does not reinforce denial.**
   2. Although this may be done later, the patient needs immediate support from a professional nurse.
   3. Leaving the room is a form of abandonment.
   4. Although this statement identifies feelings, it supports denial.

3. **TEST-TAKING TIP** The word "least" in the stem indicates negative polarity. The word "psychosocial" is the key word in the stem that directs attention to content. Option 2 is unique because it is the only option that provides physical nursing care. Options 1, 3, and 4 are interventions based on psychosocial principles of care.

   1. Calling a patient by name individualizes care and supports dignity and self-esteem.
   2. **Usually eating is an independent activity of daily living; for an adult, assistance with meals may precipitate feelings of dependence and regression.**
   3. Identifying the achievement of goals is motivating and supports independence, self-esteem, and self-actualization.

   4. Explaining care provides emotional support because it reduces fear of the unknown and involves the patient in the care.

4. 1. This is inappropriate probing and violates the patient's right to privacy or may put the patient on the defensive.
   2. This is an inappropriate question; not all the nurses on the team may want to assume this intervention.
   3. **This response identifies that the patient is considering personal spiritual needs; it provides an opportunity that the patient can accept or reject.**
   4. This is inappropriate probing and may put the patient on the defensive.

5. **TEST-TAKING TIP** The word "best" in the stem sets a priority. Option 2 is unique because it does not ask the patient to respond; it identifies behavior. Options 1, 3, and 4 are asking "What" or "Why" questions. Options 1, 3, and 4 are equally plausible because they all ask a question about something that is wrong (e.g., bothering, upset, and withdrawn).

   1. A "what....." statement is too direct; it may put the patient on the defensive and cut off communication. Also, the patient may not have the insight to answer the question.
   2. **This statement identifies behavior and provides an opportunity for the patient to verbalize further.**
   3. This statement is too direct and almost sounds like a command; it may put the patient on the defensive and cut off communication. Also, the patient may not have the insight to answer the question.
   4. "Why" questions are too direct and often patients do not have the insight to answer them. Also, this statement draws the conclusion that the patient is withdrawn, which may be inaccurate.

6. **TEST-TAKING TIP** The word "best" in the stem sets a priority. Options 1 and 2 deny the patient's feelings, concerns, or needs. Options 3 and 4 are patient-centered. Although, encouraging grief counseling is something the nurse may do in the future, it is not the best response at this time.

   1. Leaving abandons the patient at a time when emotional support may be beneficial. Abandonment is an ultimate form of denial.

2. This statement is false reassurance and denies the patient's feeling.

3. This may eventually be done, but the patient needs immediate support.

4. **This statement identifies feelings, focuses on the patient, and provides an opportunity for the patient to share feelings.**

7. **TEST-TAKING TIP** The word "most" in the stem sets a priority. The words "verbally aggressive" and "shouts" are key words in the stem that direct attention to content. Options 1, 3, and 4 deny patient feelings, concerns, or needs. Option 2 is patient-centered. Option 2 is unique because it is the only option that removes the patient from the room and does not admonish the patient's behavior.

1. This statement is a command that may demean the patient; it challenges the patient and may precipitate more aggressive behavior.

2. **This statement interrupts the behavior and protects the other patient; walking to another room uses energy, and talking promotes verbalization of feelings and concerns.**

3. This statement is judgmental; this implies the patient is not calm. An agitated patient has too much energy to sit quietly.

4. This statement is inappropriate because it challenges the patient and puts the patient on the defensive.

8. **TEST-TAKING TIP** The word "best" in the stem sets a priority. The words "nobody cares" appear in the stem and option 1; this repetition is a clang association. Options 1 and 2 are opposites. Option 2 denies patient feelings, concerns, or needs. Option 1 is patient centered.

1. **Repeating the patient's statement allows the patient to focus on what was said, validates what was said, and encourages communication.**

2. This statement is an assumption that may or may not be true and does not encourage verbalization of feelings.

3. This patient's statement reflects feelings of sadness and isolation, not anger.

4. This statement may or may not be true and does not encourage verbalization of feelings.

9. **TEST-TAKING TIP** The word "paraphrasing" is the key word in the stem that directs attention to content. Although option 3 has a clang association with the word "strict," this option denies patient feelings, concerns, or needs and should be eliminated. Option 4 is the patient-centered option.

1. This response uses reflective technique, not paraphrasing, because it identifies a feeling.

2. The patient's statement does not reflect feelings of sorrow or guilt.

3. This response denies the patient's feelings.

4. **This response restates the message using different words; paraphrasing focuses on content rather than the feeling or underlying emotional theme of the patient's message.**

10. **TEST-TAKING TIP** The word "best" in the stem sets a priority. The word "suicide" is the key word in the stem that directs attention to content. Options 1, 2, and 4 deny patient feelings, concerns, or needs. Option 3 is unique because it is the only option that addresses the patient's feelings. Option 3 is patient-centered.

1. This statement denies the patient's feelings. The patient is unable to cope, is selecting the ultimate escape, and is not capable of meeting the needs of others. This response may also precipitate feelings such as guilt.

2. This statement denies the patient's feelings; the patient must focus on the negatives before exploring the positives.

3. **Open-ended statements identify feelings and invite further communication.**

4. This response is judgmental, denies the patient's feelings, and may cut off communication. In addition, this response is too direct and the patient may not consciously know what is wrong.

11. **TEST-TAKING TIP** The word "most" in the stem sets a priority. Option 1 denies the patient's feelings, concerns, or needs. Options 3 and 4 are opposites. Option 3 is patient-centered.

1. This approach puts the focus on the nurse and cuts off communication.

2. Although this might eventually be done, it is not the priority. Also, the patient may never want to talk about a particular concern with family members.

3. **This response provides an opportunity for the patient to explore concerns and**

alternative solutions without others influencing the decision making.

4. Offering opinions is inappropriate; opinions involve judgments that are based on feelings and values that may be different from the patient's.

12. **TEST-TAKING TIP** The words "upset and agitated" are key words in the stem that direct attention to content. Option 1 denies patient feelings, concerns, or needs. It is difficult for an agitated patient to remain in bed. Option 2 is patient-centered. Although options 1 and 3 are opposites; they are distractors in this question.

1. Agitated patients may not be able to lie still. They need some outlet for energy expenditure.

2. **Agitation is a response to anxiety; the patient's feelings and concerns must be addressed to help relieve the anxiety and agitation.**

3. Keeping the patient as active as possible may increase the agitation, particularly if the cause of the agitation is ignored.

4. Pointing out the behavior to the patient is confrontational and may precipitate a defensive response by the patient.

13. **TEST-TAKING TIP** The words "reminisces extensively" are key words in the stem that direct attention to content. Options 1 and 2 deny patient feelings, concerns, or needs. Options 1 and 3 are opposites.

1. Avoiding reminiscing is inappropriate; the developmental task of older adults is to perform a life review.

2. Avoiding reminiscing is inappropriate; the developmental task of older adults is to perform a life review.

3. **The nurse is responsible for assisting the older adult to explore the past and deal with the developmental conflict of integrity versus despair.**

4 Patients should not be responsible for meeting each other's needs.

14. **TEST-TAKING TIP** The word "most" in the stem sets a priority. The words "short-term memory loss" are key words in the stem that direct attention to content. Options 2 and 3 are equally plausible because both options require the patient to remember when medications are given.

1. Although reminding the patient every time might be done, it is not the most

therapeutic intervention because it addresses only the next dose.

2. The patient probably is not capable of remembering. Too challenging a task can be frustrating.

3. The patient probably will not remember when it is time for the medication. Too challenging a task can be frustrating.

4. **A sign promotes independence and does not demean the patient; the patient can refer to the schedule when necessary.**

15. **TEST-TAKING TIP** Option 4 denies patient feelings, concerns, or needs.

1. This is too direct; the patient may not be able to put into words what is wrong.

2. **Active listening is necessary for data collection; after data are collected, feelings and concerns can be identified.**

3. When people are anxious, their conversation may ramble, but it does not necessarily mean they are confused.

4. This action denies the patient's feelings; the patient must talk further about the situation to reduce anxiety.

16. **TEST-TAKING TIP** The words "defense mechanisms" are key words in the stem that direct attention to content.

1. **Defense mechanisms are used to lower anxiety, manage stress, maintain the ego, and shelter self-esteem; they can be productive or eventually detrimental. They provide relief by releasing physical and emotional energy.**

2. Most defense mechanisms are used on an unconscious level, except for suppression, which is used by the conscious mind.

3. A somatizing behavior is identified when a patient experiences a psychological conflict as a physical symptom; physical symptoms distract the patient from the actual emotional distress as the patient internally manages the anxiety physiologically.

4. Manipulative behaviors are not known as defense mechanisms but rather as purposeful behaviors used to meet personal needs. Manipulative behaviors can be adaptive or maladaptive; they are maladaptive when they are the primary method used to meet needs, the needs of others are ignored, or others are dehumanized to meet the needs of the manipulator.

17. **TEST-TAKING TIP** The word "best" in the stem sets a priority. Options 2, 3, and

4 deny patient feelings, concerns, or needs. Options 1 and 4 are opposites. Option 1 is patient centered.

1. **This statement uses reflective technique to identify the patient's feelings regarding fear of the unknown.**
2. This statement denies the patient's feelings and cuts off communication; also, the patient's message did not indicate a need for forgiveness.
3. This statement puts the emphasis on the wrong part of the message; it ignores the patient's concern about what happens after death.
4. This statement focuses on other people's experiences rather than the patient's feelings or concerns.

18. 1. Denial is an unconscious defense mechanism; this patient consciously and voluntarily refuses to talk about the birthday.
    2. This is an assumption; there are insufficient data to reach this conclusion.
    3. This is an assumption; there are insufficient data to reach this conclusion.
    4. **This is a conscious protective mechanism in which a person actively puts anxiety-producing feelings or concerns out of the mind.**

19. **TEST-TAKING TIP** The word "most" in the stem sets a priority. Option 1 is unique. Touch is the only intervention that does not require higher intellectual functioning.

    1. **Touch is a simple form of communication that is easily understood even by confused, disoriented, or mentally incapacitated individuals.**
    2. Talking requires an interpretation of words, which is a more complex form of communication than touch.
    3. Writing requires interpretation of symbols, which is a more complex form of communication than touch.
    4. Pictures require interpretation of symbols, which is a more complex form of communication than touch.

20. **TEST-TAKING TIP** The word "best" in the stem sets a priority. Option 2 is unique. Options 1, 3, and 4 deny patient feelings, concerns, or needs; all imply that everything will get better. These responses are Pollyanna-like responses that deny the patient's feelings. Options 3 and 4 are equally plausible; both relate to getting

emotions under control or out of the system. Option 2 is patient centered.

1. This response is false reassurance.
2. **This response provides an opportunity for the patient to verbalize feelings and concerns and is patient centered.**
3. This response implies that the patient is out of control. This interferes with the patient's coping mechanisms and may not help the patient regain control.
4. This response is false reassurance; crying may or may not help this patient. Also, the use of the word *good* is a value judgment.

21. **TEST-TAKING TIP** The word "nontherapeutic" in the stem indicates negative polarity. The question is asking, "Which options are examples of inappropriate statements that the nurse should avoid when interacting with patients?"

    1. **X This statement implies that there is no reason to worry, which is a form of false reassurance.**
    2. ____ This is a therapeutic response that invites the patient to explore feelings.
    3. **X This statement takes the focus away from the patient and cuts off further communication.**
    4. ____ This is a supportive statement that focuses on what the patient may be thinking and invites an exploration of feelings and problem solving.
    5. **X This statement supports an outcome that may or may not be accomplished by physical therapy; this is false reassurance.**

22. **TEST-TAKING TIP** Options 1, 2, 4, and 5 are patient-centered options. Option 3 denies patient feelings, concerns, or needs.

    1. **X Demonstrating how to use equipment before use engages the child, helps to minimize fear of the unknown, and builds trust between the child and nurse.**
    2. **X Maintaining a smiling expression conveys that the nurse is friendly and approachable, communicates warmth and caring, and facilitates a connection between the nurse and child.**
    3. ____ Placing oneself within several inches of the child invades the child's personal space. Trust should be established first. However, positioning oneself at eye level with the child nonverbally communicates

a personal interest in the child and indicates that communication is an open channel.

4. X Encouraging the child to hold a familiar cuddly toy enhances feelings of safety and security during times of stress.

5. X Allowing the child to sit on the mother's lap enhances a feeling of safety and security during times of stress.

23. 1. X Facing the patient directly allows the patient to view the nurse's lips and facial expression, both of which improve the transmission and reception of a message.

2. X Communication can be promoted in written rather than verbal form; this reduces social isolation.

3. X Enunciating clearly presents a verbal message that should be clear and crisp; mumbling sends messages that can become distorted and misinterpreted.

4. ____ Shouting is demeaning and unnecessary.

5. ____ Communication is a two-way process: the patient is not having difficulty sending messages; the patient is having difficulty receiving messages. This intervention is more appropriate for a patient with expressive aphasia.

6. ____ The patient is having difficulty receiving messages, not sending messages.

24. **TEST-TAKING TIP** In option 3, the word "all" is understood; this option is really saying, "All patients with expressive aphasia cannot communicate." This is a specific determiner. Option 5 contains the word "all," which is a specific determiner.

1. X Personal appearance is often a reflection of how patients feel and their culture, religion, group association, and self-concept.

2. ____ Words, whether they are spoken or written, are verbal communication.

3. ____ Patients with expressive aphasia can often communicate using nonverbal behaviors, a picture board, or written messages.

4. X Touch is a form of nonverbal communication that sends a variety of messages depending on the person's

culture, sex, age, past experiences, and present situation; touch also invades a person's personal space.

5. ____ People from different cultures and people in subgroups within the same culture place different values on words.

25. **TEST-TAKING TIP** The word "depressed" is the key word in the stem that directs attention to content.

1. ____ This is future-oriented thinking and may be a form of bargaining for more time.

2. ____ This is associated with denial and bargaining.

3. X When patients are depressed, they may feel a loss of control, feel alone, and be withdrawn. With depression, there is little physical energy, a lack of concern about the activities of daily living, and a decreased interest in physical appearance.

4. X When depressed, people do not have the emotional or physical energy to attend to their appearance.

5. ____ Sarcasm generally reflects feelings of anger.

26. **TEST-TAKING TIP** The word "most" in the stem sets a priority. The words "withdrawn" and "depressed" are key words in the stem that direct attention to content. Options 1, 2, and 3 deny patient feelings, concerns, and needs.

1. ____ Explaining that the patient still can accomplish goals denies the patient's feelings.

2. ____ Assisting the patient to focus on positive thoughts denies the patient's feelings.

3. ____ It is never appropriate to offer advice; people must explore their alternatives and come to their own conclusions.

4. X Depression is the fourth stage of dying according to Kübler-Ross; patients become withdrawn and noncommunicative when feeling a loss of control and recognizing future losses. The nurse should accept the behavior.

5. X Patients who are dying become depressed when they realize that death is inevitable. The nurse should be available in case the patient wants to talk.

27. **Answer: 0.5 mL**
    Solve the problem using a formula for ratio and proportion.

    $$\frac{\text{Desire}}{\text{Have}} \quad \frac{0.5 \text{ mg}}{1 \text{ mg}} = \frac{x \text{ mL}}{1 \text{ mL}}$$

    $1 x = 0.5$

    $x = 0.5 \div 1$

    $x = 0.5 \text{ mL}$

28. **Answer: 2, 1, 4, 3**
    2. People with mild anxiety have normal or slight physiological responses (e.g., vital signs, muscle tension) because the sympathetic nervous system is barely stimulated. Their communication usually revolves around questions to obtain information.
    1. People with moderate anxiety have an increase in physiological responses (e.g., tremors, slight increase in vital signs) as a result of a greater stimulation of the sympathetic nervous system. Their communication is slightly impaired as evidenced by pitch changes and tremors of the voice, selective inattention, and focusing on one topic.
    4. People with severe anxiety have physiological reactions associated with the fight-or-flight response related to the sympathetic nervous system (e.g., increased motor activity, dilated pupils, elevated vital signs, headache, nausea, urgency, and frequency). Their mood reflects irritability.
    3. People with a panic level of anxiety have a continuation of the physiological reactions associated with the fight-or-flight response (e.g., increased motor activity, dilated pupils, elevated vital signs, headache, nausea, urgency, and frequency). Their perception is distorted and scattered and their motor activity can be erratic, combative, or withdrawn.

29. **TEST-TAKING TIP** The word "best" in the stem sets a priority. The words "gown and linens" in the stem and in option 5 comprise a clang association. Options 2, 3, and 4 deny patient feelings, concerns, or needs. Option 1 and 5 do not minimize the patient's feelings and focus on the patient; they are patient centered.
    1. X This response focuses on feelings and is supportive.

    2. ____ This response cuts off communication and puts the focus on the nurse rather than on the patient.
    3. ____ This response generalizes rather than individualizes care. It minimizes the patient's concern and may cut off communication.
    4. ____ This response generalizes rather than individualizes care. The use of the word "bad" is an assumption.
    5. X This response meets the patient's right to know who is providing care and what is to be done. This is a non-judgmental, respectful response even though it does not address the patient's feelings.

30. 1. ____ Although anticipating needs may be done occasionally, it does not increase the patient's ability to communicate.
    2. X A picture board is generally a laminated card featuring photographs or illustrations often with matching phrases associated with common personal needs. This device gives control of the conversation to the patient, which increases independence and reduces frustration when making needs known.
    3. X Communication can be both verbal and nonverbal. The use of gestures facilitates communication.
    4. X Being patient while the patient is attempting to speak demonstrates respect, allows the patient time to form the communication, and supports self-esteem.
    5. ____ Although this may be done occasionally, it does not increase the patient's ability to communicate; a yes or no response is too limited.

31. **TEST-TAKING TIP** The words "sad and withdrawn" are key words in the stem that direct attention to content. Although options 4 and 5 are opposites, option 4 abandons the patient and option 5 denies the patient's feelings. Options 4 and 5 can be eliminated. Options 1 and 2 are patient centered; they are the only responses that directly address the patient's behavior. The other options avoid the patient (option 3), abandon the patient (option 4), or deny the patient's feelings (option 5).
    1. X Using open-ended questions encourages verbalization of concerns and

allows the patient to direct the focus of the response. Open-ended statements provide a broad opening and offer a general lead. They invite the patient in a nonthreatening way to respond.

2. **X Pointing out the patient's behavior brings it to the attention of the patient and provides an opportunity to explore feelings.**

3. ____ The patient's behavior needs to be addressed more fully than only by continued observation.

4. ____ This is a form of abandonment; sad, withdrawn patients need to know that they are accepted and that the nurse is available for support.

5. ____ This response denies the patient's feelings.

32. **TEST-TAKING TIP** The word "nonverbal" in the stem and in option 1 is a clang association, and the word "verbally" in the stem and the word "verbal" in option 1 comprise a clang association. The word "behavior" in the stem and in options 1, 2, and 5 comprise clang associations. Options 1 and 5 are correct answers and option 2 is a distractor.

1. **X The patient is the primary source of information. When nonverbal communication reinforces the verbal message, the message reflects the true feelings of the patient because nonverbal behavior is under less conscious control than verbal statements.**

2. ____This abdicates the nurse's responsibility to others and obtains a response that is influenced by the family members' emotion and subjectivity.

3. **X Direct questions may ultimately be necessary if the patient's responses to open-ended questions do not clarify the nonverbal behavior.**

4. ____Nonverbal behaviors, rather than verbal statements, better reflect true feelings. Actions speak louder than words!

5. **X Pointing out behavior is a gentle way of making the patient aware of his or her behavior, which may precipitate an exploration of the patient's behavior and feelings. It is an open-ended approach because the patient is in control of the progression of the interaction.**

33. **TEST-TAKING TIP** The word "alprazolam" in the stem and in option 1 comprise a

clang association. The word "patient" in the stem and in options 3, 5, and 6 comprise clang associations.

1. **X Alprazolam can lead to dependence and abuse; therefore, the patient should be assessed for responses such as drowsiness, sedation, irritability, dizziness, blurred vision, diplopia, headache, insomnia, GI disturbances, dry mouth, tremors, confusion, slurred speech, impaired memory, and an inability to focus.**

2. ____ The antidote for alprazolam is flumazenil, not naloxone. Naloxone is an opioid antagonist that can inhibit or reverse the effects of opioids such as respiratory depression, sedation, and hypotension.

3. **X Alprazolam (Xanax) is a central nervous system depressant that can cause dizziness, drowsiness, lethargy, decreased level of alertness, confusion, mental depression, and blurred vision. The patient should be taught ways to provide for personal safety such as how to prevent falls and to avoid driving until the patient's response to the drug is determined.**

4. ____ Grapefruit juice should be avoided when receiving alprazolam. Grapefruit juice can interfere with intestinal enzymes that metabolize alprazolam, thus causing higher than normal levels of the drug in the blood and resulting in enhanced side effects.

5. **X Alprazolam should not be discontinued suddenly, to avoid signs and symptoms of withdrawal. Withdrawal should be conducted under medical supervision.**

6. **X Alprazolam should be taken only three times a day as prescribed to maintain a therapeutic blood level of the drug in the body. Extra doses can lead to toxicity or dependence and should not be taken without medical supervision.**

34. Answer: 2, 3, 1, 5, 4

2. *Denial or disbelief* is the first stage of Kübler-Ross's grieving theory. The patient is saying "No not me." The patient may be in denial, distrust the diagnosis, or seek multiple diagnostic opinions. The patient may intellectually understand the diagnosis but not emotionally integrate the diagnosis.

3. *Anger* is the second stage of Kübler-Ross's grieving theory. The patient may question "Why me?" The patient also may cite reasons why it is impossible to have the diagnosis or respond with anger and hostility.

1. *Bargaining* is the third stage of Kübler-Ross's grieving theory. The patient is saying "Yes me, but" and is attempting to gain more time.

5. *Depression* is the fourth stage of Kübler-Ross's grieving theory. The patient is saying "Yes me" as the eventual death is realized. The patient may grieve future losses, talk, withdraw, cry, or feel alone.

4. *Acceptance* is the fifth and last stage of Kübler-Ross's grieving theory. The patient is saying "OK, me." The patient may have a decreased interest in activities, be quiet and peaceful, and be involved in completing personal affairs or planning the funeral. Sometimes the patient will reach this stage before family members; the nurse should help family members to understand and allow the patient to withdraw.

35. 1. The patient's responses do not support the presence of mild anxiety. Mild anxiety is associated with increased questioning, mild restlessness, increased arousal and alertness, and the absence of physiological responses.

2. The patient's responses do not support the presence of moderate anxiety. Moderate anxiety is associated with voice tremors and pitch changes, tremors and shakiness, increased muscle tension, selective inattention, slightly increased respiratory and pulse rates, and mild gastric symptoms.

3. The patient's responses are indicative of severe anxiety. Severe anxiety is associated with tachycardia, hyperventilation, headache, dizziness, nausea, increased motor activity, and inability to relax. The person's communication may be difficult to understand, and the patient has difficulty concentrating and is easily distracted.

4. The patient's responses do not support the presence of a panic level of anxiety. Panic level anxiety is associated with agitation, trembling, poor motor coordination, dyspnea, palpitations, choking, chest pain or pressure, feeling of impending doom, paresthesia, diaphoresis, distorted or exaggerated perception, and communication that may not be understandable.

PHYSICAL ASSESSMENT OF PATIENTS

This section includes questions related to various aspects of physical and psychosocial assessment. Questions focus on temperature, pulse, respirations, blood pressure, level of consciousness, level of orientation, and principles related to specimens and the collection of specimens such as for a culture and sensitivity test. Questions also address assessments common to infection, the general adaptation syndrome, and the inflammatory process. Additional questions focus on whether assessment data are subjective or objective, whether sources are primary or secondary, responsibilities of the nurse regarding data collected during assessment, sources of data, and the use of common physical examination techniques.

QUESTIONS

1. Which is the primary source for assessing how a patient slept?
   1. Nurse
   2. Patient
   3. Patient's roommate
   4. Nursing-care assistant

   TEST-TAKING TIP Identify the key word in the stem that directs attention to content. Identify the unique option.

2. When a nurse goes into a room to take a patient's temperature, the patient is drinking a cup of coffee. How long should the nurse wait to take the patient's oral temperature?
   1. 5 minutes
   2. 7 minutes
   3. 15 minutes
   4. 30 minutes

   TEST-TAKING TIP Identify the key word in the stem that directs attention to content.

3. A nurse is assessing the vital signs of several patients. Which signs of respiratory distress should the nurse report to the primary health-care provider?
   1. Respiratory rate of 26 breaths per minute with an irregular rhythm
   2. Respiratory rate of 16 breaths per minute with an irregular rhythm
   3. Respiratory rate of 18 breaths per minute with a regular rhythm
   4. Respiratory rate of 20 breaths per minute with a regular rhythm

   TEST-TAKING TIP Identify the key word in the stem that directs attention to content. Identify duplicate facts among options.

4. The function of which part of the anatomy is reflected when the nurse obtains a radial pulse rate?
   1. Arteries
   2. Blood
   3. Heart
   4. Veins

   TEST-TAKING TIP Identify the key word in the stem that directs attention to content. Identify opposites in options.

5. A nurse is assessing the temperature of a patient. When can the nurse expect a patient's temperature to be at its lowest?
   1. 6 a.m.
   2. 10 a.m.
   3. 6 p.m.
   4. 9 p.m.

   TEST-TAKING TIP Identify the key word in the stem that directs attention to content.

6. When making rounds, the nurse finds a patient in bed with the eyes closed. Which should the nurse do?
   1. Return in a half hour to check on the patient
   2. Suspect that the patient is feeling withdrawn
   3. Allow the patient to continue sleeping
   4. Collect more data about the patient

   TEST-TAKING TIP Identify opposites in options.

7. A nurse takes the resting pulse of an older adult. Which pulse is within the expected range?
   1. 50 beats per minute and irregular
   2. 90 beats per minute and regular
   3. 105 beats per minute and irregular
   4. 120 beats per minute and regular

   TEST-TAKING TIP Identify key words in the stem that direct attention to content. Identify duplicate facts among options.

8. A nurse obtains the rectal temperature of an adult. Which rectal temperature is within the expected range?
   1. 96.4°F
   2. 97.6°F
   3. 99.8°F
   4. 101.2°F

   TEST-TAKING TIP Identify key words in the stem that direct attention to content.

9. A patient has a history of heart disease. After walking to the lounge, the patient sits in a chair, places a fist against the chest, and states, "I have a severe upset stomach." Which should the nurse do **first**?
   1. Obtain vital signs.
   2. Walk the patient back to bed.
   3. Administer an antacid to the patient.
   4. Document the patient's change in status.

   TEST-TAKING TIP Identify the word in the stem that sets a priority.

10. A nurse obtains the blood pressure of several patients. Which blood pressure reading is considered the **most** hypertensive?
   1. 90/70 mm Hg
   2. 130/86 mm Hg
   3. 160/90 mm Hg
   4. 150/115 mm Hg

   TEST-TAKING TIP Identify the word in the stem that sets a priority. Identify the key word in the stem that directs attention to content.

11. Which action is common to the collection of specimens for culture and sensitivity regardless of their source?
1. The specimen should be collected in the morning.
2. Gloves, a gown, and a mask should be worn.
3. Two specimens should always be obtained.
4. Surgical asepsis should be maintained.

TEST-TAKING TIP Identify key words in the stem that direct attention to content. Identify the option with a specific determiner.

12. When assessing the heart rate of a patient, the nurse identifies a change in rate from 88 to 56 beats per minute. Which should the nurse do **first**?
1. Wait a half hour and retake the pulse.
2. Obtain the other vital signs.
3. Ask about recent activity.
4. Tell the nurse in charge.

TEST-TAKING TIP Identify the word in the stem that sets a priority.

13. A nurse should identify a patient's health beliefs before giving care. Which should the nurse identify **first** about the patient when making this assessment?
1. Level of wellness
2. Acceptable values
3. Frame of reference
4. Use of defense mechanisms

TEST-TAKING TIP Identify the word in the stem that sets a priority.

14. The function of which part of the anatomy is primarily being assessed when a nurse obtains a patient's pedal pulse?
1. Veins
2. Heart
3. Blood
4. Arteries

TEST-TAKING TIP Identify the word in the stem that sets a priority. Identify key words in the stem that direct attention to content. Identify opposites in options.

15. Which principle of blood pressure physiology should the nurse understand when assessing a patient's cardiac function?
1. The blood pressure reaches a peak followed by a trough.
2. A peak pressure occurs when the left ventricle relaxes.
3. The pulse pressure occurs during diastole.
4. A trough pressure occurs during systole.

TEST-TAKING TIP Identify key words in the stem that direct attention to content. Identify the clang association. Identify the unique option.

16. A nurse is monitoring the results of a culture and sensitivity report from a specimen from a wound. Which does the sensitivity part of the report indicate?
1. All of the microorganisms present
2. Antibiotics that should be effective
3. Virulence of the organisms in the exudate
4. Extent of the patient's response to the pathogens

TEST-TAKING TIP Identify key words in the stem that direct attention to content. Identify the option with a specific determiner.

17. Which are examples of objective data collected during a nursing history and physical examination of a newly admitted patient? **Select all that apply.**
1. _____ Pain
2. _____ Fever
3. _____ Nausea
4. _____ Fatigue
5. _____ Hypertension

TEST-TAKING TIP Identify the key word in the stem that directs attention to content. Identify equally plausible options.

18. A patient has herpes zoster. Place an X over the site the nurse should assess because it is the **most** common site of herpes zoster lesions.

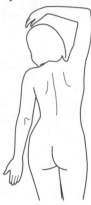

TEST-TAKING TIP Identify the word in the stem that sets a priority.

19. A nurse is assessing a patient's orientation times three. Which are nursing interventions that should be included in this assessment? **Select all that apply.**
1. _____ Asking the patient's name
2. _____ Having patients state the time of day
3. _____ Inquiring if patients know where they are
4. _____ Ascertaining if the patient can follow simple directions
5. _____ Determining if the patient follows movement with the eyes

20. A nurse is caring for a patient who has an elevated temperature. Which route should the nurse use when assessing a patient for a rapid change in core temperature?

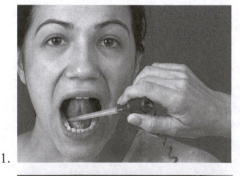

1.

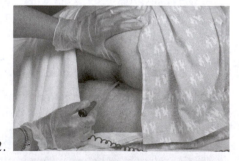

2.

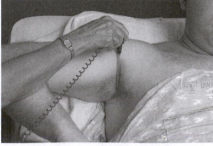

3.

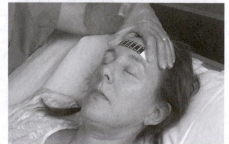

4.

TEST-TAKING TIP Identify key words in the stem that direct attention to content.

21. Which patient reactions indicate that the inflammatory response has entered the first phase? **Select all that apply.**
    1. ____ Pain
    2. ____ Heat
    3. ____ Fever
    4. ____ Exudate
    5. ____ Erythema

    TEST-TAKING TIP Identify key words in the stem that direct attention to content.

22. A nurse on the day shift is caring for a middle-aged adult admitted during the night with the flu. At 0800 the nurse identifies that the patient is lethargic and obtains the patient's vital signs, which are: oral temperature, 103.8°F; pulse, 120 beats per minute, irregular; respirations, 34, labored; oxygen saturation, 86%. The nurse compares these most recent vital signs with the values obtained previously. Which should the nurse do?
    1. Initiate the rapid response team.
    2. Administer the prescribed ibuprofen.
    3. Recheck the vital signs in 15 minutes.
    4. Change the oxygen via nasal cannula to a face mask at 6 liters.

VITAL SIGNS SHEET

Time	0200	0400	0600
Temperature	101.8°F	102.°F	102.2°F
Pulse	98	106	112
Respirations	22	24	28
SaO2	96%	95%	94%

    TEST-TAKING TIP Identify opposites in options.

23. Which information about a patient is classified as subjective data? **Select all that apply.**
    1. ____ Is experiencing palpitations
    2. ____ Reports feeling nauseated
    3. ____ Has a headache
    4. ____ Looks tired
    5. ____ Is crying

    TEST-TAKING TIP Identify the key word in the stem that directs attention to content. Identify equally plausible options.

24. A nurse is working as a triage nurse in the emergency department. Place the following patients in the order in which they should receive care.
    1. Infant having a seizure
    2. Man with acute pancreatitis
    3. Woman with acute chest pain
    4. Adolescent with a blood glucose level of 110 mg/dL
    5. Child with a non–life-threatening cut that needs stitches

    Answer: _____

25. An older adult reports shortness of breath, fever, coughing, and excessive mucus. The primary health-care provider diagnoses bronchitis and admits the patient for intravenous antibiotic therapy. The nurse assesses the patient's breath sounds as part of the admission assessment to the unit. Place an X over the site where the nurse should place the stethoscope when assessing for bronchial breath sounds.

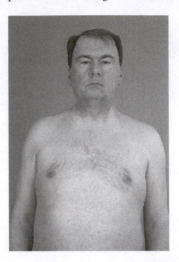

26. A patient reports a dull ache in the calf of the left leg. Identify the assessment that the nurse should **avoid** considering this information?

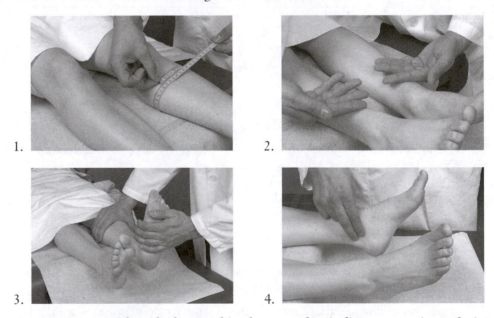

1.

2.

3.

4.

TEST-TAKING TIP Identify the word in the stem that indicates negative polarity.

27. For which is the nurse assessing when touching the patient is this manner?
    1. Appearance of reactive hyperemia
    2. Presence of sensory perception
    3. Symmetry of skin temperature
    4. Strength of the lower legs

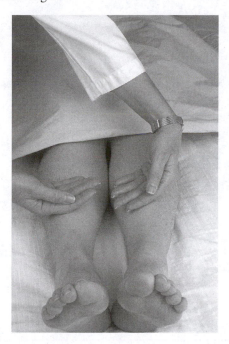

28. A nurse performing triage in the emergency department is reviewing admission data about four patients. Place the patients in the order in which departmental staff should attend to the needs of these patients.
    1. A 12-year-old child who fell off a bicycle reporting pain in the right wrist and is accompanied by a parent
    2. A 30-year-old butcher who cut off ⅓ of his right index finger and arrived with the severed finger in a clean towel
    3. A 55-year-old man who is taking warfarin daily and fell on the ice, causing a large painful bruise on the right buttock
    4. A 70-year-old woman who has a temperature of 102.4°F and respirations of 24 because of a reported worsening upper respiratory tract infection.

    Answer: _____

29. A nurse is auscultating a patient's apical heart rate. Place an X on the location where the stethoscope should be placed to access the point of maximum impulse.

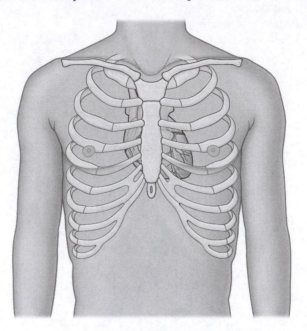

30. A nurse is obtaining an oral temperature with an electronic thermometer. Which must the nurse do? **Select all that apply.**
1. ____ Use the green probe.
2. ____ Take the temperature before breakfast.
3. ____ Use a new probe cover for each patient.
4. ____ Wipe the probe with alcohol after each use.
5. ____ Assess if the route is appropriate for the patient.

TEST-TAKING TIP Identify key words in the stem that direct attention to content.

31. A nurse is using the equipment indicated in the illustration to assess a pedal pulse. Which steps are associated with the use of this equipment? **Select all that apply.**
1. ____ Ensure that a dorsalis pedis pulse is present.
2. ____ Assess the rate and rhythm of the dorsalis pedis pulse.
3. ____ Tilt the end of the probe 45° to the dorsalis pedis artery.
4. ____ Apply a water-soluble lubricant on the end of the probe.
5. ____ Locate the groove between the great toe and first toe and move toward the top of the foot until the dorsalis pedis pulse is found.

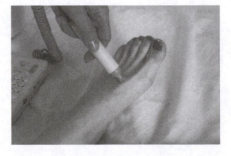

32. A nurse must obtain a blood specimen from the surface of an adult's finger using a spring-loaded lancet. Place an X on the site that is the appropriate location for the skin puncture.

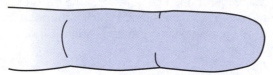

33. A nurse working in a long-term care facility is taking the blood pressures of a group of older adults. Which are the reasons why the nurse can expect an increase in blood pressure in this group of older adults? **Select all that apply.**
1. ____ Aging hearts
2. ____ Thicker blood
3. ____ Lifestyle stressors
4. ____ Less elastic vessels
5. ____ Presence of atherosclerosis

34. A nurse is caring for patient who is on contact isolation and is having temperatures taken with a non-mercury thermometer. Which temperature is indicated in the illustration?
1. 100.2°F
2. 100.6°F
3. 101.4°F
4. 102.8°F

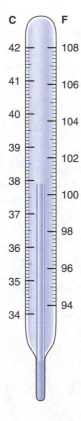

35. A nurse is caring for a patient who sustained trauma in an occupational accident. The nurse makes the following patient assessments: opens eyes when asked a question; speaks words but is disoriented to time, place, and person; and follows instructions when assisted to change position. The nurse uses the Glasgow Coma Scale (GCS) to rate the patient's level of consciousness. Which point total on the Glasgow Coma Scale should the nurse document in the patient's clinical record indicating the patient's level of consciousness?
1. 9
2. 11
3. 13
4. 15

GLASGOW COMA SCALE

	Points
Eye Opening	**Points**
Eyes open spontaneously	4
Eyes open in response to voice	3
Eyes open in response to pain	2
No eye opening response	1
Best Verbal Response	**Points**
Oriented (e.g., to person, place, time)	5
Confused, speaks but is disoriented	4
Inappropriate, but comprehensible words	3
Incomprehensible sounds but no words are spoken	2
None	1
Best Motor Response	**Points**
Obeys command to move	6
Localizes painful stimulus	5
Withdraws from painful stimulus	4
Flexion, abnormal decorticate posturing	3
Extension, abnormal decerebrate posturing	2
No movement or posturing	1
Total Points	**?**

36. A nurse is assessing the skin of an older adult. Which changes in the patient's skin should the nurse anticipate? **Select all that apply.**
1. _____ Increased pigmented spots
2. _____ Decreased thickness
3. _____ Increased elasticity
4. _____ Decreased dryness
5. _____ Increased tone

TEST-TAKING TIP Identify key words in the stem that direct attention to content.

37. A nurse is caring for a patient with a diagnosis of liver disease. Place an X over the body cavity that the nurse should assess for the presence of ascites?

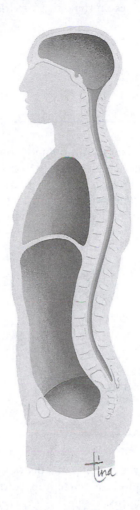

38. A nurse is palpating a patient's radial pulse and identifies that it can be obliterated with slight presure. Which words accurately reflect this assessment when documenting the information in the pateint's clinical record? **Select all that aply.**
1. _____ Bounding
2. _____ Thready
3. _____ Absent
4. _____ Weak
5. _____ Full

TEST-TAKING TIP Identify key words in the stem that direct attention to content. Identify equally plausible options. Identify opposites in options.

39. A charge nurse receives the following clinical record of a patient being sent to a medical unit from the emergency department. Which is important for the charge nurse to assess after the patient arrives on the unit from the emergency department?
1. Pulse rate
2. Blood pressure
3. Respiratory rate
4. Oxygen saturation

PATIENT'S CLINICAL RECORD

Admission History

A 75-year-old adult obtained an appointment with a primary health-care provider because of an upper respiratory infection. While entering the primary health-care provider's office the older adult fell to the ground, and the primary health-care provider called for an ambulance. Numerous tests were performed in the emergency department, and the older adult is being admitted to the hospital for management of dehydration. The patient has a 5-year history of Parkinson disease, has hypertension, has no family, and lives alone.

Vital Signs Flow Sheet

Blood pressure: 110/65 mm Hg
Pulse: 100 beats/min, thready
Respirations: 28 breaths/min, regular
Temperature: 99.6°F, orally
Oxygen saturation: 89%

Primary Health-Care Provider's Orders

1,000 mL 0.9% sodium chloride at 125 mL/hr
Encourage oral fluid intake
Oxygen 2 L via nasal cannula

40. A primary nurse assesses all the patients in a district at the beginning of a shift. Which patient responses require the nurse to perform an immediate focused assessment? **Select all that apply.**
1. _____ Suprapubic distention
2. _____ Edema of 2+ in the ankles
3. _____ Difficulty sleeping at night
4. _____ Lack of a bowel movement in 3 days
5. _____ Blanchable erythema in the sacral area

TEST-TAKING TIP Identify the word in the stem that sets a priority. Identify key words in the stem that direct attention to content.

1. **TEST-TAKING TIP** The word "primary" is the key word in the stem that directs attention to content. Option 2 is unique. Options 1, 3, and 4 involve people other than the patient.

   1. The nurse is a secondary source of data. The nurse may not be totally aware of how well the patient slept.
   2. **Patients are primary sources and the only sources able to provide subjective data concerning how they slept.**
   3. Patients should not be held responsible for other patients.
   4. A nursing-care assistant is a secondary source of information.

2. **TEST-TAKING TIP** The word "oral" is the key word in the stem that directs attention to content.

   1. Five minutes is too short a period of time for the mouth to recover from the hot fluid; the dilated vessels in the mouth and the warmth of the tissues from the hot fluid will cause an inaccurate increase in the temperature reading.
   2. Seven minutes is too short a period of time for the mouth to recover from the hot fluid; the dilated vessels in the mouth and the warmth of the tissues from the hot fluid will cause an inaccurate increase in the temperature reading.
   3. **It takes at least 15 minutes for the vessels in the mouth and the mucous membranes to recover from the hot fluid and for the mouth to return to the patient's core temperature.**
   4. This is unnecessary. Thirty minutes is too long a time period to wait for the mouth to recover from the hot fluid.

3. **TEST-TAKING TIP** The word "distress" is the key word in the stem that directs attention to content. Options 1 and 2 contain the duplicate fact that the patient's respirations are irregular. Options 3 and 4 contain the duplicate fact that the patient's respirations are regular. If you know that respirations should be regular, then options 3 and 4 are distractors. If you know that an irregular rhythm is common with respiratory distress, then you can focus on options 1 and 2.

   1. **Tachypnea, a respiratory rate greater than 24 breaths per minute, along with an irregular rhythm, indicates that the body is in respiratory distress.**
   2. This is within the expected range of 12 to 20 breaths per minute. An irregular rhythm without other signs of distress does not necessitate notifying the primary health-care provider.
   3. Breathing is usually regular and within the range of 12 to 20 breaths per minute.
   4. Although the rate is at the high end of the expected range of 12 to 20 breaths per minute, it is an acceptable rate, particularly when the rhythm is regular.

4. **TEST-TAKING TIP** The word "radial" is the key word in the stem that directs attention to content. The radial site for assessing the pulse rate and function of the heart is the most common site used for this purpose. Although options 1 and 4 are opposites, neither one is the correct answer. Arteries carry blood away from the heart; veins carry blood to the heart. In this question, these options are distractors.

   1. Elasticity and rigidity of the vessel walls and the quality and equality of pulses provide data about the status of the arteries.
   2. Blood is assessed through laboratory tests performed on blood specimens.
   3. **The heart is a pulsatile pump that ejects blood into the arterial system with each ventricular contraction; the pulse is the vibration transmitted with each contraction of the heart.**
   4. A pulse is palpated in an artery, not a vein.

5. **TEST-TAKING TIP** The word "lowest" is the key word in the stem that directs attention to content.

   1. **A person's body temperature is at its lowest in the early morning. Core temperatures vary with a predictable pattern over 24 hours (diurnal or circadian rhythms) because of hormonal variations.**
   2. Body temperature is not at its lowest at 10 a.m.; body temperature steadily increases as the day progresses.
   3. Body temperature peaks between 5 and 7 p.m.

4. Body temperature is not at its lowest at 9 p.m.; body temperature is still decreasing from its peak.

6. **TEST-TAKING TIP** Options 1 and 3 are opposite to option 4.

1. Waiting is unsafe.
2. This is an assumption based on insufficient data.
3. Assuming that the patient is sleeping is a conclusion made with insufficient information.
4. **More information must be collected to make a complete assessment and reach an accurate conclusion.**

7. **TEST-TAKING TIP** The words "resting," "older adult," and "expected" are key words in the stem that direct attention to content. Options 1 and 3 relate to an irregular pulse. Options 2 and 4 relate to a regular a pulse. If you know that a pulse should be regular, then options 1 and 3 can be eliminated. If you know that a resting pulse should be regular, focus attention on options 2 and 4. If you know that the expected range for a pulse is 60 to 100 beats per minute, focus on option 2. If you know the acceptable range for a pulse, you can still get the answer correct without knowing that the rhythm should be regular.

1. A rate of 50 is below the expected range of a pulse rate in an older adult. The rhythm should be regular, not irregular.
2. **The expected heart rate in an older adult is between 60 and 100 beats per minute and regular.**
3. A rate of 105 is too high for a heart rate taken at rest; in older adults, a decreased contractile strength of the myocardium may cause the heart rate to increase to this rate during mild exercise. The rhythm should be regular, not irregular.
4. A rate of 120 is too high for a heart rate at rest.

8. **TEST-TAKING TIP** The words "rectal" and "expected range" are key words in the stem that direct attention to content.

1. 96.4°F is below the expected range for a rectal temperature.
2. 97.6°F is below the expected range for a rectal temperature.
3. **A temperature of 99.8°F is within the expected range of 98.6°F to 100.6°F for a rectal temperature.**
4. A temperature of 101.2°F indicates a fever.

9. **TEST-TAKING TIP** The word "first" in the stem sets a priority.

1. **A further assessment is necessary; vital signs reflect the cardiopulmonary status of the patient. The patient may be experiencing a cardiac event.**
2. Activity at this time is unsafe because it will increase the demands on the heart.
3. The nurse does not have enough information to conclude that the problem is gastritis; administering an antacid is a dependent function of a nurse that requires a prescription.
4. Although this should be done eventually, it is not the priority.

10. **TEST-TAKING TIP** The word "most" in the stem sets a priority. The word "hypertensive" is the key word in the stem that directs attention to content.

1. A blood pressure reading of 90/70 mm Hg reflects hypotension.
2. This is considered prehypertension, not hypertension. Blood pressure values of 120 to 139 systolic and 80 to 89 diastolic are considered prehypertensive.
3. Although a systolic reading of 160 is high and needs to be reported to the primary health-care provider, a blood pressure with a higher diastolic reading is more dangerous.
4. **A blood pressure with a higher diastolic pressure is more hypertensive than a blood pressure with a higher systolic pressure but lower diastolic pressure. The diastolic pressure is the pressure exerted against the arterial walls when the ventricles are at rest; the higher the diastolic pressure, the more dangerous the situation.**

11. **TEST-TAKING TIP** The words "common to" and "culture and sensitivity" are key words in the stem that direct attention to content. Option 3 contains the word "always," which is a specific determiner.

1. The time of day is irrelevant for the collection of most specimens for culture and sensitivity.
2. Gloves may be worn when collecting specimens to protect the nurse, not to maintain sterility of the specimen; gowns and masks generally are unnecessary unless splashing of body fluids is likely.
3. Generally, if a specimen is collected using sterile technique, one specimen is

sufficient for testing for culture and sensitivity. However, blood cultures for a disease such as endocarditis may require several specimens over a 24- to 48-hour period.

4. **The results of a culture and sensitivity test will be inaccurate if the steps of the collection procedure and collection container are not kept sterile; a contaminated specimen container introduces extraneous microorganisms that falsify and misrepresent results.**

12. **TEST-TAKING TIP** The word "first" in the stem sets a priority.

1. Waiting is unsafe. The change in pulse may indicate an impending problem.
2. **Corroborative data should be obtained; the vital signs reflect cardiopulmonary functioning. When there is an alteration in one vital sign, there usually is a change in another.**
3. Activity will increase, not decrease, the heart rate.
4. Alerting the nurse in charge might be necessary after other more appropriate interventions.

13. **TEST-TAKING TIP** The word "first" in the stem sets a priority.

1. Assessing a patient's level of wellness should be done later.
2. Viewing a person's value system as acceptable or unacceptable is judgmental.
3. **Attitudes and beliefs influence health practices and how one perceives self-health; the nurse must always "begin care where the patient is."**
4. Assessing the use of defense mechanisms should be done later.

14. **TEST-TAKING TIP** The word "primarily" in the stem sets a priority. The words "pedal pulse" are key words in the stem that direct attention to content. Options 1 and 4 are opposites. Arteries carry blood away from the heart and veins carry blood to the heart. These opposites are more difficult to identify than most opposites. Although the function of the heart can be assessed any time an arterial pulse is monitored, pedal pulses generally are monitored to assess adequacy of blood flow to the feet.

1. Veins do not have a pulse.
2. Radial, carotid, or apical pulses, not pedal pulses, readily assess heart function.

3. Laboratory tests assess blood and its components.
4. **The presence, absence, or quality of pedal pulses reflects the adequacy of arterial circulation in the feet; peripheral pulses should be present, equal, and symmetrical.**

15. **TEST-TAKING TIP** The words "cardiac function" are key words in the stem that direct attention to content. The word "blood" in the stem and in option 1 is a clang association. Options 2, 3, and 4 each identify one factor related to blood pressure and when it occurs. Option 1 is unique because it identifies two factors related to blood pressure and does not contain the words "pressure occurs."

1. **Peak pressures occur when the ventricles contract and trough pressures occur when the ventricles relax; these occur with each contraction and relaxation of the heart.**
2. Peak pressures occur when the ventricles contract.
3. Pulse pressure is the difference between the systolic and diastolic pressures.
4. Peak pressures, not trough pressures, occur during systole.

16. **TEST-TAKING TIP** The words "sensitivity" and "indicate" are key words in the stem that direct attention to content. Option 1 contains the word "all," which is a specific determiner. This option can be eliminated from consideration.

1. Examination of a specimen under a microscope, not the sensitivity part of a culture and sensitivity test, identifies the microorganisms present.
2. **Areas of lack of growth of microorganisms surrounding an antibiotic on a culture medium indicate that the microorganism is sensitive to the antibiotic and the antibiotic is capable of destroying the microorganism.**
3. The ability to produce disease (virulence) is not determined by the sensitivity portion of a culture and sensitivity test; virulence is determined by statistical data concerning morbidity and mortality associated with the microorganisms.
4. The clinical manifestation of the disease process reflects the extent of the patient's response to the microorganism present.

17. **TEST-TAKING TIP** The word "objective" is the key word in the stem that directs attention to content. Options 2 and 5 are similar because they are measurable. Options 1, 3, and 4 are similar because these responses can be described only by the patient.

1. ____ Pain is a subjective clinical indicator; subjective data are a patient's perceptions, feelings, sensations, or ideas.

2. **X Fever is an objective clinical indicator because it can be measured with a thermometer.**

3. ____ Nausea is a subjective clinical indicator, based on a patient's feelings or perceptions.

4. ____ Fatigue is a subjective clinical indicator, based on a patient's feelings or perceptions.

5. **X Hypertension (increased blood pressure) can be measured with a sphygmomanometer and therefore is objective information.**

18. **TEST-TAKING TIP** The word "most" in the stem sets a priority. This is the most common site for herpes zoster lesions. It is a disease related to activation of the latent human herpesvirus 3. It is also known as shingles. Lesions most commonly occur along affected nerves, causing crops of vesicles over the related dermatome.

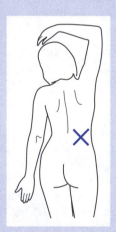

19. 1. **X Questions related to time, place, and person (assessing orientation in three ways) are essential when assessing a patient's level of orientation. When oriented, patients should know their names (person).**

2. **X When oriented, patients should know the time of day (time).**

3. **X When oriented, patients should know where they are (place).**

4. ____ Following simple directions can be done by confused, disoriented patients.

5. ____ Following movement with the eyes can be done by confused patients.

20. **TEST-TAKING TIP** The words "rapid change" and "core temperature" are key words in the stem that direct attention to content.

1.

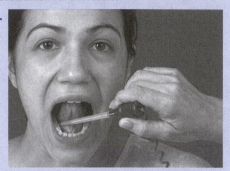

This is the oral route. It is the best route when assessing a rapid change in a patient's core temperature. When an oral thermometer is placed posteriorly into the sublingual pocket it is close to the sublingual artery, which reflects a rapid change in core body temperature.

2.

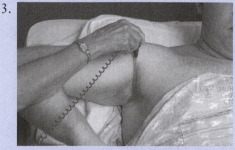

This is the rectal route. Although the rectal route is the most accurate route for measuring core body temperature, it is not the best route to assess for a rapid change in core body temperature.

3.

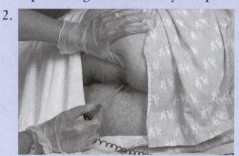

This is the axillary route. Although it is noninvasive and easily accessible, it is not the best route for this patient because the axillary temperature lags behind the core temperature during a rapid change in core temperature.

4.

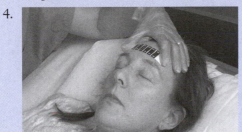

This is the skin route. This route only indicates body surface temperature. This is the least accurate and reliable route to take a core temperature

21. **TEST-TAKING TIP** The words "inflammatory response" and "first phase" are key words in the stem that direct attention to content.

1. **X Pain occurs during the first phase of the inflammatory response in reaction to the release of histamine at the injury site. Histamine promotes vessel permeability, which increases edema, causing pressure on nerve endings.**

2. **X Heat occurs during the first phase of the inflammatory response in reaction to the release of histamine at the injury site. Histamine causes dilation of capillaries resulting in blood flooding the area, which makes it warm to the touch.**

3. ____ Fever is a systemic, not a local, response and is not indicative of phase 1 of the inflammatory response.

4. ____ Phase 2, not phase 1, of the inflammatory response is characterized by the formation of an exudate; it consists of a combination of cells and fluids produced at the localized site of injury.

5. **X During the first phase of the inflammatory response, histamine is released, resulting in increased blood flow to the area. Dilation of capillaries causes the area to be flooded with blood, which makes the area appear red.**

22. **TEST-TAKING TIP** Options 1 and 3 are opposites. The intervention in option 1 does something immediately, whereas the intervention in option 3 waits 15 minutes.

1. **The patient's status indicates the need for immediate medical intervention.**

The patient's condition has continually deteriorated over the past 6 hours.

2. Although ibuprofen may be administered, another option is the priority.

3. It is unsafe to waste 15 minutes considering the patient's deteriorating condition. Another option is the priority.

4. Changing the oxygen via a nasal cannla to a face mask at 6 liters should be done after the option that is the priority is implemented. Taking the time to gather equipment to change the nasal cannula to a face mask will delay the primary action.

23. **TEST-TAKING TIP** The word "subjective" is the key word in the stem that directs attention to content. Options 1, 2, and 3 are similar because the patient is the only one who can describe palpitations, nausea, and headache. Options 4 and 5 are similar because they include assessments that can be observed by another person. The options within each group are equally plausible. You have to identify which group of options you should choose based on your understanding of the concept of objective versus subjective data.

1. **X Subjective data are data that can be described or verified only by the patient. Palpitations are the subjective symptom of an excessively rapid, irregular heart rate.**

2. **X Nausea is subjective information that can be described or verified only by the patient.**

3. **X A description of a headache is subjective information because it can be described only by the patient.**

4. ____ Looks tired is a conclusion based on an observation.

5. ____ Crying is an objective datum because it can be observed by another person.

24. **Answer: 1, 3, 2, 5, 4**

1. **An infant having a seizure should receive care first because the infant is in acute distress. A person having a seizure should never be left alone. The primary responsibilities include maintaining patient safety and observing the characteristics of the seizure.**

3. **A woman having acute chest pain should receive care second because chest pain can indicate a myocardial infarction or other potentially fatal cardiac event.**

2. **Acute pancreatitis is extremely painful, and therefore this patient should be medicated as soon as possible after patients with life-threatening problems are stabilized.**

5. **A child with a non–life-threatening cut that needs stitches can wait until the more acute patients are attended to and stabilized.**

4. **A blood glucose level of 110 mg/dL or less is considered within the expected (normal) range; therefore meeting the needs of patients with more acute problems first is appropriate.**

25. **Bronchial breath sounds are heard in the anterior neck and nape of the neck posteriorly. They are loud, high-pitched, hollow sounds with a short inspiratory phase and a long expiratory phase.**

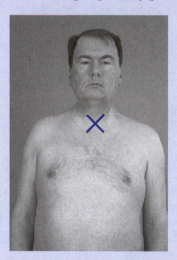

26. **TEST-TAKING TIP** The word "avoid" in the stem indicates negative polarity. The question is asking, "What should the nurse *not* do?"

1. This photograph depicts measuring the circumference of the calf. This is an acceptable objective assessment when measuring edema or inflammation of the calf.

2. This photograph depicts assessing skin temperature using the backs of the hands, which are more sensitive to skin temperature than the palms of the hands. The nurse is assessing symmetry of skin temperature. This is an acceptable assessment technique in this situation.

3. **This photograph depicts supporting the patient's leg while dorsiflexing the foot. Dorsiflexion of a foot that precipitates calf pain (Homan's sign) indicates the presence of a deep vein thrombosis. Eliciting the Homan's sign in the presence of calf pain is**

contraindicated because this action increases the risk of causing a thrombus to dislodge, which can migrate to the lung resulting in a life-threatening pulmonary embolus.

4. This photograph depicts assessment of the posterior tibial pulse. This is an acceptable assessment technique in this situation.

27. 1. The nurse is not testing for the appearance of reactive hyperemia. Reactive hyperemia is the transient increase in blood flow following a short period of ischemia. Hyperemia is often associated with the response of tissue over a bony prominence after relief of pressure when a person's position is changed.

2. The nurse is not testing for the presence of sensory perception. Sensory perception in an extremity is commonly tested for pain, vibration, and position sense, as well as other tests using various stimuli such as cotton balls and pointy and dull objects while the patient's eyes are closed.

3. **The nurse is testing the patient's skin temperature to determine if circulation is the same in both legs. If circulation is impaired in one leg, it will feel cooler than the leg with more adequate circulation. The back of the hands, rather than the palms, are more sensitive when assessing changes in skin temperature.**

4. The nurse is not testing the strength of the patient's legs. When testing for strength in the legs the nurse may flex the patient's knee while supporting the patient's lower leg and then ask the patient to press the sole of the foot against the nurse's hand.

28. Answer: 3, 2, 4, 1

3. **The patient taking warfarin (Coumadin) should be attended to first because the risk of bleeding internally as a result of the fall can be life-threatening. Once the patient's vital signs are assessed and it is determined that the patient is not bleeding internally, then another patient can be attended to next.**

2. **The 30-year-old butcher who cut off one-third of his right index finger should be attended to second. It is essential that reconstructive surgery occur quickly if the severed finger is to remain viable. Although this patient's condition is serious, a patient with a potentially life-threatening situation should be attended to first.**

4. The woman with the upper respiratory tract infection should be attended to third. The vital signs are not elevated enough to indicate imminent danger. Two other patients require more immediate attention. This patient should be attended to before the last patient because an older adult has less compensatory reserve than a younger person.

1. Although the 12-year-old child may have fractured the wrist, needing the care of an orthopedist, this situation is the least serious when compared with the other situations.

29. To assess the apical heart rate the nurse should position a stethoscope over the site of maximum impulse, the apex of the heart. Two-thirds of the heart extends to the left of the midline of the body. The widest part is called the base and is located just below the second rib. The base is where the great vessels enter and leave the heart. The blunt pointed end is called the apex and is located to the left of the patient's sternum just over the diaphragm. To find the apex of the heart find the angle of Louis (bump below the sternal notch where the manubrium and sternum meet) and slide a finger into the second intercostal space on the left side of the sternum. Place one finger in each intercostal space, moving down to the fifth intercostal space. Slide a finger to the midclavicular line over the apex of the heart. This is the location indicated by the X.

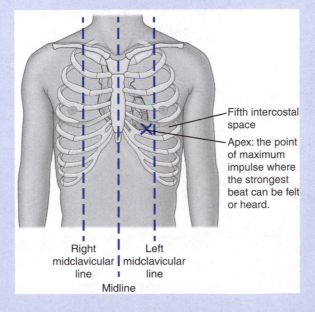

Fifth intercostal space

Apex: the point of maximum impulse where the strongest beat can be felt or heard.

Right midclavicular line | Left midclavicular line

Midline

30. **TEST-TAKING TIP** The words "oral" and "electronic thermometer" are key words in the stem that direct attention to content.

1. X A green probe is used for an oral temperature and a red probe is used for a rectal temperature.
2. ____ Taking the temperature before breakfast is unnecessary; however, daily temperatures should be taken at the same time for comparison purposes. Temperatures usually are lowest in the early morning and highest between 5 and 7 p.m.
3. X Because an electronic thermometer is used for multiple patients, a probe cover is a medical aseptic barrier technique used to prevent the spread of microorganisms.
4. ____ Wiping the probe with alcohol after each use is unnecessary because the probe is covered with a new probe cover before each use and is discarded after it is used. If the probe becomes accidentally contaminated, it must be decontaminated by wiping it with alcohol.
5. X The oral route should not be used for individuals who are unconscious, are mouth breathers, or cannot follow directions, or who have just consumed cold or hot liquids or food.

31. 1. X When using a Doppler the presence of the dorsalis pedis pulse indicates the presence of arterial circulation to the distal portion of the extremity. A Doppler machine accentuates the sounds of blood flowing through an artery.
2. ____ It is not necessary to assess the rate and rhythm of the dorsalis pedis pulse. The nurse should assess the presence and volume of the dorsalis pedis pulse. The rate and rhythm are important when assessing the radial, apical, or carotid pulses.
3. X Tilting the probe at a 45° angle to the dorsalis pedis artery helps to access the signal (e.g., pulsing, rhythmic hissing sound) indicating the presence of the dorsalis pedis pulse.
4. ____ Water-soluble lubricant should not be substituted for transmission gel when using a Doppler. Transmission gel ensures optimal contact between the probe and the patient's skin, is an excellent conducting agent, and has a gliding property that facilitates movement of the probe without losing contact with the skin.
5. X This is the best action to find the dorsalis pedis pulse. Place the Doppler probe in the groove between the great

toe and first toe and move along the top of the foot toward the ankle until the dorsalis pedis pulse is located.

32. An X within either of the two shaded areas toward the fingertip is a correct answer. Off-center toward the lateral aspect of a finger has fewer nerve endings compared with the center of the pad of the distal end of a finger.

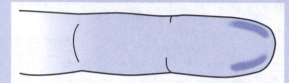

33. 1. _____ In aging hearts there is decreased contractile strength of the myocardium that results in a decreased cardiac output. The body compensates for this by increasing the heart rate, not the blood pressure.
    2. _____ Aging does not cause thicker blood. Polycythemia (greater concentration of erythrocytes to plasma), a pathological condition, can cause a higher viscosity of the blood, resulting in hypertension.
    3. _____ This is a generalization that may or may not be true. An older adult may have physical, cognitive, and social changes, and how the person perceives them and adapts to them determines whether the individual's lifestyle is stressful and whether it influences blood pressure.

4. X As people age, vascular changes and the accumulation of sclerotic plaques along the walls of vessels occur, making them more rigid. Vascular rigidity increases vascular resistance, which increases blood pressure.
5. X As people age, yellowish plaques containing cholesterol, lipoid material, and lipophages build up in the intima and inner media of large and medium-sized arteries (atherosclerosis); this pathological process narrows the lumen of vessels, increasing the pressure within the vessels.

34. 1. The illustration does not indicate a temperature of 100.2°F.
    2. **The illustration indicates a temperature of 100.6°F.**
    3. The illustration does not indicate a temperature of 101.4°F.
    4. The illustration does not indicate a temperature of 102.8°F.

35. 1. The number 9 does not reflect the patient's total points on the Glasgow Coma Scale.
    2. The number 11 does not reflect the patient's total points on the Glasgow Coma Scale.
    3. **The number 13 reflects the patient's total points on the Glasgow Coma Scale as demonstrated in the following scale.**
    4. The number 15 does not reflect the patient's total points on the Glasgow Coma Scale.

GLASGOW COMA SCALE

Eye Opening	Points
Eyes open spontaneously	4
Eyes open in response to voice	**3**
Eyes open in response to pain	2
No eye opening response	1
Best Verbal Response	**Points**
Oriented (e.g., to person, place, time	5
Confused, speaks but is disoriented	**4**
Inappropriate, but comprehensible words	3
Incomprehensible sounds but no words are spoken	2
None	1
Best Motor Response	**Points**
Obeys command to move	**6**
Localizes painful stimulus	5
Withdraws from painful stimulus	4
Flexion, abnormal decorticate posturing	3
Extension, abnormal decerebrate posturing	2
No movement or posturing	1
Total Points	**13**
Major Head Injury	≤8
Moderate Head Injury	**9–12**
Minor Head Injury	**13–15**

36. **TEST-TAKING TIP** The words "older adult" and "skin" are key words in the stem that direct attention to content.

    1. __X__ The size of pigment-containing cells (melanocytes) increases in size as one ages, particularly on skin exposed to the sun.

    2. __X__ The skin of the older adult decreases in thickness because of loss of dermal and subcutaneous mass. These loses occur in response to a flattening of the dermal-epidermal junction, reduced thickness and vascularity of the dermis, and slowing of epidermal proliferation.

    3. ____ As a person's skin ages it decreases, not increases, in elasticity because collagen fibers become coarser and more random, and there is a degeneration of elastic fibers in the dermal connective tissue.

    4. ____ As a person's skin ages it increases, not decreases, in dryness because of a reduction in moisture content, sebaceous gland activity, and circulation to the skin.

    5. ____ As a person's skin ages it decreases, not increases, in tone because of loss of dermal mass. This occurs because of flattening of the dermal-epidermal junction,

reduced thickness and vascularity of the dermis, and slowing of epidermal proliferation.

37. Venous return from the stomach, small intestine, colon, spleen, and pancreas flows via veins to the portal vein (hepatic portal circulation). The portal vein transports blood into the liver where blood is detoxified. Blood then exits the liver via hepatic veins, to the inferior vena cava, and eventually to the right atrium of the heart. With advanced liver disease there is increased pressure in liver blood flow, which in turn results in an increase in pressure in the hepatic portal circulation (portal hypertension). In addition, an impaired liver is unable to produce adequate amounts of albumin, the principal protein in blood, which is necessary to maintain blood volume. The increase in venous pressure in the hepatic portal circulation and a decrease in albumin are responsible for moving fluid from the hepatic portal circulation, a high-pressure space, to the abdominal cavity, a low-pressure space, resulting in ascites. See Figure B for an illustration of hepatic portal circulation.

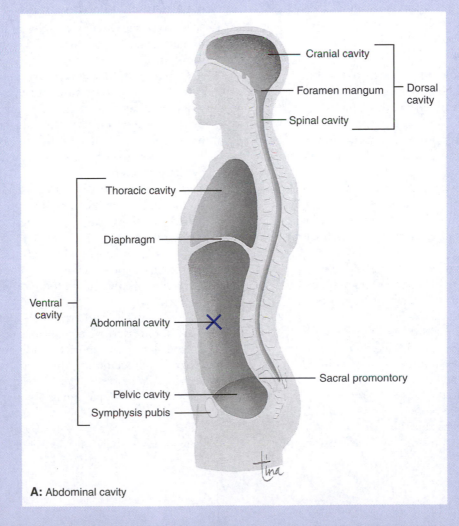

A: Abdominal cavity

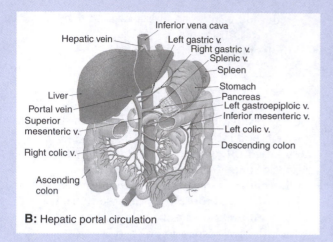

B: Hepatic portal circulation

38. **TEST-TAKING TIP** The words "obliterated with slight pressure" are key words in the stem that direct attention to content. The words "Bounding" and "Full" are equally plausible. The words "Thready" and "Weak" are equally plausible. The words "Bounding" and "Full" are opposite to the words "Thready" and "Weak." Generally a correct answer is one of the opposites. Either "Bounding" and "Full" are correct answers or "Thready" and "Weak" are correct answers. Because a multiple-response question must have at least two correct answers you can eliminate option 3 from further consideration.

1. _____ A bounding pulse is strong when palpated. The pulse is not obliterated when moderate pressure is applied to the artery.
2. **X A thready pulse is difficult to feel when palpated and is obliterated with slight pressure.**
3. _____ An absent pulse is the nonexistence of a detectable pulse.
4. **X A weak pulse is difficult to feel when palpated and is obliterated with slight pressure.**
5. _____ A full pulse is strong and easily counted when palpated. The pulse is not obliterated when moderate pressure is applied to the artery.

39. 1. A pulse rate of 100 beats per minute is within the expected range of 60 to 100 beats per minute. A pulse volume that is thready is expected when a person is dehydrated because of hypovolemia.
2. Although the blood pressure should be checked because it is low for a 75-year-old person with a history of hypertension, it is

not the priority at this time. A decreased blood pressure is consistent with dehydration.
3. Although the respiratory rate should be checked because it is increased beyond the expected range of 15 to 20 breaths per minute for an older adult, the nurse has to consider that the patient has an upper respiratory tract infection. Because an increase in respiratory rate with a respiratory tract infection is expected, it is not as critical as another assessment among the options.
4. **The patient's oxygen saturation rate of 89% is below the expected range of a healthy older adult of 95% to 100%. The primary health-care provider should be informed when the oxygen saturation decreases below the expected range because a change in the patient's oxygen orders may be necessary to meet the oxygen needs of the patient.**

40. **TEST-TAKING TIP** The word "immediate" in the stem sets a priority. The words "response requires" and "focused assessment" are key words in the stem that direct attention to content.

1. **X Suprapubic distention may indicate urinary retention; a focused assessment is required.**
2. **X Dependent edema is a response related to problems such as hypervolemia, a decreased cardiac output, or impaired kidney functioning. The patient immediately should be assessed further because these conditions can be life-threatening.**
3. _____ Although difficulty sleeping at night should be explored further, it is not a life-threatening problem and therefore is not a priority.
4. _____ Although lack of a bowel movement should be explored further, it is not a life-threatening problem and therefore is not a priority.
5. _____ Blanchable erythema in an area at risk for a pressure ulcer indicates that the area has been exposed to pressure. However, circulation to the area is not impaired. Pressure that produces non-blanchable erythema signals a potential ulceration and meets the criteria for a stage I pressure ulcer. The patient should be assessed further, but it is not a priority.

MEETING PATIENTS' PHYSICAL SAFETY AND MOBILITY NEEDS

This section includes questions related to maintaining patients' physical safety and mobility needs. In relation to patients' safety needs, this section emphasizes the concepts of the use of restraints, issues associated with smoking and fire, prevention of injury, electrical safety, protection of a patient experiencing a seizure, and safety related to oxygen use. In relation to patients' mobility needs, this section includes questions that address the maintenance and restoration of musculoskeletal function and the prevention of musculoskeletal complications. These questions focus on knowledge, principles, and devices related to the prevention of pressure (decubitus) ulcers, contractures, and other hazards of immobility. Additional questions test principles associated with body alignment, transfer, range of motion, ambulation, positioning, and dressing.

QUESTIONS

1. A nurse is examining the literature regarding the cause of accidents in the hospital setting. Which does the nurse conclude is the **main** reason for accidents in hospitals?
   1. People sneak cigarettes.
   2. Equipment breaks unexpectedly.
   3. Patients do not recognize hazards.
   4. Safety precautions always take extra time.

   TEST-TAKING TIP Identify the word in the stem that sets a priority. Identify the option with a specific determiner.

2. A nurse identifies that a patient sitting in a wheelchair begins to have a tonic-clonic (formerly called grand mal) seizure. Which should the nurse do?
   1. Transfer the patient to an empty room to provide privacy.
   2. Return the patient to bed to provide a soft surface.
   3. Move the patient to the floor to prevent injury.
   4. Secure the patient to prevent falling.

   TEST-TAKING TIP Identify key words in the stem that direct attention to content.

3. Disoriented, confused patients, who are restrained, often struggle against restraints. Which does the nurse conclude is the primary reason for this behavior?
   1. Response to discomfort
   2. Attempt to gain control
   3. Effort to manipulate the staff
   4. Inability to understand what is occurring

   TEST-TAKING TIP Identify the word in the stem that sets a priority. Identify key words in the stem that direct attention to content. Identify the clang association.

4. A nurse is working in an assisted-living facility that has designated smoking areas. Which is the **best** nursing intervention to prevent accidents associated with smoking?
   1. Supervising individuals when they want to smoke
   2. Removing cigarettes from individuals who smoke
   3. Encouraging individuals who smoke to give up smoking
   4. Asking family members of individuals who smoke not to bring cigarettes to the facility

   TEST-TAKING TIP Identify the word in the stem that sets a priority. Identify key words in the stem that direct attention to content. Identify options that deny patient feelings, concerns, or needs. Identify the unique option. Identify the patient-centered option.

5. A nurse is responding to a fire alarm within the hospital. Which should the nurse do when transporting a fire extinguisher to a fire scene on a different level of the building than the one on which the nurse is working?
   1. Use the stairs.
   2. Pull the safety pin.
   3. Keep it from touching the floor.
   4. Always run as quickly as possible.

   TEST-TAKING TIP Identify key words in the stem that direct attention to content. Identify the option with a specific determiner.

6. A primary nurse is orienting a newly admitted patient to the hospital. Which is the **most** important information that the nurse should review with the patient?
   1. Name of the nurse in charge
   2. Potential date of discharge
   3. Daily routine on the unit
   4. Use of the call bell

   TEST-TAKING TIP Identify the word in the stem that sets a priority. Use Maslow's Hierarchy of Needs to help identify the most important information that the patient should know from among the options offered.

7. A nurse on the evening shift in the hospital is caring for a slightly confused patient. Which is the **most** effective nursing intervention to prevent disorientation at night?
   1. Check on the patient regularly.
   2. Turn on a small night-light.
   3. Place a call bell in the bed.
   4. Describe the environment.

   TEST-TAKING TIP Identify the word in the stem that sets a priority. Identify key words in the stem that direct attention to content. Identify the unique option. Identify equally plausible options. Identify the clang association.

8. While walking, a patient becomes weak and the patient's knees begin to buckle. Which should the nurse do?
   1. Hold up the patient.
   2. Walk the patient to the closest chair.
   3. Call for assistance to help the patient.
   4. Lower the patient to the floor carefully.

   TEST-TAKING TIP Identify key words in the stem that direct attention to content. Identify opposites in options.

9. A nurse identifies that the electrical cord on a patient's radio is frayed near the plug. Which should the nurse do?
   1. Report the problem to the supervisor.
   2. Unplug it and put it in the patient's closet.
   3. Remove it from the patient's room and send it home with a family member.
   4. Ask the maintenance department to apply nonconductive tape to the damaged section.

10. A nurse is caring for an older adult on bedrest. Which should the nurse provide to **best** prevent a pressure (decubitus) ulcer in this patient?
    1. An air mattress
    2. A daily bed bath
    3. A high-protein diet
    4. An indwelling urinary catheter

    TEST-TAKING TIP Identify the word in the stem that sets a priority. Identify key words in the stem that direct attention to content.

11. Which is the **most** therapeutic exercise that can be done by a patient confined to bed?
    1. Isometric exercises
    2. Active-assistive exercises
    3. Active range-of-motion exercises
    4. Passive range-of-motion exercises

    TEST-TAKING TIP Identify the word in the stem that sets a priority. Identify opposites in options.

12. A nurse is transferring a patient from the bed to a chair using a mechanical lift. As the nurse begins to raise the lift off the bed, the patient begins to panic and scream. Which should the nurse do?
    1. Say, "Relax" and slowly continue the transfer.
    2. Immediately lower the patient back onto the bed.
    3. Quickly continue and say, "Be calm, it's almost over."
    4. Stop the lift from rising until the patient regains control.

    TEST-TAKING TIP Identify key words in the stem that direct attention to content. Identify opposites in options. Identify options that deny patient feelings, concerns, or needs. Identify the patient-centered option.

13. While a patient is lying in the dorsal recumbent position, the patient's legs externally rotate. Which equipment should the nurse use to prevent external rotation?
    1. Bed cradle
    2. Trochanter roll
    3. Elastic stockings
    4. High-top sneakers

    TEST-TAKING TIP Identify key words in the stem that direct attention to content.

14. A patient is afraid of falling when it is time to get out of bed to a chair. Which is the **best** action by the nurse to reduce the patient's fear?
    1. Allow the patient to decide when to get up.
    2. Inform the patient that a fall will not occur.
    3. Transfer the patient using a mechanical lift.
    4. Permit the patient to set the pace of the transfer.

    TEST-TAKING TIP Identify the word in the stem that sets a priority. Identify key words in the stem that direct attention to content. Identify the clang association. Identify the option that denies patient feelings, concerns, or needs. Identify patient-centered options.

15. A patient who had a brain attack (stroke, cerebrovascular accident) 3 days earlier has left-sided hemiparesis. Which should the nurse plan to do when dressing the patient?
    1. Put the patient's left sleeve on first.
    2. Encourage the patient to dress independently.
    3. Instruct the patient to wear clothes with zippers.
    4. Tell the patient to get clothes with buttons in the front.

    TEST-TAKING TIP Identify key words in the stem that direct attention to content. Identify the clang association. Identify equally plausible options. Identify the unique option. Identify the option that denies patient feelings, concerns, or needs.

16. Which is the **most** important principle of body mechanics when the nurse positions a patient?
1. Making the patient comfortable
2. Elevating the patient's arms on pillows
3. Maintaining the patient in functional alignment
4. Keeping the patient's head higher than the heart

TEST-TAKING TIP Identify the word in the stem that sets a priority. Identify key words in the stem that direct attention to content.

17. Warm, dry heat to be applied via an aquathermia pad to a patient's lower back is ordered to ease muscle spasms resulting from a fall. Which should the nurse do? **Select all that apply.**
1. ____ Set the pad at 98°F to 104°F.
2. ____ Apply the pad directly to the patient's skin.
3. ____ Remove the pad 20 to 30 minutes after it is applied.
4. ____ Moisten the liner between the pad and the cover of the pad.
5. ____ Put the pad under the patient after the patient is placed in the supine position.

18. A patient with one-sided weakness (hemiparesis) is ordered to be transferred out of bed to a chair twice a day. Which should the nurse plan to do? **Select all that apply.**
1. ____ Place rubber soled shoes on the patient's feet.
2. ____ Position the hands on the patient's scapulae.
3. ____ Support the patient on the affected side.
4. ____ Pivot the patient on the unaffected leg.
5. ____ Keep the patient's feet together.

TEST-TAKING TIP Identify key words in the stem that direct attention to content.

19. When the home care nurse places an egg-crate pad under a patient the spouse asks, "What is the purpose of that pad?" Which are the purposes of an egg-crate pad that should be included in a response to the spouse's question? **Select all that apply.**
1. ____ Absorbs moisture
2. ____ Limits perspiration
3. ____ Prevents pressure ulcers
4. ____ Supports the body in alignment
5. ____ Distributes pressure over a larger area

TEST-TAKING TIP Identify the key word in the stem that directs attention to content.

20. A nurse identifies the illustrated ulcer when completing a skin assessment for a newly admitted patient. Which stage ulcer should the nurse indicate on the pressure ulcer flow sheet?

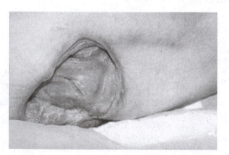

1. Stage I
2. Stage II
3. Stage III
4. Stage IV

21. A nurse is planning a turning schedule for a patient with limited mobility. Which positions that contribute to the development of a pressure ulcer in the sacral area should be avoided in this patient's plan of care? **Select all that apply.**
   1. _____ Sims
   2. _____ Prone
   3. _____ Contour
   4. _____ High-Fowler
   5. _____ Dorsal recumbent

   TEST-TAKING TIP Identify the word in the stem that indicates negative polarity. Identify key words in the stem that direct attention to content.

22. A nurse reviews a patient's clinical record. Which should the nurse do **first** in response to the change in the patient's behavior?
   1. Initiate the bed alarm on the bed.
   2. Administer the prescribed sedative.
   3. Place a vest restraint on the patient and notify the primary health-care provider.
   4. Assign a staff member to stay with the patient and notify the primary health-care provider.

PATIENT'S CLINICAL RECORD

Progress Note
Nursing Note 1800: 88-year-old adult with mild dementia admitted to the hospital for urosepsis at 1300. On admission the patient was alert and answering and asking questions appropriately. Over the past several hours the patient has become confused and is attempting to pull out the IV line and urinary catheters and climb over the bedrail. The patient's eyes are darting about the room and intermittently the patient will wring the hands and pick at the bedding.

Vital Signs Flow Sheet
Blood pressure: 160/95 mm Hg
Pulse: 110 beats/min
Respirations: 28 breaths/min
Temperature: 99.6°F

Primary Health-Care Provider's Orders
IV 1,000 mL 0.9% sodium chloride every 12 hours
Urinary retention catheter
Vital signs every 4 hours
Zolpidem 10 mg PO hs

---

23. A nurse is caring for a group of patients. Which patients are at the greatest risk of developing a pressure (decubitus) ulcer? **Select all that apply.**
   1. _____ Those who have paraplegia
   2. _____ Those who have a colostomy
   3. _____ Those who use crutches to ambulate
   4. _____ Those who use a reclining wheelchair
   5. _____ Those who are ambulatory but confused
   6. _____ Those who are on bedrest but able to move

   TEST-TAKING TIP Identify the word in the stem that sets a priority. Identify key words in the stem that direct attention to content.

24. A hospitalized patient dies after a long illness. Which should the nurse do as part of postmortem care? **Select all that apply.**
1. ____ Remove tubes if an autopsy is not required.
2. ____ Attach an identification tag to the body.
3. ____ Raise the head of the bed slightly.
4. ____ Carefully remove any dentures.
5. ____ Firmly tie the wrists together.
6. ____ Gently close the eyes.

25. A nurse is caring for a patient positioned in the left lateral position. Place an X over the bony prominence that the nurse should be most concerned about regarding development of a pressure ulcer.

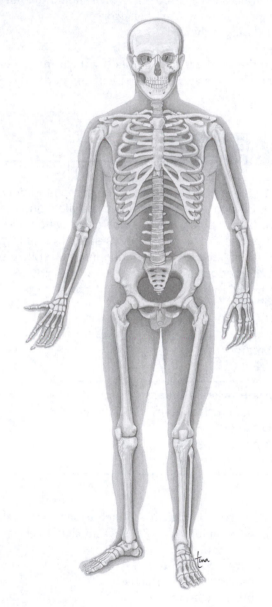

26. A nurse is caring for a patient who was newly diagnosed with a latex allergy. Which information should the nurse include in the teaching plan? **Select all that apply.**
1. ____ Wear clothing labeled hypoallergenic.
2. ____ Carry injectable epinephrine or keep it within easy reach.
3. ____ Avoid clothing with spandex because spandex contains rubber.
4. ____ Examine tags on clothing to ensure that they do not contain latex.
5. ____ Have someone remove plants such as a poinsettias, ficus, and rubber tree plants from the home.

27. A primary health-care provider orders crutches for a person who has a left lower leg injury. The nurse is teaching the person how to rise from a chair without bearing weight on the left leg. Place the following steps in the order in which they should be implemented.
    1. Put one crutch under each arm.
    2. Slide the buttocks toward the edge of the chair.
    3. Hold both crutches together on the hand bars with the left hand.
    4. Push down on the arm of the chair on the unaffected side while bearing weight on the hand bars of the crutches.
    5. Extend the right leg while keeping the right foot flat on the floor, elevate the body to a standing position, and then check balance.

    Answer: _____

28. A nurse is positioning a patient in a lateral position. Which actions by the nurse contribute to the patient's functional alignment? **Select all that apply.**
    1. ____ Utilizing a trochanter roll
    2. ____ Putting a pillow under the upper leg
    3. ____ Placing a small pillow under the waist
    4. ____ Using a pillow to support the upper arm
    5. ____ Positioning a pillow behind the patient's back

    TEST-TAKING TIP Identify key words in the stem that direct attention to content.

29. Which knot should the nurse use when attaching the strap of a restraint to a bed frame?

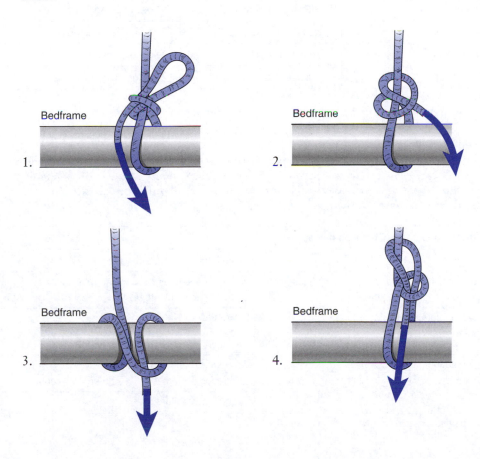

30. A nurse left a bedside rail down of a patient who was premedicated with an opioid in preparation for surgery. The patient was found on the floor. The patient was examined by the rapid response team and no injury was identified as a result of the fall. The patient was returned to bed. The nurse inserted a brief description of the event on the Unusual Occurrence Report. Place a check in the box in front of the most appropriate category in the "Occurrence Category" section of the Unusual Occurrence Report that relates to this event.

Unusual Occurrence Report

Date of Event: _____   Time of Event: _____   Department: _____

Patient Last Name:	First Name:	MI:
Patient #:	Attending Physician:	
Visitor Last Name:	First Name:	Phone #:
Employee Name:	Dept:	
Physician Name:	Specialty:	

Occurrence Category (Check most appropriate)

☐ Agency nurse-related	☐ AMA	☐ Delay in treatment
☐ Diet-related	☐ HIPAA compliance	☐ Loss of personal property
☐ Medication-related	☐ Narcotics-related	☐ Order not executed
☐ Patient injury	☐ Peer-review related	☐ Restraint-related
☐ Staff injury	☐ Supplies/Equipment	☐ Visitor injury
☐ Fall		
☐ Other (please explain):		

Description of Occurrence:

A patient was medicated with an opioid. The patient's bedside rail was left in the down position. The patient was found on the floor. The patient was examined by the rapid response team. No injury was identified as a result of the fall. The patient was returned to bed.

Contributing Factors (Check all that apply)

☐ Individual:	☐ System:
Knowledge, skills, and/or experience (please list): ☐ Unclear ☐ Incomplete	Policies/procedures not in place (please list): ☐ Unclear ☐ Outdated
Standard of care or practice (please list): ☐ Non-adherence	Environmental: ☐ Staffing ☐ Patient acuity ☐ Congestion
Documentation (please list): ☐ Incomplete ☐ Inadequate	Communications and work flow: ☐ Intradepartmental ☐ Interdepartmental
	☐ Equipment failure
Other (please explain):	

Submitted by:	Dept:	Date:

31. Which are the reasons why restraints are used when caring for patients? **Select all that apply.**
    1. ____ Limit movement
    2. ____ Reduce agitation
    3. ____ Immobilize patients
    4. ____ Prevent patient injury
    5. ____ Prohibit a patient from hurting others

32. Which events require a nurse to complete an incident (variance) report? **Select all that apply.**
    1. ____ A patient who falls in the bathroom but who is not injured
    2. ____ A nurse who refuses to be floated to a unit other than the usual unit assigned
    3. ____ A visitor who faints when seeing an ill family member in the intensive-care unit
    4. ____ A resident physician who is angry because of being awakened to examine a patient
    5. ____ A nurse's aide working in a hospital who applies a topical fungicide cream to a patient's perineal area.

33. Identify the illustration that indicates flexion and extension of the ankle.

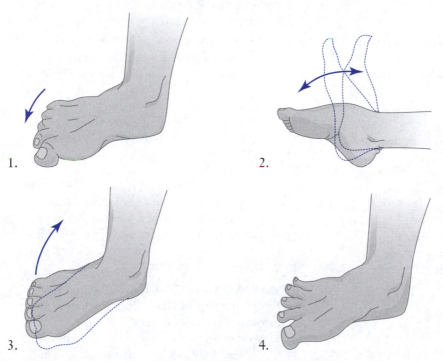

34. Which developmental factors specific to adolescents influence their ability to remain safe? **Select all that apply.**
    1. ____ Believe they are invincible
    2. ____ Use tools and household items
    3. ____ Engage in risk-taking behaviors
    4. ____ Tend not to wear seat belts in cars
    5. ____ Are exposed to increased peer relationships

    TEST-TAKING TIP Identify key words in the stem that direct attention to content.

35. An older adult has been taking 20 mg of furosemide by mouth twice a day along with an antihypertensive medication. The patient's blood pressure has progressively decreased and the patient has experienced several episodes of lightheadedness. The primary health-care provider changes the furosemide prescription to 15 mg by mouth twice a day. An oral solution is prescribed because the patient has difficulty swallowing pills. The furosemide solution states that there are 10 mg/1 mL of solution. How many milliliters of furosemide should the nurse administer over 24 hours? **Record your answer using a whole number.**

    Answer: _____ mL

MEETING PATIENT'S PHYSICAL SAFETY AND MOBILITY NEEDS ANSWERS AND RATIONALES

1. **TEST-TAKING TIP** The word "main" in the stem sets a priority. The word "always" in option 4 is a specific determiner.

    1. Statistics do not support cigarette smoking as the most common cause of hospital accidents. Most hospitals are smoke free.
    2. Equipment usually is monitored for preventive maintenance; equipment generally shows wear and tear before it breaks.
    3. **Patients can be cognitively impaired, deny their physical impairments, or have limited perception, which impedes their ability to recognize hazards.**
    4. Usually it takes the same amount of time to do something correctly as it does to do it incorrectly.

2. **TEST-TAKING TIP** The words "wheelchair" and "tonic-clonic seizure" are key words in the stem that direct attention to content.

    1. The need for privacy is not the priority. Transporting a patient in a wheelchair during a tonic-clonic (grand mal) seizure can cause muscle strain, bone fractures, or other injury and is unsafe.
    2. Attempting to return a patient to bed during a tonic-clonic (grand mal) seizure can cause muscle strain, bone fractures, or other injury. Returning the patient to bed should be done after the seizure is over.
    3. **Moving the patient to the floor is the safest action; it provides free movement on a supported surface.**
    4. Securing a patient in a wheelchair during a tonic-clonic (grand mal) seizure can cause muscle strain, bone fractures, or other injury and is an unsafe action.

3. **TEST-TAKING TIP** The word "primary" in the stem sets a priority. The words "confused" and "struggle" are key words in the stem that direct attention to content. The word "confused" in the stem and the words "inability to understand" in option 4 is an obscure clang association.

    1. A restraint should not cause discomfort if it is applied correctly and checked frequently.
    2. Confused, disoriented patients who are restrained may become agitated and respond in a reflex-like way; attempts to gain control require problem solving, which they usually are unable to perform.

    3. A patient usually struggles against a restraint to get free, not to manipulate staff.
    4. **Disoriented and confused patients do not always have the cognitive ability to understand what is happening to them and often struggle against restraints.**

4. **TEST-TAKING TIP** The word "best" in the stem sets a priority. The words "prevent accidents" are key words in the stem that direct attention to content. Options 2, 3, and 4 deny patient feelings, concerns, or needs or are equally plausible. Option 1 is unique because it is the only option that permits the individual to smoke. Option 1 is patient centered.

    1. **If a facility allows smoking, supervision provides for safety because the caregiver can intervene if the condition becomes unsafe.**
    2. Removing cigarettes from individuals who smoke is punitive and should be done only if attempts to teach safety precautions and policies fail to foster safe smoking behavior.
    3. Although this is ideal, it denies the individual's right to smoke in designated areas.
    4. Asking family members not to bring in cigarettes for individuals who smoke denies the individual's feelings, concerns, and needs and is punitive.

5. **TEST-TAKING TIP** The words "different level" are key words in the stem that direct attention to content; it should direct the test-taker to the words "stairs" in option 1. The word "always" in option 4 is a specific determiner.

    1. **Using the stairs during a fire is safe practice; elevators must be avoided because they may break down and trap a person.**
    2. The safety pin is pulled only when the extinguisher is going to be used.
    3. Often extinguishers are dragged along the floor en route to a fire because they are heavy; this is an acceptable practice.
    4. Running should be avoided; it can cause injury and panic.

6. **TEST-TAKING TIP** The word "most" in the stem sets a priority. Learning how to use the call bell system in case immediate

assistance is a necessary safety issue and takes priority over the other options, which are psychosocial according to Maslow's Hierarchy of Needs.

1. Although the patient should be told the name of the nurse in charge of the unit, this is not the priority intervention.
2. Identifying the potential date of discharge is the primary health-care provider's, not the nurse's, responsibility.
3. Although teaching the patient about the daily routine on the unit is important and should be done, safety needs come first.
4. **Explaining the use of a call bell meets basic safety and security needs; the patient must know how to signal for help.**

7. **TEST-TAKING TIP** The word "most" in the stem sets a priority. The words "minimally confused" and "prevent disorientation at night" are key words in the stem that direct attention to content. Option 2 is the only option that states an action that is unique to the night time. Options 1, 3, and 4 are equally plausible and are implemented regardless of the time of day or orientation of the patient. The word "night" in the stem and in option 2 is a clang association.

1. Although checking on the patient regularly is something the nurse should do, it will not prevent disorientation.
2. **A small night-light in the room provides enough light for visual cues for a minimally confused patient, which should help prevent or limit disorientation when the patient awakens at night.**
3. The patient has to be oriented enough to be aware of the presence of the call bell before it can be used.
4. The patient may not remember the description of the environment on awakening and may become disoriented in the dark.

8. **TEST-TAKING TIP** The words "knees begin to buckle" are key words in the stem that direct attention to content. Options 1 and 4 are opposites.

1. Trying to hold up the patient may injure the nurse and cause both the nurse and the patient to fall.
2. The patient is already falling; walking the patient to the closest chair is not an option.
3. By the time help arrives, the patient may already be on the floor; calling out can scare the patient and others.

4. **Lowering the patient to the floor is the safest action; guiding the patient to the floor helps to break the patient's fall and minimize injury, particularly to the head.**

9. 1. Reporting the frayed wire is ineffective in preventing the risk of injury.
2. Putting the radio in the patient's closet does not preclude that it may be taken out and used again.
3. **Removing the radio from the room and sending it home with a family member is the safest option; this action removes it from use.**
4. Attempting to repair an electrical cord with nonconductive tape is unsafe; it should be properly repaired by a trained person.

10. **TEST-TAKING TIP** The word "best" in the stem sets a priority. The words "bedrest," "prevent," and "pressure ulcer" are key words in the stem that direct attention to content.

1. **An air mattress distributes body weight over a larger surface and reduces pressure over bony prominences.**
2. Although bathing removes secretions and promotes clean skin, it can be drying, which can compromise skin integrity.
3. Protein does not prevent pressure (decubitus) ulcers. Protein is the body's only source of nitrogen and is essential for building, repairing, or replacing body tissue. It requires a primary health-care provider's order.
4. An indwelling urinary catheter should never be used to prevent a pressure (decubitus) ulcer; however, a catheter may be used to prevent contamination of a pressure (decubitus) ulcer after it is present in a patient who is incontinent of urine. It requires a primary health-care provider's order.

11. **TEST-TAKING TIP** The word "most" in the stem sets a priority. Options 3 and 4 are opposites.

1. Isometric exercise involves contracting and relaxing a muscle without moving the joint; this improves muscle tone but does not put joints through full range of motion.
2. In active-assistive exercise, the patient attempts active exercise and receives some support and assistance from the nurse. Active-assistive range-of-motion exercise does not provide for as much isotonic exercise as does active range-of-motion exercise.

3. **Active range-of-motion exercise is preferable because it is an isotonic exercise that causes muscle contraction and increases joint mobility, circulation, and muscle tone because the patient actively moves joints through their full range of motion.**

4. Passive range-of-motion exercise occurs when a joint is moved by a source other than the muscles articulating to the joint. Passive range-of-motion exercise puts a joint through full range and prevents contractures but does not increase muscle tone because the muscles are not contracted.

12. **TEST-TAKING TIP** The words "panic" and "scream" are key words in the stem that direct attention to content. Options 2 and 3 are opposites. Options 1, 3, and 4 deny the patient's feelings of fear. Option 2 is patient centered.

1. Continuing with the transfer ignores the patient's concern. Telling a person to relax will not necessarily precipitate a relaxation response.

2. **Lowering the patient onto the bed recognizes the cause of the fear and responds to the source.**

3. Continuing with the transfer denies the patient's fears and can intensify the patient's fearful response.

4. Leaving the patient up in the air can intensify the patient's fearful response.

13. **TEST-TAKING TIP** The words "prevent external rotation" are key words in the stem that direct attention to content.

1. A bed cradle keeps linen off the feet and legs; it supports patient comfort, but it does not prevent external rotation.

2. **A trochanter roll prevents the hip and leg from externally rotating by positioning the leg in functional alignment.**

3. Elastic stockings do not prevent external rotation; they are used to increase venous return in the lower legs.

4. High-top sneakers prevent plantar flexion, not external rotation.

14. **TEST-TAKING TIP** The word "best" in the stem sets a priority. The words "afraid," and "reduce" are key words in the stem that direct attention to content. The words "falling" in the stem and "fall" in option 2 comprise a clang association; however, this option is a distractor. Eliminate option 2 because it clearly

denies the patient's feelings. Options 1 and 4 are patient centered.

1. Waiting and thinking about the transfer can increase fear, not reduce fear; the patient may decide never to get out of bed.

2. Informing the patient that a fall will not occur is false reassurance and denies the patient's fears.

3. Using a mechanical lift may contribute to feelings of dependence and loss of control. The question identifies a fearful patient, not an immobile patient.

4. **Allowing the patient to set the pace of the transfer supports the need of the patient to be in control; the patient's concerns generally are reduced in proportion to an increase in control.**

15. **TEST-TAKING TIP** The words "left-sided hemiparesis" and "3 days earlier" are key words in the stem that direct attention to content. The word "left" in the stem and in option 1 is a clang association. Options 3 and 4 are equally plausible. Options 2, 3, and 4 are similar because they contain the verbs "encourage," "instruct," and "tell," which all require verbal interaction with the patient. Option 1 is unique because it is the only option in which the nurse is actually dressing the patient. Option 2 denies the patient's need for assistance during the acute phase of this illness.

1. **The left upper extremity on the affected side should be dressed first to avoid unnecessary strain; the unaffected side generally has greater range of motion.**

2. It is unreasonable to expect self-sufficiency during the acute phase.

3. Zippers are difficult to close with one hand. Velcro closures may be more appropriate.

4. Buttons are difficult to close with one hand. Velcro closures may be more appropriate.

16. **TEST-TAKING TIP** The word "most" in the stem sets a priority. The words "principle of body mechanics" are key words in the stem that direct attention to content.

1. A comfortable position for the patient may not provide the alignment necessary to prevent complications.

2. The arms do not have to be elevated to be in alignment.

3. **Anatomic alignment maintains physical functioning and minimizes strain and**

stress on muscles, tendons, ligaments, and joints.

4. The head can be at the same level as the heart; it does not have to be higher.

17. 1. **X The aquathermia pad should be set at 98°F to 104°F for the application of warm, dry heat. This is warm enough to cause capillary dilation without resulting in a burn.**

2. ____ A covering or towel should be placed between the pad and the patient to prevent burns.

3. **X This prevents the rebound phenomenon. Heat produces maximum vasodilation in 20 to 30 minutes; if left on beyond this, the blood vessels constrict, limiting the dissipation of heat via the blood circulation.**

4. ____ Placing a moist liner between the pad and the cover of the pad provides for moist, not dry, heat.

5. ____ Placing the pad under the patient is contraindicated because the heat cannot dissipate and may burn the patient.

18. **TEST-TAKING TIP** The words "one-sided weakness" and "hemiparesis" are key words in the stem that direct attention to content.

1. **X Rubber-soled shoes provide traction between the patient's feet and the floor supporting safety.**

2. **X Positioning the hands on the patient's scapulae prevents pulling on the patient's arms and shoulders which can injure the structures of the patient's upper extremities and shoulders.**

3. ____ When transferring this patient, the nurse should stand in front of, not next to, the patient.

4. **Pivoting avoids unnecessary movement by transferring the patient to the chair while the patient supports body weight on the unaffected leg.**

5. ____ Keeping the patient's feet together narrows the base of support and decreases stability.

19. **TEST-TAKING TIP** The word "egg-crate" is the key word in the stem that directs attention to content.

1. ____ The purpose of an egg-crate pad is not to absorb moisture. A wet egg-crate pad should not be used because moisture against the skin can contribute to skin breakdown.

2. ____ The opposite may be true. Because egg-crate pads are made of synthetic materials, they can promote, rather than limit, perspiration.

3. **X Egg-crate pads distribute body weight more evenly, limiting pressure on the integumentary system, particularly over bony prominences; this limits the development of pressure ulcers.**

4. ____ Pillows and wedges, not an egg-crate pad, are used to keep the body in functional alignment.

5. **X Intermittent raised areas on the egg-crate pad help to distribute body weight evenly over the entire body surface that is in contact with the pad.**

20. 1. This is a stage I pressure ulcer: non-blanchable erythema of intact skin.

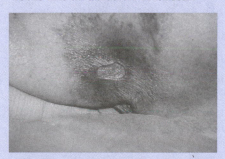

2. This is a stage II pressure ulcer: superficial partial-thickness loss involving the epidermis and dermis. It is a shallow crater and looks like an abrasion or blister.

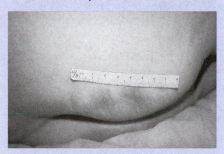

3. This is a stage III pressure ulcer: full-thickness involvement of subcutaneous tissue. It is a deep crater that may extend to but not through the fascia as well as include undermining of adjacent tissue.

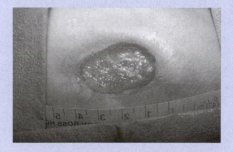

4. The question presents a stage IV pressure ulcer: full-thickness involvement that includes muscle, bone, or supporting structures. Also, it may include sinus tracts and undermining of adjacent tissue.

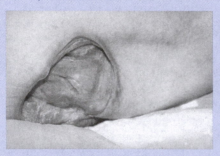

21. **TEST-TAKING TIP** The word "avoided" in the stem indicates negative polarity. The words "sacral area" and "pressure ulcer" are key words in the stem that direct attention to content.

    1. ____ The Sims position avoids pressure on the sacral area; weight is on the anterior ilium, humerus, and clavicle.
    2. ____ The prone position avoids pressure on the sacral area; prone is lying on the abdomen.
    3. X The contour position is a sitting position which places pressure on the sacral area and should be avoided when trying to prevent a sacral pressure ulcer.
    4. X In the high-Fowler position, most of the weight is placed on the sacral area; this causes sacral pressure.
    5. X In the dorsal recumbent (supine) position the majority of the weight is on the sacral area; other areas affected include the back of the head, scapulae, and heels of the feet.

22. 1. Although a bed alarm will alert the nurse to the patient's attempting to get out of bed, it will not prevent the patient from pulling out catheters.
    2. Zolpidem (Ambien) is a sedative/ hypnotic used for the induction of sleep. It is only 6 p.m. and is too early to administer the zolpidem. A prescription for a sedative/hypnotic-antianxiety agent such as lorazepam (Ativan) may be necessary to calm the patient's behavior, for which the nurse requires a prescription from a primary health-care provider. This behavior is associated with confusion and disorientation that increases during the late afternoon/evening in a patient with a history of dementia (sundowning syndrome).
    3. In this situation, a vest restraint will not fully protect the patient from self-injury. A vest restraint will not prevent the patient from pulling out the IV line or urinary retention catheter. Although a vest restraint may be used in an emergency without an order, the patient must be evaluated by a primary health-care provider within a predetermined length of time (as per protocol/state legal requirements) to rescind or provide a written order for the restraint.
    4. **Assigning a staff member to provide constant reassurance, reorientation, and monitoring is the most effective intervention and least restrictive to provide for the patient's safety. These interventions often will reassure and calm a patient experiencing sundowning syndrome (confusion and disorientation that increases during the afternoon and evening hours in a patient with dementia). The primary health-care provider should be notified of the patient's change in behavior because the primary health-care provider may want to order additional interventions.**

23. **TEST-TAKING TIP** The word "greatest" in the stem sets a priority. The words "risk" and "pressure ulcer" are key words in the stem that direct attention to content.

    1. **X Paralysis of the lower extremities (paraplegia) increases the risk of decubitus ulcers because the patient may remain in one position for prolonged periods of time. This can be prevented if a routine turning schedule is followed and skin care provided.**
    2. ____ A colostomy does not increase the risk of decubitus ulcers. However, it may increase the risk of excoriation around the stoma if special skin care is not performed.

3. ____ As long as a person can move, positioning can be changed to relieve pressure.

4. X **A patient using a reclining wheelchair has minimal lower- or upper-body control. A reclining position places excessive pressure on the sacral area.**

5. ____ A confused ambulatory patient is able to walk and therefore relieve pressure on bony prominences.

6. ____ As long as a patient on bedrest can move, pressure can be relieved by shifting the body weight or changing positions.

24. 1. X **All tubes should be removed if an autopsy is not required. If an autopsy is to be performed all tubes should be clamped and maintained in place.**

2. X **Identification tags should be attached to the patient's body (usually a toe), on the shroud or body bag, and on the patient's belongings.**

3. ____ A supine position is preferred; after rigor mortis sets in, it is difficult to reposition the body.

4. ____ Dentures should be placed in the mouth to maintain facial structure and minimize facial distortion.

5. ____ Firmly tying together the patient's wrists can cause permanent marks; wrists should be well padded and securely, yet loosely, tied so as not to cause permanent marks.

6. X **The patient's eyelids should be gently closed to avoid injury; after rigor mortis sets in, it is difficult to reposition the eyelids.**

25. **When in the left lateral position the site over the greater trochanter is most vulnerable to pressure because it is the site that bears the most body weight. Also there is little body tissue between the bone and the epidermis. Additional sites at risk include side of the head (parietal and temporal bones), ear, shoulder (acromial process), knee (medial and lateral condyles), and malleolus (medial and lateral).**

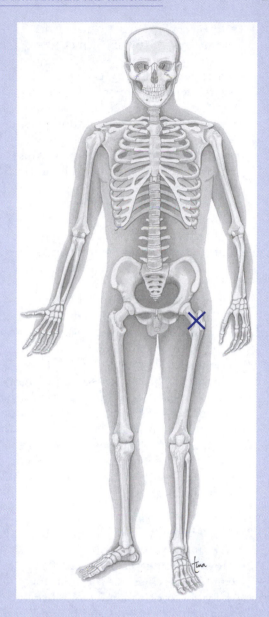

26. 1. ____ A product labeled "hypoallergenic" does not mean it is latex free. A person must examine packaging or tags to ensure that the product is free of latex.

2. X **Injectable epinephrine, such as an EpiPen, is used to manage severe allergic reactions to latex, insect bites, or foods. Its therapeutic effects are bronchodilation and maintenance of heart rate and blood pressure.**

3. ____ Spandex (generic name) was developed in 1959 by the DuPont Company and was trademarked as Lycra. Spandex

fibers are rubber-free fibers that are alternatives to latex and can be worn by a person with a latex allergy. Spandex can stretch; return to its original shape; is stronger than latex rubber fibers; is comfortable, soft, smooth, and supple; is resistant to perspiration, lotions, and body oils; blends with other fabrics; and will not pill or create static. Most important, it does not contain latex protein allergens.

4. X Latex rubber is used in the manufacture of many types of clothing to give it stretch, comfort, and freedom of movement. It is used in clothing such as leotards, athletic wear, body suits, bathing suits, socks, stockings, and elastic waistbands. Latex contains 57 allergenic proteins and more than 200 different chemicals used during its manufacture that also are known allergens. For this reason a person with a latex allergy must examine the tags of clothing to ensure that items do not contain latex.

5. X These three houseplants contain latex protein allergens and should be removed from the home of a person with a latex allergy.

27. Answer: 3, 2, 4, 5, 1

3. This frees the right hand for the next step in the procedure.

2. Moving the buttocks toward the edge of the chair allows room for the right knee to bend so that the unaffected right foot and leg are under the center of the body's mass when standing.

4. Pushing off the right arm of the chair with the right hand and extending the elbow use an upper extremity to assist the patient to a standing position.

5. Extending the right knee and hip while keeping the right foot flat on the floor while elevating the body uses the unaffected lower extremity to assist the patient to a standing position. Once standing the patient must ensure that balance is maintained. The unaffected leg can be supported against the edge of the chair, in addition to holding the hand bars of the crutches.

1. Transferring the crutches to under the arms prepares a person for crutch walking.

28. **TEST-TAKING TIP** The words "lateral" and "functional alignment" are key words in the stem that direct attention to content.

1. ____ A trochanter roll is used to prevent external rotation of the hip when the patient is in a back-lying position.

2. X Putting a pillow under the upper leg positions the upper leg and hip in functional alignment and reduces stress and strain on the hip joint.

3. ____ A pillow under the waist is used when a patient is positioned in the supine, not lateral, position.

4. X Supporting the upper arm on a pillow helps to keep the shoulder in functional alignment.

5. X A pillow behind the back will help maintain the patient in the lateral position.

29. 1. This is a quick release slip knot. The knot will immediately release when the loose end of the line is pulled. This is the appropriate knot to secure a restraint strap to a bed frame because it permits a quick release in an emergency.

2. This is a two half hitch knot. This knot cannot be released easily and should not be used to secure a restraint line to a bed frame.

3. This is a clove hitch knot. This knot cannot be released easily and should not be used to secure a restraint line to a bed frame.

4. This is a bowline knot. This knot cannot be released easily and should not be used to secure a restraint line to a bed frame.

30. The patient fell out of bed but did not sustain an injury. Therefore the section titled "Fall" is the most appropriate section to check in the Occurrence Category.

Unusual Occurrence Report

Date of Event: _____   Time of Event: _____   Department: _____

Patient Last Name:	First Name:	MI:
Patient #:	**Attending Physician:**	
Visitor Last Name:	**First Name:**	**Phone #:**
Employee Name:	**Dept:**	
Physician Name:	**Specialty:**	

Occurrence Category (Check most appropriate)

☐ Agency nurse-related	☐ AMA	☐ Delay in treatment
☐ Diet-related	☐ HIPAA compliance	☐ Loss of personal property
☐ Medication-related	☐ Narcotics-related	☐ Order not executed
☐ Patient injury	☐ Peer-review related	☐ Restraint-related
☐ Staff injury	☐ Supplies/Equipment	☐ Visitor injury
☑ Fall		
☐ Other (please explain):		

Description of Occurrence:

A patient was medicated with an opioid. The patient's bedside rail was left in the down position. The patient was found on the floor. The patient was examined by the rapid response team. No injury was identified as a result of the fall. The patient was returned to bed.

Contributing Factors (Check all that apply)

☐ Individual:	☐ System:
Knowledge, skills, and/or experience (please list): ☐ Unclear ☐ Incomplete	Policies/procedures not in place (please list): ☐ Unclear ☐ Outdated
Standard of care or practice (please list): ☐ Non-adherence	Environmental: ☐ Staffing ☐ Patient acuity ☐ Congestion
Documentation (please list): ☐ Incomplete ☐ Inadequate	Communications and work flow: ☐ Intradepartmental ☐ Interdepartmental ☐ Equipment failure

Other (please explain):

Submitted by:	Dept:	Date:

31. 1. _____ The purpose of restraints is not to limit movement.

2. _____ Restraints can increase agitation; if used when a patient is severely agitated, they can cause injury.

3. _____ Immobilization is not the purpose of restraints. Restraints should be snug, yet loose enough for some movement.

4. **X The primary reason for the use of restraints is to prevent patient**

injury; restraints are used only as a last resort to protect the patient from self- injury or from hurting others.

5. <u>X</u> In an emergency a patient may be placed in restraints when a patient's activity threatens the safety of others.

32. 1. <u>X</u> Any person who falls in an agency setting, even if not injured, requires the completion of an incident report. Documentation of the possible causes of falls collectively may help to identify trends and initiate potential corrective action.

2. _____ A nurse who refuses to float to another unit is a management problem that is handled by a nurse manager. It does not require the initiation of an incident report.

3. <u>X</u> A visitor who faints requires the initiation of an incident report. This information collectively may help to identify trends and initiate potential corrective action.

4. _____ An angry resident physician does not require the completion of an incident report. If the individual's anger impinges on the ability to provide safe and effective patient care, the nurse should step in as a patient advocate and then immediately report the event to the nursing supervisor. The nursing supervisor would then intervene, which could include an incident report if the patient was harmed. However, this scenario does not indicate that patient care was jeopardized.

5. <u>X</u> A nurse's aide who applies a topical medication has performed a function that is outside the job description of a nurse's aide. A violation of standards of nursing practice requires the initiation of an incident report. In some limited settings a nurse's aide may be trained and certified to administer medications that do not require an assessment of the patient. Assessment of the patient before and after a medication is administered is the function of the nurse who has the educational preparation to determine the significance of the patient's status.

33.

1.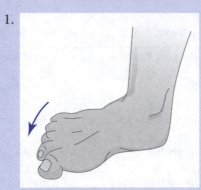

This illustration indicates flexion and extension of the toes. Flexion of the toes occurs when the joints of the toes are curled downward. Extension of the toes occurs when the toes are straightened.

2.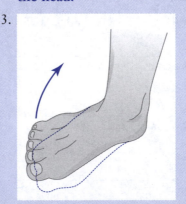

This illustration indicates flexion and extension of the ankle. Flexion of the ankle occurs when the toes of the foot are pointed upward toward the head. Extension of the ankle occurs when the toes are pointed downward away from the head.

3.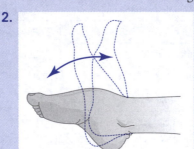

This illustration indicates eversion and inversion of athe foot. Eversion of the foot occurs when the sole of the foot is turned outward (laterally). Inversion of the foot occurs when the sole of the foot is turned inward (medially).

4.

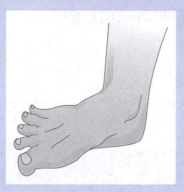

This illustration indicates abduction and adduction of the toes. Abduction of the toes occurs when the toes are are moved out to the side and spread apart. Adduction of the toes occurs when the toes are moved toward each other and brought together.

34. **TEST-TAKING TIP** The words "developmental factors," "adolescents," and "remain safe" are key words in the stem that direct attention to content.

   1. __X__ The frontal lobe of the brain that controls judgment and decision making does not fully develop until the late teenage years and early twenties. This contributes to underdevelopment of impulse control. In addition, adolescents tend to believe that adult opinions about safety are not significant or relevant.

   2. _____ Use of tools and household items as a cause of injury is related more to the school-aged child who may not have the dexterity or knowledge to use a tool safely.

3. __X__ Adolescents engage in risky behavior because of the pleasure related to a surge of epinephrine that comes with being scared and wanting to impress their friends. In addition, adolescents tend to believe that adult opinions about safety are not significant or relevant.

4. __X__ Research demonstrated that only 67% of 16 to 20 years olds use vehicle safety belts. This is lower than any other age group. The three main reasons why adolescents do not use seat belts are forgetting, wanting to be cool, and peer pressure.

5. __X__ One of the most important factors influencing adolescent behavior is the desire to belong and fit in. Adolescents will conform when pressured because they want to be a member of the group. It is believed that as adolescents move away from the family and become more independent they also feel afraid to be alone. They are too young to be too independent so they want to belong to a group that provides support and comfort.

35. Answer: 3 mL

Solve the problem using the formula for ratio and proportion.

$$\frac{\text{Desire}}{\text{Have}} \quad \frac{15 \text{ mg}}{10 \text{ mg}} = \frac{x \text{ mL}}{1 \text{ mL}}$$

10x = 15

x = 15 ÷ 10

x = 1.5 mL for each dose.

Multiply 1.5 × 2 = 3 mL over 24 hours.

MEETING PATIENTS' HYGIENE, PAIN, COMFORT, REST, AND SLEEP NEEDS

This section includes questions related to meeting patients' hygiene, comfort, rest, and sleep needs. Questions focus on theories of pain; assessment of pain; pain relief measures; rest and sleep; the backrub; making a bed; the use of heat and cold; principles associated with bed baths; preventing skin breakdown; perineal care; and care of the hair, feet, and oral cavity.

QUESTIONS

1. Which temperature should the water be when the nurse gives a patient a bed bath?
   1. 80°F to 85°F
   2. 90°F to 95°F
   3. 100°F to 105°F
   4. 110°F to 115°F

2. Which is the reason why the nurse rinses the patient after washing with soap and water during a bed bath?
   1. Increase circulation
   2. Minimize pressure ulcers
   3. Promote rest and comfort
   4. Remove residue and debris

3. A nurse identifies that a patient has offensive breath. Which is the **most** effective intervention that the nurse should encourage the patient to do?
   1. Brush the teeth and tongue after meals.
   2. Eat the foods that do not generate odors.
   3. Rinse the mouth with mouthwash every shift.
   4. Flush the mouth with peroxide and baking soda.

   TEST-TAKING TIP Identify the word in the stem that sets a priority. Identify the option with a specific determiner. Identify equally plausible options.

4. A nurse is changing the linens for a patient on bedrest. Which should the nurse do to prevent pressure (decubitus) ulcers when putting a bottom sheet on a bed?
   1. Cover it with a draw sheet.
   2. Make it with a toe pleat.
   3. Change it every day.
   4. Kept it wrinkle-free.

   TEST-TAKING TIP Identify key words in the stem that direct attention to content. Identify the option with a specific determiner.

5. A school nurse is teaching a group of high school students about health promotion and sleep. Which age group should the nurse explain requires the **least** amount of sleep?
   1. Adolescents
   2. Older adults
   3. Young adults
   4. Middle-age adults

   TEST-TAKING TIP Identify the word in the stem that indicates negative polarity.

6. A patient has a nasogastric tube. Which is a daily nursing intervention that contributes to hygiene?
   1. Instilling the system with one ounce of water
   2. Replacing the fixation device
   3. Suctioning the oral pharynx
   4. Lubricating the nares

   TEST-TAKING TIP Identify key words in the stem that direct attention to content.

7. During a clinic visit an older adult reports having cold feet at night. Which should the nurse teach the patient to do?
   1. Wear socks.
   2. Keep them elevated.
   3. Apply a heating pad.
   4. Use a hot water bottle.

   TEST-TAKING TIP Identify key words in the stem that direct attention to content. Identify equally plausible options.

8. A nurse is planning to give a patient a backrub to promote comfort and rest. Which is the reason why a backrub promotes comfort and rest?
   1. Causes vasodilation
   2. Stimulates circulation
   3. Relieves muscular tension
   4. Increases oxygen to tissues

   TEST-TAKING TIP Identify key words in the stem that direct attention to content. Identify the unique option. Identify equally plausible options.

9. A patient asks the nurse why cold compresses were ordered to treat a recent muscle sprain. Which is the reason why cold is effective in reducing the discomfort associated with a local inflammatory response that the nurse should include when answering the patient's question?
   1. Anesthetizes nerve endings and causes vasoconstriction
   2. Stimulates nerve endings and causes vasoconstriction
   3. Anesthetizes nerve endings and causes vasodilation
   4. Stimulates nerve endings and causes vasodilation

   TEST-TAKING TIP Identify duplicate facts among options.

10. Which should the nurse do to **best** promote rest and sleep in the hospital for all patients?
    1. Provide a backrub at bedtime.
    2. Turn the lights off at night.
    3. Encourage usual routines.
    4. Administer a sedative.

    TEST-TAKING TIP Identify the word in the stem that sets a priority. Identify key words in the stem that direct attention to content.

11. A nurse is planning interventions to facilitate a patient's ability to sleep. Which action minimizes the **most** common cause of insomnia?
    1. Promoting a comfortable position
    2. Decreasing environmental noise
    3. Exploring emotional concerns
    4. Regulating room temperature

    TEST-TAKING TIP Identify the word in the stem that sets a priority.

12. An order is written to apply a warm soak to a patient's extremity. Which information should the nurse include when teaching the patient how a warm soak reduces discomfort at a local inflammatory site?
    1. Decreases local circulation and limits capillary permeability
    2. Decreases tissue metabolism and increases local circulation
    3. Increases local circulation and promotes muscle relaxation
    4. Provides local anesthesia and decreases local circulation

    TEST-TAKING TIP Identify duplicate facts among options.

13. A nurse is providing oral hygiene for a patient with dentures. Which should the nurse do to support the patient's dignity?
    1. Provide a cup for the patient's teeth.
    2. Pull the curtain around the patient's bed.
    3. Support the patient in the high-Fowler position.
    4. Resist looking at the patient while the teeth are out.

    TEST-TAKING TIP Identify the key word in the stem that directs attention to content. Identify the patient-centered option.

14. When providing physical hygiene, the nurse identifies that the patient's hair is tangled and matted. Which should the nurse do?
    1. Braid the hair in sections.
    2. Use a comb instead of a hairbrush.
    3. Comb a small section of hair at a time.
    4. Brush from the roots of the hair toward the ends.

    TEST-TAKING TIP Identify key words in the stem that direct attention to content.

15. A nurse is making an occupied bed. Which is the **most** important nursing action?
    1. Place a pad on the draw sheet.
    2. Keep the patient covered.
    3. Raise both side rails.
    4. Use new linen.

    TEST-TAKING TIP Identify the word in the stem that sets a priority. Identify the patient-centered option.

16. A nurse makes the assessment that a patient's feet are dirty. Which is the **most** effective nursing intervention when planning to clean the patient's feet?
    1. Ask the patient to take a shower.
    2. Lubricate feet with lotion to soften dirt.
    3. Use an antifungal agent to prevent a fungal infection.
    4. Soak feet for a few minutes in a basin with soap and water.

    TEST-TAKING TIP Identify the word in the stem that sets a priority. Identify clang associations.

17. Which factor has the **most** significant influence on pain perception that is important for the nurse to consider when assessing a patient's pain?
    1. Duration of the stimulus
    2. Activity of the cerebral cortex
    3. Characteristics of the stimulus
    4. Level of endorphins in the blood

    TEST-TAKING TIP Identify the word in the stem that sets a priority.

18. A nurse uses a cotton blanket when bathing a patient. Which principle is the basis for using a blanket to prevent the loss of body heat during a bed bath?
    1. Evaporation
    2. Conduction
    3. Diffusion
    4. Osmosis

19. A nurse is providing a patient with a backrub after a bed bath. Which massage technique is **most** effective in promoting relaxation?
    1. Tapotement
    2. Effleurage
    3. Pétrissage
    4. Friction

    TEST-TAKING TIP Identify the word in the stem that sets a priority. Identify the key word in the stem that directs attention to content.

20. Which should the nurse do to provide emotional comfort when administering perineal care to a patient? **Select all that apply.**
1. ____ Place the patient in the supine position.
2. ____ Drape areas that are not being washed.
3. ____ Pull a curtain around the bed.
4. ____ Use warm water for washing.
5. ____ Call the patient by name.

TEST-TAKING TIP Identify key words in the stem that direct attention to content.

21. After reviewing the patient's clinical record and completing a physical assessment, which type of bath should the nurse provide?
1. Partial bath with total assistance
2. Partial bath with partial assistance
3. Complete bath with total assistance
4. Complete bath with partial assistance

PATIENT'S CLINICAL RECORD

Progress Note
A female patient has a history of a brain attack 2 years ago that caused left-sided hemiparesis. The patient is currently admitted for right flank pain and tests are scheduled to rule out renal calculus. Patient is incontinent of urine and stool.

Braden Scale
Score: 16. Responds to verbal commands and has no sensory deficit. Skin is constantly moist as detected every time patient is turned and positioned. Needs assistance to move from bed to a chair, makes frequent shifts in position but needs some assistance to turn or move up in bed. Generally eats most of every meal.

Physical Assessment
Patient is incontinent of urine and stool and is damp where skin surfaces touch (under arms, perineal area, and under the breasts). Patient is alert and responding appropriately and reports that flank pain is a level 2 since pain medication was administered 30 minutes ago. IV is running at 125 mL as ordered; IV catheter insertion site is dry and intact with no signs of infiltration or thrombophlebitis.

TEST-TAKING TIP Identify key words in the stem that direct attention to content. Identify duplicate facts in options.

22. A nurse is caring for a patient who is coping with chronic pain. Which psychological reactions to chronic pain may occur? **Select all that apply.**
1. ____ Dyspnea
2. ____ Depression
3. ____ Self-splinting
4. ____ Hypertension
5. ____ Decreased libido
6. ____ Compromised interpersonal relationships

TEST-TAKING TIP Identify key words in the stem that direct attention to content.

23. A nurse is caring for a patient who is experiencing lower back pain. The muscle relaxant cyclobenzaprine 10 mg three times a day by mouth is prescribed. Cyclobenzaprine is available in 5-mg tablets. How many tablets of cyclobenzaprine will the patient be taking in 24 hours? **Record your answer using a whole number.**

Answer: _____ tablets

24. A nurse is cleansing the perineal area of an uncircumcised male patient. Which are important actions by the nurse when performing this procedure? **Select all that apply.**
1. ____ Handling the penis always with a light touch
2. ____ Washing the shaft of the penis before the scrotum
3. ____ Repositioning the foreskin after washing the penis
4. ____ Cleansing the length of the penis down the shaft toward the glans
5. ____ Washing the glans with a circular motion from the urinary meatus outward

TEST-TAKING TIP Identify the option with a specific determiner.

25. A patient comes to the emergency department reporting pain, nausea, vomiting, and a low-grade fever. Rovsing's sign is elicited when the primary health-care provider palpates the patient's left lower quadrant. Place an X over the site where the patient felt an increase in pain.

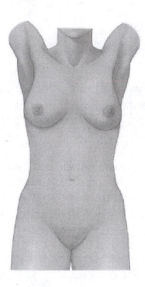

26. For which behavioral responses should the nurse assess the patient when the patient is experiencing pain? **Select all that apply.**
1. ____ Rapid, irregular breathing
2. ____ Increased muscle tension
3. ____ Facial grimacing
4. ____ Self-splinting
5. ____ Groaning
6. ____ Fatigue

TEST-TAKING TIP Identify key words in the stem that directs attention to content.

27. A nurse is caring for a patient who has a fungal infection of the feet. Which should the nurse teach the patient to employ to reduce the incidence of a fungal infection of the feet? **Select all that apply.**
1. ____ Wear flip flops to protect the feet when walking in a locker room.
2. ____ Soak the feet in a medicated solution during hygiene care.
3. ____ Apply body lotion to the feet to avoid cracks in the skin.
4. ____ Increase circulation to the feet by encouraging exercise.
5. ____ Dry well between the toes of the feet after bathing.

28. A patient says to the nurse, "Lately I've been having a hard time sleeping." Which should the nurse encourage the patient to do to promote sleep? **Select all that apply.**
   1. ____ Exercise daily.
   2. ____ Drink a cup of tea.
   3. ____ Eat only light meals.
   4. ____ Review the day's events.
   5. ____ Follow a bedtime routine.

   TEST-TAKING TIP Identify the option with a specific determiner.

29. A patient has had difficulty sleeping and the nurse secures a prescription for zolpidem 12.5 mg PO at bedtime. The medication supplied by the pharmacy is 6.25 mg/tablet. How many tablets should the nurse administer? **Record your answer using a whole number.**

   Answer: _____ tablets

30. A nurse is providing perineal care for a female patient. Which should the nurse do during this procedure? **Select all that apply.**
   1. ____ Use a new area of the washcloth for each stroke.
   2. ____ Wash from the pubis toward the rectum.
   3. ____ Always use a circular motion.
   4. ____ Clean the dirtiest area first.
   5. ____ Use only cool tap water.

   TEST-TAKING TIP Identify options with specific determiners.

31. A nurse is caring for a 6-year-old child who had abdominal surgery because of a ruptured appendix. When performing a pain assessment the nurse identifies that the child's chin is quivering and the legs are restless. The child also is squirming in the bed and whimpering softly. When the nurse hugs the child and offers verbal reassurance the child's whimpering subsides. Which is the child's pain assessment according to the FLACC Scale?

   Answer: _____

Categories	Score		
	0	**1**	**2**
Face	No particular expression or smile	Occasional grimace or frown, withdrawn, uninterested	Frequent to constant quivering chin, clenched jaw
Legs	Normal position or relaxed	Uneasy, restless, tense	Kicking, or legs drawn up
Activity	Lying quietly, normal position, moves easily	Squirming, shifting, back and forth, tense	Arched, rigid, or jerking
Cry	No cry (awake or asleep)	Moans or whimpers; occasional complaint	Crying steadily, screams or sobs, frequent complaints
Consolability	Content, relaxed	Reassured by occasional touching, hugging or being talked to, distractible	Difficult to console or comfort

FLACC behavioral scale. © 2002 The regents of the University of Michigan. All Rights Reserved.

32. A patient is experiencing interrupted sleep. For which responses associated with shortened non–rapid-eye-movement (NREM) sleep should the nurse assess the patient? **Select all that apply.**
1. ____ Fatigue
2. ____ Anxiety
3. ____ Hyperactivity
4. ____ Delayed healing
5. ____ Aggressive behavior

33. A nurse is performing oral care for a patient. Place the following illustrations in the order that they should be performed.

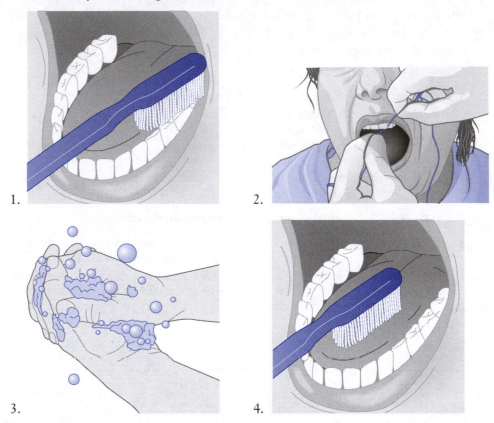

1.

2.

3.

4.

Answer: _____

34. A nurse in charge delegates the application of a cold pack to a patient. Place the following steps in the order in which they should be performed.
1. Review the order for the application of the cold pack.
2. Assess the site five minutes after application of the cold pack.
3. Place a protective barrier between the cold pack and the patient.
4. Explain the details of the application of the cold pack to the patient.
5. Assess the condition of the site where the cold pack is to be applied.

Answer: _____

35. A nurse is caring for a patient diagnosed with pediculosis *(Pediculus humanus capitis)*. Lindane shampoo is prescribed to treat this condition. Which grooming device should the nurse use after washing the patient's hair and scalp with lindane shampoo?

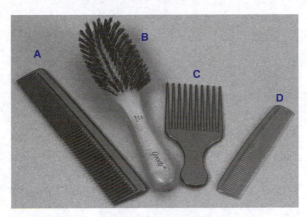

1. A
2. B
3. C
4. D

TEST-TAKING TIP Identify the key word in the stem that directs attention to content.

1. 1. 80°F to 85°F temperature range is too cool; this will promote chilling.
   2. 90°F to 95°F temperature range is too cool; this will promote chilling.
   3. 100°F to 105°F temperature range is too cool; this will promote chilling.
   4. **The temperature of bath water should be between 110°F and 115°F to promote comfort, dilate blood vessels, and prevent chilling.**

2. 1. Friction from firm, long strokes used during bathing increases circulation; it is not the reason for rinsing.
   2. Local massage and repositioning every 2 hours, not rinsing, prevent pressure ulcers.
   3. A backrub and positioning in functional alignment, not rinsing, promote rest and comfort.
   4. **Rinsing flushes the skin with clean water, which removes debris and soap residue.**

3. **TEST-TAKING TIP** The word "most" in the stem sets a priority. The word "every" in option 3 is a specific determiner. Options 3 and 4 are equally plausible.
   1. **Halitosis is often caused by decaying food particles and gingivitis; brushing the teeth and tongue cleans the oral cavity, which promotes healthy teeth and gums.**
   2. Although some foods can cause halitosis, it is more often caused by inadequate oral hygiene, a local infection, or a systemic disease.
   3. Rinsing or flushing will not remove debris caught between the teeth.
   4. Rinsing or flushing will not remove debris caught between the teeth.

4. **TEST-TAKING TIP** The words "prevent," "pressure ulcers," and "bottom sheet" are key words in the stem that direct attention to content. The word "every" in option 3 is a specific determiner.
   1. A draw sheet is an additional sheet that can add to the number of wrinkles; the purpose of a draw sheet is to keep the bottom sheet clean.
   2. A toe pleat should be placed in the top sheet and spread, not the bottom sheet. A toe pleat prevents footdrop.
   3. The bottom sheet does not have to be changed every day unless the sheet is wet or soiled.
   4. **Wrinkles exert pressure and friction against the skin, promoting the formation of pressure (decubitus) ulcers.**

5. **TEST-TAKING TIP** The word "least" in the stem indicates negative polarity.
   1. Adolescents go through a growth spurt and need more sleep than the age groups addressed in other options.
   2. **Studies demonstrate that older adults require less sleep than do people on any other developmental level.**
   3. Young adults may still be growing and are active; they need more sleep than an age group addressed in another option.
   4. Middle-age adults are usually involved with activities related to growing children and developing a career; this age requires more sleep than an age group addressed in another option.

6. **TEST-TAKING TIP** The words "daily" and "contribute to hygiene" are key words in the stem that direct attention to content.
   1. After placement is verified, instillation of solution may be done to promote catheter patency, not hygiene.
   2. This is not necessary; the fixation device should be reapplied if the nares become irritated or the device becomes soiled.
   3. Suctioning is not necessary; cleaning the oral cavity when necessary with a tooth brush, dental floss, and mouthwash followed by applying a lubricant to the lips is sufficient.
   4. **Lubricating the nares keeps the skin supple and prevents drying, which limits the development of encrustations.**

7. **TEST-TAKING TIP** The words "older adult" are key words in the stem that direct attention to content. Options 3 and 4 are equally plausible.
   1. **Wearing socks is the safest way to keep the feet warm; socks contain the heat generated by the body.**
   2. Elevation will not alter the temperature of the feet.

3. External heat produced by a heating pad can burn the feet in older adults who have reduced peripheral sensation.

4. External heat produced by a hot water bottle can burn the feet in older adults who have reduced peripheral sensation.

8. **TEST-TAKING TIP The words "comfort and rest" are key words in the stem that direct attention to content. Option 3 is unique because it addresses muscles and what is decreased (relieves) rather than what is increased ("causes" in option 1, "stimulates" in option 2, "increases" in option 4). Options 1, 2, and 4 are equally plausible because they all refer to the circulatory system.**

1. Although a backrub causes vasodilation, which improves circulation and brings oxygen and nutrients to the area, vasodilation does not promote comfort and rest.

2. Stimulation of circulation brings oxygen and nutrients to the area, but it does not promote comfort and rest.

3. **Applying long, smooth strokes while moving the hands up and down the back without losing contact with the skin has a relaxing and sedative effect. Its effect may be related to the gate-control theory of pain relief; rubbing the back stimulates large muscle fiber groups, which close the synaptic gates to pain or uncomfortable stimuli, permitting a perception of relaxation.**

4. Although a backrub ultimately does increase oxygen and nutrients to the area, oxygen and increased nutrients do not promote comfort and rest.

9. **TEST-TAKING TIP There are four hypotheses being tested in this question: cold anesthetizes nerve endings, causes vasoconstriction, stimulates nerve endings, and causes vasodilation. If you know just one of these hypotheses is wrong, then you can eliminate two distractors.**

1. **Cold is a form of cutaneous stimulation that slows the nervous conduction of impulses, thereby anesthetizing nerve endings, which relaxes muscle tension and relieves pain. Vasoconstriction decreases the flow of blood to the affected area; this limits the development of edema, which puts pressure on nerve endings, resulting in pain.**

2. Cold anesthetizes rather than stimulates nerve endings; it causes vasoconstriction.

3. Although cold does anesthetize nerve endings, it causes vasoconstriction, not vasodilation.

4. Cold anesthetizes, rather than stimulates, nerve endings and causes vasoconstriction.

10. **TEST-TAKING TIP The word "best" in the stem sets a priority. The words "all patients" are key words in the stem that direct attention to content.**

1. A backrub invades personal space and should be administered according to a patient's need and preference; a backrub may be contraindicated in certain clinical situations, such as myocardial infarction or back surgery.

2. In an unfamiliar environment, turning the lights off can precipitate confusion or disorientation; a small light provides visual cues if a person awakens at night.

3. **Usual routines meet self-identified needs and reduce anxiety because they provide a familiar pattern.**

4. Sleeping medication should not be administered until all nondrug approaches fail to achieve sleep.

11. **TEST-TAKING TIP The word "most" in the stem sets a priority.**

1. **An inability to find a position of comfort is the main reason why patients have difficulty sleeping in the hospital.**

2. Although environmental noise can interfere with sleep, it is not the factor that has been proved most often to interfere with sleep.

3. Emotional concerns have not been proved to be the factor that most often interferes with sleep.

4. Room temperature has not been proved to be the factor that most often interferes with sleep.

12. **TEST-TAKING TIP The words "increases local circulation" in options 2 and 3 and "decreases local circulation" in options 1 and 4 are examples of duplicate facts among the options. If you know that one or the other is true, the chances of selecting the correct answer has improved to 50%.**

1. Heat increases, rather than decreases, local circulation, capillary vasodilation, and permeability.

2. Although heat increases local circulation, it increases, rather than decreases, tissue metabolism. Heat causes vasodilation,

facilitating the exchange of nutrients and waste products and increasing cellular metabolism.

3. Heat increases circulation because of its vasodilating effect. Heat is known to relax muscle spasms and the discomfort associated with muscle spasm; this mechanism is unknown.

4. Cold, not heat, provides local anesthesia and decreases local circulation.

13. **TEST-TAKING TIP** The word "dignity" is the key word in the stem that directs attention to content. Option 2 is patient-centered.

1. This is used to store the dentures when the patient is sleeping and addresses the patient's safety and security needs.

2. This provides privacy while the dentures are out of the mouth and supports the patient's dignity and self-esteem.

3. This supports the patient's physical needs.

4. This is unsafe; the nurse must look at the patient to inspect the oral cavity.

14. **TEST-TAKING TIP** The words "tangled and matted" are key words in the stem that direct attention to content.

1. Braiding the hair in sections should be done after the hair is combed and untangled. Not all patients want their hair to be braided.

2. Either a comb or brush can be used.

3. Separating the hair into small sections promotes ease in combing and limits discomfort.

4. When removing tangles, the hair should be grasped at the scalp and the loose ends combed; each stroke should start progressively higher than the preceding stroke up the shafts of hair strands.

15. **TEST-TAKING TIP** The word "most" in the stem sets a priority. Option 3 is the patient-centered option because it focuses on the patient rather than on steps in a procedure.

1. This promotes the formation of pressure ulcers; it should be used only during perineal care or for patients who are incontinent.

2. This supports privacy and dignity and prevents chilling.

3. This does not support correct body mechanics when working and puts excessive stress on the nurse; the side rail may be lowered on the side where the nurse is working.

4. This is unnecessary unless the linens are wet or soiled.

16. **TEST-TAKING TIP** The word "most" in the stem sets a priority. The word "feet" in the stem and options 2 and 4 are clang associations.

1. Showering is not as effective as submerging the feet in soapy water.

2. A lubricant should be applied after the feet are clean.

3. The application of an antifungal agent requires a prescription from a primary health-care provider.

4. Soaking the feet for a few minutes in soap and water softens debris on the skin, between the toes, and under the toenails, facilitating cleaning.

17. **TEST-TAKING TIP** The word "most" in the stem sets a priority. All of the options address factors that influence pain, but option 2 is the "most" significant.

1. Duration is one component of a description of pain after it is perceived.

2. The cerebral cortex controls the higher levels of the perceptual aspects of pain.

3. The characteristics of pain are the components of the description of pain after it is perceived.

4. Although endorphin levels influence pain perception, it is not the most influential factor that affects the perception of pain.

18. **1. Evaporation (vaporization) is the transfer of heat through the conversion of water to a gas. This occurs when there is fluid on the skin from either perspiration or bath water.**

2. Conduction is the transfer of heat from one molecule to another while in direct physical contact.

3. Diffusion is a process whereby molecules move through a membrane from an area of higher concentration to an area of lower concentration without the expenditure of energy.

4. Osmosis is the movement of water across a membrane from an area of lesser concentration to an area of greater concentration.

19. **TEST-TAKING TIP** The word "most" in the stem sets a priority. The word

"relaxation" is the key word in the stem that directs attention to content.

1. The technique of *tapotement* is the gentle rhythmic tapping or percussion over tense muscles. The technique of tapotement is not as relaxing as another backrub technique.

2. **The technique of *effleurage* uses long, smooth, circular strokes that slide over the skin to produce muscle relaxation. The French word *effleurage* means "to touch lightly." It is performed at the beginning of a backrub before pétrissage and again at the end of the backrub.**

3. The technique of *pétrissage* kneads the skin and underlying muscles. This technique targets specific muscles to reduce muscle tension and promote circulation to peripheral capillaries. The technique of pétrissage is not as relaxing as another backrub technique.

4. The technique of *friction* uses small circular strokes that move the surface of the skin as well as underlying tissue. This stroke is used to promote circulation to peripheral capillaries. The technique of friction is not as relaxing as another backrub technique.

20. **TEST-TAKING TIP** The words "perineal" and "emotional comfort" are key words in the stem that direct attention to content.

   1. ____ Correct positioning provides for physical, not emotional, comfort.

   2. **X All areas of the body below the neck not being washed should be covered with a bath blanket to provide for privacy and to avoid chilling.**

   3. **X Perineal care is a private activity, and measures should be taken to provide for privacy.**

   4. ____ Warm water provides physical, not emotional, comfort.

   5. **X Calling the patient by name is a respectful, individualized approach that provides emotional support during invasive care.**

21. **TEST-TAKING TIP** The key words in the scenario are "incontinent of urine and stool," "constantly moist skin," "needs some assistance to turn," and "pain level 2." If you know that a person who is incontinent of urine and stool and has constantly damp skin surfaces needs a

complete bath, options 1 and 2 can be eliminated. If you know that individuals with tolerable pain and the ability to engage in some movement generally prefer to be as independent as possible, then you can eliminate options that provide total assistance. Options 1 and 3 provide total assistance and can be eliminated. Even if you know only one fact you can eliminate two options from consideration.

1. A partial bath is inappropriate. Because the patient has damp skin where skin surfaces touch, the patient needs the entire body washed, rinsed, and dried, not just the face, hands, back, perineal area, and axillae, which are cared for during a partial bath. Total assistance is inappropriate. Patients should be as independent as possible within their level of ability.

2. Although partial assistance is appropriate because independence should be supported within the patient's ability level, a partial bath is inappropriate. Because the patient has damp skin surfaces, the patient needs the entire body washed, rinsed, and dried, not just the face, hands, back, perineal area, and axillae, which are cared for during a partial bath.

3. Although a complete bath is appropriate, total assistance is unnecessary. The patient's pain is tolerable and the patient has the ability to move the right side of the body and some limited ability to move the left side (hemiparesis).

4. **A complete bath is necessary because the patient has damp skin surfaces where skin surfaces touch and is incontinent of urine and stool. Partial assistance should be provided. The patient should be set up to bathe as many areas as possible independently; then the nurse should wash, rinse, and dry those areas that the patient is unable to reach.**

22. **TEST-TAKING TIP** The words "psychological" and "chronic" are key words in the stem that direct attention to content.

1. ____ Dyspnea is a physiological, not a psychological, response to stress.

2. **X Patients with chronic pain commonly experience depression; this is a psychological response to lack of control over relentless pain.**

3. ____ Self-splinting is a behavioral attempt to minimize pain.

4. ____ Hypertension is a physiological, not a psychological, response to stress.

5. **X** Interest in sexual activity decreases when one is depressed and coping with pain. The desire for an absence of pain is one of the most basic physiological needs. Some consider sexual activity a physiological need but others consider it a love/belonging need.

6. **X** Compromised interpersonal relationships may occur as the patient with chronic pain depletes emotional energy and resources needed to sustain relationships.

23. **Answer: 6 Tablets in 24 hours.** Solve the problem using ratio and proportion.

$$\frac{\text{Desire}}{\text{Have}} \qquad \frac{10 \text{ mg}}{5 \text{ mg}} = \frac{x \text{ tablets}}{1 \text{ tablet}}$$

Cross-multiply $5x = 10$

Divide each side by 5 $x = 10 \div 5$

                        $x = 2$ tablets

Multiply 2 tablets by three times a day = 6 tablets in 24 hours.

24. **TEST-TAKING TIP** Option 1 contains the word "always," which is a specific determiner.

1. ____ A light touch is stimulating and may precipitate a penile erection; a firm but gentle touch should be used.

2. **X** Washing the shaft of the penis before the scrotum reflects the principle of working from clean to dirty. The tip of the penis at the urethral meatus should be washed first then the nurse should progress down the shaft of the penis toward the perineum and then the scrotum.

3. **X** Repositioning the foreskin protects the head of the penis and prevents drying and irritation; if it is allowed to remain retracted, it may cause local edema and discomfort.

4. ____ Cleaning should occur in the opposite direction, starting at the urinary meatus and then progressing down the shaft of the penis away from the urinary meatus.

5. **X** Cleaning with a circular motion beginning at the urinary meatus and moving outward moves secretions and debris away from the urinary meatus; this lessens potential contamination of the urinary tract.

25. Palpation of the left lower quadrant in a patient with appendicitis precipitates pain at McBurney's point (Rovsing's sign). McBurney's point is in the lower right quadrant half the distance from the anterior iliac crest to the umbilicus.

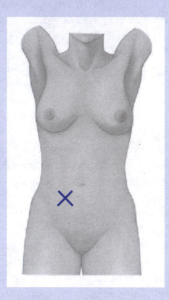

26. **TEST-TAKING TIP** The word "behavioral" is the key word in the stem that directs attention to content.

1. ____ Rapid, irregular breathing is a physiological response to pain; pain generally activates the fight-or-flight mechanism of the general adaptation syndrome.

2. ____ The general adaptation syndrome stimulates the sympathetic branch of the autonomic nervous system, which results in increased muscle tension; it is a physiological response that prepares muscles for action.

3. **X** Facial grimacing (e.g., compressing lips together, squeezing the eyes shut, contracting facial muscles) is a voluntary behavioral response to pain.

4. **X** Self-splinting is a behavioral attempt to protect the area in pain and minimize stress and strain to the area, such as supporting the area or leaning in the direction of the pain.

5. **X** Groaning is a behavioral response to pain.

6. ____ Fatigue is a physiological response to pain; physical and emotional responses to pain can use a great deal of physical

and emotional energy and leave a person fatigued.

27. 1. X Fungi grow and are transmitted to others in areas where there is moisture and the feet are not protected.
    2. ____ Medicated footbaths generally are ordered for ingrown toenails, not fungal infections; they require a primary health-care provider's order.
    3. ____ Moisturizers should be avoided between the toes because they keep the area moist, which supports fungal growth.
    4. ____ Exercise does not minimize fungal growth.
    5. X Moist, dark, warm areas facilitate the growth of microorganisms, especially fungi in the area of the feet.

28. TEST-TAKING TIP Option 3 contains the word "only," which is a specific determiner.
    1. X Exercise contributes to physical and mental relaxation, which reduces tension and promotes sleep.
    2. ____ Tea contains caffeine, which contributes to wakefulness.
    3. ____ The opposite is true. Moderate to heavy meals promote sleep; the body's energy is engaged in the process of digestion.
    4. ____ Reviewing the day's events can cause an increase in tension, which can prevent a person from falling asleep.
    5. X A bedtime routine sets a pattern of behaviors that are familiar; the routine should promote relaxation and set an expectation that rest and sleep will follow.

29. Answer: 2 tablets.
    Solve the problem using ratio and proportion.

    $$\frac{\text{Desired}}{\text{Have}} \quad \frac{12.5 \text{ mg}}{6.25 \text{ mg}} = \frac{\text{x Tab}}{1 \text{ Tab}}$$

    $6.25x = 12.5$

    $x = 12.5 \div 6.25$

    $x = 2 \text{ tablets}$

30. TEST-TAKING TIP The words "always" in option 3 and "only" in option 5 are specific determiners. Options with specific determiners rarely are correct answers.

Eliminate options 3 and 5 from further consideration.

1. X This is a basic principle of medical asepsis. This should be done so that contaminated material will not be carried by the washcloth to another area of the perineum.
2. X Cleaning from the pubis toward the rectum prevents contaminating the urinary meatus and vagina with fecal material.
3. ____ A circular motion should not be used because it will move debris from more soiled areas to less soiled areas.
4. ____ The area closest to the urinary meatus and vagina is cleaned first because it is considered the cleanest area of the perineum.
5. ____ Warm water should be used to clean the perineal area; cool water will feel uncomfortable, and hot water can injure the perineal area.

31. Answer: 6
    A quivering chin is awarded 2 points, and restlessness, squirming, whimpering, and the ability to be consoled are awarded 1 point each, for a total of 6 points. Factors that are assessed are face, legs, activity, cry, and consolability. Each can receive 0, 1, or 2 points based on the child's response to the pain. "No Pain" is equal to 0 points and "Worst Pain" is equal to 10 points.

32. 1. X During non–rapid-eye-movement (NREM) sleep the parasympathetic nervous system dominates. The heart rate, respirations, and blood pressure decrease as the body physically restores and regenerates itself. NREM sleep accounts for 75% to 80% of sleep. When NREM sleep is interrupted a person experiences fatigue and lethargy.
    2. ____ Rapid-eye-movement (REM) sleep is essential for maintaining mental and emotional equilibrium and, when interrupted, results in anxiety, irritability, excitability, confusion, and suspiciousness.
    3. ____ Interrupted REM, not NREM, sleep is associated with hyperactivity and excitability.
    4. X During NREM sleep, growth hormone is consistently secreted, which provides for protein synthesis, anabolism, and tissue repair. A lack of

NREM sleep results in delayed wound healing and immunosuppression.
5. ____ Interrupted REM, not NREM, sleep is associated with excitability, emotional lability, and suspiciousness. Interrupted NREM sleep is associated with apathy, withdrawal, and hyporesponsiveness.

33. Answer: 3, 1, 4, 2
  3. The nurse must wash his or her hands before performing any direct patient care. This limits the presence of microorganisms on the nurse's hands and prevents cross contamination.
  1. All teeth surfaces should be brushed: the biting and chewing surfaces of teeth and the inner and outer surfaces of teeth including the gum line.
  4. Brushing the tongue removes accumulated debris and dried mucus, which provide a reservoir for bacteria and produces bad breath.
  2. Moving dental floss up and down between teeth removes food particles. The mouth should be rinsed with water at the end of the procedure. Oral suction may be necessary if the patient is at risk for aspiration or is unconscious.

34. Answer: 1, 4, 5, 3, 2
  1. The application of a cold pack is a dependent function of the nurse. The order will include the type of cold delivery device to be used, the site where it should be applied, and the length of time it should remain in place.
  4. Patients have a right to know the details of a procedure to be performed and by whom. They also have the right to accept or refuse the treatment.
  5. Assessing the condition of the site (appearance of skin such as color, edema, temperature, and integrity of skin, and presence of discomfort

or pain) provides baseline information to which the patient's response to the procedure can be compared. The primary health-care provider should be notified if a contraindication (e.g., sensory impairment) for the procedure exists.
  3. Placing a protective barrier (e.g., washcloth, towel, fitted cloth sleeve) between the cold device and the patient limits the intensity of the cold application, preventing tissue trauma.
  2. Five minutes after the application of the cold pack the site should be assessed for signs such as pallor and mottling and to check if the patient feels it is too cold. The ice pack should be removed if these occur to prevent a progression to frostbite.

35. TEST-TAKING TIP The word "pediculosis" is the key word in the stem that directs attention to content.
  1. The distance between the teeth of this comb is appropriate for combing thin, straight, or slightly curly hair, not for removing nits (eggs) associated with head lice *(Pediculus humanus capitis)*.
  2. This brush is appropriate for grooming thick or thin, straight, or slightly curly hair, not for removing nits (eggs) associated with head lice *(Pediculus humanus capitis)*.
  3. This comb is not appropriate to use after shampooing with lindane to remove nits (eggs). The distance between the teeth of this comb is appropriate for thick, very curly hair because it allows the comb to gently detangle this type of hair.
  4. This comb is appropriate for removing nits (eggs) attached to hair shafts close to the scalp after shampooing for head lice infestation (pediculosis). The teeth are extremely close together, which uses friction to loosen nits attached to hair shafts.

MEETING PATIENTS' FLUID AND NUTRITIONAL NEEDS

This section includes questions related to basic fluid balance and nutrition. Specific questions focus on principles associated with therapeutic diets, enteral feedings, fluid and electrolyte balance, intake and output (I&O), dehydration, feeding patients, vitamins, parenteral nutrition, intralipids, and medications associated with meeting patients' nutritional needs.

QUESTIONS

1. A nurse is caring for an obese patient who is receiving a 1000-calorie diet. Which is **least** therapeutic when providing nursing care?
   1. Telling the patient about low-calorie snacks that can be eaten
   2. Teaching the patient to avoid starches on the meal tray
   3. Encouraging the patient to eat meals slowly
   4. Praising the patient when weight is lost

   TEST-TAKING TIP Identify the word in the stem that indicates negative polarity. Identify the unique option.

2. A nurse is monitoring a patient's intake and output. Which is an accurate way for the nurse to measure the amount of urine from the patient's urinary retention catheter?
   1. With a urometer
   2. With a marked graduate
   3. By emptying it into a bedpan
   4. By the markings on the collection bag

3. A nurse is planning for the nutritional needs of patients and is concerned about the influence of age on energy requirements. Which age group has the highest energy requirement?
   1. Birth to 1 year of age
   2. 3 to 5 years of age
   3. 13 to 19 years of age
   4. Older than 65 years of age

   TEST-TAKING TIP Identify the word in the stem that sets a priority.

4. Which should the nurse do to avoid trauma to the oral mucous membranes from hot food being served to a cognitively impaired patient?
   1. Request a menu that includes many cold foods.
   2. Always touch the food to test its temperature.
   3. Mix hot food with appropriate cold food.
   4. Wait for the hot food to cool slightly.

   TEST-TAKING TIP Identify the option with a specific determiner. Identify options that deny patient feelings, concerns, or needs.

5. A nurse is caring for an easily confused patient. Which is the **most** appropriate nursing intervention to meet the nutritional needs of this patient?
   1. Feed the patient each meal.
   2. Provide supervision when the patient eats.
   3. Explain to the patient where everything is on the tray.
   4. Encourage family members to take turns feeding the patient.

   TEST-TAKING TIP Identify the word in the stem that sets a priority.

6. A patient had a heart attack because of atherosclerotic plaques. Which is the **best** nutrient that the nurse should encourage the patient to eat to increase protein in the diet?
   1. White meats
   2. Whole milk
   3. Legumes
   4. Shrimp

   TEST-TAKING TIP Identify the word in the stem that sets a priority.

7. Which loss should be identified by the nurse as being **most** significant when caring for a patient with a draining pressure (decubitus) ulcer?
   1. Fluid
   2. Weight
   3. Protein
   4. Leukocytes

   TEST-TAKING TIP Identify the word in the stem that sets a priority. Identify key words in the stem that direct attention to content.

8. Which of the following does the nurse expect of all patients on a low-calorie diet?
   1. Breakdown of adipose tissue for energy
   2. Need for vitamin supplements
   3. Reduced body metabolism
   4. Decreased energy levels

   TEST-TAKING TIP Identify key words in the stem that direct attention to content. Identify equally plausible options.

9. Which patient response occurs when the amount of calories ingested is not sufficient for the patient's basal metabolic rate?
   1. Thready pulse
   2. Loss of weight
   3. Dependent edema
   4. Need for more sleep

10. A patient with the diagnosis of dehydration is hospitalized for intravenous rehydration therapy. Which should the nurse do immediately after the patient drinks 8 ounces of apple juice?
    1. Record the amount on the intake and output form.
    2. Assess the patient's skin turgor.
    3. Offer the patient a bedpan.
    4. Provide oral hygiene.

    TEST-TAKING TIP Identify the word in the stem that sets a priority.

11. Which should the nurse encourage a patient on a low-sodium diet to ingest?
    1. Milk
    2. Fruit
    3. Bread
    4. Vegetables

    TEST-TAKING TIP Identify key words in the stem that direct attention to content.

12. A patient has a pressure (decubitus) ulcer. Which breakfast food should the nurse encourage the patient to eat?
    1. French toast and oatmeal
    2. Oatmeal and orange juice
    3. French toast and poached eggs
    4. Poached eggs and orange juice

    TEST-TAKING TIP Identify duplicate facts among options.

13. A patient has anemia. Which vitamin should the nurse expect the primary health-care provider to prescribe?
    1. Ascorbic acid
    2. Riboflavin
    3. Folic acid
    4. Thiamin

    TEST-TAKING TIP Identify the key word in the stem that directs attention to content.

14. How should the nurse administer intralipids when a patient is receiving total parenteral nutrition (TPN) and intralipids?
    1. After the TPN infusion is completed
    2. Give the intralipids via an infusion pump
    3. Piggybacked into the proximal port of the TPN catheter
    4. Administer the intralipids through a separate intravenous line

    TEST-TAKING TIP Identify key words in the stem that direct attention to content. Identify opposites in options. Identify clang associations.

15. Which responses may occur if a patient's ordered flow rate of total parenteral nutrition (TPN) solution is administered faster than the ordered rate?
    1. Osmotic diuresis and hypoglycemia
    2. Hypoglycemia and dumping syndrome
    3. Electrolyte imbalance and osmotic diuresis
    4. Dumping syndrome and electrolyte imbalance

    TEST-TAKING TIP Identify duplicate facts among options.

16. A nurse is caring for a group of patients. Which group of patients has the **most** need for supplemental iron?
    1. Menstruating women
    2. School-age children
    3. Active adolescents
    4. Older men

    TEST-TAKING TIP Identify the word in the stem that sets a priority.

17. Which is the **most** important nutrient to provide patients to maintain life?
    1. Carbohydrates
    2. Vitamins
    3. Proteins
    4. Fluids

    TEST-TAKING TIP Identify the word in the stem that sets a priority.

18. Which group of individuals has the greatest need for calcium?
    1. Postmenopausal women
    2. School-age children
    3. Pregnant women
    4. Working men

    TEST-TAKING TIP Identify the word in the stem that sets a priority. Identify the key word in the stem that directs attention to content.

19. Which can the nurse expect the patient to do when urine output is less than fluid intake?
    1. Experience nausea
    2. Become jaundiced
    3. Void frequently
    4. Gain weight

20. A nurse is assessing a patient's pulse. Which should the nurse do if the patient's pulse is full and bounding?
    1. Check the flow rate of the patient's intravenous fluids.
    2. Measure the patient's urine specific gravity.
    3. Monitor the patient's serum glucose level.
    4. Lower the head of the patient's bed.

    TEST-TAKING TIP Identify key words in the stem that direct attention to content.

21. Iron supplements are ordered for a patient with the diagnosis of anemia. The nurse teaches the patient that the absorption of iron is facilitated by the ingestion of foods high in a particular vitamin. Which vitamin should the nurse include in this discussion?
    1. D
    2. C
    3. A
    4. K

    TEST-TAKING TIP Identify key words in the stem that direct attention to content.

22. A patient with lung cancer is concerned about having had a rapid weight loss and asks why this occurred. Which information should the nurse use as a basis for a response when answering this patient's question?
    1. Anabolism exceeds catabolism.
    2. Nutrients are unable to be absorbed.
    3. Cancer increases metabolic demands.
    4. Cell division causes an altered nitrogen balance.

    TEST-TAKING TIP Identify the clang association. Identify opposites in options.

23. Which patient statement indicates a misconception about vitamins?
    1. "My need for vitamins will change as I get older."
    2. "Some vitamins can be manufactured by the body."
    3. "I don't need vitamins because I eat a balanced diet."
    4. "Vitamins can be taken without the fear of toxic effects."

    TEST-TAKING TIP Identify the word in the stem that indicates negative polarity.

24. A patient who is receiving chemotherapy is nauseated. Which should the nurse include in the plan of care when addressing the nutritional needs of this patient? **Select all that apply.**
    1. ____ Encourage the avoidance of extremely hot or cold foods.
    2. ____ Serve the ordered diet in small quantities frequently.
    3. ____ Provide oral liquid supplements between meals.
    4. ____ Obtain an order for a full liquid diet.
    5. ____ Teach avoidance of fluids with meals.

25. A patient drinks 9 oz of milk with breakfast. How many milliliters of fluid should the nurse enter on the I&O record? **Record your answer using a whole number.**

    Answer: _____ mL

26. A nurse is caring for a patient with a vitamin K deficiency. For which responses should the nurse monitor the patient? **Select all that apply.**
1. ____ Anemia
2. ____ Muscle cramps
3. ____ Cardiac dysrhythmias
4. ____ Increased temperature
5. ____ Bleeding irregularities

TEST-TAKING TIP Identify key words in the stem that direct attention to content.

27. Intermittent tube feedings are ordered for a patient with a percutaneous endoscopic gastrostomy tube in place. Place the following steps in the order in which they should be performed.
1. Provide privacy.
2. Cleanse the hands.
3. Raise the head of the bed.
4. Collect all appropriate equipment.
5. Explain the procedure to the patient.
6. Verify the order (e.g., formula, amount, times to be administered).

Answer: _____

28. A nurse is feeding a patient with hemiparesis as the result of a brain attack. Which interventions by the nurse are important when feeding this patient? **Select all that apply.**
1. ____ Ensure that food is pureed.
2. ____ Provide foods that require chewing.
3. ____ Offer fluids with each mouthful of food.
4. ____ Elevate the head of the bed during the feeding.
5. ____ Allow time to empty the mouth of food between spoonfuls.

TEST-TAKING TIP Identify the key word in the stem that directs attention to content.

29. Based on the information on the patient's clinical record and the electrocardiogram, which should the nurse do **first**?
1. Initiate the rapid response team.
2. Discontinue the intravenous infusion.
3. Remove the milk from the patient's lunch tray.
4. Encourage the patient to use salt to season food on the lunch tray.

PATIENT'S CLINICAL RECORD

Nurse's Progress Note
1200: Patient receiving IV 1,000 mL of 0.9% sodium chloride with 40 mEq of KCl at 125 mL/hr. IV insertion site dry and intact with no signs or symptoms of infiltration or thrombophlebitis. Pulse: 70 beats/min, irregular; patient had two episodes of diarrhea and is irritable and slightly confused.

Electrocardiogram
T waves are narrow and peaked; ST-segment shows depression; QT interval is shortened.

Laboratory Findings
Serum sodium: 140 mEq/L
Serum potassium: 6.9 mEq/L
Total serum calcium: 9.0 mg/dL

30. A patient is experiencing diarrhea and needs to replace potassium. Which nutrients selected by the patient indicate that additional teaching is necessary regarding nutrients high in potassium? **Select all that apply.**
    1. ____ Beef bouillon
    2. ____ Orange juice
    3. ____ Poached egg
    4. ____ Warm tea
    5. ____ Bananas
    6. ____ Raisins

    TEST-TAKING TIP Identify the words in the stem that indicate negative polarity.

31. A patient is receiving a full-liquid diet. Which foods should the nurse remove from the patient's tray? **Select all that apply.**
    1. ____ Ice cream
    2. ____ Prune juice
    3. ____ Cream of wheat
    4. ____ Mashed potatoes
    5. ____ Raspberry gelatin

    TEST-TAKING TIP Identify the word in the stem that indicates negative polarity. Identify key words in the stem that directs attention to content.

32. A nurse is caring for a patient who is receiving chemotherapy that is nephrotoxic. The primary health-care provider orders 1000 mL of IV fluid in the immediate 4 hours before the infusion of the chemotherapeutic agent. At how many milliliters per hour should the nurse set the infusion pump? **Record your answer using a whole number.**

    Answer: _____ mL/hr

33. Which can the nurse expect to identify when a patient had a fluid intake of only 500 mL over 48 hours? **Select all that apply.**
    1. ____ Small amounts of urine at each voiding
    2. ____ Development of an atonic bladder
    3. ____ Decreased tissue turgor
    4. ____ Low specific gravity
    5. ____ Dark amber urine
    6. ____ Rapid pulse

34. After reviewing the patient's clinical record, which position should the nurse encourage the patient to assume when going to sleep?
    1. Left side-lying with head slightly elevated
    2. Prone with a small pillow under the abdomen
    3. Sims with the upper leg supported on a pillow
    4. Supine with a small pillow under the small of the back

PATIENT'S CLINICAL RECORD

Nurse's Progress Note
Reports frequent episodes of epigastric discomfort, slight difficulty swallowing, and excessive salivation. States the presence of a persistent cough, sore throat, and hoarseness.

Vital Signs Flow Sheet
Temp: 99°F, oral route
Pulse: 84 beats/min, regular
Respirations: 18 breaths/min, unlabored

Primary Health-Care Provider's Orders
Dietitian consultation
Esomeprazole 20 mg PO once daily
Magnesium/aluminum hydroxide 20 mL PO, four times a day between meals and at bedtime

35. When assessing a patient for the extent of edema, the nurse depresses the edematous area as indicated in the illustration. Place an X in front of the information that should be documented in the patient's progress notes when using the 4-point scale for grading edema.
    1. ____ Barely detectable
    2. ____ 1+
    3. ____ 2+
    4. ____ 3+
    5. ____ 4+

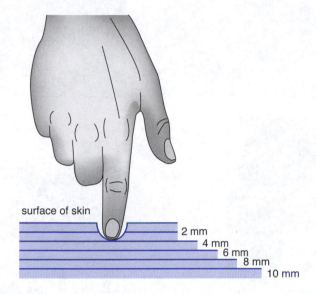

surface of skin
2 mm
4 mm
6 mm
8 mm
10 mm

TEST-TAKING TIP Identify the key word in the stem that directs attention to content.

36. A patient on a telemetry unit reports muscle weakness and extreme fatigue. The patient's ECG tracing is below. Which additional patient response should the nurse assess for that can be clustered with the results of the ECG tracing?
    1. Thirst
    2. Tremors
    3. Weak, rapid pulse
    4. Severe constipation

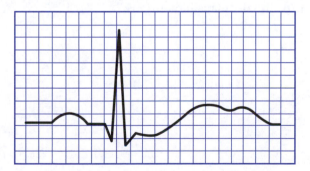

37. A nurse is working in a nursing home with a large population of older adults. Which factors related to aging influence the nutritional status of older adults that the nurse should consider? **Select all that apply.**
    1. ____ Additional need for milk products
    2. ____ Increased need for kilocalories
    3. ____ Decreased saliva production
    4. ____ Reduced sense of smell
    5. ____ Atrophy of taste buds

TEST-TAKING TIP Identify key words in the stem that direct attention to content.

38. Which photograph illustrates a technique that will elicit information about a patient's hydration status?

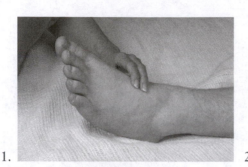

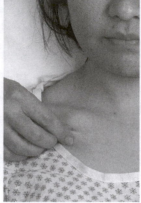

1.

2.

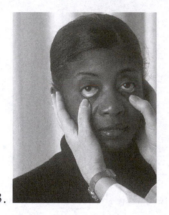

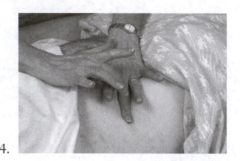

3.

4.

39. An order is written to keep a patient NPO. Which are the important actions by the nurse? **Select all that apply.**

1. _____ Allow the patient to sip clear fluids with medication.
2. _____ Remove the water pitcher from the patient's bedside.
3. _____ Give the patient mouth care every four hours.
4. _____ Measure the patient's intake and output.
5. _____ Permit the patient to suck on ice chips.

TEST-TAKING TIP Identify the key word in the stem that directs attention to content. Identify equally plausible options.

40. A nurse is caring for a patient who has a history of gastroesophageal reflux and
reports burning pain in the epigastric region after eating spicy food brought to the
hospital by a relative. Place an X on the location that the nurse expects the patient to
identify as the site of the pain.

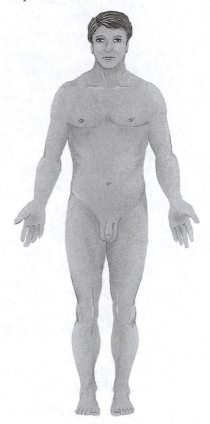

1. **TEST-TAKING TIP** The word "least" in the stem indicates negative polarity. Option 2 is the unique option; it is the only option that tells the patient to avoid something. The other options are positive statements.

   1. Identifying low-calorie snacks helps reduce caloric intake.
   2. **The patient is receiving a special diet that is carefully calculated, and all food on the tray should be eaten.**
   3. Encouraging the patient to eat meals slowly makes a meal take longer to eat and allows more time for the body to feel full.
   4. Progress should be identified to provide motivation.

2. 1. A urometer is used to measure the specific gravity of urine, not the volume of urine.
   2. **A graduate is a special container with volume markings on the side for measuring fluid; of all the options offered, it is the most accurate way to measure urine.**
   3. Bedpans are designed to collect excreta when a person cannot use a toilet or commode, not to measure urine volume.
   4. Using the markings on a urine collection bag is not accurate because the plastic that the bag is made of often stretches.

3. **TEST-TAKING TIP** The word "highest" in the stem sets a priority.

   1. **During the first year of life, the infant grows at a faster pace than at any other developmental stage; infants double their birth weight by 6 months and triple their birth weight during the first year.**
   2. The preschool (3- to 5-year-old) child's growth rate is slower than the age identified in another option. The preschool child gains only another 7 to 12 pounds in addition to the four times the birth weight gained during the first 3 years.
   3. Although the adolescent goes through a dramatic physical growth spurt that reflects significant changes in height, weight, dentition, and skeletal and sexual development, it is not as spectacular as the growth rate reflected in another option.
   4. No physical growth occurs when a person is older than 65 years of age; different

   parts of the body begin to degenerate and function slowly.

4. **TEST-TAKING TIP** The word "always" in option 2 is a specific determiner. Options 1 and 3 deny patient feelings, concerns, or needs. The patient has a right to ingest foods of different temperatures. The word "avoid" in the stem does not indicate negative polarity. The question is asking what the nurse "should do" to prevent trauma to the mouth.

   1. Patients have a right to a variety of foods, textures, and temperatures within the ordered diet.
   2. Touching the patient's food will contaminate the food.
   3. Foods should not be mixed; they should be served separately so that they retain their own flavor, texture, and temperature.
   4. **Waiting for hot foods to cool slightly is the safest and most practical action; food should be warm, rather than hot, to be safe to eat.**

5. **TEST-TAKING TIP** The word "most" in the stem sets a priority.

   1. Feeding the patient when only supervision is necessary contributes to feelings of dependence.
   2. **Supervision best keeps the patient focused on the task of eating while supporting independence.**
   3. Although this is something the nurse may do to orient the patient, the patient may forget or not understand the explanation.
   4. Although family members can be helpful, it is the responsibility of the staff, not the family members, to care for the patient.

6. **TEST-TAKING TIP** The word "best" in the stem sets a priority.

   1. White meat contains less fat than red meat but more fat than another option.
   2. Whole milk contains fat, which contributes to plaque formation in atherosclerosis.
   3. **Legumes, such as beans, peas, and lentils, contain the least amount of cholesterol and fat of the options presented and are high in protein, which is necessary for tissue regeneration.**
   4. Although shrimp is a protein source, it is high in cholesterol, which should be avoided because it contributes to plaque formation.

7. **TEST-TAKING TIP** The word "most" in the stem sets a priority. The words "loss" and "draining" are key words in the stem that direct attention to content.

   1. Although fluid is lost from a draining pressure ulcer, it does not have the most serious implication.
   2. Weight loss is related to inadequate caloric intake, not the presence of a draining pressure ulcer.
   3. **A patient can lose as much as 50 g of protein daily from a draining pressure ulcer; this is a large percentage of the usual daily requirement of 60 g of protein for women and 70 g of protein for men. Patients with draining pressure ulcers should ingest two to four times the usual daily requirements of protein to rebuild epidermal tissue.**
   4. If a pressure ulcer is infected, the leukocyte count increases, not decreases.

8. **TEST-TAKING TIP** The words "all" and "low-calorie diet" are key words in the stem that direct attention to content. Options 3 and 4 are equally plausible because decreased energy levels are often associated with a decrease in the metabolic rate.

   1. **When the number of calories ingested does not meet the body's energy requirements, the patient catabolizes body fat for energy and loses weight.**
   2. A well-balanced low-calorie diet should contain adequate vitamins, requiring no supplementation.
   3. Metabolism increases and decreases in response to the energy demands placed on the body, not as a result of a low-calorie diet.
   4. Age, body size, body and environmental temperatures, growth, gender, nutritional state, and emotional state affect energy levels.

9. 1. A thready pulse occurs with dehydration and hemorrhage. Dehydration occurs when fluid, not caloric, intake is insufficient.
   2. **When calories are insufficient to meet metabolic needs, the body catabolizes fat, resulting in weight loss.**
   3. Dependent edema occurs with decreased cardiac output.
   4. Sleeping is not related directly to a decreased caloric intake; however, a patient who is anemic may tire easily from an inadequate intake of iron or folic acid.

10. **TEST-TAKING TIP** The word "immediately" in the stem sets a priority.

    1. **Nursing care should be documented immediately after it is provided. There are 30 mL in each ounce; therefore, the patient ingested 240 mL.**
    2. Assessing skin turgor immediately after a patient drinks 8 ounces of fluid is too early to evaluate the patient's response to fluid intake.
    3. Offering a bedpan immediately after a patient drinks 8 ounces of fluids is too early to expect the patient to void.
    4. Mouth care usually is not required after drinking fluid; mouth care should be provided routinely on awakening, after meals, and at bedtime.

11. **TEST-TAKING TIP** The words "low-sodium" are the key words in the stem that direct attention to content.

    1. Whole milk, depending on the brand, has approximately 130 mg of sodium per 8 oz.
    2. **Fresh fruits contain the least amount of sodium per serving of the options presented; most fresh fruits such as apples, pears, bananas, peaches, and cantaloupe contain less than 10 mg of sodium per serving.**
    3. White bread, depending on the brand, has 55 to 225 mg of sodium per slice.
    4. Fresh vegetables, such as peas, beans, carrots, broccoli, cauliflower, corn, and celery, contain approximately 40 mg of sodium per serving.

12. **TEST-TAKING TIP** Four different foods that contribute to healing are offered. If you can identify one food that most contributes to healing (eggs or orange juice), you can narrow the correct answer to two options. If you can identify one food that is least beneficial to the healing process (oatmeal or French toast), you can narrow the correct answer to two options.

    1. Although French toast contains some egg coating, which has protein, it does not contain the amount of protein in another option. Oatmeal does not contain protein or vitamin C.
    2. Although orange juice contains vitamin C, which contributes to wound healing, oatmeal does not contain protein or vitamin C.
    3. Each poached egg contains 6 to 8 g of protein; protein contains the amino acids necessary for building cells and therefore for wound healing. Although French toast

contains some egg coating, which has protein, it does not contain vitamin C.

4. **This is the best combination of foods in the options offered. Each egg contains 6 to 8 g of protein; protein contains the amino acids necessary for building cells and therefore for wound healing. Orange juice contains vitamin C, which promotes collagen formation, enhances iron absorption, and maintains capillary wall integrity.**

13. **TEST-TAKING TIP** The word "anemia" is the key word in the stem that directs attention to content.

1. Ascorbic acid (vitamin C) is not used to treat anemia. Ascorbic acid promotes collagen formation, enhances iron absorption, and maintains capillary wall integrity.
2. Riboflavin (vitamin B_2) is not used to treat anemia. Riboflavin functions as a coenzyme in the metabolism of carbohydrates, fats, amino acids, and alcohol.
3. **Folic acid (vitamin B_9, folate) promotes the maturation of red blood cells. When red blood cells decrease below the expected range of 4.2 million/mm³ for women and 4.7 million/mm³ for men, a person is considered anemic.**
4. Thiamin (vitamin B_1) is not used to treat anemia. Thiamin performs as a coenzyme in the metabolism of carbohydrates, fats, amino acids, and alcohol.

14. **TEST-TAKING TIP** The words "intralipids" and "total parenteral nutrition (TPN)" are key words in the stem that direct attention to content. Options 3 and 4 are opposites. The word "intralipids" in the stem and the word "intralipids" in options 2 and 4 are clang associations. Although "TPN" in the stem and in options 1 and 3 are clang associations, they are distractors because this question is asking about intralipids. Examine options 2 and 4 carefully. Option 4 is the correct answer.

1. The solutions can be run at the same time but through different lines.
2. Because an intralipid solution is a concentrated source of nonprotein kilocalories, it is desirable for an infusion pump to be used; however, an infusion pump does not have to be used because the solution can flow via gravity.
3. If an intralipid solution is mixed with a dextrose/amino acid solution, the fat emulsion breaks down; the solutions must not be administered through the same line.
4. **Administering intralipids through a separate intravenous line ensures that the intralipid solution is NOT mixed with a dextrose/amino acid solution. If they are mixed, the fat emulsion breaks down.**

15. **TEST-TAKING TIP** Four clinical findings are offered as undesirable results associated with an increase in the flow rate of TPN above the ordered rate: osmotic diuresis, hypoglycemia, dumping syndrome, and electrolyte imbalance. If you are able to identify one response that is unrelated to an increased TPN rate, you can eliminate two distractors. If you are able to identify one response that is related to an increase in a TPN rate above the ordered rate, you can narrow the correct answer to two options.

1. Although osmotic diuresis does occur, hyperglycemia, not hypoglycemia, may result.
2. Hyperglycemia, not hypoglycemia, may result. Dumping syndrome, the rapid entry of food from the stomach into the jejunum, can occur with an intermittent tube feeding, not TPN.
3. **The hypertonic TPN solution pulls intracellular and interstitial fluid into the intravascular compartment; the increased blood volume increases circulation to the kidneys, raising urinary output (osmotic diuresis). Potassium and sodium imbalances are common among patients receiving TPN. Therefore, TPN rates must be carefully controlled.**
4. Potassium and sodium imbalances are common among patients receiving TPN. However, dumping syndrome can occur with an intermittent tube feeding, not TPN.

16. **TEST-TAKING TIP** The word "most" in the stem sets a priority.

1. **Iron is essential to the formation of hemoglobin, a component of red blood cells, which is lost in menstrual blood.**
2. Supplemental iron is unnecessary in growing children (1 to 13 years). However, infants (birth to 1 year) who are breast-fed need some iron supplementation from 4 to 12 months of age, and formula-fed

infants need iron supplementation throughout the first year of life.

3. Supplemental iron is unnecessary for active adolescents.

4. Supplemental iron is unnecessary for healthy older men.

17. **TEST-TAKING TIP** The word "most" in the stem sets a priority.

1. Although carbohydrates are important, the body can survive longer without this nutrient than it can without the nutrient in the correct answer.

2. Although vitamins are important, the body can survive longer without this nutrient than it can without the nutrient in the correct answer.

3. Although proteins are important, the body can survive longer without this nutrient than it can without the nutrient in the correct answer.

4. **The most basic nutrient needed is water because all body processes require an adequate fluid balance in the body.**

18. **TEST-TAKING TIP** The word "greatest" in the stem sets a priority. The word "calcium" is the key word in the stem that directs attention to content.

1. Although postmenopausal women can benefit from an increase in calcium to prevent osteoporosis, the need is not as high as the group of individuals in the correct answer.

2. School-age children do not have the highest need for calcium. An adequate intake of milk and dairy products meets minimum daily requirements of calcium for school-age children.

3. **Calcium should be increased 50% to an intake of 1.2 gram per day to provide calcium for fetal tooth and bone development; this is essential during the third trimester when fetal bones are mineralized.**

4. Working men do not have the highest need for calcium. An adequate intake of milk and dairy products meets minimum daily requirements of calcium for working men.

19. 1. Nausea is not a common symptom of fluid volume excess.

2. Jaundice is related to impaired liver and biliary function, not fluid volume excess.

3. The opposite is true; the patient will void infrequently.

4. **Fluid weighs 1 kg (2.2 lb) per liter. A patient can gain 6 to 8 pounds before edema can be identified through inspection.**

20. **TEST-TAKING TIP** The phrase "full and bounding" are key words in the stem that direct attention to content.

1. **Intravenous solutions are administered directly into the intravascular compartment; if the intravenous flow rate is excessive, it will cause a full, bounding pulse related to hypervolemia.**

2. The specific gravity of urine reflects the concentrating ability of the kidneys, not the cardiovascular system.

3. A full, bounding pulse is not related to hyperglycemia or hypoglycemia; a weak, thready pulse is a late sign of diabetic ketoacidosis.

4. A full, bounding pulse may indicate hypervolemia; in this compromised patient, lowering the head of the bed may impede respirations and is therefore contraindicated.

21. **TEST-TAKING TIP** The words "absorption of iron is facilitated by" are key words in the stem that direct attention to content.

1. Vitamin D is essential for adequate absorption and utilization of calcium in bone and tooth growth; it does not facilitate the absorption of iron.

2. **Ascorbic acid (vitamin C) helps to change dietary iron to a form that can be absorbed by the body.**

3. Vitamin A is essential for the growth and maintenance of epithelial tissue, maintenance of night vision, and promotion of resistance to infection.

4. Vitamin K is essential for the formation of prothrombin, which prevents bleeding.

22. **TEST-TAKING TIP** The word "cancer" in both the stem and option 3 is a clang association. Options 1 and 3 are obscure opposites.

1. With cancer, catabolism exceeds anabolism.

2. The ability to utilize nutrients is not impaired with cancer.

3. **The energy required to support the rapid growth of cancerous cells increases the metabolic demands 1.5 to 2 times the resting energy expenditure.**

4. The by-products of cell breakdown cause a negative nitrogen balance.

23. **TEST-TAKING TIP** The word "misconception" in the stem indicates negative polarity. This question is asking, "Which option contains inaccurate information?"
    1. The National Academy of Sciences, National Academy Press, Washington, DC, publishes the Recommended Dietary Allowance (RDA) of vitamins. The list reflects age, gender, and physical status differences.
    2. Vitamin D can be synthesized by the body. In addition to dietary intake, vitamin D is manufactured in the skin.
    3. Ordinarily, healthy persons who eat a variety of foods that reflect a balanced diet should not need vitamin supplements.
    4. **This is an inaccurate statement. Megadoses of vitamins can cause hypervitaminosis and result in toxicity.**

24. **TEST-TAKING TIP** The word "all" in option 2 is a specific determiner. Options 1 and 2 are opposites. The word "nausea" in the stem and the words "nauseated" in option 1 and the word "nausea" in option 2 are clang associations. Examine options 1 and 2 carefully. Option 1 is the correct answer.
    1. **X Extremely hot or cold foods can precipitate nausea.**
    2. **X Small quantities of food frequently offered establish small, realistic goals for the patient without being overwhelming.**
    3. ____ Supplements may interfere with the intake of regularly scheduled meals.
    4. ____ A full-liquid diet does not reduce nausea and it does not meet nutritional needs.
    5. **X Fluids with meals can excessively fill the stomach, which can precipitate nausea.**

25. **Answer: 270 mL**
    One ounce is equal to 30 mL; therefore, 9 ounces × 30 mL = 270 mL.

26. **TEST-TAKING TIP** The words "vitamin K deficiency" are key words in the stem that direct attention to content.
    1. **X Anemia is caused by bleeding that can occur with vitamin K deficiency.**
    2. ____ Vitamin K deficiency is unrelated to muscle cramps. Calcium contributes to neuromuscular excitability, and therefore lowered calcium levels can result in muscle cramps and tetany.

    3. ____ Vitamin K deficiency is unrelated to cardiac dysrhythmias. A deficiency of vitamin B_1 (thiamin) can result in tachycardia and cardiac enlargement; deficiencies in calcium, magnesium, and potassium can also contribute to cardiac problems.
    4. ____ A deficiency in vitamin K does not contribute to the occurrence of infection, which will cause an increase in temperature. Vitamins A and C help build resistance to infection.
    5. **X Vitamin K is essential for prothrombin formation and blood clotting; if a patient is deficient in vitamin K, the patient experiences a prolonged clotting time and is prone to bleeding.**

27. **Answer: 6, 5, 2, 4, 1, 3**
    6. Administering a tube feeding is a dependent function of the nurse. The primary health-care provider's order must be verified.
    5. Explaining the procedure to the patient should be done before equipment is brought to the bedside. Bringing equipment to the bedside without a prior explanation may cause anxiety.
    2. Hand hygiene (e.g., washing with soap and water or using an alcohol-based gel) removes microorganisms from the nurse's skin that may contaminate clean equipment.
    4. Collecting all equipment at the same time prevents the need to interrupt the procedure to collect forgotten equipment.
    1. Providing privacy (e.g., pulling the curtain, closing the door) should be done to maintain patient confidentiality and emotional comfort. A tube feeding is an invasive procedure.
    3. Raising the head of the bed helps to keep the formula in the stomach via gravity; it limits the risks of formula passing into the esophagus and aspiration.

28. **TEST-TAKING TIP** The word "hemiparesis" is the key word in the stem that directs attention to content.
    1. ____ Pureed food may not be necessary; the patient may only need more time to thoroughly manage the food.
    2. ____ This may be unsafe and possibly unreasonable because the patient has a reduced ability to move the muscles on

one side of the face necessary for chewing. A mechanical soft diet may be necessary.

3. ____ Fluids with each mouthful will increase the risk of aspiration; fluid is more difficult to control than food when swallowing.

4. **X Elevating the head of the bed reduces the risk of aspiration.**

5. **X Allowing time to empty the mouth of food between spoonfuls minimizes food buildup in the mouth; also it does not rush the patient.**

29. 1. **The electrocardiogram tracing and patient responses indicate a medication-induced hyperkalemia, which can cause a life-threatening cardiac dysrhythmia. The patient's electrocardiogram and the patient's responses (irregular pulse, diarrhea, irritability and confusion) are signs of hyperkalemia and indicate an emergency. Initiating the rapid response team is the priority.**

2. If the nurse discontinues the IV infusion, intravenous access will not be available for emergency intravenous medications. The second action of the nurse is to replace the IV bag that is hanging with 0.9% sodium chloride after initiating the first action, which has priority.

3. Removing milk from the patient's lunch tray is unnecessary. The patient's total serum calcium level is within the expected range of 8.5 to 10.5 mg/dL.

4. Encouraging the patient to use salt to season food on the lunch tray is unnecessary. The patient's serum sodium level is within the expected range of 135 to 145 mEq/L.

30. **TEST-TAKING TIP** The words "additional teaching is necessary" in the stem indicate negative polarity. This question is asking, "Which food or drink contains the least amount of potassium?"

1. **X One cup (one package) of beef bouillon contains approximately 27 mg of potassium and is not a good choice because it is low in potassium.**

2. ____ One cup of orange juice is a good choice because it contains approximately 475 mg of potassium.

3. **X A poached egg contains approximately 65 mg of potassium and is not a good choice because it is low in potassium.**

4. **X One cup of tea contains approximately 35 mg of potassium and is not a good choice because it is low in potassium.**

5. ____ One banana is a good choice because it contains approximately 450 mg of potassium.

6. ____ One ounce (1/8 cup) of raisins is a good choice because it contains approximately 200 mg of potassium.

31. **TEST-TAKING TIP** The word "remove" in the stem indicates negative polarity. This question is asking, "Which food is *not* permitted on a full-liquid diet?" The words "full-liquid diet" are key words in the stem that direct attention to content.

1. ____ Ice cream changes its state from a solid to a liquid at room temperature.

2. ____ Prune juice is a fluid and is permitted on a full-liquid diet.

3. **X Cream of wheat is considered solid food and is not permitted on a full-liquid diet.**

4. **X Mashed potatoes are considered solid food and are not permitted on a full-liquid diet.**

5. ____ Raspberry gelatin changes its state from a solid to a liquid at room temperature.

32. **Answer: 250 mL/hr**
Infusion pumps are set at milliliters per hour.
1000 mL ÷ 4 hours = 250 mL/hr.

33. 1. ____ The bladder still fills to the patient's usual capacity before there is a perceived need to void.

2. ____ An atonic bladder is caused by a neurological problem; it is a loss of the sensation of fullness that leads to distention from overfilling.

3. **X As fluid in the intravascular compartment decreases, fluid is pulled from the intracellular and interstitial compartments in an attempt to maintain cardiac output.**

4. ____ Reduced fluid intake produces a concentrated urine with a specific gravity more than 1.030. The expected range for urine specific gravity is 1.001 to 1.029.

5. **X Dark amber is the color of urine when fluid intake is less than 1500 to 2000 mL/day; the urine is concentrated.**

6. **X The heart rate increases when hypovolemia occurs in an attempt to increase cardiac output.**

34. 1. The patient is receiving esomeprazole (Nexium) and magnesium/aluminum hydroxide (Mylanta) for upper gastrointestinal issues. The patient's responses indicate gastroesophageal reflux disease. The respiratory responses are most likely because of respiratory aspiration of gastric contents causing irritation and inflammation and the resulting cough, sore throat, and hoarseness. A left side-lying position with the head slightly elevated uses gravity to keep gastric contents in the stomach as well as facilitate esophageal emptying along the normal left to right anatomical curve into the stomach. In a home, the head of the bed can be raised on 4- to 6-inch blocks. Gravity helps to keep gastric contents in the stomach when sleeping.

2. The patient's responses indicate gastroesophageal reflux disease. The prone position increases intra-abdominal pressure, which will increase the risk of gastroesophageal reflux and aspiration of gastric contents.

3. The patient's responses indicate gastroesophageal reflux disease. The Sims position will increase intra-abdominal pressure, which will increase the risk of gastroesophageal reflux and aspiration of gastric contents.

4. The patient's responses indicate gastroesophageal reflux disease. The supine position allows gastric contents to reflux easily into the esophagus and pharynx, placing the patient at risk for aspiration.

35. TEST-TAKING TIP The word "edema" is the key word in the stem that directs attention to content.

1. ____ Barely detectable: Barely detectable and 1+ edema are synonymous and are characterized by a 2 mm or less depression when edematous tissue is compressed.

2. ____ 1+ edema: 1+ and barely detectable are synonymous.

3. X 2+ edema: 2+ edema is characterized by a 2- to 4-mm depression when compressing edematous tissue.

4. ____ 3+ edema: 3+ edema is characterized by a 5- to 10-mm depression when compressing edematous tissue depending on the reference source. Some sources say 5 to 10 mm and some say 6 to 8 mm.

5. ____ 4 + edema: 4 + edema is characterized by more than an 8- or 10-mm depression when compressing edematous tissue depending on the reference source. Some sources say more than 8 mm and some say more than 10 mm.

36. 1. Thirst is associated with hypernatremia, which is not this patient's clinical situation as indicated by the ECG tracing. In addition, hypernatremia is indicated by an elevated temperature, tachycardia, elevated blood pressure, nausea and vomiting, increased reflexes, restlessness, and seizures.

2. Tremors are associated with hyponatremia, which is not this patient's clinical situation as indicated by the ECG tracing. In addition, hyponatremia is indicated by anorexia, nausea, vomiting, headache, lethargy, nonelastic skin turgor, and confusion, and seizures as a result of an increase in intracranial pressure.

3. A weak, rapid pulse is associated with hypokalemia, which is confirmed by the ECG tracing; with hypokalemia there is ST-segment depression, a flattened T wave, and the presence of a U wave. In addition to the characteristic ECG tracing, a weak, rapid pulse, muscle weakness, and fatigue, a patient with hypokalemia may experience nausea and vomiting, decreased gastrointestinal motility, decreased reflexes, abdominal distention, and dysrhythmias.

4. Severe constipation is associated with hypercalcemia, which is not this patient's clinical situation as indicated by the ECG tracing. In addition hypercalcemia is indicated by deep bone pain, flank pain from renal calculi, vomiting, decreased reflexes, increased urine calcium, osteoporosis, increased hyperparathyroid hormone (PTH) levels, and decreased PTH levels with malignancy.

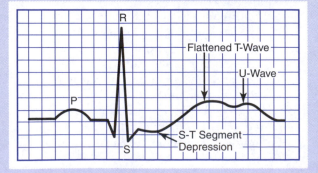

37. **TEST-TAKING TIP The words "aging" and "nutritional status" are key words in the stem that direct attention to content.**

   1. ____ The daily recommended need for dairy intake according to the MyPlate diet for healthy individuals is 3 cups from 9 years of age to 51+ years of age. It also recommends that fat-free or 1% milk be substituted for whole milk. An increase in dairy products may be needed by older adults who are at risk for osteoporosis.

   2. ____ The need for kilocalories decreases because of a lower metabolic rate and reduction in physical activity associated with older adults.

   3. **X Saliva production decreases by approximately 66% when one ages. Salivary ptyalin decreases, interfering with the breakdown of starches.**

   4. **X Practically all body systems decline slightly with aging, including the senses. The sense of smell is interrelated to the sense of taste.**

   5. **X Taste perception decreases because of atrophy of the taste buds; sweet and salty tastes are lost first.**

38. 1. In this photograph the nurse is palpating the patient's dorsalis pedis pulse. This assessment provides information about the patient's distal arterial circulation.

   2. **In this photograph the nurse is testing the patient's skin turgor. The nurse gently pinches the patient's skin and assesses how long it takes to return to its pre-pinched state. If it takes more than several seconds to return to its pre-pinched state (tenting), it indicates that the patient may be dehydrated.**

   3. In this photograph the nurse is assessing the patient's conjunctiva for a blue discoloration (cyanosis – blue discoloration from excessive deoxyhemoglobin in the blood) or yellow discoloration (jaundice—yellow discoloration from deposition of bile pigments). Normally the conjunctiva should be pink.

   4. In this photograph the nurse is performing indirect palpation. This technique elicits a sound when one of the nurse's fingers strikes another finger positioned over a site. The sound elicited may indicate that air, fluid, or solid tissue is under the area that is being tapped.

39. **TEST-TAKING TIP "NPO" is the key word in the stem that directs attention to content. Options 1 and 5 are equally** plausible. Both are either correct answers or incorrect answers.

   1. ____ Fluids of any kind are contraindicated when a patient is NPO; NPO means *non per os*, which means "nothing by mouth."

   2. **X Removing the water pitcher from the patient's bedside prevents the patient from accidently drinking fluid.**

   3. **X When people are NPO, they tend to have dry mucous membranes and thick secretions on the tongue and gums; mouth care cleans the oral cavity.**

   4. **X A patient who is NPO generally is receiving intravenous fluids. The intake and output should be measured when a patient is NPO to ensure that the patient is receiving adequate fluid intake via the intravenous route and is in fluid balance.**

   5. ____ Ice chips are considered fluids; fluids of any kind are contraindicated when a patient is NPO. NPO *(non per os)* means "nothing by mouth."

40. **The epigastric region is over the stomach, liver, pancreas, and right and left kidneys. A patient who has burning pain indicative of gastroesophageal reflux generally will point to the epigastric region as the site of the pain, indicated by the X.**

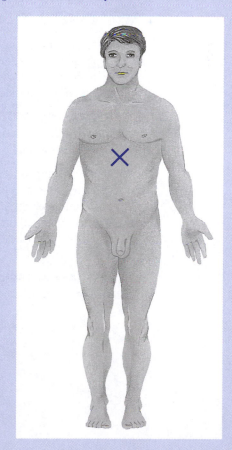

MEETING PATIENTS' ELIMINATION NEEDS

This section includes questions related to bowel and bladder needs. Topics associated with intestinal elimination include incontinence, constipation, diarrhea, enemas, bowel retraining, and medications. Questions also focus on patient needs associated with urinary elimination and include topics such as incontinence, bladder retraining, toileting, and external and indwelling urinary catheters.

QUESTIONS

1. A patient reports being constipated. Which should the nurse encourage the patient to eat?
   1. Fresh fruit and whole-wheat bread
   2. Whole-wheat bread and chicken
   3. Plain yogurt and fresh fruit
   4. Chicken and plain yogurt

   TEST-TAKING TIP Identify the key word in the stem that directs attention to content. Identify duplicate facts among options.

2. A patient scheduled for bowel surgery asks the nurse why a tap-water enema was ordered. Which information is important for the nurse to include in a response to the patient's question?
   1. Minimizes intestinal gas
   2. Cleanses the bowel of stool
   3. Reduces abdominal distention
   4. Decreases the loss of electrolytes

   TEST-TAKING TIP Identify the key word in the stem that directs attention to content. Identify equally plausible options. Identify the clang association.

3. A confused patient asks to use the bathroom even though the patient was toileted only 30 minutes earlier. Which should the nurse do?
   1. Explain that this is unnecessary because of the patient's recent trip to the bathroom.
   2. Request an order for an indwelling urinary catheter for the patient.
   3. Persuade the patient to try to hold it for at least an hour.
   4. Assist the patient to the bathroom.

   TEST-TAKING TIP Identify options that deny patient feelings, concerns, or needs. Identify the patient-centered option. Identify clang associations. Identify opposites in options.

4. A 750-mL tap-water enema is ordered for a patient. Which should the nurse do to **best** promote acceptance of the volume ordered?
   1. Administer the fluid slowly, and have the patient take shallow breaths.
   2. Place the patient in the left lateral position, and slowly administer the fluid.
   3. Have the patient take shallow breaths, and keep the fluid at body temperature.
   4. Keep the fluid at body temperature, and place the patient in the left lateral position.

   TEST-TAKING TIP Identify the word in the stem that sets a priority. Identify duplicate facts among options.

5. A nurse collected information from several patients. Which information indicates the patient who has the highest risk for developing diarrhea?
   1. Is physically active
   2. Drinks a lot of fluid
   3. Eats whole-grain cereal
   4. Is experiencing emotional problems

   TEST-TAKING TIP Identify the word in the stem that sets a priority. Identify the unique option.

6. A nurse is caring for a debilitated patient who is constipated and unable to tolerate a large volume of enema solution. Which solution should the nurse anticipate that the primary health-care provider will order?
   1. Hypertonic fluid
   2. Normal saline
   3. Soapy water
   4. Tap water

   TEST-TAKING TIP Identify the key word in the stem that directs attention to content.

7. In which position should a nurse place a patient when administering an enema?
   1. Dorsal recumbent
   2. Right lateral
   3. Back lying
   4. Left Sims

   TEST-TAKING TIP Identify equally plausible options. Identify opposites in options.

8. A patient has a loose, watery stool in the morning. What question should the nurse ask the patient to determine if the patient has diarrhea?
   1. "What did you have for dinner last night?"
   2. "Are you experiencing abdominal cramping?"
   3. "Have you been drinking a lot of fluid lately?"
   4. "When was the last time you had a similar stool?"

   TEST-TAKING TIP Identify the obscure clang association.

9. A patient has a full body cast and is experiencing diarrhea. Which potential patient response is a primary concern associated with this situation?
   1. Pressure ulcers
   2. Wound infection
   3. Urinary incontinence
   4. Hip flexion contracture

   TEST-TAKING TIP Identify the word in the stem that sets a priority.

10. A nurse is caring for a patient diagnosed with stress incontinence. Which is the common underlying cause of stress incontinence that the nurse needs to consider when caring for this patient?
    1. Response to a specific volume of urine in the bladder
    2. Results from an increase in intra-abdominal pressure
    3. Results from a urinary tract infection
    4. Response to an emotional strain

11. A rectal tube is ordered for a postoperative patient. Which is the main purpose for the tube that the nurse should discuss with the patient before inserting the tube?
1. Administer an enema
2. Dilate the anal sphincters
3. Relieve abdominal distention
4. Visualize the intestinal mucosa

TEST-TAKING TIP Identify the word in the stem that sets a priority. Identify key words in the stem that direct attention to content.

12. Which aspect of urine should the nurse evaluate when assessing the patency of a urinary retention (Foley) catheter?
1. Color
2. Clarity
3. Volume
4. Constituents

TEST-TAKING TIP Identify the unique option.

13. Which is the **most** common concern of patients who have a colostomy that the nurse should anticipate?
1. Maintenance of skin integrity
2. Frequency of defecation
3. Consistency of feces
4. Presence of odor

TEST-TAKING TIP Identify the word in the stem that sets a priority. Identify the unique option.

14. A nurse observes that a newborn's urine is very light yellow. Which factor related to newborns supports the nurse's conclusion that this observation is expected?
1. Ingest only fluids
2. Cannot control urination
3. Are unable to concentrate urine
4. Always void more frequently than adults

TEST-TAKING TIP Identify key words in the stem that direct attention to content. Identify options with specific determiners. Identify clang associations.

15. A culture and sensitivity test of a patient's urine is ordered. Which should the nurse do to ensure accurate results of a urine culture and sensitivity test?
1. Obtain two urine specimens.
2. Collect a midstream urine sample.
3. Use only the first voiding of the day.
4. Use a twenty-four-hour urine collection.

TEST-TAKING TIP Identify key words in the stem that direct attention to content. Identify clang associations. Identify the option with a specific determiner.

16. A nurse is assessing a patient for the presence of dysuria. Which question should the nurse ask the patient?
1. "Does pain or burning occur when you urinate?"
2. "Can you start and stop the flow of urine with ease?"
3. "Do you pass a little urine when you cough or sneeze?"
4. "Are you able to empty your bladder fully each time you void?"

17. A patient is admitted with a diagnosis of upper gastrointestinal bleeding. Which should the nurse expect the color of this patient's stool to be?
    1. Red
    2. Pink
    3. Black
    4. Brown

18. A nurse is caring for a female patient who has to go home with an indwelling urinary catheter (Foley catheter). Which should the nurse teach the patient about the urine collection system? **Select all that apply.**
    1. ____ Prevent dependent loops in the tubing.
    2. ____ Keep it below the level of the pelvis.
    3. ____ Carry it at waist level when walking.
    4. ____ Secure the tubing to the thigh.
    5. ____ Change it at least once a week.
    6. ____ Clamp it when out of bed.

19. A nurse is applying a condom catheter (external catheter) after perineal care for an uncircumcised patient. Which should the nurse do? **Select all that apply.**
    1. ____ Lubricate around the glans.
    2. ____ Replace the foreskin over the glans.
    3. ____ Secure the condom directly behind the glans.
    4. ____ Retract the foreskin behind the head of the glans.
    5. ____ Leave an inch space between the condom sheath and the tip of the glans.

    TEST-TAKING TIP Identify key words in the stem that direct attention to content. Identify opposites in options.

20. A nurse is caring for a patient who has an order for insertion of a catheter for continuous bladder irrigation. Identify the catheter that should be inserted by the nurse.

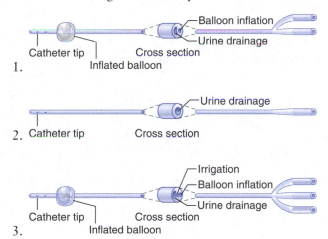

1.

2.

3.

21. A urinary retention catheter is ordered for a female patient. Place an arrow pointing to the area where a urinary retention catheter should be inserted.

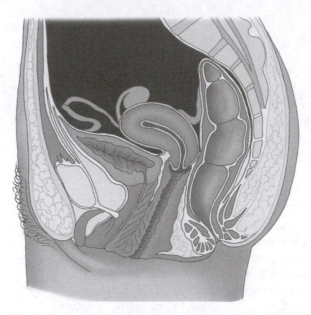

22. A primary health-care provider prescribes 500 mg of an antibiotic to be administered by the intravenous piggyback (IVPB) method to a patient with urosepsis. The label on a 1-gram vial of the medication states, "Add 2.7 mL of sterile water to yield 3 mL." How much solution should the nurse add to the 50-mL bag of sterile water when preparing the IVPB medication? **Record your answer using one decimal place.**

Answer: _____mL

23. A nurse makes the inference that a patient may be experiencing urinary retention. Which patient clinical manifestations support this inference? **Select all that apply.**
1. ____ Painful micturition
2. ____ Concentrated urine
3. ____ Abdominal distention
4. ____ Functional incontinence
5. ____ Urinating small amounts frequently

24. Which patients are at the greatest risk for developing constipation? **Select all that apply.**
1. ____ Toddler
2. ____ Adolescent
3. ____ Older adult
4. ____ Middle-age man
5. ____ Pregnant woman

TEST-TAKING TIP Identify the word in the stem that sets a priority.

25. A nurse is caring for a patient who had general anesthesia for surgery 6 hours ago. Place an X over the area of the abdomen that the nurse should palpate when determining if the urinary bladder is distended with urine.

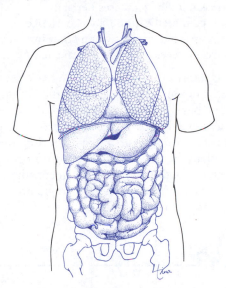

26. A nurse is interviewing an older adult patient who came to the health clinical reporting the problem of frequent constipation. Which questions by the nurse will provide significant data that indicate that the patient is experiencing perceived constipation rather than just constipation? **Select all that apply.**
1. ____ "Do you experience prolonged straining to expel hard stool?"
2. ____ "How often do you use an enema to stimulate a bowel movement?"
3. ____ "Do you use laxatives and cathartics to precipitate daily bowel movements?"
4. ____ "How many servings of vegetables, fruits, and whole-grain foods do you eat daily?"
5. ____ "Do you have dry stool that requires you to hold your breath and bear down to defecate?"

   TEST-TAKING TIP Identify equally plausible options.

27. A nurse is engaged in the following activity. Which actions should be implemented by the nurse? **Select all that apply.**
1. ____ Don sterile gloves.
2. ____ Cleanse the port with an antiseptic swab.
3. ____ Ensure tubing is empty of urine before clamping the tubing.
4. ____ Unclamp the tubing just before collecting the urine specimen.
5. ____ Clamp the tubing distal to the port 30 minutes before collecting the specimen.

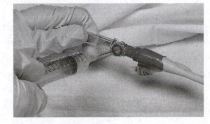

28. Which should the nurse consider when planning for the elimination needs of a patient? **Select all that apply.**
   1. ____ Peristalsis increases after ingestion of food.
   2. ____ Emotional stress initially decreases peristalsis.
   3. ____ Patients taking pain medication may experience constipation.
   4. ____ Intrathoracic pressure decreases when straining during defecation.
   5. ____ Daytime control of feces generally is achieved by 2.5 years of age.

29. A home health nurse is interviewing a patient who has been receiving physical therapy in the home because of muscular weakness of the left upper arm and left leg (hemiparesis) resulting from a brain attack (cerebrovascular accident, stroke). The nurse obtains the patient's vital signs, collects data from the patient, and reviews the patient's diet. Which is the primary nursing intervention for this patient?
   1. Discuss with the patient the importance of performing more physical exercise.
   2. Teach the patient about foods that can result in constipation.
   3. Refer the patient to the primary health-care provider.
   4. Encourage the patient to drink more fluid.

PATIENT'S CLINICAL RECORD

Vital Signs
Temperature: 97.8°F, oral
Pulse: 90 beats/minute, regular rhythm
Respirations: 22 breaths/minute, unlabored
Blood pressure: 142/90 mm Hg

Patient Interview
Patient states that physical therapy can be tiring at times but that the exercises are conscientiously carried out several times a day in addition to a half-mile walk daily. Reports feeling bloated and has to strain to have a bowel movement about twice a week. States voiding sufficient quantities of yellow urine 3 to 4 times a day.

Dietary History
Usually eats yogurt and a banana for breakfast, a cheese omelet for lunch, and meat with rice and one vegetable for dinner. Patient has a chocolate candy bar or chocolate ice cream for dessert with dinner. Patient states, "I eat to live. I do not live to eat." Consumes approximately 8 cups of fluid a day, mostly water.

---

30. A patient's urinary retention catheter collection bag must be emptied at the end of a shift. The nurse washes the hands with soap and water and dons clean gloves. Place the following steps in the order in which they should be performed.
   1. Drain urine in the urinary tubing into the bag.
   2. Calculate the volume of urine and discard the urine into the toilet.
   3. Reclamp the drainage spout just as the last of the urine exits the collection bag.
   4. Unclamp the drainage spout and direct the flow of urine into the measuring device.
   5. Place a calibrated container on a clean Chux on the floor just under the collection bag.
   6. Wipe the drainage spout with an alcohol swab and replace it into the slot on the collection bag.

Answer: _____

31. Which are natural physiological functions of the body that help prevent infection? **Select all that apply.**
1. ____ The low pH of urine
2. ____ An increased temperature
3. ____ The flushing action of urine flow
4. ____ The high pH of gastric secretions
5. ____ A rapid expulsion of stool from the intestine

TEST-TAKING TIP Identify key words in the stem that direct attention to content.

32. A patient experiencing urinary retention requires the insertion of the catheter that is in the illustration. Which is an essential nursing action associated with the use of this urinary catheter?
1. Empty the urine collection bag at the end of each shift.
2. Prevent dependent loops in the urine collection tubing.
3. Use a sterile catheter kit when inserting the catheter.
4. Secure the catheter to the patient's thigh.

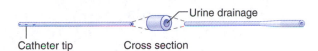

Catheter tip   Cross section

33. Which actions should the nurse include in all bladder-retraining programs? **Select all that apply.**
1. ____ Toilet the patient every 2 hours.
2. ____ Provide 3000 mL of fluids a day.
3. ____ Use adult incontinence underwear.
4. ____ Toilet the patient first thing in the morning.
5. ____ Document the time and amount of each voiding.

TEST-TAKING TIP Identify key words in the stem that direct attention to content. Identify the option with a specific determiner.

34. A colostomy can be surgically created in a variety of places along the length of the large intestine. Which colostomy site will result in stool that is pasty in consistency?

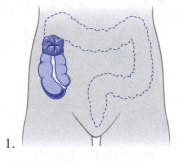
1.

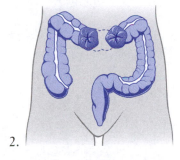
2.

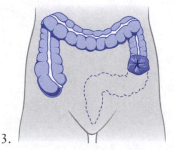
3.

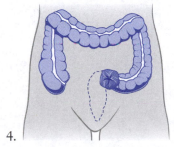
4.

35. A nurse is caring for a patient receiving a continuous bladder irrigation after prostate surgery. At the completion of a 12-hour shift the patient received a total of 1000 mL of fluid via the oral route, 900 mL via the intravenous route, and 4050 mL of bladder irrigant. The volume of fluid emptied from the urinary collection bag totaled 5600 mL. Which was the actual urine output for the 12 hours the nurse cared for the patient? **Record your answer using a whole number.**

Answer: _____ mL

1 **TEST-TAKING TIP** The word "constipated" is the key word in the stem that directs attention to content. Four different foods are offered that help a patient who is constipated. If you are able to identify one food that contributes to increasing peristalsis and the relief of constipation, you can narrow the correct answer to two options. If you are able to identify one food that is not beneficial for the relief of constipation, you can delete two options.

1. **Fresh fruit and whole-wheat bread contain roughage, which adds bulk to stool, increasing peristalsis.**
2. Although whole-wheat bread contains roughage, chicken does not contain much roughage.
3. Although fresh fruit contains roughage, plain yogurt contains yeast, not roughage.
4. Chicken does not contain much roughage, and plain yogurt contains yeast, not roughage.

2. **TEST-TAKING TIP** The word "bowel" is the key word in the stem that directs attention to content because surgeons performing abdominal surgery generally prefer that the bowel be free of stool. Options 1 and 3 are equally plausible because abdominal distention is often caused by intestinal gas. The word "bowel" in the stem and in option 2 is a clang association.

1. A Harris drip (Harris flush), not a tap-water enema, helps evacuate intestinal gas.
2. **A tap-water enema introduces a hypotonic fluid into the intestinal tract; distention and pressure against the intestinal mucosa increase peristalsis and evacuation of stool.**
3. Reducing intestinal gas is a secondary gain because flatus and stool are evacuated along with enema solution.
4. A tap-water enema increases, not decreases, loss of electrolytes because it is a hypotonic solution.

3. **TEST-TAKING TIP** Options 1 and 3 deny patient feelings, concerns, or needs. Option 4 is patient-centered. The word "bathroom" in the stem and in options 1 and 4 are clang associations. Options 1 and 4 are opposites.

1. Reminding the patient that voiding occurred 30 minutes earlier denies the patient's need to void now.
2. Indwelling urinary catheters should not be used to avoid incontinence or the inconvenience of frequently toileting a patient.
3. The patient has a need to void now; 1 hour is too long to postpone urination.
4. **Immediate toileting meets the patient's need to void and promotes continence. Regardless of whether the patient is confused, the patient should be taken to the bathroom.**

4. **TEST-TAKING TIP** The word "best" in the stem sets a priority. Four different interventions are offered as actions that help a patient retain a 750-mL tap-water enema. If you can identify one action that is based on a scientific principle associated with tap-water enema administration, you can narrow the correct answer to two options. If you can identify one action that is not based on a scientific principle associated with tap-water enema administration, you can delete two options from consideration.

1. Although the slow administration of enema fluid is appropriate, encouraging shallow breaths, versus deep breaths, may contribute to an increase in intra-abdominal pressure, which can interfere with the retention of enema fluid.
2. **Both of these actions contribute to retention of enema fluid. In the left lateral position, the sigmoid colon is below the rectum, facilitating the instillation of fluid. The slow administration of enema fluid minimizes the probability of intestinal spasms and premature evacuation of the enema fluid before a therapeutic effect is achieved.**
3. Encouraging shallow breaths and using a 98.6°F enema fluid interfere with the instillation and retention of enema fluid. Encouraging deep breaths, not shallow breaths, helps to prevent patients from holding their breath, which increases intra-abdominal pressure; increased intra-abdominal pressure can interfere with the instillation and retention of

enema fluid. A water temperature of 98.6°F is too cool and can contribute to intestinal muscle spasm and discomfort.

4. Although placing the patient on the left side is appropriate, a water temperature of 98.6°F is too cool and can contribute to intestinal muscle spasm and discomfort. Enema water temperature should be between 105°F and 110°F because warm fluid promotes muscle relaxation and comfort.

5. **TEST-TAKING TIP** The word "highest" in the stem sets a priority. Option 4 is unique because it is the only option that is *not a healthy* activity.

1. Being physically active helps to prevent constipation. It does not precipitate diarrhea.
2. Drinking a lot of fluid helps to prevent constipation. It does not precipitate diarrhea.
3. Eating whole-grain cereal helps to prevent constipation. It does not precipitate diarrhea.
4. **Psychological stress initially increases intestinal motility and mucus secretion, promoting diarrhea.**

6. **TEST-TAKING TIP** The word "debilitated" is the key word in the stem that directs attention to content.

1. **A hypertonic enema solution uses only 120 to 180 mL of solution. Hypertonic solutions expend osmotic pressure that draws fluid out of interstitial spaces; fluid pulled into the colon and rectum distend the bowel, causing an increase in peristalsis, resulting in bowel evacuation.**
2. A normal saline enema is isotonic and requires a volume of 500 to 750 mL to be effective; the volume of fluid, not its saline content, causes an evacuation of the bowel.
3. A soapsuds enema requires a volume of 750 to 1,000 mL of fluid to effectively evacuate the bowel.
4. A tap-water enema usually requires a minimum of 750 mL of water to effectively evacuate the bowel.

7. **TEST-TAKING TIP** Options 1 and 3 are equally plausible. Options 2 and 4 are basically opposites.

1. The dorsal recumbent position does not use the natural curve of the rectum and sigmoid colon to facilitate instillation of enema solution.

2. The right lateral position does not use the natural curve of the rectum and sigmoid colon to facilitate instillation of enema solution.
3. Back-lying position does not use the natural curve of the rectum and sigmoid colon to facilitate instilation of enema solution.
4. **The left Sims position permits enema solution to flow downward via gravity along the natural curve of the rectum and sigmoid colon, promoting instillation and retention of the solution.**

8. **TEST-TAKING TIP** The word "diarrhea" in the stem is an obscure clang association with the words "similar stool" in option 4.

1. Although this answer may help determine if food influenced the patient's intestinal elimination, it does not further assess the presence of diarrhea.
2. Cramping is not specific to diarrhea; it also is associated with constipation and intestinal obstruction.
3. Excessive fluid intake is excreted through the kidneys, not the intestinal tract.
4. **Diarrhea is the defecation of liquid feces and increased frequency of defecation. The patient's recent pattern of bowel elimination should be determined.**

9. **TEST-TAKING TIP** The word "primary" in the stem sets a priority.

1. **In addition to being warm and moist, feces contain enzymes that promote tissue breakdown. A full-body cast limits mobility, which may result in prolonged compression of capillaries in dependent tissues promoting the development of a pressure ulcer.**
2. There is no wound present to become infected; fecal material may cause a vaginal or urinary tract infection, not a wound infection.
3. Immobility may precipitate urinary retention rather than incontinence; diarrhea will not promote urinary incontinence.
4. With a full-body cast, the hips usually are in extension.

10. 1. Incontinence in response to a specific volume of urine in the bladder occurs in reflex, not stress, incontinence.
2. **When intra-abdominal pressure increases, the person with stress**

incontinence usually experiences urinary dribbling, or an approximate loss of 50 mL of urine or less. In some patients once urination begins it continues until the bladder is empty.

3. Urinary tract infections often cause frequency as a result of irritation of the mucosal wall of the bladder, not stress incontinence.

4. Emotional strain may cause frequency, not stress incontinence.

11. **TEST-TAKING TIP** The word "main" in the stem sets a priority. The words "rectal tube" are key words in the stem that direct attention to content.

1. An enema tube is used to administer an enema.

2. This is not the purpose of a rectal tube.

3. **A rectal tube is inserted past the anal sphincters (6 inches in an adult and 2 to 4 inches in a child) and left in place for 30-minute intervals every 2 to 3 hours; rectal tubes are used to promote the passage of flatus, reducing abdominal distention.**

4. A rectal tube is not used to visualize the intestinal mucosa. A proctoscope is an instrument designed to visualize the rectum; a sigmoidoscope is an instrument designed to visualize the sigmoid colon and the rectum; and a colonoscope is an instrument designed to visualize the entire large intestine.

12. **TEST-TAKING TIP** Option 3 is the unique option. It is the only option that does not begin with the letter "C." Also, options 1, 2, and 3 address the concept of *what is in urine*. The word "volume" in option 3 addresses the concept of *quantity*.

1. The color of urine reflects urine concentration, blood in the urine (hematuria), or a reaction to a specific drug or food, not catheter patency.

2. A cloudy urine indicates the presence of such products as red or white blood cells, bacteria, prostatic fluid, or sperm. Clarity will not indicate catheter patency.

3. **If urine volume is minimal or nonexistent, it indicates that the catheter is obstructed, the ureters are obstructed, or the kidneys are not producing urine.**

4. Abnormal constituents of urine such as pus or blood indicate a possible pathological process, not catheter patency.

13. **TEST-TAKING TIP** The word "most" in the stem sets a priority. Option 4 is unique; option 1, 2, and 3 are related to physical concerns, whereas option 4 relates to a psychological concern.

1. Although maintenance of skin integrity is important, it is not the most common concern of patients with a colostomy.

2. Although frequency of defecation may be a concern of some patients, it is not the most common concern of patients with a colostomy.

3. Consistency of the feces is not as major a concern as another factor. The consistency of feces varies according to the location of the stoma along the intestinal tract.

4. **The ability to control odor is a major psychological concern of people with a colostomy, because the odor can be offensive if not controlled.**

14. **TEST-TAKING TIP** The words "infant," "urine," and "expected outcome" are key words in the stem that direct attention to content. The words "only" in option 1 and "always" in option 4 are specific determiners. The words "urine" in the stem and "urination" in option 2 and "urine" in option 3 are clang associations. Carefully examine both these options. Option 3 is the correct answer.

1. Infants void very light yellow urine because of immature kidney function, not because they ingest only fluids.

2. Although it is true that infants have not developed neuromuscular control of urination, the inability to control micturition voluntarily has no impact on the color of urine voided.

3. **An infant's kidneys are unable to concentrate urine and reabsorb water efficiently. When the body is too immature to concentrate urine, urine is diluted and very light yellow.**

4. Although this is a correct statement by itself, it is not related to the content in the stem. Infants' bladders are smaller than bladders of adults and they can retain only a small volume of urine. Frequency is not related to the color of urine.

15. **TEST-TAKING TIP** The words "culture and sensitivity" are key words in the stem that direct attention to content. The word "urine" in the stem and in options 1, 2, and 3 are clang associations. The word "only" in option 3 is a specific determiner.

1. Two specimens are unnecessary.
2. **A midstream urine sample contains a specimen that is relatively free of microorganisms from the urethra. After perineal care, cleansing of the urethral opening, and the initiation of urination, a specimen is collected during the midportion of the stream. This technique avoids collection of urine during the initial stream that may be contaminated with bacteria from the urethra.**
3. Specimens collected from the first voiding of the morning should be avoided; stagnant urine does not reflect urine that is recently produced by the urinary system.
4. Twenty-four hours of urine is needed for special tests such as the measurement of levels of adrenocortical steroids, hormones, and creatinine clearance tests, not for a urine culture and sensitivity test.

16. 1. **This question relates to painful or difficult urination (dysuria). It is most often caused by bladder or urethral inflammation or trauma.**
2. This question might be asked if there is a concern that the person is experiencing difficulty initiating urination (hesitancy) or urge incontinence.
3. This question relates to stress incontinence, which is the immediate involuntary loss of urine during an increase in intra-abdominal pressure.
4. This question might be asked if there is a concern that the person is retaining urine in the bladder after urinating (residual urine).

17. 1. Red stools indicate lower, not upper, gastrointestinal bleeding.
2. Pink stools, although uncommon, may indicate lower gastrointestinal bleeding mixed with mucus or intestinal fluid.
3. **Black (tarry) stools indicate upper gastrointestinal bleeding. Enzymes acting on the blood turn it black. In addition, iron supplements, excessive intake of red meat, and dark green vegetables can cause greenish-black stools.**
4. Brown is the expected color of stool. The brown color is caused by the presence of

stercobilin and urobilin, which are derived from a pigment in bile (bilirubin).

18. 1. **X Eliminating dependent loops in the tubing prevents urine from inadvertently flowing back into the bladder; gravity allows the urine to flow from the urinary bladder to the collection bag without staying in dependent loops for prolonged periods of time.**
2. **X Positioning the catheter collection bag below the level of the pelvis prevents urine from flowing back into the bladder; urine flows out of the bladder by gravity.**
3. ____ Carrying the bag at waist level allows urine to flow back into the bladder, which can contribute to a urinary tract infection.
4. **X Securing the tubing to the thigh will limit trauma to the urinary meatus.**
5. ____ An indwelling urinary catheter and collection bag constitute a closed system and should be changed only every 4 to 6 weeks unless crusting or sediment collects on the inside of the tubing.
6. ____ It is unnecessary to clamp an indwelling urinary catheter when a patient is out of bed.

19. **TEST-TAKING TIP** The words "uncircumcised" and "after perineal care" are key words in the stem that direct attention to content. Options 2 and 4 are opposites.

1. ____ The area around the glans of the penis should not be lubricated; this will prevent the condom device from staying securely in place.
2. **X Perineal care should be provided when changing a condom catheter; in uncircumcised men, if the foreskin is not replaced to over the distal portion of the penis, it can tighten around the shaft of the penis, causing local edema and pain.**
3. ____ A condom catheter (external catheter) should be secured farther up the shaft of the penis, not immediately behind the glans.
4. ____ If the foreskin is not returned over the glans, it can tighten around the shaft of the penis, causing local edema and pain.
5. **X This space prevents irritation of the tip of the penis; in addition, the 1-inch space allows urine to flow unimpeded and is not long enough to permit the condom sheath to twist.**

20. 1. This is a double-lumen urinary retention catheter. One lumen is used to inflate the balloon and one lumen is used for urine drainage, which is connected to a collection bag.

2. This is a single-lumen (straight) urinary catheter generally used to drain the bladder of urine or to obtain a sterile urine specimen.

3. **This is a triple-lumen urinary catheter. One lumen is used to inflate the balloon, one lumen is used for the introduction of the irrigation solution and is connected to a 3000 mL bag of irrigant, and one lumen is used for drainage that accumulates in a collection bag.**

21. A urinary retention catheter is inserted into the meatus of the urethra, which leads to the urinary bladder. The urethra is directly behind the pubic symphysis and anterior to the vagina. The urinary meatus is between the clitoris and vaginal opening.

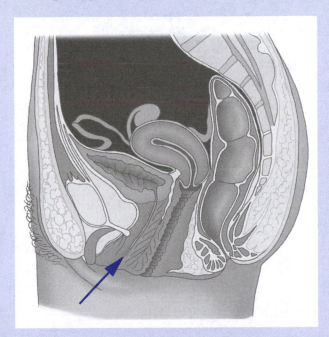

22. Answer: 1.5 mL.
Use ratio and proportion to solve for x. Five hundred milligrams is equal to 0.5 gram.

$$\frac{\text{Desired dose}}{\text{Have dose}} \quad \frac{0.5 \text{ g}}{1.0 \text{ g}} = \frac{x \text{ mL}}{3 \text{ mL}}$$

$$1x = 3 \times 0.5$$

$$x = 1.5 \text{ mL}$$

23. 1. ____ Painful micturition (dysuria) generally is caused by infection, inflammation, or injury, not urinary retention.

2. ____ Concentrated urine is caused by inadequate fluid intake and indicates dehydration, not urinary retention.

3. **X Abdominal distention occurs as a result of the buildup of urine in the bladder. Outlet obstruction, decreased bladder tone, neurological dysfunction, opioids, and trauma can precipitate urinary retention.**

4. ____ Functional incontinence is unrelated to retention. Functional incontinence occurs when a person who is aware of the need to void is unable to reach the toilet in time.

5. **X Voiding small amounts of urine along with a distended bladder is indicative of urinary retention with overflow; the bladder fills until pressure builds within the bladder to the point that the urinary sphincters release enough urine to relieve the pressure.**

24. **TEST-TAKING TIP The word "greatest" in the stem sets a priority.**

1. ____ A toddler usually drinks adequate fluids, eats a regular diet, and is very active; these activities contribute to bowel elimination.

2. ____ An adolescent usually eats more food than at earlier developmental stages and may report indigestion, not constipation; indigestion is a response to increased gastric acidity that occurs during adolescence.

3. **X Older adults have a decrease in peristalsis and many older adults engage in less physical activity. Some older adults have dental/gum problems that result in their eating a soft diet; a soft diet usually is low in fiber.**

4. ____ As people advance through middle adulthood, they are at risk for gaining weight, not developing constipation.

5. **X The growing size of the fetus exerts pressure on the rectum and bowel, which impinges on intestinal functioning, contributing to constipation; the decreased motility causes increased absorption of water, promoting constipation.**

25. Answer: Hypogastric region
Two transverse (horizontal) planes and two sagittal planes divide the abdomen into nine areas. When a urinary bladder fills with urine, it will rise upward into the abdominal cavity (shaded). In assessing a distended urinary bladder, palpation will reveal a round, firm mass above the symphysis pubis. Percussion will elicit a hollow, drum-like sound.

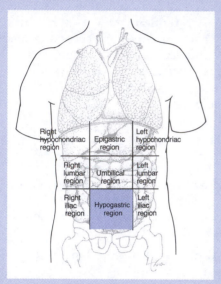

26. TEST-TAKING TIP Options 1 and 5 are questions that seek the same information; they are equally plausible. Option 1 is no better than option 5. Eliminate both from further consideration.

1. ____ This question does not identify the behavior that indicates perceived constipation; it does address a behavior that is associated with constipation.

2. X A form of constipation considered to be "perceived" is when a person diagnoses oneself as being constipated and routinely uses enemas to produce a daily bowel movement.

3. X A form of constipation considered to be "perceived" is when a person diagnoses oneself as being constipated and routinely uses medications such as laxatives or cathartics to produce a bowel movement every day.

4. ____ An inadequate intake of fiber is not a behavior indicating perceived constipation; it may identify a precipitating cause of constipation.

5. ____ This question does not identify a behavior that indicates perceived constipation; it does attempt to collect information associated with constipation.

27. 1. ____ Sterile gloves are not necessary to maintain sterile technique when collecting a urine specimen from a urinary retention catheter. Clean gloves are worn to protect the nurse from exposure to the patient's urine.

2. X Cleansing the port with an antiseptic swab prevents the introduction of pathogens into the closed urinary drainage system.

3. X Making sure that the tubing is empty of urine before clamping the tubing ensures that the urine collected is fresh, newly excreted urine and not urine that has been lying in the tubing for an excessive period of time.

4. ____ The clamp should be unclamped after, not before, collection of the urine specimen. If the clamp is unclamped before the urine is collected, urine will flow by gravity into the collection bag and there may not be enough urine in the tubing for an adequate volume of urine for a specimen.

5. X The tube should be clamped distal to the port. This allows recently excreted urine to accumulate at and above the level of the port.

28. 1. X Food or fluid that enters and fills the stomach or the duodenum stimulates peristalsis; this is called the "gastrocolic reflex" or "duodenocolic reflex."

2. ____ Emotional stress initially increases peristalsis because the bowel evacuates its contents to prepare for the "fight." When the sympathetic nervous system increases its control in response to stress, the action of the parasympathetic nervous system decreases. The parasympathetic nervous system initially stimulates peristalsis, and as its action decreases, peristalsis also decreases.

3. X Opioid analgesics depress the central nervous system slowing peristalsis, which places the patient at risk for constipation.

4. ____ Straining at defecation increases, not decreases, intrathoracic pressure. Forcible exhalation against a closed glottis (Valsalva maneuver) increases intrathoracic pressure, which impedes venous return. When the breath is released, blood is propelled through the heart, causing tachycardia and an increased blood

pressure; a reflex bradycardia immediately follows. With an increase in intrathoracic pressure, immediate tachycardia and bradycardia occur in succession; patients with heart problems can experience a cardiac arrest.

5. X At 2.5 years of age muscles and nerves have matured to where a child can typically gain daytime bowel control after a program of toilet training.

29. 1. The patient does not have to perform more exercises. The patient is physically active doing physical therapy exercises several times a day as well as taking a half-mile walk daily. The patient also has indicated that the exercises can be tiring at times.

2. The patient is experiencing constipation, a human response the nurse is legally permitted to treat. Constipation is infrequent (less than three stools weekly) fecal elimination or the passage of hard, dry feces. The patient is consuming foods low in fiber (e.g., yogurt, eggs, cheese, and rice) and high in fat (dairy products, chocolate, and meat). Low-fiber foods leave little residue after they are digested. High-fiber foods leave residue after they are digested that promotes the formation of feces as well as peristalsis. Foods high in fat take longer to pass through the gastrointestinal system, allowing more fluid to be reabsorbed before being eliminated. Unripe bananas can cause constipation because they contain approximately 80% starch and a small amount of pectinase. Ripe bananas do not cause constipation because they contain approximately 5% starch and a large amount of pectinase, which breaks down the pectin between the cells in bananas, making them easier to digest. The nurse must explore what type of bananas the patient is consuming.

3. Referring the patient to the primary health-care provider is not necessary. The nurse has the legal responsibility and expertise to address this patient's problem. The nurse would be abdicating nursing responsibilities to another health-care professional.

4. Increasing fluid intake is not necessary. Two liters of fluid a day is an adequate fluid intake to maintain metabolic functions.

30. Answer: 1, 5, 4, 3, 6, 2
1. Draining urine in the urinary tubing into the bag ensures that all the urine excreted within a specified time frame is included in the amount of urinary output.
5. A clean Chux on the floor provides a barrier between the calibrated container and the floor, which prevents contamination of the container. Placing the container on the floor provides a firm surface for collecting the urine, which prevents accidental spilling of urine. Placing the container just under the collection bag allows the urine to flow into the container without contaminating the drainage spout.
4. Unclamping the drainage spout allows urine to flow out of the collection bag and into the container by gravity.
3. A urinary retention catheter system is a closed, sterile system. The clamp on the drainage spout should be reclamped just as the last amount of urine exits the system. This prevents microorganism from entering the system.
6. Wiping the drainage spout with an alcohol swab reduces the amount of bacteria present, limiting the risk of a urinary infection.
2. Patients with a urinary retention catheter are on intake and output. All urinary output must be calculated as part of the patient's output. Discarding urine into a toilet eliminates exposure of the patient's urine to others.

31. TEST-TAKING TIP The words "physiological" and "prevent infection" are key words in the stem that direct attention to content.

1. X Freshly voided urine is slightly acidic; this medium is unfavorable to microorganisms.
2. ____ An increased temperature results from released toxins in the presence of infection; it may help to limit an already existing infection, but it does not prevent an infection.
3. X Microorganisms congregate at the urinary meatus because it is warm, moist, and dark; when urine flows down the urethra and out of the

urinary meatus, the force of urine carries away microorganisms, which minimizes ascending infections.

4. ____ Gastric secretions are acidic and have a low pH.

5. ____ Rapid peristalsis results in diarrhea; this is not a usual physiological function of the body but rather a response to an irritant or a pathogen.

32. 1. This type of urinary catheter (straight catheter) is not attached to a collection bag. The straight catheter in the illustration is left in the urinary bladder just long enough to empty the bladder of urine and then immediately is removed.

    2. There is no urine collection tubing used with this type of urinary catheter (straight catheter). The urine usually is collected in the container associated with the catheterization kit.

    3. **Using sterile technique when inserting a straight catheter reduces the risk of introducing a pathogen into the bladder.**

    4. A straight urinary catheter does not remain in the bladder once the bladder is emptied of urine. A double-lumen catheter used with an indwelling urinary catheter should be secured to the patient to prevent tension on the catheter that has been left in place.

33. **TEST-TAKING TIP** The words "all bladder-retraining programs" are key words in the stem that direct attention to content. The word "every" in option 1 is a specific determiner.

    1. ____ Toileting is not automatically implemented every 2 hours but is based on the individual needs of the patient.

    2. ____ The volume of scheduled fluid intake is based on the individual needs of the patient.

    3. ____ Incontinence pads generally are not encouraged when implementing a bladder-retraining program; however, devices used depend on individual needs and preferences of the patient.

4. X Toileting a patient first thing in the morning is done for all patients on a bladder retraining program; it empties the urinary bladder in the morning before other activities of daily living. When one moves from a lying down to a vertical position, urine moves toward the trigone and urinary meatus. The increased pressure of urine in this area stimulates the desire to void.

5. X The nurse should document the time and amount of each voiding. This will provide information that may reflect a pattern to the patient's voiding; this information should influence the toileting scheduling.

34. 1. This site is the ascending colon, which contains the most liquid stool because it is at the beginning of the large intestine, where little fluid has yet to be reabsorbed.

    2. **This site is the transverse colon with a double-barreled colostomy. The stool produced will be soft and pasty because just a little fluid has been reabsorbed. Eighty percent of the fluid that enters the bowel is reabsorbed eventually as fecal material progresses through the large intestine.**

    3. This site is the descending colon, where stool is soft but formed. More fluid has been reabsorbed than in the transverse colon but less fluid has been reabsorbed than in the sigmoid colon.

    4. This site is the sigmoid colon. The stool produced will be formed and firm because it is the final small segment of the large intestine. The sigmoid colon is the intestinal section just before the rectum, anal canal, and anus.

35. **Answer: 1550 mL**
    The nurse should deduct the volume of bladder irrigant from the total output in the urinary collection bag (5600 − 4050 = 1550 mL) to arrive at the patient's total urine output for 12 hours. The oral and intravenous intake is unrelated to calculating the actual urine output.

MEETING PATIENTS' OXYGEN NEEDS

This section includes questions related to assessments and interventions associated with expected and abnormal respiratory and circulatory function. Questions focus on topics such as preventing aspiration, providing emergency care for aspiration, techniques and devices that assess or increase respiratory or circulatory function, and assessments and interventions associated with the administration of oxygen.

QUESTIONS

1. Oxygen therapy via nasal cannula is ordered for a patient. Which should the nurse do **first?**
   1. Lubricate the nares with water-soluble jelly.
   2. Explain the rules of fire safety to the patient.
   3. Post the fire safety rules on the door to the room.
   4. Adjust the flow rate before applying the nasal prongs.

   TEST-TAKING TIP Identify the word in the stem that sets a priority.

2. A patient with a history of chronic respiratory disease begins to have difficulty breathing. For which **most** serious responses should the nurse assess the patient?
   1. Orthostatic hypotension when rising and the need to sit in the orthopneic position
   2. Wheezing sounds on inspiration and the need to sit in the orthopneic position
   3. Mucus tinged with frank red streaks and wheezing sounds on inspiration
   4. Chest pain and mucus tinged with frank red streaks

   TEST-TAKING TIP Identify the word in the stem that sets a priority. Identify duplicate facts among options.

3. A patient is receiving oxygen through a nasal cannula. Which should the nurse do to prevent skin breakdown around the patient's nares?
   1. Provide the patient with oral hygiene whenever necessary.
   2. Remove the tubing for 15 minutes every 2 hours.
   3. Adjust the cannula so it is comfortable.
   4. Reposition the patient every 2 hours.

   TEST-TAKING TIP Identify key words in the stem that direct attention to content. Identify options with specific determiners. Identify clang associations.

4. While eating, a male patient clutches the upper chest with the hands, appears unable to breathe, and has a frightened facial expression. Which should the nurse do **first?**
   1. Start artificial respirations.
   2. Perform abdominal thrusts.
   3. Slap the patient on the back.
   4. Ask the patient if he is choking.

   TEST-TAKING TIP Identify the word in the stem that sets a priority. Identify the unique option.

5. A nurse is monitoring a patient with a respiratory problem for the presence of cyanosis. Which are the **most** appropriate sites to assess?
   1. Lower legs and around the mouth
   2. Around the mouth and fingernail beds
   3. Conjunctiva of the eyes and lower legs
   4. Fingernail beds and conjunctiva of the eyes

   TEST-TAKING TIP Identify the word in the stem that sets a priority. Identify duplicate facts among options.

6. A patient has moderate chronic impaired peripheral arterial circulation. For which responses should the nurse assess the patient?
   1. Cool extremities and yellow toenails
   2. Cyanosis of the feet and yellow toenails
   3. Cool extremities and continuous leg discomfort
   4. Cyanosis of the feet and continuous leg discomfort

   TEST-TAKING TIP Identify key words in the stem that direct attention to content. Identify duplicate facts among options.

7. A protocol in the postanesthesia care unit is that all patients must have pulse oximetry monitoring. Which does pulse oximetry monitor?
   1. Heart rate
   2. Vital signs
   3. Blood pressure
   4. Oxygen saturation

   TEST-TAKING TIP Identify the obscure clang association.

8. Which individual should the nurse identify as having the **most** dramatic increase in the need for oxygen?
   1. Person with a fever
   2. Individual exercising
   3. Woman who is pregnant
   4. Patient receiving general anesthesia

   TEST-TAKING TIP Identify the word in the stem that sets a priority. Identify key words in the stem that direct attention to content. Identify the clang association.

9. A nurse identifies that a patient has excessive sputum. Which intervention is **most** effective for maintaining a patent airway in this patient?
   1. Active coughing
   2. Incentive spirometry
   3. Nebulizer treatments
   4. Abdominal breathing

   TEST-TAKING TIP Identify the word in the stem that sets a priority.

10. A nurse is caring for a patient who is experiencing respiratory difficulty. Which **most** accurately measures the adequacy of tissue oxygenation that the nurse should monitor?
    1. Hematocrit values
    2. Hemoglobin levels
    3. Arterial blood gases
    4. Pulmonary function tests

    TEST-TAKING TIP Identify the word in the stem that sets a priority. Identify the key word in the stem that directs attention to content.

11. A nurse identifies that a patient with an infection has tachypnea. Which should the nurse consider is the reason for this response?
    1. Increase in the metabolic rate
    2. Need to retain carbon dioxide
    3. Decrease in carbon dioxide levels
    4. Attempt to compensate for respiratory alkalosis

12. A patient comes to the emergency department in respiratory distress and the nurse identifies the presence of wheezing breath sounds. Which does the nurse determine is the cause of these sounds?
    1. Fluid in the lung.
    2. Sitting in the orthopneic position.
    3. Air moving through a narrowed airway.
    4. Pleural surfaces that rub against each other.

13. A nurse determines that a patient is experiencing Kussmaul respirations. Which description of the patient's respirations supports the nurse's conclusion?
    1. Recurring pattern of quick, shallow respirations alternating with irregular periods of apnea
    2. Repeating pattern of increasing rate and depth of respirations alternating with apnea
    3. Labored respirations, with breathlessness, that are possibly painful
    4. High rate and depth of respirations that are regular

    TEST-TAKING TIP Identify opposites in options.

14. A nurse is caring for a patient with a diagnosis of anemia. Which physiological activity is altered as a result of the pathophysiology of anemia?
    1. Perfusion of oxygen
    2. Diffusion of oxygen
    3. Exchange of oxygen
    4. Transport of oxygen

15. A patient in respiratory distress is coughing excessively. The nurse assesses whether the cough is productive or nonproductive. Which is associated with a productive cough?
    1. Causes pain
    2. Results in sputum
    3. Interferes with breathing
    4. Gets progressively worse

    TEST-TAKING TIP Identify the key words in the stem that direct attention to content.

16. A patient is newly diagnosed with hypertension. An antihypertensive medication once a day in the morning and a 2-gram sodium diet are ordered. Which is **most** important for the nurse to teach the patient?
    1. "Avoid adding salt to cooked foods."
    2. "Use less salt when preparing foods."
    3. "Take your medication exactly as prescribed."
    4. "Measure your blood pressure every morning."

    TEST-TAKING TIP Identify the word in the stem that sets a priority. Identify equally plausible options. Identify the clang association.

17. A nurse must obtain a pulse oximetry reading of a female patient who is experiencing shortness of breath and has a history of peripheral vascular disease. The patient has acrylic fingernails, nail polish on the toenails, and pierced earrings. Which is the **most** appropriate site to attach the pulse oximetry probe?
    1. Earlobe
    2. Large toe
    3. Index finger
    4. Bridge of nose

    TEST-TAKING TIP Identify the word in the stem that sets a priority.

18. A nurse is providing oropharyngeal suctioning with a Yankauer (tonsil-tip) suction device for a patient with dysphagia. During the procedure the patient begins to gag and vomit. Which should the nurse do?
    1. Raise the head of the bed.
    2. Turn the patient onto a lateral position.
    3. Give the patient oxygen via nasal cannula.
    4. Continue the procedure to patient's oral cavity.

19. A hospitalized patient has difficulty swallowing. Which should the nurse do to help prevent this patient from aspirating? **Select all that apply.**
1. _____ Ensure a small amount of food is included with each mouthful.
2. _____ Encourage that fluids be mixed with food in the mouth.
3. _____ Allow time between spoonfuls for chewing.
4. _____ Promote conversation during meals.
5. _____ Cut up meat into small pieces.

20. Ampicillin 100 mg/kg/day PO divided into 4 doses daily is prescribed for a child. The child weighs 31 pounds. Ampicillin is supplied in an oral solution of 125 mg/5 mL. How much solution should the nurse administer for each dose? **Record your answer using a whole number.**

Answer: _____ mL

21. A nurse is educating a patient who has impaired circulation to the lower extremities. Which actions should the nurse include in the teaching program about how to care for the feet? **Select all that apply.**
1. _____ Apply moisturizing lotion to the toes daily.
2. _____ Use a mirror to check the under-surfaces of the feet every day.
3. _____ Limit walking barefoot to carpeted surfaces when in the home.
4. _____ Use warm socks rather than a heating pad when the feet are cold.
5. _____ Report breaks in the skin of the feet to the primary health-care provider.

TEST-TAKING TIP Identify clang associations.

22. A nurse is auscultating a patient's breath sounds. Place an X over the site where the nurse should place the stethoscope when assessing breath sounds in the right middle lobe via the lateral approach.

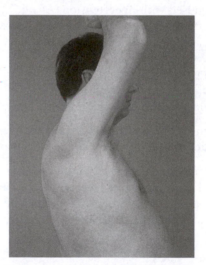

23. A patient ambulating in the hall reports having sudden chest pain. Which should the nurse do? **Select all that apply.**
1. _____ Obtain vital signs.
2. _____ Perform a pain assessment.
3. _____ Walk the patient back to bed slowly.
4. _____ Return the patient to bed via a wheelchair.
5. _____ Have the patient stand still until the discomfort subsides.

TEST-TAKING TIP Identify opposites in options. Identify the clang association.

24. A nurse identifies the following deformity of the fingers of both hands when performing a physical assessment of a patient. Which body systems commonly are involved with the development of this human response? **Select all that apply.**
1. ____ Skeletal
2. ____ Endocrine
3. ____ Respiratory
4. ____ Cardiovascular
5. ____ Gastrointestinal

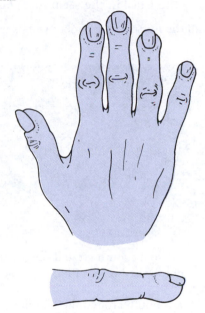

25. A patient with the diagnosis of pneumonia is transferred from the emergency department to a medical unit at 4:30 p.m. The patient arrives on a stretcher in the low-Fowler position. The primary health-care provider writes the following orders and prescription: chest radiograph, sputum for culture and sensitivity, oxygen via nasal cannula at 2 L/min, bedrest, regular diet, and ciprofloxacin 400 mg IVPB every 12 hours. In what order should the nurse perform the following activities?
1. Obtain vital signs.
2. Administer the antibiotic.
3. Order a regular diet dinner.
4. Place in the high-Fowler position.
5. Obtain sputum for culture and sensitivity.
6. Begin oxygen via nasal cannula at 2 L/min.

Answer: _____

26. A patient has dysphagia. Which should the nurse do to prevent aspiration after meals? **Select all that apply.**
1. ____ Position the patient in the low-Fowler position.
2. ____ Keep the head of the bed elevated for an hour.
3. ____ Administer mouth care when necessary.
4. ____ Place a pitcher of water at the bedside.
5. ____ Inspect the mouth for pocketed food.

TEST-TAKING TIP Identify key words in the stem that direct attention to content.

27. Which individuals are **most** likely to have life-threatening complications when experiencing a respiratory infection? **Select all that apply.**
1. _____ Infant
2. _____ Older adult
3. _____ Adolescent
4. _____ Young adult
5. _____ School-age child

TEST-TAKING TIP Identify the word in the stem that sets a priority.

28. Which instruction should the nurse give a patient who is using the device in the illustration?

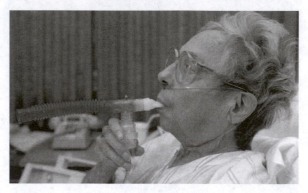

1. Breathe out normally, seal your mouth around the mouthpiece, breathe in slowly and deeply as possible, hold your breath at least 3 seconds, and remove the mouthpiece and exhale.
2. Hold the device, seal your mouth around the mouthpiece, and breathe in and out slowly and deeply.
3. Seal your mouth around the mouthpiece and breathe in and out normally.
4. Take a deep breath and forcefully exhale through the mouthpiece.

29. When obtaining the vital signs of a patient a nurse identifies that the patient has bradypnea. Which pattern reflects bradypnea?

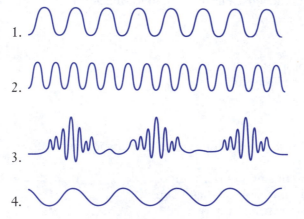

30. Based on the data in the patient's clinical record, which should the nurse do **first** when the condition of the patient changed suddenly?
1. Call the respiratory therapist, and obtain a pulse oximetry reading.
2. Initiate the rapid response team, and notify the primary health-care provider.
3. Elevate the head of the bed to 45 degrees, and start oxygen via nasal cannula.
4. Take the patient's blood pressure, and start an IV line with 0.9% sodium chloride.

PATIENT'S CLINICAL RECORD

Nurse's Progress Note 0900
Patient 4 days postoperative for a right total hip replacement. Alert, oriented times 3. Reports dull ache in operative site on a level 2 that increases to a level 4 with movement. Right lower extremity peripheral pulses are present and strong. Capillary refill of toes is 2 sec. Suture line dry, edges approximated with no signs of inflammation or dehiscence. Abduction maintained. Underactive bowel sounds noted in upper right quadrant. Voiding sufficient quantity. No adventitious breath sounds. Patient reports a slight ache in calf of right extremity. No swelling or heat observed at site. Encouraged patient to remain in bed with entire right extremity supported on 1 pillow; primary health-care provider's office notified and awaiting orders.

Vital Signs 0900
Blood pressure: 140/75 mm Hg
Pulse: 84 beats/min, regular rhythm
Respirations: 18 breaths/min

Change in patient's condition when turning and positioning patient at 0930
When assisting the patient to turn on the left side based on the turning and positioning schedule, the patient reported sudden severe substernal chest pain, became diaphoretic, and appeared very anxious. Pulse 110, weak and rapid; respirations 32, labored.

TEST-TAKING TIP Identify the word in the stem that sets a priority.

31. A nurse teaches a patient how to self-administer a corticosteroid via a metered-dose inhaler with an extender. Which behaviors indicate that the patient understands the teaching? **Select all that apply.**
1. _____ Rinses the mouth with water after the treatment
2. _____ Waits at least 1 minute before taking the next puff
3. _____ Rolls the canister between the hands slowly before using the device
4. _____ Positions the mouthpiece directly in front of the mouth while inhaling
5. _____ Assumes the semi-Fowler position with the head supported on a pillow

32. Oseltamivir 45 mg twice a day for 5 days is prescribed for a child with influenza. The package insert states to loosen powder from side of bottle, and add 55 mL of water to yield 6 mg/mL. How much oral suspension should the nurse administer for each dose? **Record your answer using one decimal place.**

Answer: _____ mL

33. Place an X on the site that the nurse **most** commonly assesses for the presence of a pulse when administering cardiopulmonary resuscitation to an adult.

TEST-TAKING TIP Identify the word in the stem that sets a priority.

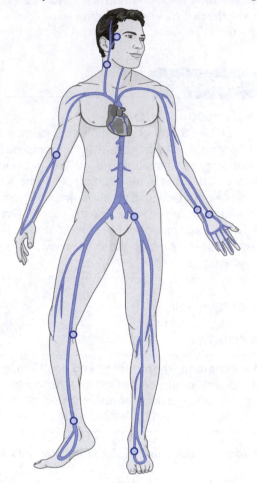

34. Which are nursing interventions that increase both circulation and respiration in a patient? **Select all that apply.**
1. _____ Encourage the use of a spirometer.
2. _____ Reposition the patient every 2 hours.
3. _____ Massage the bony prominences with lotion.
4. _____ Assist the patient with ambulating in the hall.
5. _____ Teach the patient to cough after breathing deeply every 4 hours.

TEST-TAKING TIP Identify the key word in the stem that directs attention to content.

35. A nurse is administering physical hygiene to a patient receiving a continuous nasogastric tube feeding. Which should the nurse do to prevent aspiration when giving this patient a bed bath and changing the linens? **Select all that apply.**
1. _____ Lower the height of the bag containing the feeding formula.
2. _____ Slow the rate of flow on the infusion pump.
3. _____ Maintain elevation of the head of the bed.
4. _____ Obtain additional assistance.
5. _____ Shut off the infusion pump.

TEST-TAKING TIP Identify key words in the stem that direct attention to content. Identify clang associations.

1. **TEST-TAKING TIP** The word "first" in the stem sets a priority.

   1. Lubricating the nares with water-soluble jelly is unnecessary; the nares should be cleaned only with soap and water daily and whenever necessary.
   2. **Safety is a priority; patients must understand the rules related to oxygen use and that oxygen supports combustion.**
   3. Although putting an oxygen-in-use sign with fire safety rules on the door to the room is important, it is not as important as another intervention.
   4. Although adjusting the oxygen level before applying the nasal prongs is important, it is not the priority.

2. **TEST-TAKING TIP** The word "most" in the stem sets a priority. Five patient responses are offered in different combinations for you to choose from as being the most serious in this situation. If you are able to identify one response that appears in two options that is most serious, you can narrow the choice to two options. If you can identify one response that appears in two options that is least significant, you can eliminate two distractors from consideration.

   1. Orthostatic hypotension when rising and the need to sit in the orthopneic position are common clinical findings of individuals with chronic respiratory disease and are not as serious as another option. Rising slowly permits the circulation to adjust to the change in position, thereby minimizing orthostatic hypotension. Elevating the head helps breathing by lowering the abdominal organs via gravity, which allows the diaphragm to contract more efficiently on inspiration.
   2. Wheezing sounds on inspiration and the need to sit in the orthopneic position are common responses associated with respiratory disease and are not as serious as another option. Raising the head of the bed helps breathing by lowering the abdominal organs by gravity, which allows the diaphragm to contract more efficiently on inspiration. Wheezing on inspiration is a response to an increase in airway resistance.
   3. Although mucus tinged with frank red streaks and wheezing are common responses to respiratory disease, this combination of responses is not as serious as another combination of responses among the options.
   4. **Mucus tinged with frank red streaks is a common response to chronic respiratory disease, and chest pain may indicate a pneumothorax; these are the two most serious responses and should be reported to the primary health-care provider immediately.**

3. **TEST-TAKING TIP** The words "prevent" and "nares" are key words in the stem that direct attention to content. The word "every" in options 2 and 4 is a specific determiner. The word "cannula" in the stem and in option 3 is a clang association.

   1. Although oral hygiene is important, it is mainly pressure that causes skin breakdown; oral hygiene alone does not prevent skin breakdown.
   2. Fifteen minutes is too long to remove oxygen from a patient who needs oxygen.
   3. **If the cannula comfortably rests in the nares, it avoids pressure on the nares that can cause skin breakdown.**
   4. Repositioning the patient prevents pressure ulcers of dependent areas of the body but does not prevent skin breakdown around the nares.

4. **TEST-TAKING TIP** The word "first" in the stem sets a priority. Option 4 is unique because it is the only option that is an assessment. Options 1, 2, and 3 are all actions.

   1. Action before assessment is inappropriate. The patient is not in respiratory arrest; food is lodged in the respiratory passages.
   2. Action before assessment is inappropriate. Abdominal thrusts may be done after it is determined that the patient cannot speak because of a totally obstructed airway.
   3. Action before assessment is inappropriate. Slapping the patient on the back may cause the aspirated object to lodge deeper in respiratory passages.
   4. **If the patient can speak, the airway is partially obstructed. If the patient cannot speak, the airway is totally obstructed. Assessment is the priority because each of the situations requires a different intervention.**

5. **TEST-TAKING TIP** The word "most" in the stem sets a priority. Four different sites are presented as preferred sites to assess for the presence of cyanosis. If you are able to identify one site that is the least desirable to use for the assessment of cyanosis, you can eliminate two distractors and narrow the choice to two options. If you are able to identify one site that is desirable to use for the assessment of cyanosis, you can narrow the choice to two options.

1. Although the lips and mucous membranes of the mouth are a primary site to assess for early signs of oxygen deprivation, the lower legs are not the first sites to assess for systemic oxygen deprivation.
2. **Nail beds, lips, and mucous membranes of the mouth are the primary sites to assess for signs of oxygen deprivation. The mucous membranes of the mouth are highly vascular and the presence of an excessive concentration of deoxyhemoglobin in the blood is observable.**
3. Pallor of the conjunctiva of the eyes, not cyanosis, reflects reduced oxyhemoglobin. The lower legs are not the first sites to assess for systemic oxygen deprivation.
4. Although the nail beds are a primary site to assess for signs of oxygen deprivation, pallor of the conjunctiva of the eyes, not cyanosis, reflects reduced oxyhemoglobin.

6. **TEST-TAKING TIP** The words "moderate chronic" and "peripheral arterial" are key words in the stem that direct attention to content. Four different responses are offered as common responses to prolonged impaired peripheral arterial circulation. If you are able to identify one response that is common to this situation, you can narrow the choice to two options. If you are able to identify one response that is unrelated to prolonged impaired peripheral arterial circulation, you can eliminate two distractors and narrow the choice to two options.

1. **Yellow toenails and cool extremities both indicate impaired arterial circulation; there is a decrease in oxygen and nutrients to the area.**
2. Although yellow toenails indicate prolonged tissue hypoxia of the extremity, it is ascending pallor from the toes and descending rubor from the knees, not cyanosis, that reflect impaired peripheral arterial perfusion.
3. Although cool extremities reflect inadequate peripheral arterial perfusion, leg pain on

activity (intermittent claudication), not continuous leg discomfort, is a clinical manifestation of chronic peripheral arterial disease.
4. Leg discomfort related to decreased peripheral arterial perfusion is usually intermittent and associated with activity (intermittent claudication). Pallor ascending from the toes and rubor descending from the knees, not cyanosis, reflect moderate chronic impaired peripheral arterial perfusion.

7. **TEST-TAKING TIP** The "ox" in "oximetry" in the stem and the word "oxygen" in option 4 are similar because they both begin with the letters "ox." This is an obscure clang association.

1. The heart rate is obtained by palpating a peripheral pulse or auscultating the apical pulse.
2. Temperature is measured by a thermometer, pulse by palpation, respirations by observation, and blood pressure by a sphygmomanometer.
3. Blood pressure is measured by a sphygmomanometer.
4. **Oxygen saturation via pulse oximetry measures the degree to which hemoglobin is saturated with oxygen; it provides some indication of the efficiency of lung ventilation.**

8. **TEST-TAKING TIP** The word "most" in the stem sets a priority. The words "dramatic increase" are key words in the stem that direct attention to content. The word "individual" in the stem and in option 2 is a clang association.

1. A fever causes an increase in a person's metabolic rate; however, a fever does not place as high a demand on the body's need for oxygen as a factor in another option.
2. **Most exercise dramatically increases the metabolic rate, which, in turn, increases the body's demand for oxygen.**
3. Although a pregnant woman's metabolic rate is increased, pregnancy does not place as high a demand on the body's need for oxygen as a factor in another option.
4. General anesthesia relaxes the muscles of the body; when muscles are relaxed, the metabolic rate decreases and the demand for oxygen also decreases.

9. **TEST-TAKING TIP** The word "most" in the stem sets a priority.

1. **A cough forcefully expels air from the lungs and is an effective self-protective**

reflex to clear the trachea and bronchi of secretions.

2. An incentive spirometer is a device used to encourage voluntary deep breathing, not to clear an airway; it is used to prevent or treat atelectasis.

3. A nebulizer treatment does not clear an airway; it adds moisture or medication to inspired air to alter the tracheobronchial mucosa. After the respiratory passages are dilated or mucolytic agents have reduced the viscosity of secretions, the patient can cough more productively.

4. Abdominal breathing does not clear the air passages. It helps to decrease air trapping and reduce the work of breathing.

10. **TEST-TAKING TIP The word "most" in the stem sets a priority. The word "accurately" is the key word in the stem that directs attention to content.**

1. Although the hematocrit is the percentage of red blood cell mass in proportion to whole blood, it is not an accurate test for adequacy of tissue oxygenation; a low hematocrit may indicate possible water intoxication, and an increased hematocrit may indicate dehydration.

2. Although hemoglobin is the red pigment in red blood cells that carries oxygen, it is not an accurate test for adequacy of tissue oxygenation; a decreased hemoglobin value is evidence of iron-deficiency anemia or bleeding.

3. **Arterial blood gases include the levels of oxygen, carbon dioxide, bicarbonate, and pH. Blood gases determine the adequacy of alveolar gas exchange and the ability of the lungs and kidneys to maintain acid-base balance of body fluids.**

4. Pulmonary function tests measure lung volume and capacity; although these tests provide valuable information, they do not provide specific data about tissue oxygenation.

11. 1. **Because of the energy required to "fight" an infection, the basal metabolic rate increases, resulting in an increased respiratory rate (tachypnea).**

2. The body has a need to exhale, not retain, carbon dioxide.

3. Tachypnea occurs in the presence of increased levels of carbon dioxide and

carbonic acid, not decreased carbon dioxide levels.

4. The patient with an infection is more likely to be experiencing metabolic acidosis; tachypnea that progresses to hyperventilation causes respiratory alkalosis.

12. 1. Sounds caused by fluid in the alveoli of the lung are called *crackles* or *rales*, and sounds caused by fluid or resistance in the bronchi of the lung are called *rhonchi* or *gurgles*.

2. Positioning is unrelated to adventitious breath sounds (abnormal breath sounds).

3. *Wheezes* occur as air passes through airways narrowed by secretions, edema, or tumors; these high-pitched squeaky musical sounds are best heard on expiration and usually are not changed by coughing.

4. A *pleural friction rub* is a superficial grating sound heard particularly at the height of inspiration and not relieved by coughing; it is caused by the rubbing together of inflamed pleural surfaces.

13. **TEST-TAKING TIP Options 1 and 4 are opposites. In option 1 respirations are shallow and irregular. In option 4 respirations have a high depth and are regular.**

1. Recurring pattern of quick, shallow respiration alternating with irregular periods of apnea is characteristic of Biot's respiration. Biot's respiration is associated with neurological problems such as damage to the pons as a result of brain attack, trauma, or uncal or tentorial herniation.

2. Repeating pattern of increasing rate and depth of respiration alternating with apnea is characteristic of Cheyne-Stokes respiration. The breathing cycle begins with shallow breaths that gradually increase to an abnormal depth and rate, and then the breaths gradually become slower and shallower until there is a period of apnea, and the cycle begins again. Cheyne-Stokes respiration is associated with heart failure; and chronic pulmonary edema; and events that damage the respiratory center of the brain such as brain attack, encephalitis, and tumors or metastatic disease causing increased intracranial pressure.

3. Labored respiration, with breathlessness, that is possibly painful is known as dyspnea. Various medical conditions that

impair the ability of the lungs to exchange oxygen and carbon dioxide such as asthma; emphysema; tumors, interstitial lung disease; congestive heart failure; cardiac ischemia; and infections such as bronchitis, pneumonia, or tuberculosis can precipitate dyspnea.

4. **A high rate and depth of respiration is known as Kussmaul respiration. It is the body's effort to correct severe metabolic acidosis, particularly diabetic ketoacidosis (DKA), by blowing of excess carbon dioxide. Kussmaul respirations also are associated with renal failure.**

14. 1. Perfusion relates to the extent of inflow and outflow of air between the alveoli and pulmonary capillaries or the extent of blood flow to the pulmonary capillary bed; perfusion is not related to red blood cell levels.
    2. Diffusion occurs at the alveolar capillary beds and is not related to anemia.
    3. Exchange of oxygen occurs in the capillary beds of the alveoli via the process of diffusion; this is unrelated to anemia.
    4. **The hemoglobin portion of red blood cells transports oxygen from the alveolar capillaries in the lungs to distant tissue sites.**

15. **TEST-TAKING TIP** The words "productive cough" are the key words in the stem that direct attention to content.
    1. A productive cough may or may not produce pain, depending on the patient's underlying condition.
    2. **A productive cough is a cough accompanied by expectorated secretions. When a patient raises respiratory secretions and expectorates them, breathing usually improves.**
    3. Although coughing does interfere with breathing, this is not the definition of a productive cough.
    4. When a cough is productive, it does not indicate that it is progressive.

16. **TEST-TAKING TIP** The word "most" in the stem sets a priority. Options 1 and 2 are equally plausible. Both options address using less salt when preparing food. The word "medication" in the stem and in option 3 is a clang association.
    1. Although advising that salt should not be added to cooked foods is important, it is not the priority information. Salt promotes fluid retention, which will

increase the circulating blood volume and thus the blood pressure.
    2. Although advising that salt should not be added during food preparation is important, it is not the priority information. Restricting salt in the diet will help limit fluid retention and thus reduce the blood pressure. However, it is not as effective as another intervention.
    3. **The most effective way to lower the blood pressure is to take the prescribed antihypertensive medication daily.**
    4. It is not necessary to take daily blood pressure measurements unless specifically ordered to do so by the primary healthcare provider.

17. **TEST-TAKING TIP** The word "most" in the stem sets a priority.
    1. **The earlobe has adequate circulation to obtain an accurate oxygen saturation reading. Earrings can be removed.**
    2. A toe is an inappropriate site to obtain an accurate oxygen saturation reading in a patient who has peripheral vascular disease. An extremity must have adequate blood flow and be clean and dry for an accurate reading to be obtained. Recent studies indicate that most nail polish does not significantly interfere with accurate results in healthy individuals. Many facilities have nail polish remover pads to remove nail polish before applying a pulse oximetry probe.
    3. Acrylic nails interfere with signal transmission, resulting in inaccurate oxygen saturation results.
    4. The bridge of the nose is an inappropriate site to obtain an oxygen saturation reading in a patient who is experiencing shortness of breath.

18. 1. Raising the head of the bed should be done when the patient is finished vomiting. Raising the head of the bed will facilitate respirations by allowing the abdominal contents to drop by gravity, thereby not exerting pressure against the diaphragm.
    2. **Turning the patient to a side-lying position will permit the vomitus to exit the mouth by gravity. This will prevent the vomitus from flowing to the back of the oropharynx, where it can enter the respiratory tract when the patient inhales (aspiration).**
    3. Giving oxygen may or may not be done when the patient is done vomiting. The

use of oxygen will depend on the patient's respiratory status.

4. Continuing suctioning the patient's oral cavity while the patient is gagging and vomiting is unrealistic and traumatic. The vomitus can still enter the respiratory tract when the patient inhales (aspiration).

19. 1. **X The act of chewing (mastication) is facilitated by taking smaller portions of food at a time in the mouth. The risk for aspiration increases when the mouth is overwhelmed by a large volume of food at one time.**

2. _____ Fluids before swallowing can flush food into the breathing passages rather than down the esophagus.

3. **X Well-chewed food is broken down and mixed with saliva, forming a bolus of food; a bolus of food that is well chewed is easier to swallow, causing less risk for aspiration.**

4. _____ Talking while eating can increase the risk for aspiration. People should not talk with food in their mouths; people need to inhale before talking and this action may cause aspiration of food when food is in the mouth.

5. **X Cutting meat into small pieces provides food that may be easier to chew; the patient still must take the time to chew the food adequately before attempting to swallow.**

20. Answer: 14 mL
One kilogram is equal to 2.2 pounds; therefore, divide 31 pounds by 2.2 kilograms to determine the child's weight in kilograms (31 pounds ÷ 2.2 kilograms = 14 kilograms). To determine the child's daily dose multiply the child's weight in kilograms by the prescribed dose per kilogram (14 kilograms × 100 mg = 1400 mg total daily dose). To determine the amount of mg per dose divide the total daily dose by 4 (1400 mg total daily dose ÷ 4 doses daily = 350 mg per dose). Solve the rest of the problem using ratio and proportion.

$$\frac{\text{Desire}}{\text{Have}} \quad \frac{350 \text{ mg}}{125 \text{ mg}} = \frac{x \text{ mL}}{5 \text{ mL}}$$

$125 \text{ x} = 350 \times 5$

$125 \text{ x} = 1750$

$x = 1750 \div 125$

$x = 14 \text{ mL per dose}$

21. **TEST-TAKING TIP The word "feet" in the stem and in options 2, 4, and 5 are clang associations.**

1. _____ Applying moisturizing lotion to the feet keeps skin supple. However, moisturizing lotion should not be applied between the toes because doing so supports fungal and bacterial growth. Also, it can macerate the skin.

2. **X Checking the feet using a mirror to monitor all surfaces daily is an excellent way to identify problems early.**

3. _____ People with impaired circulation to the feet should always wear sturdy, well-fitting, closed-toe shoes to protect the feet from injury.

4. **X Warm socks and blankets should be used when the feet are cold because heating pads and hot water bottles may cause burns. Often people with impaired circulation to the feet also have reduced sensation, which predisposes them to failing to identify injury to the feet.**

5. **X Reporting a break in the skin or injury to feet to a primary health-care provider ensures that the patient receives appropriate medical intervention in the way of topical or systemic treatment to prevent infection and/or to facilitate healing.**

22. The right lung has three lobes: the right upper lobe (RUL), right middle lobe (RML), and right lower lobe (RLL). Using the lateral approach, the right middle lobe is auscultated above the eighth rib in front of the anterior axillary line.

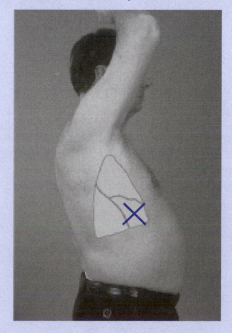

23 **TEST-TAKING TIP** Options 3 and 4 are opposite to option 5. The word "pain" in the stem and in option 2 is a clang association.

1. <u>X</u> The patient's vital signs should be taken and compared with baseline data. Alterations in vital signs may reflect a cardiopulmonary event (e.g., angina, myocardial infarction, pulmonary embolus).

2. <u>X</u> A detailed pain assessment (e.g., description, intensity, location, precipitating activity) will help the primary health-care provider to establish a diagnosis.

3. ____ Walking should be avoided; activity increases the demand on the heart and will increase the pain.

4. <u>X</u> Reducing activity and bedrest decreases the oxygen demand on the heart; this, in turn, will limit the pain. After the activity is interrupted, the nurse should obtain the vital signs and conduct a thorough pain assessment.

5. ____ Standing still will continue to place a demand on the heart and should be avoided. The pain may take a long time to subside.

24. 1. ____ Skeletal changes do not occur with clubbing of the fingers.

2. ____ The endocrine system commonly is not related to the development of clubbing of the fingers. However, hyperthyroidism is associated with about 1% of individuals who develop clubbing of the fingers.

3. <u>X</u> Diseases of the respiratory system and another system account for 80% of individuals who develop clubbing of the fingers. Clubbing of the fingers generally is caused by chronic hypoxia. Clubbing of the fingernails involves the loss of the normal Lovibond angle between the nail bed and the cuticle, a softening of the nail bed, and convexity of the nail. In addition, the finger develops a "drumstick" appearance resulting from proliferation of soft tissue around the terminal phalanges of the fingers.

4. <u>X</u> Diseases of the cardiovascular system and another system account for 80% of individuals who develop clubbing of the fingers. Clubbing of the fingers generally is caused by chronic

hypoxia. Clubbing of the fingers involves the loss of the normal Lovibond angle between the nail bed and the cuticle, a softening of the nail bed, and convexity of the nail. In addition, the finger develops a "drumstick" appearance resulting from proliferation of soft tissue around the terminal phalanges of the fingers.

5. ____ Diseases of the gastrointestinal system are the cause in only about 5% of individuals who develop clubbing of the fingernails. Diseases include inflammatory bowel disease; sprue; and neoplasms of the esophagus, liver, and bowel.

25. Answer: 4, 6, 1, 5, 2, 3

4. Place in the high-Fowler position. The patient's respiratory status should be supported initially and then the other orders can be implemented in order of importance. The high-Fowler position allows the abdominal organs to drop by gravity, which promotes expansion of the thorax on inhalation.

6. Begin oxygen via nasal cannula at 2 L/min. The administration of exogenous oxygen increases the amount of oxygen being delivered to the alveoli.

1. Obtain vital signs. Obtaining the vital signs collects information that provides critical baseline information about the patient. The time it takes to obtain the vital signs may compromise the patient's respiratory status and should be done after other more important interventions. This follows the ABCs (Airway, Breathing, Circulation) of meeting a patient's basic needs.

5. Obtain sputum for culture and sensitivity. After the patient's respiratory status is supported and assessed, then the sputum can be collected for the culture and sensitivity test. This specimen should be collected before the administration of any antibiotic that may alter test results.

2. Administer the ciprofloxacin (Cipro). Administering the ciprofloxacin after the sputum specimen for culture and sensitivity is obtained prevents erroneous test results.

3. Order a regular diet dinner. Finally, the regular diet can be ordered; this is the least critical intervention for this patient.

26. **TEST-TAKING TIP** The words "after meals" are key words in the stem that direct attention to content.

    1. _____ A high-Fowler, not a low-Fowler, position facilitates food retention by gravity.
    2. **X Keeping the head of the bed elevated promotes retention of food in the stomach rather that permitting regurgitation, which increases the risk for aspiration.**
    3. _____ Frequent mouth care provides comfort, but it does not reduce the risk of aspiration.
    4. _____ Fluids can be easily aspirated by a patient who has difficulty swallowing; fluid intake should be supervised.
    5. **X Patients who have difficulty swallowing do not recognize that food can become trapped in the buccal cavity and eventually be aspirated.**

27. **TEST-TAKING TIP** The word "most" in the stem sets a priority.

    1. **X Because of the small lumens of their respiratory passages, infants and toddlers are at serious risk for airway obstruction as a result of a respiratory tract infection. Obstruction may occur because of edema and/or mucus plugs.**
    2. **X As the respiratory system undergoes changes during the aging process there is a decline in respiratory function (e.g., less thoracic expansion, less alveoli and thoracic recoil, larger dead space). In addition, older adults have less efficient immune systems.**
    3. _____ Healthy adolescents usually do not encounter any serious event in response to respiratory infections.
    4. _____ Healthy young adults usually do not encounter any serious event in response to respiratory infection.
    5. _____ Healthy school-age children usually do not encounter any serious event in response to respiratory infections; however, school-age children generally have respiratory infections more frequently because of exposure to other children.

28. 1. These are the instructions for using an incentive spirometer. An incentive spirometer is designed to have a person deep breathe and expand the lungs to help prevent respiratory complications of immobility.

    2. These are the instructions for using a nebulizer, which is the device in the photograph. A nebulizer is a medication delivery system that produces an aerosol spray, which is inhaled via a mouthpiece. Breathing deeply and slowly facilitates contact of the medication with the respiratory tract mucosa.
    3. These are instructions for assessing tidal volume. Tidal volume is the volume of air inhaled and exhaled with each normal breath, which is approximately 500 mL.
    4. These are the instructions for using a peak expiratory flow meter (PEFM), which measures the peak expiratory flow rate (PEFR). A peak expiratory flow rate is the volume of air that can be forcefully exhaled after taking in a deep breath.

29. 1. This pattern represents eupnea. Eupnea is easy, normal respirations that are equal in depth and have a regular rhythm. The expected respiratory rate of a healthy individual is between 12 to 20 breaths per minute.
    2. This pattern represents tachypnea. Tachypnea is a respiratory rate that exceeds 20 breaths per minute.
    3. This pattern represents Cheyne-Stokes respirations. Cheyne-Stokes respirations are slow, shallow respirations that gradually increase in depth and frequency and then gradually decrease in depth and frequency until they once again are slow and shallow.
    4. **This pattern represents bradypnea. Bradypnea is a respiratory rate that is less than 12 breaths per minute.**

30. **TEST-TAKING TIP** The word "first" in the stem sets a priority.

    1. These actions waste critical minutes when interventions that support respirations should be implemented.
    2. Although both these actions are important, the patient's immediate oxygen needs should be met first.
    3. **These are the two actions that should be implemented immediately. The patient's responses indicate a pulmonary embolus, which can be life threatening. Elevating the head of the bed facilitates ventilation by lowering abdominal structures, permitting easier expansion of the lungs on inspiration. The head of the bed should not be elevated**

higher than 60 degrees to prevent excessive hip flexion that can cause dislocation of the hip prosthesis. Oxygen can be provided without a primary health-care provider's order in an emergency.

4. Although these actions are important, the actions in other options should be implemented first. The nurse needs a primary health-care provider's order to initiate an IV infusion.

31. 1. **X Rinsing the mouth removes any remaining medication. This prevents irritation to the oral mucosa and tongue as well as oral fungal infections.**

2. **X Waiting between puffs of the inhaler allows time for the medication from the first puff to be absorbed.**

3. ____ Rolling the canister between the hands slowly before using the inhaler may not mix the medication adequately and result in an inadequate dose. The canister should be shaken several times before use.

4. ____ When an extender (spacer) is used with a metered-dose inhaler the mouthpiece of the extender should be placed in the mouth over the tongue with the teeth and lips tightly around the mouthpiece.

5. ____ The patient should be in an upright (standing, sitting, or high-Fowler) position to promote lung expansion when inhaling.

32. Answer: 7.5 mL
Solve the problem using ratio and proportion.

$$\frac{\text{Desire}}{\text{Have}} \quad \frac{45 \text{ mg}}{6 \text{ mg}} = \frac{x \text{ mL}}{1 \text{ mL}}$$

6 x = 45

x = 45 ÷ 6

x = 7.5 mL

33. **TEST-TAKING TIP The word "most" in the stem sets a priority.**

The carotid artery should be assessed during CPR because a person in cardiac arrest reduces circulation to the extremities in an attempt to perfuse core organs. Therefore, a carotid artery may have a pulse while the pulses at other sites are weak or absent.

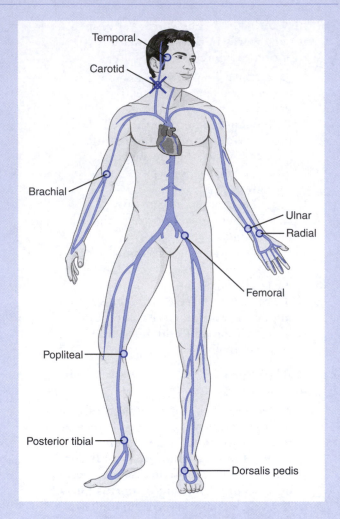

34. **TEST-TAKING TIP The word "both" is the key word in the stem that directs attention to content. The interventions chosen must increase both circulation and respiration.**

1. ____ The use of a spirometer only helps to prevent respiratory complications.

2. **X Repositioning the patient every 2 hours helps prevent fluid from collecting in lung fields, which can contribute to infection and interfere with respiration. Repositioning the patient also relieves pressure and increases activity, thereby promoting circulation.**

3. ____ Massaging bony prominences with lotion only increases local circulation.

4. **X Ambulation requires the upright position that relieves pressure against body tissues. The activity of walking increases cardiac output that will increase circulation. Also, the activity of walking increases the oxygen demands on the body that will increase the depth and rate of respirations.**

5. ____ Coughing and deep breathing only help to prevent respiratory complications. Also, coughing and deep breathing should be performed hourly when awake.

35. **TEST-TAKING TIP The words "prevent aspiration" are key words in the stem that direct attention to content. The word "bed" in the stem and in option 3 is a clang association. The word "feeding" in the stem and in option 5 is a clang association.**

1. ____ Lowering the height of the bag containing the feeding formula only slows the rate of the feeding if it is infusing by gravity; it does not halt its flow. Continuing the feeding adds a volume of fluid that may be aspirated. Lowering the height of the bag containing the feeding formula will have no effect on the rate of flow of the formula if it is being regulated by an infusion pump.

2. ____ The administration of a volume of feeding may promote aspiration.

3. **X The head of the bed should remain elevated during the bath and linen change. The bed can be made from the top of the bed to the foot of the bed rather than from side to side. Elevation of the head of the bed keeps the feeding in the stomach by gravity.**

4. ____ Seeking additional assistance does not reduce the risk of aspiration.

5. **X Shutting off the feeding reduces the risk of aspiration by temporarily halting the administration of a volume of feeding.**

ADMINISTRATION OF MEDICATIONS

This section includes questions related to the principles associated with the administration of medications via the oral, parenteral (intravenous, intramuscular, intradermal, and subcutaneous injections), topical, ear, eye, vaginal, and rectal routes. The questions focus on allergies, untoward effects, toxic effects, developmental considerations associated with medications, the Z-track method, peak and trough levels of medications, pain assessment before administering medication for pain, and computation of dosage.

QUESTIONS

1. A nurse changes the needle of the syringe after drawing up the required dose of a caustic medication. Which factor about the needle necessitates changing the needle after drawing up the caustic medication?
   1. It is too long for the required route.
   2. It is coated with the medication.
   3. It is no longer sterile.
   4. It is not sharp.

   TEST-TAKING TIP Identify the clang association. Identify the unique option.

2. A nurse must administer a 2-mL intramuscular injection to an adult patient who is in severe pain and lying in the supine position. Which muscle is the safest for the nurse to use to administer an intramuscular injection to this patient?
   1. Deltoid
   2. Dorsogluteal
   3. Ventrogluteal
   4. Vastus lateralis

   TEST-TAKING TIP Identify the word in the stem that sets a priority. Identify the key word in the stem that directs attention to content. Identify equally plausible options.

3. At which angle should the nurse insert a ½-inch needle when administering insulin?
   1. 30 degrees
   2. 45 degrees
   3. 90 degrees
   4. 180 degrees

   TEST-TAKING TIP Identify key words in the stem that direct attention to content.

4. A nurse is administering oral medications to children. Which is the **most** important factor that the nurse must consider?
   1. Age
   2. Weight
   3. Level of anxiety
   4. Developmental level

   TEST-TAKING TIP Identify the word in the stem that sets a priority. Identify the key word in the stem that directs attention to content.

5. A patient is receiving an intravenous piggyback (IVPB) medication every 4 hours. Because the medication has a narrow therapeutic window, a peak blood level is ordered. When should the nurse plan to obtain a blood specimen for this test?
   1. Three hours after administering a dose
   2. One hour before administering a dose
   3. Halfway between two scheduled doses
   4. One hour after administering a dose

   TEST-TAKING TIP Identify opposites in options. Identify equally plausible options.

6. Besides inhibiting microbial growth, an antibiotic may also depress the bone marrow. In which category is the depression of bone marrow classified?
   1. Overdose
   2. Side effect
   3. Habituation
   4. Idiosyncratic effect

7. Which route of administration is used only for its local therapeutic effect?
   1. Rectum
   2. Nose
   3. Skin
   4. Eye

   TEST-TAKING TIP Identify key words in the stem that direct attention to content.

8. A nurse plans to inject an intravenous medication via an existing intravenous line. Which should the nurse do **first?**
   1. Determine the patency of the intravenous line.
   2. Select the port closest to the needle entry site.
   3. Pinch the tubing above the port being used.
   4. Clean the injection port with an antiseptic.

   TEST-TAKING TIP Identify the word in the stem that sets a priority. Identify the clang association.

9. A nurse is filling a syringe with medication from a multiple-dose vial. Which should the nurse do?
   1. Keep the needle above the level of the liquid and maintain sterile technique.
   2. Keep the needle below the level of the liquid and record the date and time on the vial when opened.
   3. Keep the needle below the level of the liquid and change the needle after withdrawing the solution.
   4. Keep the needle above the level of the liquid and inject air at 1.5 times the volume of the prescribed dose.

   TEST-TAKING TIP Identify duplicate facts among options. Identify the clang association.

10. A nurse is administering an intradermal injection to a patient. For which response is this patient at the highest risk?
    1. Interaction with other drugs
    2. Idiosyncratic reaction
    3. Allergic response
    4. Overdose

    TEST-TAKING TIP Identify the word in the stem that sets a priority. Identify the key word in the stem that directs attention to content.

11. A nurse is preparing to instill a vaginal cream. Which position should the nurse instruct the patient to assume?
    1. Dorsal recumbent position
    2. Low-Fowler position
    3. Left-lateral position
    4. Supine position

12. Which does the nurse conclude is the **most** dangerous route of administering medication?
    1. Intravenous push
    2. Piggyback infusion
    3. Subcutaneous injection
    4. Intramuscular injection

    TEST-TAKING TIP Identify the word in the stem that sets a priority.

13. A nurse is administering a drug via the Z-track injection method. Which action is unique to this procedure?
1. The injection sites are rotated along a "Z" pattern on the abdomen.
2. A "Z" is formed when dividing the buttocks into quadrants.
3. An air lock is established behind the bolus of medication.
4. The skin is pulled laterally before needle insertion.

TEST-TAKING TIP Identify key words in the stem that direct attention to content.

14. Peak and trough levels are ordered to monitor the plasma profile of an antibiotic. When should the nurse plan for a blood specimen to be drawn when measuring the trough level of the drug?
1. First thing in the morning
2. Halfway between scheduled doses
3. A half hour before a scheduled dose
4. A half hour after drug administration

TEST-TAKING TIP Identify the key word in the stem that directs attention to content. Identify opposites in options.

15. Via which area of the body should the nurse administer a medication that is in the form of a troche?
1. Rectal vault
2. Buccal cavity
3. Vaginal vault
4. Auditory canal

16. A nurse concludes that a transdermal patch is the **most** effective method for the delivery of an analgesic for a patient with cancer. Which rationale supports the nurse's conclusion?
1. Releases controlled amounts of medication over time
2. Produces fewer side effects than other routes
3. Affects only the area covered by the patch
4. Has an immediate systemic effect

TEST-TAKING TIP Identify the word in the stem that sets a priority. Identify opposites in options. Identify the option with a specific determiner.

17. Which route is considered to be the **most** desirable when administering medications?
1. Via injection
2. Intravenous
3. By mouth
4. Topical

TEST-TAKING TIP Identify the word in the stem that sets a priority.

18. Which site should the nurse use for a subcutaneous injection to ensure its **most** rapid absorption?
1. Abdomen
2. Buttock
3. Thigh
4. Arm

TEST-TAKING TIP Identify the word in the stem that sets a priority.

19. Medication is prescribed for an infant that must be administered via an intramuscular injection. Which muscle should the nurse use to administer the injection?
1. Deltoid
2. Dorsogluteal
3. Ventrogluteal
4. Rectus femoris

TEST-TAKING TIP Identify the unique option.

20. Which route of delivery for medication should be administered cautiously by the nurse if the patient is an older adult who is cachectic?
1. Intradermal
2. Intravenous
3. Subcutaneous
4. Intramuscular

TEST-TAKING TIP Identify the key word in the stem that directs attention to content. Identify the unique option.

21. A nurse is caring for a 2-year-old child who has an order for intravenous (IV) fluids. The nurse is unable to obtain an intravenous volume control device and decides to administer the IV via gravity. An IV administration set with which drop factor is **most** appropriate for the nurse to use when initiating this IV?
1. 10
2. 15
3. 20
4. 60

TEST-TAKING TIP Identify the word in the stem that sets a priority.

22. A patient is admitted to the hospital with a diagnosis of congestive heart failure and pulmonary edema. Furosemide 30 mg IM STAT is prescribed for a patient. The available Lasix is 10 mg/mL. Indicate how much solution of Lasix the nurse should administer by shading in the area on the syringe.

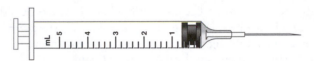

23. An antihypertensive agent is prescribed for a patient. Place the following steps in the order in which they should be performed by the nurse.
1. Verify the order.
2. Perform hand hygiene.
3. Obtain the patient's blood pressure.
4. Assist the patient to take the medication.
5. Place single-dose packages in a medication cup.
6. Check the patient's identification and allergy bands.

Answer: _____

24. Ear drops are prescribed for an adult patient. Which should the nurse do when instilling ear drops into the patient's ear? **Select all that apply.**
1. _____ Press a cotton ball gently into the ear canal.
2. _____ Pull the pinna of the ear upward and backward.
3. _____ Tug the pinna of the ear downward and backward.
4. _____ Direct the flow of fluid against the wall of the ear canal.
5. _____ Hold a dropper approximately two inches above the ear canal.

TEST-TAKING TIP Identify the key word in the stem that directs attention to content. Identify opposites in options.

25. Which question should the nurse ask a female patient before administering a medication that is teratogenic?
1. _____ "Have you ever had an anaphylactic reaction?"
2. _____ "Have you been using birth control?"
3. _____ "Were you ever addicted to drugs?"
4. _____ "Do you have any allergies?"
5. _____ "Are you pregnant?"

26. Place an X where the nurse should look along a primary administration set to determine if an IV solution, infusing by gravity, is running at the rate ordered.

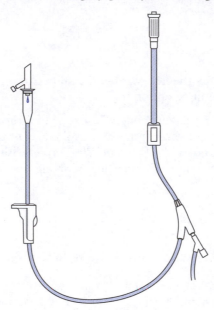

27. A nurse is checking medication prescriptions written by a primary health-care provider. Identify the prescriptions that the nurse should consult with the provider about to clarify the prescription because components of the orders do not meet standards identified by The Joint Commission. **Select all that apply.**
    1. ____ Morphine sulfate 2 mg IV every 2 hours prn for severe incisional pain
    2. ____ Gentamicin ophthalmic solution 2 gtts AU qid
    3. ____ Regular insulin 5 units sub-Q STAT
    4. ____ Docusate sodium 100 mg PO qd
    5. ____ Alprazolam .5 mg PO tid

    TEST-TAKING TIP Identify the words in the stem that indicate negative polarity.

28. Which statements indicate to the nurse that the patient understands teaching regarding the self-administration of eye medication? **Select all that apply.**
    1. ____ "I can wipe away excess ointment on my eyelid."
    2. ____ "I should gaze upward while instilling eye drop medication."
    3. ____ "I should close my eyes tightly after the medicine is in my eye."
    4. ____ "I should place one drop of the medication inside my lower eyelid."
    5. ____ "I can easily transmit the infection from one eye to the other if I do not use precautions."

29. A nurse is administering an oral medication to a patient. Which should the nurse do to **best** protect the patient from aspiration? **Select all that apply.**
    1. ____ Offer extra water.
    2. ____ Put crushed tablets in applesauce.
    3. ____ Give the patient one tablet at a time.
    4. ____ Position the patient in a sitting position.
    5. ____ Inspect the mouth after the patient swallows.

    TEST-TAKING TIP Identify the word in the stem that sets a priority.

30. Ibuprofen 400 mg PO twice a day is prescribed for a patient. On hand is ibuprofen 200 mg per tablet. How many tablets should the nurse administer? **Record your answer using a whole number.**

    Answer: _____ tablets

31. A patient has a prescription for regular insulin 20 units subcutaneously STAT. Which syringe should the nurse use to administer this medication?

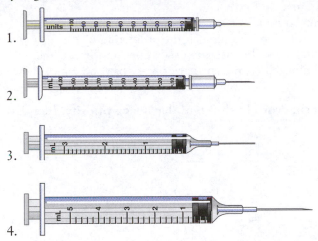

1.

2.

3.

4.

32. A nurse is administering medications to a group of older adults. For which responses specifically related to aging should the nurse assess these patients? **Select all that apply.**
1. ____ Toxicity
2. ____ Side effects
3. ____ Drug interactions
4. ____ Allergic reactions
5. ____ Teratogenic effects

TEST-TAKING TIP Identify key words in the stem that direct attention to content.

33. A nurse is evaluating a mother's ability to administer nose drops to her child. Which actions indicate that the mother is administering the nose drops correctly? **Select all that apply.**
1. ____ Encouraging sniffing the medication into the lungs
2. ____ Allowing the sitting position after the medication is given
3. ____ Tilting the head backward before instilling the medication
4. ____ Putting the remaining medication in the dropper back into the bottle
5. ____ Positioning the dropper a third of an inch inside the nares without touching the sides of the nostril

TEST-TAKING TIP Identify key words in the stem that direct attention to content.

34. A nurse must administer a prescribed medication via the rectal route. Place the following steps in the order in which they should be implemented.
1. Position the patient in the Sims position.
2. Use water-soluble jelly to lubricate the suppository.
3. Instruct the patient to remain in a side-lying position for at least 10 minutes.
4. Determine if there are any contraindications to the insertion of a suppository.
5. Insert the suppository 1 to 3 inches past the internal sphincter using an index finger.

Answer: _____

35. When making rounds the nurse identifies the following situation with an intravenous secondary (intravenous piggy back, IVPB) infusion that is attached to a primary infusion. What should the nurse do **first**?
1. Document that the secondary infusion is completed.
2. Ensure that the primary infusion is running at the ordered rate.
3. Remove the secondary infusion administration set from the primary line.
4. Document what was administed via the current primary bag and hang a new primary bag.

TEST-TAKING TIP Identify the word in the stem that sets a priority. Identify clang associations.

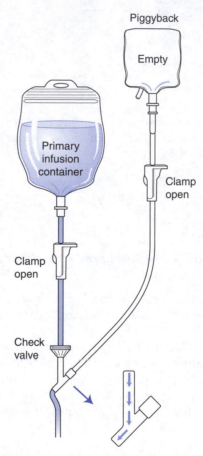

36. A liquid medication is prescribed for a patient who has the diagnosis of dementia. The medication has an unpleasant taste and the manufacturer recommends that it be stored in a refrigerator. What should the nurse plan to do when administering this medication? **Select all that apply.**
1. _____ Warm it to room temperature before the medication is administered.
2. _____ Provide oral hygiene after the medication is administered.
3. _____ Use a needleless syringe to administer the medication.
4. _____ Check the mouth after administering the medication.
5. _____ Offer ice chips before administering the medication.

37. A nurse is caring for a patient with cancer who is experiencing pain at 7 p.m. (1900 hour). The nurse assesses the patient and reviews the patient's prescribed medications and the medication administration record. Which nursing intervention is **most** appropriate for this patient?
1. Notify the prescribing provider about the patient's status.
2. Wait 1 hour to give the prescribed hydromorphone 4 mg.
3. Administer the prescribed acetaminophen 650 mg.
4. Reassess the patient in 30 minutes.

PATIENT'S CLINICAL RECORD

Primary Health-Care Provider's Orders
Acetaminophen 325 mg PO every 6 hours for mild pain
Acetaminophen 650 mg PO every 4 hours for moderate pain
Hydromorphone 4 mg PO every 4 hours for severe pain

Medication Administration Record
0200: Acetaminophen 325 mg PO for mild abdominal pain (3 on 0 to 10 scale)
0800: Acetaminophen 650 mg PO for moderate abdominal pain (7 on 0 to 10 scale)
1200: Hydromorphone 4 mg PO for severe abdominal pain (8 on 0 to 10 scale)
1600: Hydromorphone 4 mg PO for severe abdominal pain (8 on 0 to 10 scale)

Patient Assessment
Patient reporting sharp abdominal pain of 9 on a scale of 0 to 10. Vital signs are: Pulse, 68 beats/min, regular rhythm; Respirations, 9 breaths/min, shallow, unlabored; BP, 106/72 mm Hg.

38. A patient has a prescription for albuterol 90 mcg/spray, 2 puffs via a metered-dose inhaler with a spacer every 12 hours. Place the following steps in the order in which they should be implemented by the nurse.
1. Breathe in deeply and slowly after activating the canister.
2. Seal the lips around the mouthpiece of the spacer.
3. Remove the cap and shake the canister well.
4. Rinse the mouth with water and spit it out.
5. Exhale fully through the mouth.

Answer: _____

39. Which parts of a syringe must remain sterile when drawing up medication from a vial and administering an injection? **Select all that apply.**
1. _____ Flange
2. _____ Plunger
3. _____ Needle hub
4. _____ Needle shaft
5. _____ Outside barrel

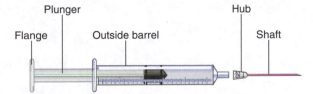

40. A nurse teaches a patient to self-administer eye drops. The nurse identifies that further teaching is needed when the patient says, "I should:
1. _____ Wipe my eye moving from the outer corner toward my nose."
2. _____ Hold the eyedropper about a half inch above my eye."
3. _____ Close my eyes gently after instilling the medication."
4. _____ Put the fluid in a pocket in the lower lid of my eye."
5. _____ Hold my upper eyelid up."

TEST-TAKING TIP Identify the word in the stem that indicates negative polarity.

1. **TEST-TAKING TIP** The word "medication" in the stem and option 2 is a clang association. Option 2 is unique. Options 1, 3, and 4 are all negative statements. In option 1, "too long" indicates that the needle is "not" the correct length.

   1. There is not enough information to come to this conclusion. There is no information in relation to whether the medication should be administered subcutaneously or intramuscularly.
   2. **Changing to a new needle prevents tracking the medication through the subcutaneous tissue and skin.**
   3. If all of the principles of sterile technique are followed when preparing an injection, the needle is still considered sterile.
   4. Most needles are made of stainless steel with a beveled tip that makes them sharp; they do not need to be replaced due to dullness after drawing up medication because they remain sharp.

2. **TEST-TAKING TIP** The word "safest" is the word in the stem that sets a priority and is the key word in the stem that directs attention to content. Options 2 and 3 are equally plausible because they both require repositioning the patient.

   1. The deltoid is not well developed in many adults and children. The radial and ulnar nerves and brachial artery lie in the upper arm along the humerus. The deltoid should not be used for intramuscular injections unless other sites are unavailable.
   2. To access the dorsogluteal site, the patient must be repositioned, which may increase pain. Historically, the dorsogluteal was the preferred site for an intramuscular injection; however, there is a higher risk of hitting the sciatic nerve, blood vessels, or greater trochanter. Hitting the sciatic nerve can cause partial or permanent paralysis of the leg.
   3. To access the ventrogluteal site, the patient must be repositioned, which may increase pain. The ventrogluteal is the preferred site after the vastus lateralis; it is safe to use in cachectic patients and children older than 18 months.
   4. **The vastus lateralis is the preferred site for this patient because this muscle has no major nearby nerves and blood vessels and absorbs drugs rapidly. In addition, using this muscle does not require the patient, who is in pain, to be moved and repositioned.**

3. **TEST-TAKING TIP** The words "½-inch needle" are key words in the stem that direct attention to content.

   1. A 30-degree angle is too shallow an angle for a subcutaneous injection.
   2. A 45-degree angle is too shallow for the administration of a subcutaneous injection with a needle that is only ½-inch long. A 45-degree angle is appropriate if the needle is ⅝-inch or 1-inch long.
   3. **A 90-degree angle is appropriate for a subcutaneous injection with a ½-inch needle; it injects the insulin into the loose connective tissue under the dermis.**
   4. To use a 180-degree angle for any injection is impossible. Various injection methods are from 15 degrees to 90 degrees, not 180 degrees.

4. **TEST-TAKING TIP** The word "most" in the stem sets a priority. The word "children" is the key word in the stem that directs attention to content.

   1. Age is not reliable for calculating a pediatric dose of medication.
   2. **Children's body sizes are different, necessitating calculation of drug dosage by weight, rather than by age or developmental level. Weight is an objective, specific, and accurate way to calculate appropriate medication dosages for children.**
   3. Level of anxiety does not influence calculation of dosage of medication for a child.
   4. Developmental level does not influence calculation of dosage of medication for a child.

5. **TEST-TAKING TIP** Options 2 and 4 are opposites. Options 1 and 2 are equally plausible because they both refer to 1 hour before administering a dose.

   1. A blood test taken 3 hours after administering a dose that is given every 4 hours will not provide an accurate peak blood level. A blood level 3 to 3½ hours after administration of a drug given every 4 hours provides information about a trough level.

2. A blood specimen taken 1 hour before administering a dose will not provide an accurate peak blood level. A blood level at 30 to 60 minutes before the next dose measures a trough level.

3. A blood level specimen taken halfway between two scheduled doses will not provide an accurate result when testing for a peak blood level for a drug administered every 4 hours.

4. **Most medications administered every 4 hours have a peak concentration about 1 hour after administration.**

6. 1. An overdose occurs when a person receives a dose larger than the usual recommended dose; this rarely is planned and usually is an accident/error.

2. **A side effect is a secondary effect. Side effects can be harmless or can cause injury; if injurious, the drug is discontinued.**

3. Habituation is an acquired tolerance from continued exposure to a substance.

4. An idiosyncratic effect is an unexpected effect; it can be an overreaction, an underreaction, or an unusual reaction.

7. **TEST-TAKING TIP** The words "only" and "local" are key words in the stem that direct attention to content.

1. Medication can be administered via the rectum for either a local or systemic effect; medications can be absorbed through the rich vascular bed in the mucous membranes.

2. Medication can be administered via the nose for either a local or systemic effect.

3. Medications can be administered via the skin for either a local or systemic effect.

4. **Medications are instilled into the eye only for their local effect; part of the procedure for instillation of eye drops is to apply gentle pressure to the naso-lacrimal duct for 10 to 15 seconds to prevent absorption of the medication into the systemic circulation.**

8. **TEST-TAKING TIP** The word "first" in the stem sets a priority. The words "intravenous line" in the stem and in option 1 is a clang association.

1. **For medication to enter a vein, the intravenous line must be unobstructed; therefore, the nurse should determine the patency of the intravenous line. The nurse must also ensure that the medication is administered into a vein, not into subcutaneous tissue.**

2. Although selecting the port closest to the catheter insertion site is part of the procedure, it is not what the nurse should do first.

3. Although pinching the tubing above the port being used is part of the procedure, it is not what the nurses should do first.

4. Although cleaning the injection port is part of the procedure, it is not what the nurse should do first.

9. **TEST-TAKING TIP** Options 1 and 4 contain a duplicate fact and options 2 and 3 contain a duplicate fact. If you know whether a needle should be kept above or below the level of fluid in a vial, you can reduce your final selection to two options. The word "vial" in the stem and in option 2 is a clang association.

1. Although sterile technique should be maintained, the bevel of the needle should be kept below the level of the fluid to prevent the syringe from filling with air.

2. **The bevel of the needle must be kept below the level of the fluid to prevent air from entering the syringe. Once opened, medications should be marked with the date and time of opening because medications generally have a recommended period of viability before they should be discarded.**

3. Although the bevel of the needle should be kept below the level of the fluid, changing the needle is unnecessary. The needle needs to be changed only when the solution is caustic to tissues.

4. The bevel of the needle should be kept below the level of the fluid or the syringe will fill with air. The amount of air injected into the vial should equal the amount of solution to be withdrawn; extra air will result in excessive pressure within the closed space of the vial.

10. **TEST-TAKING TIP** The word "highest" in the stem sets a priority. The word "intradermal" is the key word in the stem that directs attention to content.

1. A drug interaction occurs when one drug alters the action of another drug; this is not a possible response to a single intradermal injection.

2. Idiosyncratic reactions are unpredictable effects; they are usually underreactions, overreactions, or reactions that are different from the expected reaction. Idiosyncratic reactions are less likely to

occur than allergic reactions with intradermal injections.

3. **An intradermal injection is given under the skin to test for such things as tuberculosis and allergies; these drugs can cause an anaphylactic reaction if absorbed by the circulation too quickly or if the person has a hypersensitivity to the solution.**

4. Overdoses are a risk with all types of injections, but the highest risk of overdose is via the intravenous, not intradermal, route.

11. 1. **The dorsal recumbent position (supine position with the hips and knees bent) allows easy access to and exposure of the vaginal orifice. Lying in this position for 10 minutes after administration of the vaginal cream prevents its drainage from the vaginal canal.**

2. The low-Fowler position does not thoroughly expose the vaginal orifice.

3. The left-lateral position does not thoroughly expose the vaginal orifice. This position is used for the administration of enemas and rectal suppositories.

4. The supine position does not expose the vaginal orifice.

12. **TEST-TAKING TIP** The word "most" in the stem sets a priority.

1. **An IV push or bolus administration of medication is the instillation of a medication directly into a vein; this rapid administration of an entire dose of medication places the patient at highest risk for adverse effects.**

2. Although an intravenous piggyback is a dangerous route, the medication is diluted and it is infused over a longer time period than in an IV push.

3. A solution injected into subcutaneous tissue is absorbed over a longer period of time than an IV push.

4. A solution injected into a muscle is absorbed over a longer period of time than an IV push.

13. **TEST-TAKING TIP** The words "Z-track" and "unique" are key words in the stem that direct attention to content.

1. An intramuscular site, preferably the dorsogluteal, is used for Z-track, not the abdomen, which is used for subcutaneous injections.

2. The buttocks are not divided by a "Z." When the buttocks (dorsogluteal) are used for intramuscular injections, the usual bony landmarks must be used to identify the correct insertion site. The dorsogluteal site is no longer recommended because of its proximity to the sciatic nerve.

3. The air-lock technique also can be done with intramuscular injections. When air is injected behind the medication, the air clears the needle of medication. This technique is controversial and is being researched for evidenced-based practice.

4. **The "Z" in the Z-track method refers to pulling the skin to the side before and during an intramuscular injection. This technique alters the position of skin layers so that after the skin is released and the needle is removed, the injected fluid is kept within the muscle tissues and does not rise in the needle tract, which can irritate subcutaneous tissues.**

14. **TEST-TAKING TIP** The word "trough" is the key word in the stem that directs attention to content. Options 3 and 4 are opposites.

1. The peak and trough of a blood plasma level depend on the time the last dose was administered.

2. Halfway between scheduled doses will not be a time period when a drug is at its lowest concentration in the blood.

3. **"Trough level" refers to when a drug is at its lowest concentration in the blood in response to biotransformation; this usually occurs during the time period just before the next scheduled dose.**

4. Many variables affect the time when a drug reaches its peak plasma level within an individual; however, a half hour after the administration of an antibiotic, one can safely plot the antibiotic plasma level on the rising side of the curve of the plasma level profile, not within the trough.

15. 1. A suppository is designed for administering medication into the rectum.

2. **A troche (lozenge) is placed in the space between the upper or lower molar teeth and gums (buccal cavity)**

so that it can release medication as it dissolves.

3. A suppository, solution, or cream can be delivered to the vaginal vault by a vaginal applicator.

4. Medication in a suspension can be administered via a dropper into the auditory canal.

16. **TEST-TAKING TIP** The word "most" in the stem sets a priority. Options 1 and 4 are opposites. Option 3 contains the word "only," which is a specific determiner.

1. **Transdermal disks or patches have semipermeable membranes that allow medication to be absorbed through the skin slowly over a long period of time (usually 24 to 72 hours).**

2. The medication, not the route of delivery, produces side effects.

3. Transdermal disks or patches deliver medications that produce systemic effects.

4. The systemic effect depends on the amount of time it takes for the drug to be absorbed through the skin; this takes longer with a transdermal route than with parenteral routes.

17. **TEST-TAKING TIP** The word "most" in the stem sets a priority.

1. Administering a medication via an injection is not the most desirable route for medication administration. An injection carries a higher risk than medication administered via many other routes because the medication is rapidly absorbed and a needle enters the skin.

2. The intravenous route is not the most desirable route for medication administration. The intravenous route carries the highest risk because a needle enters the skin and the medication is delivered directly into the bloodstream.

3. **Using the oral route is the safest way to administer medication because it is convenient, it does not require piercing the skin, it usually does not cause physical or emotional stress, and the medication is absorbed slowly.**

4. Because absorption is affected by a variety of factors, such as the extent of the capillary network and condition of the skin, the topical route is not the most accurate and

therefore not the most desirable method of administration.

18. **TEST-TAKING TIP** The word "most" in the stem sets a priority.

1. **Subcutaneous tissue of the abdomen has a large capillary bed that facilitates absorption of injected medication.**

2. Medication injected into the buttocks is absorbed at a slower rate than medication injected into the abdomen.

3. Medication injected into the thigh is absorbed at the slowest rate.

4. Medication injected into the arm is absorbed at a slower rate than medication injected into the abdomen.

19. **TEST-TAKING TIP** Option 4 is unique because it is the only option with two words.

1. The deltoid muscle is contraindicated for intramuscular injections in infants and children. This site has a small amount of muscle mass and it lies close to the radial nerve and brachial artery.

2. The dorsogluteal muscle is contraindicated for an intramuscular injection in children younger than 18 months of age because the muscle mass is inadequate to allow a safe injection. Also, the sciatic nerve and gluteal artery lie close to the site.

3. An infant or toddler should not receive an intramuscular injection into the ventrogluteal muscle; the muscle is not well developed until the child begins to walk.

4. **The rectus femoris muscle, which belongs to the quadriceps muscle group, is the site of choice for intramuscular injections in infants and children. It is the largest and most well-developed muscle in infants, is easy to locate, and is away from major blood vessels and nerves.**

20. **TEST-TAKING TIP** The word "cachectic" is the key word in the stem that directs attention to content. Option 3 is unique because it begins with a word with "S" as the first letter, not with the prefix "Intra-."

1. An intradermal injection is administered by inserting the needle of a syringe through the epidermis into the dermis where the fluid is injected. This is a safe procedure in an older adult who is cachectic.

2. Intravenous medications can be administered safely to cachectic older adults.

3. **Older adults and cachectic individuals have a decrease in subcutaneous tissue. When a subcutaneous injection is administered to a patient with insufficient subcutaneous tissue, the medication usually is absorbed faster; this may be unsafe.**

4. Although muscle mass may be smaller in older adults and cachectic individuals, an intramuscular injection can be administered safely by using a 1-inch rather than a 1½-inch needle.

21. **TEST-TAKING TIP** The word "most" in the stem sets a priority.

1. Intravenous tubing with a drop factor of 10 represents 10 drops per 1 mL and is considered a macrodrip. It is difficult to regulate the rate of an IV with 10 drops per mL to children.

2. Intravenous tubing with a drop factor of 15 represents 15 drops per 1 mL and is considered a macrodrip. It is difficult to regulate the rate of an IV with 15 drops per mL to children.

3. Intravenous tubing with a drop factor of 20 represents 20 drops per 1 mL and is considered a macrodrip. It is difficult to regulate the rate of an IV with 20 drops per mL to children.

4. **Intravenous tubing with a drop factor of 60 represents 60 drops per 1 mL and is considered a microdrip. It is easier to regulate the rate of an IV with 60 drops per mL than it is to regulate tubing that requires fewer drops to deliver 1 mL, especially to children. Children usually receive less mL per hour than adults.**

22. **Answer: 3 mL**
Solve the problem using ratio and proportion.

$$\frac{\text{Desire}}{\text{Have}} \quad \frac{30 \text{ mg}}{10 \text{ mg}} = \frac{x \text{ mL}}{1 \text{mL}}$$

10x = 30

x = 30 ÷ 10

x = 3 mL

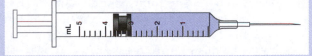

23. **Answer: 1, 2, 5, 6, 3, 4**
1. **Administering medication is a dependent function of the nurse. The nurse must verify the primary health-care provider's original prescription.**

2. **Verifying the prescription requires the nurse to touch a computer or a clinical record, both of which are considered contaminated objects. Hand hygiene reduces the number of microorganisms on the nurse's hands before touching a unit dose package that will be given to a patient.**

3. **A medicine cup permits the nurse to carry the medication to the patient without contaminating the medication; also, the single-dose package will not be wasted if the medication is not administered to the patient.**

4. **The identity of the patient must be verified before administering the medication to ensure that it will be given to the correct patient. The allergy band also should be checked to ensure that the patient is not allergic to the prescribed medication.**

5. **An antihypertensive agent is administered to decrease blood pressure. The patient's blood pressure should be obtained before administration and routinely after administration to determine if there has been a therapeutic response. Also, frequently the primary health-care provider or a protocol will indicate that the medication be held if the blood pressure is below a certain level.**

6. **The patient should be assisted to take the medication. The nurse may just open the package, drop the tablet into the medication cup, and hand the cup to the patient with a glass of water. Depending on the patient's needs, the nurse may use the medication cup to place the tablet in the patient's mouth followed by a sip of water or crush the tablet (if not enteric coated) and mix it with a teaspoonful of applesauce before administering it to the patient.**

24. **TEST-TAKING TIP** The word "adult" is the key word in the stem that directs attention to content. Options 2 and 3 are opposites.

1. _____ A cotton ball may be placed in the outermost part of the ear; it should not be pressed into the ear canal.

2. <u>X</u> **Pulling the pinna of the ear upward and backward straightens the ear canal of an adult. This action facilitates the distribution of the medication into the external ear canal.**

3. ____ The pinna of the ear should be pulled downward and backward to straighten the ear canal of a child younger than 3 years of age, not an adult.

4. <u>X</u> **Directing the flow of fluid against the wall of the ear canal prevents fluid from falling against the eardrum, which can cause trauma.**

5. ____ The force exerted by a drop falling from the height of 2 inches can injure the eardrum. The dropper should be held ½ inch (1 cm) above the ear canal, and the drop should fall against the wall of the canal and then flow toward the eardrum.

25. 1. ____ This question is unrelated to the concept of teratogenic. An anaphylactic reaction is a severe, systemic hypersensitivity to a drug, food, or chemical.

2. <u>X</u> **A drug that is teratogenic can cause adverse effects in an embryo or fetus. The prescribing of a drug that is teratogenic may be delayed until a pregnancy test confirms that the patient is not pregnant.**

3. ____ This question is unrelated to the concept of teratogenic. Drug addiction refers to an uncontrollable craving for a chemical substance because of a physical or psychological dependence.

4. ____ This question is unrelated to the concept of teratogenic. Allergies are unpredictable hypersensitive reactions to allergens such as drugs.

5. <u>X</u> **"Teratogenic," when used in the context of medication, refers to a drug that can cause adverse effects in an embryo or fetus.**

26. **The nurse should count the drops per minute falling in the drip chamber to determine if the intravenous solution is running at the rate ordered. The administration set indicates the number of drops per 1 mL (drop factor). The following formula can be used to determine the ordered rate, and then the product of that formula can be compared with the actual rate being delivered to the patient. Discrepancy between these rates indicates an inaccurate flow rate.**

$$\frac{\text{Total mL ordered} \times \text{the drop factor}}{\text{Total time in minutes}}$$

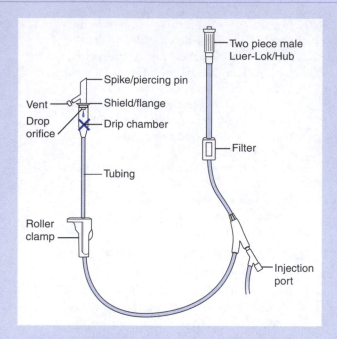

27. **TEST-TAKING TIP The words "do not meet standards" are the words in the stem that indicate negative polarity.**

1. ____ This is a correctly written prescription. It contains the medication spelled out (morphine sulfate). It contains the dose (2 mg), the route (IV), the frequency (every 2 hours), and a parameter for administration (for severe incisional pain).

2. <u>X</u> **There is an error in this prescription. AU indicates both ears, and gentamicin ophthalmic solution is a medication that is administered to the eyes. Although the abbreviation AU has not been disallowed by The Joint Commission, many agencies require AU to be written out (i.e., both ears).**

3. ____ This is a correctly written prescription. It contains the medication spelled out (regular insulin). It contains the dose (5 units) and the term "units" is spelled out. It contains the route (sub-Q), and frequency (STAT, now). The Joint Commission has not disallowed the use of sub-Q, SQ, or SC. However, many agencies require that these abbreviations be avoided and the word subcutaneously be spelled out.

4. <u>X</u> **The abbreviation "*qd*" for *daily* is disallowed by The Joint Commission. The prescription should state *daily*, meaning *every day*. When *qd* is written it may be misinterpreted as *qid* which is four times the dose.**

5. <u>X</u> The dosage for alprazolam should contain a "0" before the decimal point (0.5). This is done so that the decimal point is not overlooked. If 5 mg is given instead of .5 mg the patient will receive 10 times the prescribed dose. This must be clarified with the prescribing provider.

28. 1. <u>X</u> Excess medication is unneeded and can be wiped away; also, it promotes comfort.

2. <u>X</u> Gazing upward moves the cornea upward and away from the conjunctival sac where medication should be instilled.

3. ____ Closing eyes tightly will force medication out of the eye, reducing the dose of the medication being delivered. Eyes should be closed gently to disperse medication and not force medication out of the eye.

4. <u>X</u> The conjunctival sac, the correct location to instill eye drops, is inside the lower eyelid.

5. <u>X</u> Eye infections can be easily transmitted from one eye to the other; however, it must be stressed that if aseptic principles are followed, cross-infection can be minimized.

29. **TEST-TAKING TIP The word "best" in the stem sets a priority.**

1. ____ Excessive water may promote aspiration.

2. <u>X</u> Crushed medications should be mixed in a soft food such as applesauce to make the bolus easy to swallow; the applesauce allows for more control of swallowing.

3. <u>X</u> One tablet at a time promotes safety when swallowing. Attempting to swallow several tablets at the same time may precipitate the gag reflex, which predisposes the patient to aspiration.

4. <u>X</u> The sitting position allows the patient to control the flow of fluid to the back of the oropharynx and promotes the flow of fluid down the esophagus via gravity.

5. <u>X</u> Inspecting the mouth after administering medication is important to ensure that the patient does not retain unswallowed medication in the mouth that can be aspirated.

30. Answer: 2 tablets
Solve the problem using ratio and proportion.

$$\frac{\text{Desire}}{\text{Have}} \quad \frac{400 \text{ mg}}{200 \text{ mg}} = \frac{\text{x Tab}}{1 \text{ Tab}}$$

$$200x = 400$$
$$x = 400 \div 200$$
$$x = 2 \text{ tablets}$$

31. 1. This syringe is an insulin syringe marked in units. It has a small-gauge (27- to 29-gauge) needle and ¼- to ⅜-inch length needle. This syringe is used to administer insulin via the subcutaneous route.

2. This syringe is inappropriate to administer insulin via the subcutaneous route. This is a 1-mL tuberculin syringe marked in 0.01-mL increments. It has a small-gauge (26- to 27-gauge) needle and ¼-inch length needle. This syringe is used to administer a TB skin test (tuberculin purified protein derivative [PPD]) via the intradermal route.

3. This is the appropriate syringe to use when administering medications via the intramuscular route. It has a 21-gauge needle and it is 1.5 inches long to penetrate tissue to the level of a muscle.

4. This is the appropriate syringe to use when preparing medications with a volume of 5 mL or less that is being reconstituted or added to a larger volume of solution. Although this 5-mL syringe is marked in whole milliliters, has a 20- to 21-gauge needle, has a 1.5-inch length needle, and can be used to administer an intramuscular injection, a 3-mL volume syringe with an appropriate needle gauge and length is used more often for an intramuscular injection.

32. **TEST-TAKING TIP The words "specifically" and "older adults" are key words in the stem that direct attention to content.**

1. <u>X</u> Biotransformation of drugs is less efficient in older adults than during younger developmental ages; when drugs are not fully metabolized, degraded, or excreted, toxic levels can accumulate.

2. ____ Harmless or injurious side effects (secondary effects) are common to people of all ages, not just older adults.

3. <u>X</u> Drug interactions are common to people of all ages, but more so in older

adults. Older adults tend to have chronic health problems that require a multiplicity of medications. Also, older adults may take over-the-counter medications to address problems, such as insomnia and constipation, that occur with aging.

4. ____ Allergic reactions are common to people of all ages, not just older adults.

5. ____ Teratogenic refers to agents that cause physical defects in a developing fetus. This is a concern in women of childbearing age.

33. **TEST-TAKING TIP** The words "administering nose drops correctly" are key words in the stem that direct attention to content.

1. ____ Sniffing the medication is contraindicated because sniffing pulls the medication to the oropharynx, where it will be swallowed rather than inhaled into the upper respiratory tract. Nose drops should be directed toward the midline of the superior concha of the ethmoid bone as the patient breathes through the mouth.

2. ____ Sitting upright after administering nose drops is contraindicated because sitting up allows the fluid to drain from the nares rather than be inhaled into the upper respiratory tract. The patient should remain with the head and neck hyperextended for 1 minute.

3. **X Tilting the head backward allows the instilled drops to flow well back into the nostril.**

4. ____ Returning the remaining fluid in the dropper to the bottle is a violation of medical asepsis.

5. **X Holding the dropper approximately a third of an inch inside the nares ensures that the entire drop enters the nostril. Not touching the mucous membranes prevents contamination of the dropper and limits precipitating a sneeze.**

34. **Answer: 4, 1, 2, 5, 3**

4. **Assessing for any contraindications protects the patient from a complication, such as stimulation of vagal nerves in the rectal area, is inappropriate when a patient has a cardiac problem, or from trauma if a patient is already experiencing rectal bleeding.**

1. **Placing the patient in the Sims position provides access to and visualization of**

the patient's perianal area. The left Sims position is preferred because the suppository will follow the natural curve of the rectum and sigmoid colon.

2. **Lubricating the suppository reduces friction, which eases insertion of the suppository and limits trauma to the anal and rectal mucosa.**

5. **Inserting the suppository 1 to 3 inches positions the suppository past the internal rectal sphincter, which facilitates the retention of the suppository.**

3. **Remaining in the side-lying position facilitates retention and absorption of the medication.**

35. **TEST-TAKING TIP** The word "first" in the stem sets a priority. The word "secondary" in the stem and in options 1 and 3 comprise clang associations. The word "primary" in the stem and in options 2 and 4 comprise clang associations. Unfortunately, using clang associations is not helpful in answering this question.

1. Although the nurse should document that the secondary infusion has completed, it is not the priority.

2. **Ensuring that the primary infusion is running at the ordered rate is the priority. Frequently the flow rate of a secondary infusion is much faster than the primary infusion. When the secondary infusion is completed the check valve in the primary infusion set will allow the primary infusion to flow at the rate set for the secondary infusion.**

3. Although the nurse should remove the empty secondary infusion bag and set, it is not the priority.

4. A new primary bag of solution is hung when the current primary bag is empty.

36. 1. ____ Unpleasant-tasting medication usually is more palatable if administered cold rather than at room temperature.

2. **X Oral hygiene removes residual medication from the mouth and clears the palate of the unpleasant taste.**

3. **X Using a needleless syringe deposits medication on the back of the tongue avoiding stimulation of taste buds in the front of the mouth.**

4. **X It is essential to check the mouth of a patient with dementia after administering an oral medication. This action ensures that the medication was swallowed.**

5. X Ice chips help to numb the taste buds minimizing the objectionable taste of an unpleasant medication.

37. 1. Notifying the prescribing provider of the patient's status is the appropriate intervention. The patient's pain has become progressively more intense over the course of the day and the medication protocol must be examined and possibly revised to adequately relieve this patient's pain. Opioids depress the central nervous system, resulting in depressed respirations, heart rate, and blood pressure. The rapid response team should be notified if the patient's respirations, heart rate, and blood pressure are very depressed or the patient is excessively sedated.
   2. Waiting 1 hour to administer hydromorphone is an inappropriate intervention. The patient will unnecessarily be in severe pain for 1 hour. Also, the patient's pain has become progressively more intense over the course of the day. The patient's respirations are depressed and may become further depressed if hydromorphone is administered.
   3. Administering acetaminophen 650 mg is an inappropriate intervention. The patient is experiencing severe, not moderate, pain.
   4. Reassessing the patient in 30 minutes is inappropriate. The patient will continue to be in severe pain during this time.

38. Answer: 3, 5, 2, 1, 4
   3. Shaking the canister ensures that the ingredients in the medication are well mixed.
   5. Exhaling through the mouth efficiently clears air from the lungs. The goal of an inhaler is to have medication reach deep into the lungs. When a person efficiently exhales a large lung surface is made available to come into contact with the subsequent inhaled medication.
   2. Sealing the lips around the mouthpiece prevents medication from escaping from around the mouth and mouthpiece and allows delivery of an accurate dose.
   1. Breathing in deeply delivers medication deep into the lungs. Inhaling slowly allows for prolonged contact of the medication with the lining of the respiratory tract.
   4. Medication in a metered-dose inhaler may cause irritation of the oral mucosa

or a fungal infection of the oral cavity. A swish and spit with water after the procedure reduces exposure of the oral mucosa to the medication, reducing the risk of irritation to or a fungal infection of the oral cavity.

39. 1. ____ The flange does not have to be kept sterile. It is pulled back with the hands when drawing up air or medication and depressed when injecting air into a vial or when administering medication to the patient.
   2. X The plunger must remain sterile because the plunger comes into contact with the sterile inside of the barrel when the plunger is depressed as air is injected into the medication vial. Then, the plunger is withdrawn, pulling sterile medicated solution into the sterile inside of the barrel.
   3. X The needle hub must remain sterile because it may come into contact with the break in the skin caused by insertion of the needle into the patient's body.
   4. X When the shaft of a needle is sterile it will not insert pathogens into the patient's body when the skin is pierced.
   5. ____ The outside of the barrel does not come into contact with sterile medication solution and therefore does not have to be sterile.

40. **TEST-TAKING TIP** The word "further" in the stem indicates negative polarity. What should the patient "not do?"

   1. X The eye should be wiped moving from the inner to the outer canthus; this promotes comfort, prevents trauma, and moves excess medication away from the nasolacrimal duct, minimizing systemic absorption and infection.
   2. ____ It is desirable to hold the dropper ½ to ¾ inch above the conjunctival sac. Holding it higher may injure the eye because of the force exerted by the drop; holding it lower increases the risk of contaminating the dropper or injuring the eye.
   3. ____ Closing the eyes gently after administering eye drops is acceptable because it distributes medication across the eye.
   4. ____ This is appropriate because it permits medication to remain in the eye and promotes an even distribution of medication.
   5. X It is unnecessary to hold the upper eyelid up.

MEETING THE NEEDS OF PERIOPERATIVE PATIENTS AND PATIENTS WITH WOUNDS

This section includes questions related to meeting the needs of patients before, during, and after surgery (perioperative period). The questions focus on physical assessment and on prevention and care related to common complications associated with the perioperative period, such as hemorrhage, wound dehiscence, atelectasis, infection, and thrombophlebitis. The principles of perioperative teaching, meeting patients' emotional needs, sterile technique, and types of dressings and wounds are also tested. In addition, assessment and care of postoperative tubes and wound drainage systems are addressed.

QUESTIONS

1. When a patient is brought to the postanesthesia care unit, the nurse is told that the patient lost 2 units of blood during surgery. For which responses significant to this information should the nurse assess the patient?
   1. Rapid, deep breathing and increased blood pressure
   2. Rapid, deep breathing and decreased blood pressure
   3. Slow, shallow breathing and increased blood pressure
   4. Slow, shallow breathing and decreased blood pressure

   TEST-TAKING TIP Identify duplicate facts among options. Identify opposites in options.

2. While a preoperative patient is being transferred to a stretcher to be taken to the operating room, the nurse attempts to have the patient remove dentures. The patient states, "I do not want to be seen without my dentures in my mouth." Which should the nurse do?
   1. Explain the importance of this rule.
   2. Allow the patient to keep them in the mouth.
   3. Explore the patient's feelings regarding not wearing dentures.
   4. Remove the dentures before anesthesia and replace them as soon as the patient awakens.

   TEST-TAKING TIP Identify the option that denies the patient's feelings, concerns, or needs. Identify patient-centered options. Identify clang associations. Identify opposites in options.

3. A patient is exhibiting difficulty coping with postoperative psychological stress. Which can the nurse do to **best** help this patient cope?
   1. Teach the use of imagery.
   2. Encourage ventilation of feelings.
   3. Promote intellectual adaptive responses.
   4. Obtain a prescription for an antianxiety medication.

   TEST-TAKING TIP Identify the word in the stem that sets a priority.

4. A nurse is caring for a group of patients in the postanesthesia care unit. Which intervention **best** prevents atelectasis immediately after surgery?
   1. Humidification of oxygen
   2. Diaphragmatic breathing
   3. Progressive activity
   4. Postural drainage

   TEST-TAKING TIP Identify the word in the stem that sets a priority. Identify the key word in the stem that directs attention to content.

5. A nurse on a surgical unit routinely assesses patients' incisions as part of postoperative care. After surgery, when should the nurse be alert for clinical signs of wound infection?
   1. Between days 3 and 5 after surgery
   2. Between days 1 and 2 after surgery
   3. Within 24 hours after surgery
   4. 7 days after surgery

   TEST-TAKING TIP Identify key words in the stem that direct attention to content.

6. Which intervention is unique to a Hemovac or Jackson-Pratt drain, that is different from a T-tube or an indwelling urinary catheter?
   1. Assess characteristics of the effluent.
   2. Maintain patency of the conduit.
   3. Ensure negative pressure.
   4. Measure output.

   TEST-TAKING TIP Identify the key word in the stem that directs attention to content.

7. An enema is ordered for a patient scheduled for bowel surgery. For which potential event associated with surgery is the enema primarily designed to prevent?
   1. Intraoperative peristalsis
   2. Postoperative constipation
   3. Contamination of the operative field
   4. Fecal incontinence during the procedure

   TEST-TAKING TIP Identify the word in the stem that sets a priority.

8. When talking with a hospitalized preoperative patient, a nurse discovers that the patient smokes two packs of cigarettes a day. This information was not documented in the patient's clinical record. Which should the nurse do?
   1. Inform the surgeon about the patient's smoking.
   2. Ask the patient to stop smoking until after surgery.
   3. Remove the patient's cigarettes at midnight before surgery.
   4. Advise the patient to join a smoking cessation group after discharge.

   TEST-TAKING TIP Identify options that deny patient feelings, concerns, or needs. Identify the unique option.

9. After a patient has a procedure that uses the femoral artery as an access, a pressure dressing is applied at the catheter insertion site. Which is the primary purpose of this pressure dressing?
   1. Prevents pain
   2. Limits infection
   3. Decreases drainage
   4. Promotes hemostasis

   TEST-TAKING TIP Identify the word in the stem that sets a priority. Identify the unique option.

10. After concerns about pain, the **most** commonly asked question by preoperative patients is, "When will I be able to:
    1. Eat?"
    2. Shower?"
    3. Go home?"
    4. Have visitors?"

    TEST-TAKING TIP Identify the word in the stem that sets a priority. Use Maslow's Hierarchy of Needs to establish the priority.

11. A nurse is caring for a patient who just had thoracic surgery. Which is the **most** specific assessment related to this type of surgery?
    1. Blood pressure
    2. Urinary output
    3. Intensity of pain
    4. Rate and depth of respirations

    TEST-TAKING TIP Identify the word in the stem that sets a priority. Identify key words in the stem that direct attention to content. Identify the unique option.

12. A nurse is caring for a patient with a nasogastric tube to low continuous suction. Which is the **most** effective way for the nurse to prevent dislodgment of the nasogastric tube?
    1. Pin it to the patient's pillow.
    2. Attach it to the patient's gown.
    3. Secure the tube to the patient's nose.
    4. Instruct the patient not to touch the tube.

    TEST-TAKING TIP Identify the word in the stem that sets a priority. Identify equally plausible options. Identify clang associations.

13. Which is the **most** therapeutic statement by the nurse when assessing a patient's knowledge of surgery?
    1. "Have you ever had surgery before?"
    2. "Tell me about your surgical experiences."
    3. "Surgery can be a frightening experience."
    4. "Do you have any concerns about surgery?"

    TEST-TAKING TIP Identify the word in the stem that sets a priority. Identify the global option.

14. A nurse is caring for a postoperative patient who had abdominal surgery. Which should the nurse do to help prevent postoperative wound dehiscence?
    1. Keep the area clean and dry.
    2. Change the dressing every eight hours.
    3. Medicate the patient for pain around the clock.
    4. Encourage the patient to support the incision during activity.

    TEST-TAKING TIP Identify key words in the stem that direct attention to content. Identify equally plausible options.

15. A postoperative patient has a history of heart disease. Which nursing assessment is **most** significant when monitoring this patient?
    1. Pain at the site of the incision
    2. Alterations in fluid balance
    3. Irregular pulse rhythm
    4. Dependent edema

    TEST-TAKING TIP Identify the word in the stem that sets a priority. Identify equally plausible options. Identify the obscure clang association.

16. A nurse is assessing a postoperative patient who has just been extubated. Which patient response indicates mild postoperative laryngeal spasm after extubation?
    1. Wheezing
    2. Crackles
    3. Gurgles
    4. Rales

    TEST-TAKING TIP Identify key words in the stem that direct attention to content. Identify equally plausible options.

17. A primary health-care provider orders a wound to be packed with a wet-to-damp gauze dressing. Which should the nurse explain to the patient is the primary reason for this type of dressing?
    1. "It minimizes the loss of protein."
    2. "It facilitates the healing process."
    3. "It increases the resistance to infection."
    4. "It prevents the entry of microorganisms."

18. A patient has a portable wound drainage system after resection of a tumor in the neck. When should the nurse empty the portable wound drainage system?
    1. After it is full
    2. Every 2 hours
    3. Every 4 hours
    4. When it is half full

19. A surgical patient is transferred from the postanesthesia care unit to a medical-surgical unit and the nurse reviews the surgeon's orders. Which vitamin should the nurse be alert for that is commonly prescribed postoperatively?
    1. Vitamin C
    2. Vitamin A
    3. Vitamin K
    4. Vitamin B

20. A nurse is caring for a patient with a nasogastric tube attached to suction. Which is an essential nursing action in relation to the nasogastric tube?
    1. Using sterile technique when irrigating the line
    2. Recording the intake and output every 2 hours
    3. Maintaining suction at the prescribed level
    4. Providing oral hygiene every 4 hours

21. Which nursing interventions are related to the prevention of postoperative thrombophlebitis? **Select all that apply.**
    1. _____ Walking regularly
    2. _____ Massaging the legs
    3. _____ Increasing fluid intake
    4. _____ Providing a diet high in fiber
    5. _____ Applying antiembolism stockings

    TEST-TAKING TIP Identify key words in the stem that direct attention to content.

22. Identify the nursing actions that maintain sterile technique? **Select all that apply.**
    1. _____ Always hold wet gauze upward until ready for use.
    2. _____ Change gloves if they are positioned below the waist.
    3. _____ Clean edges of the wound before the center of the wound.
    4. _____ Wipe the wound in a circular motion from the outside inward.
    5. _____ Sterile equipment should remain inside a 1-inch border of the sterile field.

    TEST-TAKING TIP Identify the clang association.

23. A nurse is applying the dressing depicted in the illustration. Place the following steps in the order in which they should be implemented.
1. Peel paper backing from the dressing.
2. Place your hand on the dressing for approximately ten seconds.
3. Document the date, time, and your initials on the edge of the dressing.
4. Place the dressing over the wound and gently use a hand to smooth it toward the edges.

Answer: _____

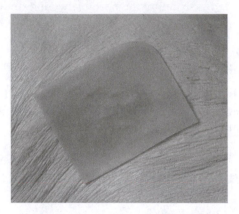

24. A patient who received spinal anesthesia is transferred to the postanesthesia care unit. Which are the **most** important postoperative nursing assessments of this patient? **Select all that apply.**
1. ____ Peripheral circulation
2. ____ Level of consciousness
3. ____ Orientation to time and place
4. ____ Sensation in the legs and toes
5. ____ Ability to move the lower extremities

TEST-TAKING TIP Identify the word in the stem that sets a priority. Identify the key word in the stem that directs attention to content.

25. A postoperative patient voids for the first time after surgery. The nurse measures the amount of urine in a graduate as indicated in the illustration. How many milliliters should the nurse document that the patient voided? **Record your answer using a whole number.**

Answer: _____ mL

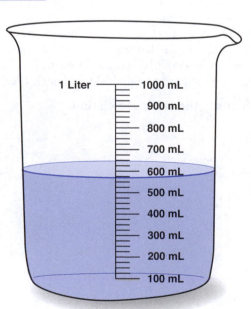

26. Which factors place an older adult at greater risk during surgery than a younger person? **Select all that apply.**
    1. ____ Increased glomerular filtration rate
    2. ____ Decreased rigidity of arterial walls
    3. ____ Elevated basal metabolic rate
    4. ____ Lowered hepatic functioning
    5. ____ Reduced cardiac reserve

    TEST-TAKING TIP Identify the word in the stem that sets a priority. Identify key words in the stem that direct attention to content.

27. A nurse is caring for patients with a variety of wounds. Which type of wounds heal by primary intention? **Select all that apply.**
    1. ____ Surgical incision
    2. ____ Excoriation
    3. ____ Deep burn
    4. ____ Paper cut
    5. ____ Abrasion

    TEST-TAKING TIP Identify the key word in the stem that directs attention to content.

28. A nurse compares a patient's current status with the patient's previous information. Based on this analysis and protocols established for the postanesthesia care unit, what should the nurse do first before notifying the surgeon?
    1. Reinforce the dressing.
    2. Increase the flow rate of the IV infusion.
    3. Raise the oxygen flow rate to 12 L/minute.
    4. Elevate the head of the bed to a high-Fowler position.

POSTANESTHESIA CLINICAL RECORD

Admitting Note
0800: Patient accepted from circulating nurse and anesthesiologist after having a 2-cm noncancerous tumor removed from right side of neck. Oral airway in place. Oxygen face tent set at 10 L/min. Dressing dry and intact. IV of 1,000 mL of 0.9% sodium chloride at 125 per/hr in progress with 400 mL left in bag. IV insertion site dry and intact, no signs of infiltration or inflammation.

Vital Signs
Blood pressure: 140/75 mm Hg
Pulse: 78 beats/min, regular rhythm
Respirations: 22 breaths/min
Oxygen saturation: 97%

Nurse's Progress Note
0900: Airway in place. Patient still unresponsive. Moderate amount of blood identified on linen under patient's neck. Blood pressure 100/60; pulse 90 beats/min; respirations 24 breaths/min, unlabored.

29. A nurse is caring for four patients with abdominal wounds. Identify the wound that should cause the most concern.

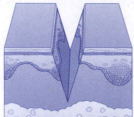

1.

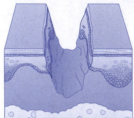

2.

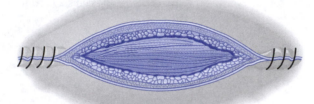

3.

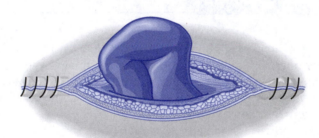

4.

30. A nurse is providing preoperative instruction for a patient who is to have abdominal surgery. Which patient statements indicate that further preoperative teaching is needed? **Select all that apply.**

1. ____ "I should anticipate that I will have a bowel movement the day after surgery."
2. ____ "It will hurt less if I apply pressure against the incision when coughing."
3. ____ "I will be in the postanesthesia care unit for several hours."
4. ____ "It is important for me to lie still while I am on bedrest."
5. ____ "I can ask for medication when I have severe pain."

TEST-TAKING TIP Identify the word in the stem that indicates negative polarity. Identify the clang association.

31. A nurse is caring for a patient with the type of wound dressing depicted in the illustration. Which type of wound should the nurse generally expect to see under this dressing?
    1. Wound with a Hemovac drain
    2. Wound with copious secretions
    3. Wound with negative pressure therapy
    4. Wound with approximated wound edges

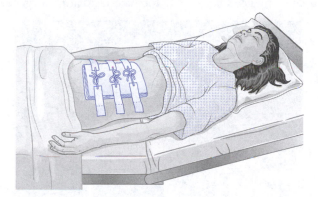

32. A nurse is assessing a patient's wound postoperatively. Place an X on the section of this wound that causes the **most** concern?

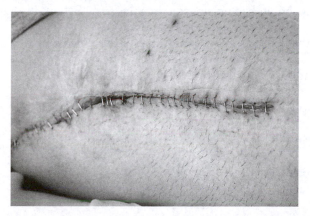

33. A child has a surgical repair of an inguinal hernia and acetaminophen 192 mg PO every 4 hours × four doses is prescribed. Liquid acetaminophen is available 160 mg/5 mL. How many milliliters should the nurse administer? **Record your answer using a whole number.**

    Answer: _____ mL

34. The device in the photograph is ordered for a postoperative patient. The patient asks the nurse, "Why do I have to wear these things?" Which information should the nurse include in the response to the patient's question? **Select all that apply.**
    1. _____ Keeps the lower extremities warm
    2. _____ Helps prevent deep vein thromboses
    3. _____ Accelerates the rate of wound healing
    4. _____ Promotes circulation of blood back to the heart
    5. _____ Eliminates the need for leg and foot exercises after surgery

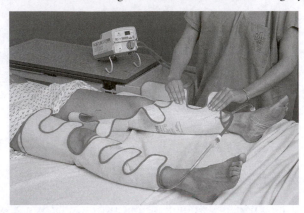

35. A nurse is caring for a patient with the wound therapy portrayed in the illustration. Which actions should be implemented by the nurse? **Select all that apply.**
    1. _____ Apply a skin protectant around wound edges.
    2. _____ Cut the dressing to the approximate size of the wound.
    3. _____ Pack the deep crevices of the wound gently with the dressing.
    4. _____ Irrigate the wound as prescribed moving from the dirty to clean end of the wound.
    5. _____ Compress the dressing with a transparent occlusive film dressing 2 inches beyond wound edges.

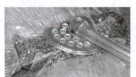

1. **TEST-TAKING TIP** The question is testing your knowledge about the type of breathing and the type of blood pressure associated with hypovolemia secondary to blood loss. If you know just one of these facts related to hypovolemia, you can reduce your final selection to two options. Options 1 and 4 are opposites, and options 2 and 3 are opposites. Although there are two sets of opposites in this item, it is easier and more productive to focus instead on the duplicate facts to help you eliminate distractors.

   1. Although rapid, deep breathing is associated with hypovolemia, the blood pressure decreases, not increases.
   2. **With a decrease in circulating red blood cells, respiration increases in rate and depth to meet oxygen needs. With a reduction in blood volume, there is a decrease in blood pressure.**
   3. With hypovolemia, the breathing is rapid and deep, not slow and shallow, and the blood pressure decreases, not increases.
   4. Although the blood pressure decreases with hypovolemia, the respirations are rapid and deep, not slow and shallow.

2. **TEST-TAKING TIP** Option 1 denies the patient's feelings, concerns, or needs and should be eliminated. Options 2, 3, and 4 appear to be patient centered. The word "dentures" in the stem and options 3 and 4 comprise clang associations. Options 2 and 3 do not address the fact that the dentures need to be removed for safety. Options 2 and 4 are opposites. An analysis of options leaves option 4 as the correct answer. Option 4 is patient centered, contains a clang association, and is a safe action that takes into consideration the feelings of the patient. Also, it is one of the options that is an opposite. More often than not the correct answer is one of the options that are opposites.

   1. Explaining the importance of this rule denies the patient's feelings and cuts off communication; care can be individualized while still meeting safety needs.
   2. It is unsafe to allow dentures to be in the mouth during surgery because dentures may be aspirated while the patient is unconscious.

   3. Although exploring the patient's feelings might be done, it does not address safety needs.
   4. **Removing the dentures immediately before surgery and returning them as soon as possible after surgery meets the patient's self-esteem needs while providing for physical safety.**

3. **TEST-TAKING TIP** The word "best" in the stem sets a priority.

   1. Teaching imagery may reduce anxiety temporarily, but it does not address the underlying concerns.
   2. **This provides open-ended communication and allows the patient to explore concerns.**
   3. Intellectual adaptive responses take place in the cognitive domain (which addresses intellectual/knowledge needs), not the affective domain (which addresses psychological needs).
   4. Medication may be unnecessary if the patient's psychological needs are addressed effectively.

4. **TEST-TAKING TIP** The word "best" in the stem sets a priority. The word "immediately" is the key word in the stem that directs attention to content.

   1. Humidification of oxygen keeps the mucous membranes of the respiratory tract moist; it does not prevent atelectasis.
   2. **Diaphragmatic breathing expands the alveoli, which prevents atelectasis; it also precipitates coughing, which prevents the accumulation and stagnation of secretions.**
   3. Activity promotes cardiopulmonary and circulatory functioning in general; it does not specifically prevent atelectasis. Progressive activity, such as ambulation, is not performed in the postanesthesia care unit.
   4. Postural drainage promotes the flow of mucus out of segments of the lung; it is not done routinely after surgery to prevent atelectasis.

5. **TEST-TAKING TIP** The words "wound infection" in the stem direct attention to content.

   1. **Microorganisms in a wound can precipitate an infection, which manifests itself in 3 to 5 days; erythema, pain, edema,**

chills, fever, and purulent drainage indicate infection.

2. One to 2 days is too short a time for an infectious process to develop from a surgical incision; a contaminated, traumatic wound may precipitate an infection this early.

3. Within 24 hours after surgery is too short a time for an infectious process to develop from a surgical incision; a contaminated, traumatic wound may precipitate an infection this early.

4. An infectious process generally manifests itself before 7 days; wound dehiscence or evisceration may occur 5 to 10 days after surgery before collagen formation occurs.

6. **TEST-TAKING TIP The word "unique" is the key word in the stem that directs attention to content.**

   1. All drainage must be assessed for quantity, color, consistency, and odor.
   2. All conduits (e.g., tubes, catheters) must be patent for drainage to occur.
   3. **Portable wound drainage systems work by continuous low negative pressure as long as the suction bladder is less than half full; T tubes and indwelling urinary catheters work via gravity.**
   4. The volume of fluid over specific time periods must be measured for all drainage.

7. **TEST-TAKING TIP The word "primarily" in the stem sets a priority.**

   1. Although an enema may reduce bowel peristalsis intraoperatively (during surgery) because the bowel will be empty of stool, it is not the purpose of an enema before bowel surgery.
   2. Postoperative constipation is prevented by activity and adequate fluid intake.
   3. **If feces are present in the bowel when the intestine is incised, the excrement spills into the abdominal cavity, causing contamination and increasing the risk of peritonitis.**
   4. Although an enema prevents fecal incontinence during surgery, it is not the purpose of thorough bowel preparation for intestinal surgery.

8. **TEST-TAKING TIP Options 2, 3, and 4 deny patient feelings, concerns, or needs. Option 1 is unique because it involves communicating information to the surgeon. Options 2, 3, and 4 involve interacting with the patient.**

   1. **The surgeon should be informed of this fact because it may influence the**
   type of anesthesia to be administered and the perioperative medical regimen.

   2. If the patient is willing to stop smoking, it should be discontinued before and after surgery to prevent respiratory complications. The nurse should recognize that the patient may need to continue to smoke because it may be a coping mechanism.
   3. The nurse does not have a right to take a patient's belongings; the patient should be told where and when smoking is permitted or if the facility is "smoke free."
   4. Discussing a Smoke Enders Club is inappropriate at this time because the patient is concerned with the present situation; this may eventually be done after surgery.

9. **TEST-TAKING TIP The word "primary" in the stem sets a priority. Option 4 is unique because it is from a positive perspective, expressed by the word "promote." Options 1, 2, and 3 are from a negative perspective, expressed by the words *prevent, limit,* and *decrease.***

   1. Although a pressure dressing may help prevent the accumulation of interstitial fluid, thereby limiting pain, it does not prevent pain; also, this is not the primary purpose of a pressure dressing.
   2. Surgical asepsis, not a pressure dressing, limits infection.
   3. Dressings usually do not decrease drainage.
   4. **Pressure causes the constriction of peripheral blood vessels, which prevents bleeding; it also eliminates dead space in underlying tissue so that healing can progress.**

10. **TEST-TAKING TIP The word "most" in the stem sets a priority. Meeting nutritional needs is a physiological need, a first level need according to Maslow's Hierarchy of Needs theory.**

    1. **After concerns about pain, eating is the most common concern of postoperative patients. Food intake is essential for life and is a physiological need. It has the highest priority of the options offered according to Maslow.**
    2. Although knowing when one can shower may be important to some patients, it is not the most basic, common concern of the majority of patients. Showering refers to microbiological safety, which is a second-level need according to Maslow.

3. Although wanting to know when one can go home may be important to some patients, it is not the most basic, common concern of the majority of patients. Going home refers to love and belonging, which is a third-level need according to Maslow.

4. Although having visitors may be important to some patients, it is not the most basic, common concern of the majority of patients. Having visitors is related to love and belonging needs, which is a third-level need according to Maslow.

11. **TEST-TAKING TIP** The word "most" in the stem sets a priority. The words "thoracic" and "specific" are key words in the stem that direct attention to content. Option 4 is unique because it is the only option with two assessments.

1. Monitoring the blood pressure is important after any surgery but is not specific to thoracic surgery.

2. Monitoring fluid intake and urinary output is important after all types of surgery; it is not unique to thoracic surgery.

3. Monitoring the characteristics of pain is required after all types of surgery but is not specific to thoracic surgery.

4. **Thoracic surgery involves entering the thoracic cavity; respiratory function becomes a priority.**

12. **TEST-TAKING TIP** The word "most" in the stem sets a priority. Options 1 and 2 are equally plausible. The word "tube" in the stem and in options 3 and 4 comprise clang associations.

1. Pinning the tubing to the patient's bed linen is unsafe; tension on the tube will increase with patient movement, which may result in displacement of the tube.

2. Attaching the tubing to the gown is unsafe. Patient movement will increase tension on the tubing and may result in displacement of the tube.

3. **Attaching a nasogastric tube to the patient's nose via tape or a tube fixation device anchors the tube and helps prevent the tube from becoming dislodged.**

4. Although the patient should be instructed not to touch the tube, this is not the most effective way to prevent dislodgment of the tube because patients tend to touch foreign objects that irritate the body.

13. **TEST-TAKING TIP** The word "most" in the stem sets a priority. Options 1 and 4 ask direct questions that require a "yes" or "no" answer. Option 2 is global in that the question in option 1 is included under the more open-ended question in option 2. Option 3 should be eliminated immediately because it unnecessarily introduces the concern "surgery is frightening."

1. This statement is a direct question that can be answered with a "yes" or a "no."

2. **This statement is an open-ended question that invites the patient to discuss past experiences. The patient's past experiences may be less anxiety producing than the present situation, and they provide a database for future teaching.**

3. This statement may precipitate unnecessary anxiety; feelings should be raised by the patient, not by the nurse.

4. This statement is a direct question that the patient may be unable or unwilling to answer or can be answered with a "yes" or "no" response. Concerns generally focus on feelings rather than knowledge.

14. **TEST-TAKING TIP** The words "prevent" and "dehiscence" are key words in the stem that direct attention to content. Options 1 and 2 are equally plausible; they both reflect actions that are associated with the dressing and prevent infection.

1. Keeping the wound clean and dry should prevent infection, not wound dehiscence.

2. Changing the wound dressing every 8 hours should prevent infection, not wound dehiscence.

3. Pain medication promotes comfort; it does not limit the occurrence of dehiscence.

4. **Pressure against the incision supports the integrity of the approximation of the edges of the wound.**

15. **TEST-TAKING TIP** The word "most" in the stem sets a priority. Options 2 and 4 are equally plausible; they both relate to problems with fluid balance. The words "heart" in the stem and "pulse" in option 3 is an obscure clang association. Left ventricular contraction of the heart precipitates the pulse.

1. Pain at the incisional site is common to postoperative patients and not specific to a postoperative patient with a history of heart disease.

2. Although changes in fluid balance are an important assessment, an alteration in fluid balance is not immediately life threatening.

3. An irregular pulse rhythm may indicate a life-threatening dysrhythmia.

4. Although assessment of dependent edema is important, it is not as critical as another assessment.

16. **TEST-TAKING TIP** The words "mild" and "laryngeal spasm" are key words in the stem that direct attention to content. Options 2 and 4 are equally plausible. Rales and crackles both describe the same adventitious lung sound heard on auscultation caused by air passing over retained secretions or the abrupt opening of collapsed airways.

1. **Wheezing, which consists of high-pitched whistling sounds, is caused by air moving through a narrowed or partially obstructed airway.**

2. Crackles, also known as rales, are sounds caused by air passing through respiratory passages containing excessive moisture.

3. Gurgles, formerly known as rhonchi, are sounds caused by air moving through tenacious mucus or narrowed bronchi.

4. Rales, more commonly known as crackles, are sounds caused by air passing through respiratory passages containing excessive moisture.

17. 1. Wet-to-damp packing of a wound is not done to minimize the loss of protein from a wound. Protein loss occurs until the wound heals.

2. Packing a wound with wet-to-damp dressings allows epidermal cells to migrate more rapidly across the bed of the wound surface than dry dressings, thereby facilitating wound healing.

3. Although packing a wound with wet-to-damp dressings will wick exudate up and away from the base of the wound and therefore help to increase resistance to a wound infection, it is not the primary reason for its use.

4. This is not the primary purpose of a wet-to-damp gauze dressing. Dry sterile dressings are used to prevent the entry of microorganisms into a wound.

18. 1. After the device is full is undesirable because of the reduced effectiveness of the system's negative pressure.

2. Depending on the amount of drainage 2 hours may be too soon or not long enough

to maintain adequate suction. Opening the device increases the risk of infection and should be done only when necessary.

3. Opening the device increases the risk of infection and should be done only when necessary.

4. The force of the vacuum within the system reduces as the collection chamber fills. Therefore, the collection chamber should be emptied when it is half full to ensure the effectiveness of suction.

19. 1. **Vitamin C (ascorbic acid) is essential for collagen formation, the single most important protein of connective tissue. The recommended daily dose is 60 mg; however, a postoperative patient may need up to 1000 mg of vitamin C for tissue repair, necessitating supplementation.**

2. Although vitamin A is associated with epithelial tissue, usually it is not prescribed individually but rather as part of a multivitamin.

3. Although vitamin K promotes blood clotting by increasing the synthesis of prothrombin by the liver, usually it is not prescribed unless the patient has liver disease or a bleeding tendency.

4. Although the B-complex vitamins are related to protein synthesis and cross-linking of collagen fibers, they usually are not prescribed individually but rather as part of a multivitamin.

20. 1. Medical, not surgical, asepsis is necessary. The gut is not considered a sterile space.

2. It is unnecessary to monitor the intake and output this frequently. The I&O must be recorded at routine intervals as per hospital policy, such as at the end of each shift and every 24 hours.

3. The level of suctioning is part of the order for nasogastric decompression. Low suction pressure is between 80 and 100 mm Hg, and high suction pressure is between 100 and 120 mm Hg. Suctioning must be maintained continuously with a Salem sump to prevent reflux of gastric secretions into the vent lumen, which will obstruct its functioning and result in mucosal damage. A single-lumen tube requires low intermittent suction to prevent the tube from adhering to the stomach mucosa.

4. Oral hygiene should be provided more frequently than every 4 hours. Because

there is no food or fluid to stimulate salivary gland secretion and the tube in the nose may interfere with breathing, precipitating mouth breathing, the mouth becomes dry.

21. **TEST-TAKING TIP** The words "prevent" and "thrombophlebitis" are key words in the stem that direct attention to content.
    1. X Ambulating increases circulation in the lower extremities, which helps prevent thrombus formation.
    2. ____ Massaging the legs can traumatize the vessels, contributing to the formation of thrombi.
    3. X Increasing fluid intake promotes hemodilution, which limits thrombus formation.
    4. ____ A high-fiber diet will help prevent constipation, not thrombophlebitis.
    5. X Antiembolism stockings promote venous return, which prevents the formation of thrombi.

22. **TEST-TAKING TIP** The word "sterile" in the stem and in option 5 is a clang association.
    1. ____ Fluid from the wet gauze can run down the upraised hand. When the hand is repositioned with the fingers downward, the fluid that runs back down the hand may be contaminated, which, in turn, contaminates the gauze.
    2. X When sterile gloves are accidentally positioned below the waist they are considered out of the line of the nurse's sight and must be changed because the gloves may have inadvertently become contaminated.
    3. ____ Cleaning the edges of the wound before the center of the wound can move contaminated material from a more contaminated section to a less contaminated section of the wound. The center of a wound is considered less contaminated than the edges of the wound or the surrounding skin; therefore, the nurse should wipe a wound moving from the center outward using one gauze pad per stroke.
    4. ____ Wiping the wound in a circular motion from the outside inward can move contaminated material from a more contaminated section to a less contaminated section of a wound. The center of a wound is considered less contaminated than the edges of the wound or the surrounding skin; therefore, the nurse should

wipe a wound moving from the center outward using one gauze pad per stroke.
    5. X The outer 1-inch boarder of a sterile field is considered contaminated. All sterile equipment must remain inside this border to be considered sterile.

23. Answer: 3, 1, 4, 2
    3. Documenting important information on this hydrocolloid dressing before it is applied prevents unnecessary pressure over the wound when documenting the information on the dressing after it is applied. Pressure against a dressing after it is applied may be uncomfortable or painful for the patient. Documenting important information on the outside of the dressing ensures that others know the date and time the dressing was applied and the identity of the nurse applying the dressing.
    1. Removing the paper exposes the adhesive backing of this hydrocolloid dressing before the dressing is applied.
    4. Placing this hydrocolloid dressing gently on the wound and smoothing it toward the edges ensures that the dressing is against the wound. Working gently avoids undue pressure against the wound.
    2. Placing a hand on this hydrocolloid dressing for approximately 10 seconds uses body heat to mold the dressing to the skin. This action improves adherence of the dressing to the patient's skin.

24. **TEST-TAKING TIP** The word "most" in the stem sets a priority. The word "spinal" is the key word in the stem that directs attention to content.
    1. ____ Spinal anesthesia does not alter peripheral circulation.
    2. ____ General anesthesia, not spinal anesthesia, acts on the cerebral centers to produce loss of consciousness.
    3. ____ General anesthesia, not spinal anesthesia, acts on the cerebral centers and alters orientation to time, place, and person.
    4. X Spinal anesthesia causes loss of sensation in the toes, perineum, legs, and abdomen. When sensations in the legs and toes return, the patient is considered to have recovered from the effects of the spinal anesthetic.
    5. X Spinal anesthesia causes loss of motion in the lower extremities. When

mobility of the legs and toes return the patient is considered to have recovered from the effects of the spinal anesthetic.

25. **Answer: 575**
    Each line represents 25 mL of urine.

26. **TEST-TAKING TIP The word "greater" in the stem sets a priority. The words "older adult" are key words in the stem that direct attention to content.**

    1. ____ Older adults have a decreased, not increased, glomerular filtration rate.
    2. ____ Older adults have an increased, not decreased, rigidity of arterial walls.
    3. ____ Older adults have a lowered, not elevated, basal metabolic rate.
    4. **X The size of the liver, blood flow in the liver, and enzyme production by the liver decrease; the half-life of anesthetic agents and medications increase, which may result in toxicity.**
    5. **X As one ages, cardiac output and strength of cardiac contractions decrease and the heart rate takes longer to return to the resting rate. Sudden physical or emotional stresses may result in cardiac dysrhythmias and heart failure.**

27. **TEST-TAKING TIP The word "primary" is the key word in the stem that directs attention to content.**

    1. **X Primary intention is the healing process that consists of the stages of defensive, reconstructive, and maturative healing; it involves a clean wound that has edges that are closely approximated.**
    2. ____ An excoriation is an abrasion, a loss of superficial skin layers caused by trauma, friction, chemicals, or digestive enzymes. An excoriation heals by secondary intention.
    3. ____ A burn has wound edges that are not approximated and the wound usually is wide and open. A burn heals by secondary intention.
    4. **X A paper cut is a slice or sliver-like wound with very close approximated edges. It heals by primary intention.**
    5. ____ An abrasion, like an excoriation, is the loss of superficial skin layers caused by trauma, friction, chemicals, and digestive enzymes. An abrasion heals by secondary intention.

28. 1. Reinforcing the dressing should be done eventually, but it is not the priority.
    2. **Protocols generally permit the nurse to increase the flow rate of an IV infusion when a postoperative patient in the postanesthesia care unit demonstrates signs of hemorrhage until the surgeon can be notified. The decrease in blood pressure, the increase in pulse and respiratory rates, and blood on the linen under the patient's neck support the conclusion that the patient may be hemorrhaging.**
    3. The suggested flow rate for a face tent is 8 to 10 L/min.
    4. Elevating the head of the bed higher than the semi-Fowler position is too high for an unresponsive patient. A high-Fowler position may be assumed after recovery from anesthesia.

29. 1. This is the least serious wound of the wounds presented. This wound appears to be clean with edges that can be approximated with sutures. This wound will heal by primary intention.

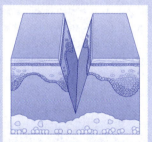

    2. This wound is less serious than two other wounds presented. This wound has irregular wound edges that will heal by secondary intention.

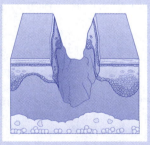

    3. This wound has wound edges that have separated and the muscle layer is visible (dehiscence). Although this is a serious complication of wound healing it is not as serious as another wound presented in the question. Dehiscence occurs in approximately 0.3% to 3% of patients with abdominal surgery with studies

documenting mortality rates of 14% to 30%. Dehiscence generally occurs between the 5th and 12th day postoperatively.

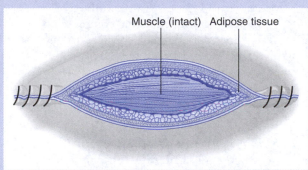

Muscle (intact)   Adipose tissue

4. **This illustration exhibits evisceration, which is a life-threatening condition. Evisceration occurs when abdominal contents protrude through separated wound edges precipitating necrosis of the intestines or overwhelming sepsis. Evisceration occurs in approximately 1% to 2% of patients with abdominal surgery with the largest number appearing between the 7th and 10th day postoperatively. Evisceration has a mortality rate of 30% to 37%.**

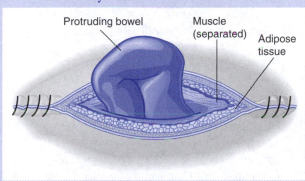

Protruding bowel   Muscle (separated)   Adipose tissue

30. **TEST-TAKING TIP The word "further" in the stem indicates negative polarity. The question is asking, "Which statements by the patient are *not accurate?*" The word "surgery" in the stem and in option 1 is a clang association.**

1. **X It takes a minimum of 2 to 3 days for peristalsis to return after abdominal surgery because of the effects of anesthesia and manipulation of the abdominal organs, particularly the intestines.**

2. ____ Applying pressure against an incision is an acceptable practice to minimize incisional pain and help prevent dehiscence when performing any activity that increases intra-abdominal pressure.

3. ____ Patients are kept in the postanesthesia care unit until reactive and stable.

4. **X Remaining immobile after surgery is unacceptable because it promotes cardiopulmonary, vascular, and gastrointestinal complications; the patient needs further preoperative teaching. There are many types of exercises that can be performed when on bedrest.**

5. **X Pain relief is more effective when analgesics are administered before pain becomes severe; this prevents excessive peaks and troughs in the pain experience.**

31. 1. The illustrated dressing generally is not necessary for a wound with a Hemovac drain. In addition, a drainage tube exiting the dressing and terminating in a Hemovac collection container would be visible when examining the patient's abdominal area, which is not present.

2. **An open wound with copious (i.e., large, profuse, abundant) amounts of secretions requires frequent changing. This minimizes drainage coming into contact with intact tissue, avoiding maceration of skin. The Montgomery straps dressing in the illustration does not require the constant removal and reapplication of tape when frequent dressing changes are necessary. The nurse unties the straps, removes the soiled dressing, cleanses the wound, applies a sterile dressing, and reties the straps to hold the dressing in place.**

3. This is not an illustration of a wound with negative pressure therapy. A wound with negative pressure therapy has a transparent dressing with a tube leading from the center of the dressing to a machine that maintains negative pressure and collects drainage.

4. A wound with approximated wound edges does not need the dressing in the illustration. A wound with approximated wound edges generally has only small amounts of serosanguineous drainage requiring a dry sterile dressing for 1 to 2 days.

32. **The section indicated by the X identifies wound edges that are separating. A partial or complete parting of the outer layers of a wound (dehiscence) occurs in approximately 3% of patients with abdominal**

surgery. Between the 5th and 12th post-operative days is the critical time when dehiscence commonly occurs. Sutures or staples that are too close together, too far apart, or removed prematurely can contribute to dehiscence. In addition, edema or infection at the incisional site or obesity may also contribute to dehiscence.

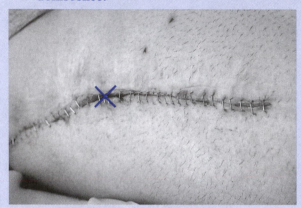

33. **Answer: 6 mL**
Solve the problem using ratio and proportion.

$$\frac{\text{Desire}}{\text{Have}} \quad \frac{192 \text{ mg}}{160 \text{ mg}} = \frac{\text{x mL}}{5 \text{ mL}}$$

$$160x = 192 \times 5$$
$$160x = 960$$
$$x = 960 \div 160$$
$$x = 6 \text{ mL}$$

34. 1. ____ Keeping the lower extremities warm is not the purpose of sequential compression devices.
2. **X Sequential compression devices help prevent venous pooling by facilitating venous return to the heart. Venous stasis contributes to deep vein thrombosis, which can be minimized with the use of sequential compression devices and foot and leg exercises.**
3. ____ Sequential compression devices do not accelerate the rate of wound healing.
4. **X Sequential compression devices inflate and deflate chambers in the** device, moving from distal to proximal, promoting venous blood return to the heart. This action helps prevent venous stasis, which is associated with the development of deep vein thromboses.
5. ____ The use of a sequential compression device does not eliminate the need to implement foot and leg exercises after surgery. Both interventions should be employed to reduce the risk of deep vein thromboses associated with postoperative recovery.

35. 1. **X This is a photograph of negative pressure wound therapy. Applying a skin protectant around wound edges helps reduce the risk of skin breakdown.**
2. **X This is a photograph of negative pressure wound therapy. Cutting the dressing to the approximate size of the wound prepares the equipment for the dressing change.**
3. ____ This is a photograph of negative pressure wound therapy. The dressing should be gently placed into the wound cavity. Packing the dressing into deep crevices or overfilling the wound is contraindicated because it compresses tissue, which may impair circulation.
4. ____ This is a photograph of negative pressure wound therapy. When irrigating a wound, the nurse should always move from the clean to the dirty end of the wound because doing so reduces the risk of contaminating the clean end of the wound.
5. ____ This is a photograph of negative pressure wound therapy. Although a transparent occlusive film dressing should be applied so that it extends 1 to 2 inches beyond wound edges, it should be done lightly so as not to compress the underlying dressing. Compression of the underlying dressing can impair circulation to the wound bed and local tissue hindering healing.

MEETING PATIENTS' MICROBIOLOGICAL SAFETY NEEDS

This section includes questions on concepts and principles related to topics such as medical asepsis, surgical asepsis, types of isolation, and the chain of infection. Particular emphasis is placed on nursing actions that protect the nurse and the patient from microorganisms, including questions on hand hygiene and disposal of contaminated equipment and linen. The questions also address risk factors for infection, common clinical findings related to infection, and patient teaching/learning of infection control practices.

QUESTIONS

1. A nurse is teaching a patient about ways to prevent infection. Which **best** increases a patient's defense against microorganisms?
   1. Covering a cough
   2. Maintaining intact skin
   3. Changing bed linen daily
   4. Using an antiseptic mouthwash

   TEST-TAKING TIP Identify the word in the stem that sets a priority.

2. Which can the nurse do to prevent fungal infections in a hospitalized patient?
   1. Apply moisturizing lotion to the patient's body.
   2. Provide a daily bath for the patient.
   3. Dry the folds of the patient's skin.
   4. Keep the patient's room cool.

3. A nurse initiates contact precautions for a patient with a wound infection. Which should the nurse do to help the patient cope with the psychological aspects of these precautions?
   1. Draw a smiley face on the mask.
   2. Don gloves when providing direct care.
   3. Explain the importance of contact precautions.
   4. Wear a gown only when interaction between the patient and nurse's uniform is likely.

   TEST-TAKING TIP Identify the key word in the stem that directs attention to content. Identify the option with a specific determiner. Identify the clang association.

4. A nurse irrigates the wound of a patient on contact precautions. Which should the nurse do **first** to remove personal protective equipment when leaving this patient's room?
   1. Untie the gown at the waist.
   2. Untie the gown at the neck.
   3. Remove the gloves.
   4. Remove the mask.

   TEST-TAKING TIP Identify the word in the stem that sets a priority.

5. A nurse is planning care for patients who are diagnosed with acquired immunodeficiency syndrome (AIDS). For which complication are all these patients at the greatest risk?
   1. Environmental disorientation
   2. Acquired infections
   3. Secondary cancer
   4. Pressure ulcers

   TEST-TAKING TIP Identify the word in the stem that sets a priority. Identify the key word in the stem that directs attention to content. Identify the clang association.

6. A nurse is caring for a patient with an infection. For which **most** common response to infection should the nurse assess the patient?
   1. Fever
   2. Anorexia
   3. Headache
   4. Dehydration

   TEST-TAKING TIP Identify the word in the stem that sets a priority. Identify the key word in the stem that directs attention to content.

7. Which question should the nurse ask a patient with an infection when taking a nursing history as opposed to a medical history?
   1. "Have you done any traveling lately?"
   2. "How long has the infection been present?"
   3. "When did you first notice your symptoms?"
   4. "How does the infection affect your daily routine?"

   TEST-TAKING TIP Identify equally plausible options. Identify the clang association.

8. An adult man is admitted to the hospital with a medical diagnosis of fever of unknown origin. Which laboratory result should the nurse report to the primary health-care provider?
   1. White blood cell count of 20,000/μL
   2. Urine specific gravity of 1.020
   3. Hemoglobin of 14.5 g/dL
   4. Hematocrit of 42%

9. A nurse observes a nursing assistant violate aseptic technique when removing soiled gloves. Which did the nursing assistant do that was incorrect?
   1. Grasped the outer surface of the left glove below the thumb with the gloved right hand
   2. Contained the removed glove from the left hand within the fingers of the gloved right hand
   3. Discarded the right glove that had been inverted containing the left glove into an appropriate waste container
   4. Used the left ungloved thumb and forefinger to grasp the inside and outside of the cuff of the gloved right hand

   TEST-TAKING TIP Identify words in the stem that indicate negative polarity.

10. When removing protective gloves that were worn to start an intravenous solution, a female nurse notices that there is a small amount of the patient's blood on two sections of her forearm. Which should the nurse do **first**?
    1. Flush from the elbow to the fingers with hot water.
    2. Clean soiled areas with gauze moistened with alcohol.
    3. Wash blood-exposed areas with warm water and soap.
    4. Absorb blood with a paper towel and don clean gloves.

    TEST-TAKING TIP Identify the word in the stem that sets a priority. Identify clang associations.

11. A nurse is changing a patient's bed linens. Where should the nurse place soiled linen when it is removed from the bed?
    1. In a soiled linen hamper
    2. On the overbed table
    3. Into the laundry chute
    4. On a chair

    TEST-TAKING TIP Identify the clang association. Identify equally plausible options.

12. In which environment do bacteria rapidly multiply?
1. Hot
2. Cool
3. Cold
4. Warm

TEST-TAKING TIP Identify opposites in options.

13. Linens that are still clean are often reused by the same patient. Which article of linen is **least** likely to be reused by the nurse when making the bed?
1. Top sheet
2. Bedspread
3. Pillowcase
4. Cotton blanket

TEST-TAKING TIP Identify the word in the stem that indicates negative polarity. Identify the unique option.

14. A patient on contact precautions needs a blood pressure reading taken every shift. Which is the **most** practical intervention by the nurse to keep the sphygmomanometer from spreading microorganisms?
1. Place it in a protective bag.
2. Keep it in the patient's room.
3. Soak it in a germicidal solution.
4. Store it in the dirty utility room.

TEST-TAKING TIP Identify the word in the stem that sets a priority. Identify the key word in the stem that directs attention to content.

15. Which has the greatest impact on limiting the spread of microorganisms?
1. Disposable equipment
2. Double-bagging
3. Wearing gloves
4. Hand hygiene

TEST-TAKING TIP Identify the word in the stem that sets a priority.

16. A nurse is cleaning an emesis basin containing purulent material. Which should the nurse do **first?**
1. Spray the basin with a disinfectant.
2. Wash the basin with hot, soapy water.
3. Rinse the basin with cold running water.
4. Clean the basin with an antiseptic agent.

TEST-TAKING TIP Identify the word in the stem that sets a priority.

17. A nurse is assessing a patient's wound. Which characteristic of the wound's exudate indicates to the nurse that the wound may be infected?
1. Serous
2. Purulent
3. Sanguineous
4. Serosanguineous

TEST-TAKING TIP Identify the unique option.

18. Penicillin 2.4 million units IM × 1 is prescribed for a patient with an infection. The medication comes in the form of a powder of 5 million units per vial with instructions for reconstitution. The directions state to add 3.2 mL of sterile diluent to yield 3.5 mL of solution. How many milliliters should the nurse administer? **Record your answer using one decimal place.**

Answer: _____ mL

19. A nurse is observing a student nursing assistant practice activities associated with exiting the room of a patient on contact isolation. Which photograph indicates that further teaching is necessary?

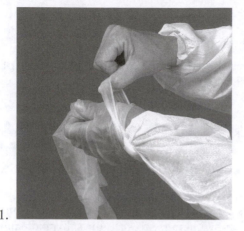

1.

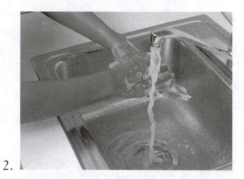

2.

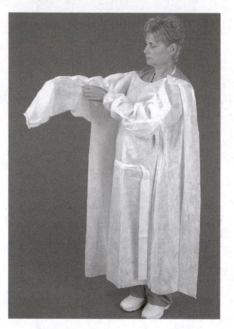

3.

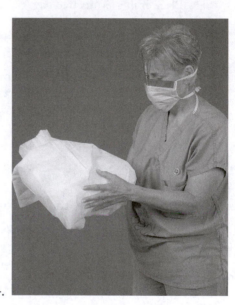

4.

20. Which actions break the chain of infection from a portal of exit from a reservoir? **Select all that apply.**
1. _____ Washing the hands
2. _____ Disposing of soiled linen
3. _____ Disinfecting used equipment
4. _____ Covering the mouth when coughing
5. _____ Avoiding breastfeeding when HIV positive

TEST-TAKING TIP Identify key words in the stem that direct attention to content.

21. Airborne precautions are ordered for a patient with the diagnosis of tuberculosis. Which nursing actions are specific to caring for the patient on airborne precautions? **Select all that apply.**
1. _____ Keeping the patient's door closed
2. _____ Donning a gown when administering medications
3. _____ Wearing disposable gloves when delivering a meal
4. _____ Wearing a high-efficiency particulate air filter respirator
5. _____ Instructing the patient to wear a mask when receiving care

TEST-TAKING TIP Identify key words in the stem that direct attention to content.

22. A nurse must change a patient's sterile dressing. Place the following steps in the order in which they should be performed.
1. Don the first glove with the fingers held downward toward the floor.
2. Open the outer glove package, grasp the inner package, and lay it on a waist-high, clean surface.
3. Interlock the fingers of both hands to ensure that the gloves and its fingers are securely in place.
4. Grasp the inside cuff of the glove of the dominant hand with the thumb and first two fingers of the nondominant hand.
5. Pick up the glove for the nondominant hand from the outside of the cuff with the gloved dominant hand and insert the nondominant hand.

Answer: _____

23. A nurse is making rounds at the beginning of a shift and identifies the following sources of infection. Which situations require the nurse to intervene to reduce the risk of infection? **Select all that apply.**
1. _____ An intravenous tubing labeled as being changed 5 days previously
2. _____ A urinal with urine hanging from the side rail of the patient's bed
3. _____ A urinary retention catheter collection bag containing 1500 mL of urine
4. _____ A closed bottle of sterile normal saline labeled as being opened 20 hours earlier
5. _____ An opened container of pudding on the bedside table being saved for a snack in the afternoon

24. Postoperatively a patient has an order for the incision to be cleansed with normal saline and the application of a dry sterile dressing. Which stroke should the nurse perform first when cleansing the wound?
1. A
2. B
3. C

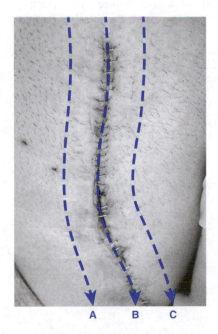

A   B   C

25. A 75-year-old man is transferred from a nursing home to the emergency department of the hospital. Which type of isolation precautions should the nurse initiate after reviewing the transfer form supplied by the nursing home and the results of the initial physical assessment in the hospital?
1. Droplet
2. Contact
3. Airborne
4. Protective

PATIENT'S CLINICAL RECORD

Laboratory Results
RBC: 4.5×10^6
WBC: 18,000/mm^3
Hb: 16 g/dL
Hct: 45%

Patient History
MRSA positive
Type 1 diabetes
Brain attack with residual left hemiparesis

Physical Assessment
Full-thickness skin loss including subcutaneous tissue in the sacral area; area is 3×4 cm with a small amount of yellow drainage. Vital signs: Temperature 100°F (oral); Pulse 92 beats per minute; Respirations 22 breaths per minute. Incontinent of urine and feces.

---

26. A patient with a vertical abdominal wound that is healing by secondary intention has an order for the wound to be irrigated with 0.9% sodium chloride twice a day. The nurse places the patient in the low-Fowler position. Place an X where the nurse should direct the stream of solution when irrigating the patient's wound.

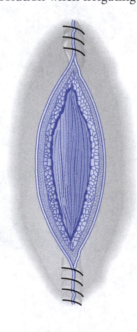

27. A patient with gonorrhea is to receive ceftriaxone 250 mg IM STAT. The vial contains 1 gram of ceftriaxone with the instructions to add 3.5 mL of diluent to yield 4 mL of solution. How much solution of ceftriaxone should the nurse prepare to administer the prescribed dose? **Record your answer using a whole number.**

   Answer: _____ **mL**

28. Which should the nurse do when engaged in hand hygiene using soap and water? **Select all that apply.**
    1. ____ Wash the hands for a minimum of fifteen seconds.
    2. ____ Wash with the hands held higher than the elbows.
    3. ____ Rinse with the hands held lower than the elbows.
    4. ____ Turn the faucet on with a clean paper towel.
    5. ____ Adjust the water to a warm temperature.

    TEST-TAKING TIP Identify the clang association.

29. Which factors identified by the nurse create the greatest risk for a patient to develop a respiratory tract infection? **Select all that apply.**
    1. ____ Gastric surgery
    2. ____ Urinary catheter
    3. ____ Long hospital stay
    4. ____ Painful chest injury
    5. ____ Nasogastric tube to suction

    TEST-TAKING TIP Identify the word in the stem that sets a priority. Identify the clang association.

30. A nurse is irrigating a wound of a patient who is on contact precautions. Which nursing actions are appropriate when caring for this patient? **Select all that apply.**
    1. ____ Donning goggles for the irrigation
    2. ____ Wearing a respirator device when giving care
    3. ____ Washing the hands immediately after removing soiled gloves
    4. ____ Ensuring that negative air pressure in the room is maintained
    5. ____ Removing the gown before the gloves when leaving the room

    TEST-TAKING TIP Identify key words in the stem that direct attention to content. Identify the clang association.

1. **TEST-TAKING TIP** The word "best" in the stem sets a priority.

   1. Covering a cough protects others from the patient's microorganisms.
   2. **The skin is a barrier to pathogens and, if pierced or broken, serves as a portal of entry for microorganisms.**
   3. Although changing bed linen daily may reduce the number of microorganisms present, it does not best protect the patient from microorganisms.
   4. Although using an antiseptic mouthwash may reduce the number of microorganisms present, it does not best protect the patient from microorganisms.

2. 1. Moisturizers soften skin; they do not protect the skin from fungal infection.
   2. Although bathing daily is helpful in preventing infection, it is not the best way to prevent the growth of fungi.
   3. **Fungi multiply rapidly in places where moisture content is high, such as in skin folds. Careful drying of skin folds, especially under the breasts and arms, between the toes, and in the perineal area, helps prevent the development of fungal infections.**
   4. A cool room may reduce perspiration; however, it is not the best way to prevent the growth of fungi.

3. **TEST-TAKING TIP** The word "psychological" is the key word in the stem that directs attention to content. Option 4 contains the word "only," which is a specific determiner. The words "contact precautions" in the stem and option 3 is a clang association.

   1. A mask is necessary only if splashing of blood or body fluids is expected. The patient may interpret a smiley face as an attempt to minimize the gravity of the illness; humor must be used carefully.
   2. Gloves must be worn by everyone who enters the room of a patient on contact precautions; it does not address the psychological needs of the patient.
   3. **Explanations support understanding, acceptance, and compliance with isolation precautions. When people understand the reason for a procedure, fear of the unknown and anxiety usually are reduced.**

   4. Wearing a gown does not address the psychological needs of the patient. A gown is necessary if there is a possibility of contact with infected surfaces or items; in addition, it is necessary if the patient is incontinent or has diarrhea, a colostomy, or wound drainage not covered and contained by a dressing.

4. **TEST-TAKING TIP** The word "first" in the stem sets a priority.

   1. **The waist is considered contaminated and should be untied with a gloved hand.**
   2. Ties at the neck are considered clean and should be untied after the gloves are removed.
   3. Gloves are removed after waist ties are untied.
   4. After the gloves are removed, the mask is removed by touching only the ties. This is done to prevent contamination of the nurse's head, hair, and hands.

5. **TEST-TAKING TIP** The word "greatest" in the stem sets a priority. The word "all" is the key word in the stem that directs attention to content. The correct answer must address something that is common to all patients with AIDS. The word "acquired" in the stem and option 2 is a clang association.

   1. Not all patients who have AIDS have central nervous system involvement that may cause cognitive impairment.
   2. **All patients who have AIDS are immunosuppressed and have a decreased ability to fight infection; this places them at the greatest risk for acquired infections.**
   3. Not all patients with AIDS develop cancer.
   4. Not all patients with AIDS are bed bound or cachectic, which places them at risk for pressure ulcers.

6. **TEST-TAKING TIP** The word "most" in the stem sets a priority. The word "common" modifies the word "response" and is the key word in the stem that directs attention to content.

   1. **Fever is the most common response of the hypothalamus (thermoregulatory**

center) to pyrogens that are released when phagocytic cells respond to the presence of pathogens.

2. Anorexia is a nonspecific manifestation of infection and is not as commonly exhibited by a patient with an infection as a response in another option.

3. A headache is a nonspecific manifestation of infection and is not as commonly exhibited by a patient with an infection as a response in another option.

4. Although dehydration can occur in response to a fever or an inadequate intake of fluid, it is not as common a response to infection as a response in another option.

7. **TEST-TAKING TIP Options 2 and 3 both ask questions that identify a time frame in relation to symptoms; these options are equally plausible and should be eliminated. The word "infection" in the stem and option 4 is a clang association.**

1. Although the nurse may ask about traveling, this statement relates to the medical diagnosis and to planning of the medical treatment regimen.

2. Although the nurse may ask about the length of the infection, this statement relates to the medical diagnosis and to planning of the medical treatment regimen.

3. Although the nurse may ask when symptoms were first noticed, this statement relates to the medical diagnosis and to planning of the medical treatment regimen.

4. **The nurse is mostly concerned with how the infection affects a person's functional health patterns. Many nurse practice acts recognize that nurses diagnose and treat human responses.**

8. 1. **A white blood cell count of 20,000/μL is higher than the expected range of 4,500 to 11,000/μL and generally indicates the presence of an infection.**

2. This is within the expected range of urine specific gravity of 1.001 to 1.029 and is unrelated to infection.

3. This is within the expected range for hemoglobin in an adult male, which is 13.2 to 17.3 g/dL; hemoglobin is unrelated to infection.

4. This is within the expected range for hematocrit in an adult male, which is 37% to 49%; hematocrit is unrelated to infection.

9. **TEST-TAKING TIP The words "violate" and "incorrect" in the stem indicate negative polarity. The question is asking, "Which action is *not an acceptable practice* when removing soiled gloves?"**

1. The outer surfaces of both gloves are contaminated; this action keeps the soiled parts of the gloves from contaminating the skin of the left wrist or hand.

2. This action contains the soiled glove within a small area and prevents inadvertent self-contamination.

3. This action safely disposes of both contaminated gloves; the most contaminated surfaces are inside the inverted right glove and they are contained in an appropriate receptacle for removal from the patient's unit.

4. **This is a violation of aseptic technique. The outer surface of a soiled glove is contaminated and should not be touched by an ungloved hand. While holding the removed left glove in the right hand, the individual should insert two fingers of the left, ungloved hand inside the cuff of the right glove. The individual then pulls the right glove off, turning it inside out, thereby containing the left glove inside the inverted right glove.**

10. **TEST-TAKING TIP The word "first" in the stem sets a priority. The word "blood" in the stem and options 3 and 4 comprise clang associations.**

1. Hot water does not disinfect and is unnecessary; it also may injure the tissue.

2. The disinfectant isopropyl alcohol can kill bacteria but cannot kill spores, viruses, or fungi.

3. **Washing includes the action of wetting, rubbing, and rinsing; soap reduces the surface tension of water; friction mechanically disturbs microorganisms; and rinsing flushes microorganisms from the skin.**

4. Absorbing blood with a paper towel does not adequately remove the contaminated material from the surface of the skin.

11. **TEST-TAKING TIP The words "soiled linen" in the stem and option 1 is a clang association. Options 2 and 4 are equally plausible because they are both furniture in the room and one is not better than the other.**

1. **Depositing soiled linen in a soiled linen hamper is a safe and acceptable way to contain microorganisms.**

2. Placing soiled linen on the overbed table contaminates the overbed table and is an undesirable practice; the overbed table is considered a clean surface and should not be used to hold soiled linen.

3. Placing soiled linen into a laundry chute without first placing it in a soiled linen laundry bag is an undesirable practice because it will contaminate the chute. Soiled linen must be bagged to contain microorganisms before it is deposited in a laundry chute.

4. Placing soiled linen on a chair contaminates the chair and is an undesirable practice; a chair is considered a clean surface and should not be used to hold soiled linen.

12. **TEST-TAKING TIP** Options 1 and 3 and options 2 and 4 are opposites. Unfortunately, the test-taking tip "identify opposites in options" is not helpful in eliminating options in this question.

1. Hot temperatures are used to destroy bacteria (e.g., sterilization).
2. Bacteria do not multiply rapidly in cool environments.
3. Bacteria do not multiply rapidly in cold environments.
4. **Bacteria grow most rapidly in dark, warm, moist environments, particularly when the environment is close to body temperature (98.6°F).**

13. **TEST-TAKING TIP** The word "least" in the stem indicates negative polarity. Options 1, 2, and 4 are all similar because they are articles of linen that are generally placed over the patient. Option 3 is unique because it is the only article of linen of the options offered that is positioned under the patient.

1. A top sheet is often used again if it is still clean.
2. A bedspread is often used again if it is still clean.
3. **The pillowcase comes in contact with the hair, exudate from the eyes, mucus from the nose, and saliva from the mouth. A pillowcase is easily soiled and usually needs to be replaced more often than other linen.**
4. A cotton blanket is often used again if it is still clean.

14. **TEST-TAKING TIP** The word "most" in the stem sets a priority. The word "practical"

is the key word in the stem that directs attention to content.

1. Placing it in a protective bag is unsafe. The outer surface of the bag is also contaminated and, if taken out of the room, will contaminate any surface on which it is placed.
2. **Keeping it in the patient's room is the most practical action; when isolation is discontinued, all of the equipment can be terminally disinfected.**
3. Soaking it in a germicidal solution is impractical and will harm the sphygmomanometer.
4. The sphygmomanometer is contaminated and must be disinfected before it is removed from the patient's room.

15. **TEST-TAKING TIP** The word "greatest" in the stem sets a priority.

1. Using disposable equipment is not the most effective method to reduce the spread of microorganisms; not all equipment is disposable.
2. Although double-bagging limits the spread of microorganisms, it is not the most effective method to reduce the spread of microorganisms.
3. Although gloves protect the nurse and limit the spread of microorganisms, it is not the most effective method to reduce the spread of microorganisms.
4. **Hand hygiene is the most effective measure to reduce the spread of microorganisms because it removes them from the hands that come in contact with other patients and objects.**

16. **TEST-TAKING TIP** The word "first" in the stem sets a priority.

1. Spraying the basin with a disinfectant is unnecessary.
2. Washing the basin in hot, soapy water should not be the initial intervention. Hot water coagulates the protein of organic material and causes it to stick to a surface.
3. **Rinsing the basin with cold running water is a correct action because it does not coagulate the protein of organic material, permitting it to be flushed from the surface of the basin.**
4. Antiseptics are used to limit bacteria on the skin or in wounds, not for cleaning objects.

17. **TEST-TAKING TIP** The first word in options 1, 3, and 4 all begin with the letter "S."

Option 2 is unique because it begins with the letter "P."

1. Serous exudate is watery in appearance, is composed of mainly serum, and does not indicate an infection.
2. **Purulent exudate contains material such as dead and living bacteria and dead tissue; it indicates the possibility of an infection.**
3. Sanguineous exudate indicates damage to capillaries that allows escape of red blood cells from plasma.
4. Serosanguineous exudate consists of clear and blood-tinged drainage as seen in surgical incisions.

18. **Answer: 1.7 mL**
    Solve the problem by using ratio and proportion.

    $$\frac{\text{Desire}}{\text{Have}} \quad \frac{2.4 \text{ million units}}{5 \text{ million units}} = \frac{x \text{ mL}}{3.5 \text{ mL}}$$

    $5x = 2.4 \times 3.5$

    $5x = 8.4$

    $x = 8.4 \div 5$

    $x = 1.68$; round 1.68 up to 1.7 mL

19. 1. Once the first soiled glove is removed, the photograph reflects the correct way to remove a soiled glove from the second gloved hand. The clean hand is touching the inside of the soiled glove and not the contaminated outside of the soiled glove.
    2. Once protective equipment is removed, the hands are washed again before the caregiver leaves the patient's room.
    3. **Clean hands should not touch the contaminated outer surface of the gown as it is being removed. The illustration at right indicates how the nurse should peel the gown from one shoulder and then the other in the direction of the hands while keeping the hands inside the gown. Doing so will turn the gown inside out. While keeping the hands inside the gown, the gown should be rolled so that the exterior of the gown is wrapped inside the rest of the gown so that the clean inner surface encircles and contains the contaminated outer surface.**
    4. The photograph demonstrates the correct way to hold a contained soiled gown away from the body so as not to contaminate the uniform. The rolled gown is then discarded into the appropriate waste receptacle.

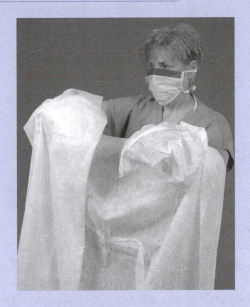

20. **TEST-TAKING TIP** The words "portal of exit" are key words in the stem that direct attention to content.

    1. ____ Hand hygiene is an important means of controlling the transmission of microorganisms from one person or object to another; it does not limit the number of microorganisms directly exiting from a reservoir.
    2. ____ Disposing of soiled linen is an important means of controlling the transmission of microorganisms from one person or object to another; it does not limit the number of microorganisms directly exiting from a reservoir.
    3. ____ Disinfecting used equipment is an important means of controlling the transmission of microorganisms from one person or object to another; it does not limit the number of microorganisms directly exiting from a reservoir.
    4. X Covering a cough limits the number of microorganisms that exit from the respiratory tract. The respiratory tract is one portal of exit from the human reservoir (source of microorganisms). Other human portals of exit include the gastrointestinal, urinary, and reproductive tracts and blood and body fluids.
    5. X Breast milk can transmit the human immunodeficiency virus from an infected mother to an infant. Breast milk is a portal of exit from the human reservoir.

21. **TEST-TAKING TIP** The words "specific to" and "airborne precautions" are key

words in the stem that direct attention to content.

1. **X** Keeping the door closed prevents the spread of microorganisms that can be transmitted via air currents. The patient should be in a room with negative air pressure.

2. ____ It is not necessary for a nurse to wear a gown when administering medications to a patient with airborne precautions.

3. ____ It is not necessary for a caregiver to wear gloves when delivering a meal tray to a patient with airborne precautions.

4. **X** Wearing a high-efficiency particulate air filter respirator (HEPA) prevents transmission of droplet nuclei less than or equal to 5 μm or dust particles containing the pathogen; these particles remain suspended in the air for extended periods of time.

5. ____ The nurse, not the patient, wears a high-efficiency particulate air filter respirator for self-protection.

22. **Answer: 2, 4, 1, 5, 3**

2. **Touching the outside package of sterile equipment with ungloved hands is an acceptable practice. A clean, dry surface prevents contamination of the wrapper; objects below the waist are considered contaminated.**

4. **The ungloved hand is permitted to touch the inner surface of a sterile glove; both surfaces are considered contaminated.**

1. **By donning the gloves with the fingers facing downward prevents the fingers of the sterile glove from folding over onto the ungloved hands and becoming contaminated.**

5. **Putting on the second glove by inserting the gloved fingers under the everted cuff of the second glove maintains sterile to sterile contact.**

3. **Sterile to sterile contact maintains sterility of the gloves. Interdigital pressure ensures that the fingers of the gloves are fully in place over the fingers.**

23. 1. **X** Most protocols require that IV tubing be changed every 72 to 96 hours. Extending use beyond the time indicated in a protocol places the patient at risk for infection. Inflammation of a vein (phlebitis) can progress to an infection.

2. **X** Urinals should be emptied as soon as they are used. Clean urinals should be stored in the lowest drawer of a bedside table or in a designated area in a patient's bathroom. The urinal should be labeled with the patient's initials.

3. ____ A urinary collection bag containing 1500 mL is not an infection risk. Although 1500 mL is a large amount of urine, most urinary collection bags can hold 2000 mL of urine. Ideally urinary collection bags should be emptied when half full to minimize stress on the tubing that can cause tension on the catheter entering the urinary meatus. To prevent infection a urinary collection bag should hang below the level of the patient's pelvis, not rest on the floor, be emptied carefully to prevent contamination of the exit port, and standard precautions followed by the caregiver at all times.

4. ____ A bottle of sterile normal saline can be used if it is tightly closed and the label indicates that it was opened within the previous 24 hours.

5. **X** Uncovered food should not be kept at the bedside because it can spoil and/or attract insects. Some health-care facilities will permit a piece of fruit wrapped in plastic or a snack in a labeled container to be kept at the bedside for a short period of time.

24. 1. Cleansing the skin on the left side of the incision first may drag microorganisms on the skin into the incision, possibly contaminating the incision.

2. **The first cleansing stroke should be over the center of the incision following line "B." The next stroke can be either on the left or right side of the incision with the final stroke being the side of the incision that has not already been cleansed. Cleaning the center of the incision first follows the concept of clean to dirty. The incision is considered "clean," whereas the skin is considered "dirty." Cleaning the skin first will draw microorganisms on the skin into the incision, possibly contaminating the incision.**

3. Cleansing the skin on the right side of the incision first may draw microorganisms on the skin into the incision, possibly contaminating the incision.

25. 1. There is no sputum culture result indicating a respiratory infection that requires droplet precautions. Increased vital signs indicate an infection, but there are no clinical findings (e.g., dyspnea, cough, increase in respiratory secretions, labored breathing, crackles/rhonchi) indicating a respiratory infection that requires a need for droplet precautions.
    2. **The patient must have contact precautions instituted because of the history of the patient's being methicillin-resistant *Staphylococcus aureus* (MRSA) positive, experiencing urine and fecal incontinence, and having a wound with yellow drainage. Contact precautions prevent the spread of pathogens from the patient to the nurse and others. The WBCs are increased above the expected range, indicating an infectious/inflammatory process. Patients with diabetes are at risk for infection because of a decreased immune response and the high glucose in tissues, which supports the growth of microorganisms. Yellow drainage from a pressure ulcer is suggestive of an infection. The increase in vital signs above the expected range reflects the stimulation of the general adaptation syndrome in response to the presence of a pathogen (e.g., MRSA).**
    3. There is no sputum culture result, indicating a respiratory infection that requires airborne precautions. The increased vital signs indicate an infection, but there are no clinical findings (e.g., dyspnea, cough, increase in respiratory secretions, labored breathing, crackles/rhonchi) indicating a respiratory infection that requires a need for airborne precautions.
    4. Protective precautions are unnecessary. Protective precautions would be necessary if the WBCs were low, not high, putting the patient at risk for infection.

26. The irrigating solution should begin flowing from the top inside edge of the wound. Initiating the flow of solution inside of the wound prevents microorganism on the skin from being carried into the wound, possibly contaminating the wound. This follows the principle of clean to dirty. The wound itself is considered "clean" and the skin is considered "dirty." By beginning at the top of the wound the solution will flow by gravity into a container held by the nurse at the bottom of the wound.

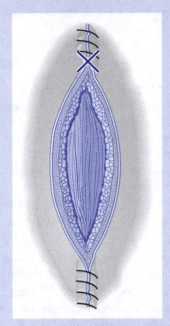

27. Answer: 1 mL
    To answer the question, first convert milligrams to grams.

    $$\frac{\text{Desire}}{\text{Have}} \quad \frac{250 \text{ mg}}{1000 \text{ mg}} = \frac{x \text{ gram}}{1 \text{ gram}}$$

    $$1000 x = 250$$
    $$x = 250 \div 1000$$
    $$x = 0.25 \text{ gram is equal to } 250 \text{ mg}$$

    Next use ratio and proportion to determine the amount of solution to administer.

    $$\frac{\text{Desire}}{\text{Have}} \quad \frac{0.25 \text{ gram}}{1 \text{ gram}} = \frac{x \text{ mL}}{4 \text{ mL}}$$

    $$1 x = 0.25 \times 4$$
    $$x = 1 \text{ mL}$$

28. **TEST-TAKING TIP The word "water" in the stem and in option 5 is a clang association.**
    1. <u>X</u> When the hands are visibly soiled, the Centers for Disease Control and Prevention recommend washing the hands with a nonantimicrobial or antimicrobial soap and water for a minimum of 15 seconds.
    2. ____ The hands should be held lower, not higher, than the elbows. The hands are more contaminated than the arms; water should flow from clean to contaminated surfaces.

3. X Rinsing with the hands lower than the elbows is correct technique; the hands are more contaminated than the arms. Water washes away debris and microorganisms and prevents recontamination of the cleaner surfaces.

4. ____ The hands and the faucet are both considered contaminated and therefore it is not necessary to use a clean paper towel to turn on the faucet. A clean paper towel should be used to turn the faucet off after the hands are washed and dried.

5. X The nurse should adjust the water to a warm, not hot, temperature; hot water removes protective oils from the skin, which causes chapping.

29. **TEST-TAKING TIP** The word "greatest" in the stem sets a priority. The words "respiratory" in the stem and "chest" in option 4 comprise an obscure clang association. "Respiratory" refers to lungs and the lungs are located in the "chest."

1. X The stomach is anatomically just below the diaphragm. Deep breathing and coughing after high abdominal surgery frequently results in pain and therefore is avoided by patients; this predisposes the patient to a respiratory infection because of the stasis of respiratory secretion and the development of atelectasis.

2. ____ A urinary catheter contributes to the risk for a urinary, not respiratory, tract infection.

3. ____ The hospital environment contains many pathogens; however, a person has to be susceptible to contract an infection.

4. X Coughing and deep breathing are often avoided by people with painful chest injuries in an effort to self-splint

and minimize pain; this allows pooling of respiratory secretions and contributes to an environment that supports the growth of microorganisms in the respiratory tract.

5. ____ A nasogastric tube decompressing the stomach removes fluid from the body, which does not increase the risk for a respiratory tract infection. A nasogastric tube used as a feeding tube may place the patient at risk for aspiration pneumonia.

30. **TEST-TAKING TIP** The words "contact precautions" are key words in the stem that direct attention to content. The words "irrigating" in the stem and "irrigation" in option 1 comprise a clang association.

1. X The nurse should wear a gown, gloves, and a face shield or goggles when splashing of body fluids may occur when a patient has a condition that requires contact precautions.

2. ____ A respirator device is not necessary for a patient on contact precautions; a regular mask with a face shield or goggles is necessary when the splashing of body fluids may occur.

3. X Hands should be washed before donning gloves and immediately after removing them.

4. ____ A room with negative air pressure is not necessary for contact precautions; a room with negative pressure is necessary with airborne precautions.

5. ____ Gloves are removed before, not after, the gown.

MEETING THE NEEDS OF PATIENTS IN THE COMMUNITY SETTING

This section encompasses questions related to caring for an individual, a family, a subgroup, or the population within a community. The questions include topics such as health-care delivery settings (e.g., nursing homes, day-care centers, assisted-living residences, occupational settings, and private homes), the focus of nursing actions (e.g., prevention of illness, health promotion, maintenance of safe environments, protection and restoration of health), and specific nursing activities (e.g., screening, health education). The questions also focus on levels of health-care services (e.g., primary, secondary, and tertiary health-care delivery), levels of disease prevention (e.g., primary, secondary, and tertiary levels of prevention), and community-focused examples related to nursing intervention (e.g., developmental stresses, common health problems, crisis intervention, and the needs of individuals in the community based on Maslow's Hierarchy of Needs).

QUESTIONS

1. A nurse is caring for a patient recently discharged from the hospital. Which nursing intervention takes priority?
   1. Providing opportunities to make choices concerning the plan of care
   2. Exploring the need to modify the home environment to prevent falls
   3. Teaching a family member how to feed a patient who has a decreased gag reflex
   4. Encouraging the patient to ventilate negative feelings about loss of independence

   TEST-TAKING TIP Identify the word in the stem that sets a priority. Use Maslow's Hierarchy of Needs to identify the priority.

2. Which trend in health care is receiving the **most** attention?
   1. Tertiary care
   2. Early diagnosis
   3. Health promotion
   4. Restorative rehabilitation

   TEST-TAKING TIP Identify the word in the stem that sets a priority.

3. Which is an essential aspect of community health nursing?
   1. Interdisciplinary nature
   2. Practice within the home setting
   3. Focus on the needs of individuals
   4. Emphasis mainly on health promotion

   TEST-TAKING TIP Identify the word in the stem that sets a priority.

4. Which group is covered by Medicare?
   1. People who receive Aid to Families with Dependent Children
   2. Women who need nurse midwife services
   3. Individuals with just a low income
   4. Adults 65 years and older

   TEST-TAKING TIP Identify the option with a specific determiner. Identify the unique option.

5. A person is exposed to an individual diagnosed with severe acute respiratory syndrome (SARS). Which method should the nurse expect to be implemented to control the spread of infection?
   1. Isolation
   2. Quarantine
   3. Segregation
   4. Surveillance

6. Which statement reflects the concept of prevalence?
   1. "On Monday morning, the school nurse identified that six children had measles."
   2. "During the last 5 years, 1% of the population of the United States had tuberculosis."
   3. "Last year, of the people at risk for developing breast cancer, 9% actually developed the disease."
   4. "On the first day of June this year, 10% of the population of Middletown had cardiovascular disease."

7. Which statement **most** accurately reflects the principle of providing for a patient's nutritional needs in the home?
   1. The patient should eat whatever is preferred as long as adequate protein is ingested.
   2. The patient should plan to eat meals at the same time as other family members.
   3. Supplements should be taken whenever the patient is hungry between meals.
   4. Support groups may be used to ensure adequate nutrition for the patient.

   TEST-TAKING TIP Identify the word in the stem that sets a priority. Identify the clang association.

8. Which is the priority when the nurse cares for an older adult in the community?
   1. Maintaining quality of life
   2. Supporting rehabilitation needs
   3. Helping with bureaucratic paperwork
   4. Encouraging interaction within the family

   TEST-TAKING TIP Identify the word in the stem that sets a priority. Identify the global option.

9. Which categories of health-care delivery are mainly associated with community-based nursing?
   1. Primary and tertiary
   2. Secondary and primary
   3. Tertiary and rehabilitation
   4. Rehabilitation and secondary

   TEST-TAKING TIP Identify the word in the stem that sets a priority. Identify duplicate facts among options.

10. Which statement is accurate about health perception and health status?
    1. Assuming the sick role generally is maladaptive and harmful to recovery.
    2. Disability is related to the extent one is able to carry out behaviors of a chosen role.
    3. The ability to tolerate illness and disability is the same for one person as for another.
    4. Anticipation of the future has minimal impact on the understanding of one's well-being.

11. Which sociological trend in the United States is predicted to have the **most** impact on the delivery of health care in the community in the next 20 years?
    1. Decrease in the number of people living in poverty
    2. Increase in the number of multiple-birth deliveries
    3. Increase in the number of graying individuals
    4. Decrease in the number of immigrants

    TEST-TAKING TIP Identify the word in the stem that sets a priority.

12. Which phrase is **most** accurately associated with the concept of community coalition?
    1. Wellness programs
    2. Growing diversity
    3. Shared purpose
    4. Home care

    TEST-TAKING TIP Identify the word in the stem that sets a priority. Identify the key word in the stem that directs attention to content.

13. A visiting nurse is caring for a bed-bound patient with a pressure ulcer. Which nursing intervention associated with providing pressure ulcer care in the home is often different from providing pressure ulcer care in the acute-care setting?
    1. Measuring a wound weekly versus daily
    2. Employing medical asepsis versus sterile technique
    3. Changing dressings every day versus three times a day
    4. Using a bulb syringe versus a piston syringe when irrigating

    TEST-TAKING TIP Identify the key word in the stem that directs attention to content. Identify the option with a specific determiner.

14. Which action by the nurse in the occupational setting reflects the lowest-level need according to Maslow?
    1. Identifying hazards in the environment
    2. Assessing the health status of employees
    3. Initiating an ordered immunization program
    4. Promoting the social adjustment of employees

    TEST-TAKING TIP Identify key words in the stem that direct attention to content.

15. Which population variable is assessed in a community profile inventory when the nurse asks, "How many people live within a square mile in the community?"
    1. Size
    2. Density
    3. Mobility
    4. Composition

16. A nurse is conducting a screening program for the leading cause of death associated with adults age 60 years or older. Which assessment by the nurse is **most** appropriate?
    1. Apical pulse
    2. Breath sounds
    3. Liver palpation
    4. Respiratory rate

    TEST-TAKING TIP Identify the word in the stem that sets a priority. Identify equally plausible options.

17. An older adult who needs minimal help with activities of daily living and who takes prescription medication twice a day is to be discharged from the hospital. Which facility **most** appropriately meets this individual's needs?
    1. Group home
    2. Nursing home
    3. Day-care center
    4. Assisted-living facility

    TEST-TAKING TIP Identify the word in the stem that sets a priority. Identify the clang association.

18. Which populations should a community health nurse anticipate to experience a maturational/developmental crisis? **Select all that apply.**
    1. _____ Recently divorced women
    2. _____ Homosexual adolescents
    3. _____ Critically ill children
    4. _____ Unemployed adults
    5. _____ New parents

    TEST-TAKING TIP Identify key words in the stem that direct attention to content.

19. Which nursing activities in the community address the **most** basic needs according to Maslow's Hierarchy of Needs? **Select all that apply.**
    1. ____ Arranging for Meals on Wheels
    2. ____ Exploring the meaning of one's life
    3. ____ Encouraging the patient to visit with friends
    4. ____ Teaching a family member to remove throw rugs
    5. ____ Supervising a patient performing a colostomy irrigation

    TEST-TAKING TIP Identify the word in the stem that sets a priority. Identify key words in the stem that direct attention to content.

20. A home health-care nurse has had several visits with an older adult who previously had type 2 diabetes mellitus and is now insulin dependent. The patient has a prescription for a mixture of NPH and regular insulin in the morning. The patient also has an order for self-monitoring of blood glucose before each meal and at bedtime with insulin coverage. The nurse has been providing teaching about blood glucose monitoring and injections of insulin. In the most recent home visit the nurse identifies that the patient has appropriate knowledge about diabetes, insulin, and how to perform self-monitoring of blood glucose and insulin injections safely, but occasionally forgets to perform glucose monitoring before lunch. The patient's blood glucose levels have been within acceptable limits. Occasionally the patient requires insulin coverage before a meal, which is effective. The home health-care nurse uses the Omaha Problem Rating Scale for Outcomes to document the patient's knowledge, behavior, and status. Which is the patient's total score?

    Answer: _____

Omaha Problem Rating Scale for Outcomes

Concepts	1	2	3	4	5
Knowledge: Ability of the client to remember and interpret information	No knowledge	Minimal knowledge	Basic knowledge	Adequate knowledge	Superior knowledge
Behavior: Observable responses, actions, or activities of the client fitting the occasion or purpose	Not appropriate behavior	Rarely appropriate behavior	Inconsistently appropriate behavior	Usually appropriate behavior	Consistently appropriate behavior
Status: Condition of the client in relation to objective and subjective defining characteristics	Extreme signs/ symptoms	Severe signs/ symptoms	Moderate signs/ symptoms	Minimal signs/ symptoms	No signs/ symptoms

21. "Upstream thinking" is a conceptual approach used in public health efforts. Which actions implemented by a community health nurse demonstrate "upstream thinking"? **Select all that apply.**

1. ____ Teaching a person with diabetes how to perform self-monitoring of blood glucose
2. ____ Conducting screening programs for the presence of hypertension in older adults
3. ____ Encouraging parents who live in old buildings to test for lead-based paint
4. ____ Urging parents to ensure that their children's vaccinations are up to date
5. ____ Facilitating support groups for people who are giving up smoking

22. Based on the information identified during the home visit, which should the nurse do **first?**

1. Administer insulin coverage as prescribed.
2. Implement the dressing change as per the order.
3. Immediately call 911 for an ambulance to transport the patient to the hospital.
4. Ask the home care supervisor to notify the primary health-care provider of the patient's status.

PATIENT'S HOME CARE CLINICAL RECORD

Admission History
A 65-year-old adult who lives alone with diagnosis of type 1 diabetes manages with diet, twice-a-day insulin doses, and insulin coverage ac and hs as prescribed. Currently receiving home care for a stage II pressure ulcer on the lateral malleolus of the right extremity. The primary health-care provider has ordered daily dressing changes and evaluation of the patient's ability to implement self blood glucose monitoring and self-administration of insulin.

Vital Signs During Home Visit
Blood pressure: 100/65 mm Hg
Pulse: 110 beats/min, thready
Respirations: 24 breaths/min

Nursing Assessment
Patient answered the door using a walker but walked slowly and reported feeling weak and fatigued. The patient verbalized experiencing an increase in urination, blurred vision, and nausea. The patient also stated, "I don't remember what my last blood glucose was or when I had insulin last." Vital signs were taken and the blood glucose level was 350 mg/dL. There was no dressing on the wound.

TEST-TAKING TIP Identify the word in the stem that sets a priority.

23. A nurse is assessing adolescents in the community. For which problems **most** commonly associated with this age group should the nurse include in a focused assessment? **Select all that apply.**

1. _____ Mumps
2. _____ Measles
3. _____ Scoliosis
4. _____ Child abuse
5. _____ Substance abuse
6. _____ Motor vehicle accidents

TEST-TAKING TIP Identify the word in the stem that sets a priority. Identify the key word in the stem that directs attention to content.

24. Which nursing actions provide support during a situational stress? **Select all that apply.**

1. _____ Counseling a parent experiencing the empty nest syndrome
2. _____ Reporting a person to the authorities for child abuse
3. _____ Encouraging an older adult to visit the senior center
4. _____ Conducting sex education classes for adolescents
5. _____ Providing pain relief for a woman with cancer

TEST-TAKING TIP Identify the key word in the stem that directs attention to content.

25. When a nurse is caring for patients in the home, it is important to incorporate principles related to community health nursing. Place the following principles in order of priority.

1. Listen attentively
2. Examine own beliefs and values
3. Remain open to other peoples' views
4. Elicit the support of community resources
5. Assist patients and family members to problem solve

Answer: _____

1. **TEST-TAKING TIP** The word "priority" in the stem requires the nurse to identify what should be done first. Option 3 is an intervention to help maintain a patent airway, a first level need according to Maslow's Hierarchy of Needs. Options 1, 2, and 4 are related to higher-level needs according to Maslow. Option 2 is a second-level need: safety and security. Options 1 and 4 are interventions that support fourth-level needs: self-esteem.

    1. Allowed choices supports self-esteem and the need to feel more empowered over one's situation (fourth-level needs). According to Maslow, this is a higher-level need than physiological needs.
    2. Modifying the home environment to prevent falls addresses safety (a second-level need), which is not as great a priority as physiological needs according to Maslow's Hierarchy of Needs.
    3. **Preventing aspiration and meeting a patient's physiological need to ingest adequate nutrition take priority over higher-level needs according to Maslow.**
    4. Exploring feelings supports self-esteem and the need to feel more empowered over one's situation (fourth-level needs). According to Maslow, this is a higher-level need than physiological needs.

2. **TEST-TAKING TIP** The word "most" in the stem sets a priority.

    1. Tertiary care involves helping patients adapt to limitations caused by illness; historically, this always has been a focus of health care.
    2. Early diagnosis and treatment to prevent complications of illness is a part of secondary care; historically, this always has been a focus of health care.
    3. **Health promotion activities, including exercise programs and low-cholesterol diets, that assist patients to maintain their present levels of health or to enhance their health in the future are a focus of primary care. Health promotion and illness prevention are receiving increased importance.**
    4. Restorative rehabilitation services are a part of tertiary care; historically, this always has been a focus of health care.

3. **TEST-TAKING TIP** The word "essential" in the stem sets a priority.

    1. **Community health nurses must develop collaborative relationships with other health-care professionals as well as with individuals and groups in the community.**
    2. Community health nurses practice in many different settings, including clinics, schools, centers of all kinds, mobile units, and places of employment, not just in the home.
    3. Community health nursing focuses on the health-care needs of groups and families within the community, not just individuals.
    4. Community health nursing focuses on illness prevention, health education, providing support services, hospice care, and rehabilitation, not just health promotion.

4. **TEST-TAKING TIP** The word "just" in option 3 is a specific determiner. Option 4 is unique; it is the only option with a numerical entry "65" as well as the inclusion of the word "and."

    1. Aid to Families with Dependent Children is unrelated to Medicare. It provides assistance to people during the childbearing years, particularly divorced or single women with children.
    2. Midwife services are unrelated to Medicare.
    3. Income is unrelated to Medicare. In 1965, Medicaid was established under Title 19 of the Social Security Act. Medicaid is a federal public assistance program for people who require financial assistance, such as low-income groups.
    4. **In 1965 the Medicare amendments (Title 18) to the Social Security Act provided a national and state health insurance program for people age 65 years and older.**

5. 1. Isolation is used to separate an infected person during the time the person is communicable. The person in the question has been exposed to the severe acute respiratory disease (SARS) pathogen but is not yet infected.
    2. **Quarantine is used to prevent further transmission of the disease in case the person should become infected as a result of exposure to the SARS**

pathogen. The exposed person is kept separate for the duration of the longest incubation period known for the disease.

3. Segregation is used to keep separate a group of infected individuals to control the spread of a disease. In the early 1900s, sanitoriums were established to separate infected individuals with tuberculosis from the general population. In China, in the spring of 2003, a separate hospital was built to segregate and treat individuals diagnosed with SARS.

4. Surveillance is associated with either personal or disease surveillance. Personal surveillance is supervision without limitations on movement. Disease surveillance is the continuing investigation of the incidence and spread of disease relevant to effective control.

6. 1. This statement represents a simple count of the number of people with a disease.

2. Calculating the prevalence rate over a period of time is called a period prevalence rate. It is calculated with the formula:

$$\text{Period Prevalence Rate} = \frac{\text{Number of Persons with a Characteristic During Period of Time}}{\text{Total Number in the Population}}$$

3. This reflects an incidence rate. It is calculated with the formula:

$$\text{Incidence} = \frac{\text{Number of Persons Developing a Disease}}{\text{Total Number at Risk per Unit of Time}}$$

4. **Prevalence refers to all people with a health condition existing in a given population at a given point in time. It is calculated with the formula:**

$$\textbf{Prevalence Rate} = \frac{\textbf{Number of Persons with a Characteristic on a Particular Day}}{\textbf{Total Number in the Population}}$$

7. **TEST-TAKING TIP** The word "most" in the stem sets a priority. The words "nutritional" in the stem and "nutrition" in option 4 is a clang association.

1. Although a diet should be designed with a patient's food preferences in mind, the diet chosen must address all nutritional components associated with the patient's needs, not just protein.

2. Although eating is considered a social activity and patients may be encouraged to eat with family members, this may not meet the nutritional needs of the patient. A variety of issues should be considered: a family meal may be too confusing and distracting; the patient may be on a restricted diet that may make the patient feel uncomfortable when eating with the family; the patient may be receiving a tube feeding and prefer not to be with the family at meal time; or the odor of food may be difficult to tolerate.

3. Supplements should be taken only if nutritional needs cannot be met with the ordered diet. Supplements are rich in calories, vitamins, and/or minerals and, if taken whenever a patient is hungry, they may exceed the patient's metabolic needs. This may contribute to complications such as excessive weight gain.

4. **Meeting the nutritional needs of a patient living at home requires the nurse to consider all phases of achieving adequate nutritional intake, such as the patient's and family's knowledge about nutrition and the ability to shop for, buy, prepare, cook, and eat food. Community support such as home-delivered meals, senior center lunch programs, meals provided by missions and shelters, school lunch programs, and community food pantries help people in need.**

8. **TEST-TAKING TIP** The word "primary" in the stem sets a priority. Option 1 is a global option that inherently includes the interventions identified in options 2, 3, and 4.

1. "Maintaining quality of life" is an option that is broad in scope and addresses improvement in all aspects of the life of the older adult.

2. "Supporting rehabilitation needs" is only one part of caring for an older adult.

3. "Helping with bureaucratic paperwork" is only one part of caring for an older adult.

4. "Encouraging interaction with the family" is only one part of caring for an older adult.

9. **TEST-TAKING TIP** The word "mainly" in the stem sets a priority. Four concepts of health-care delivery are being associated with community-based nursing: primary, secondary, tertiary, and rehabilitation. If you know one concept (either primary or tertiary) that is associated with health-care

delivery in the community setting, two options can be deleted from consideration. If you know one concept (either secondary or rehabilitation) that is not related to health-care delivery in the community setting, two options can be deleted from consideration.

1. **Primary care is associated with health promotion, screening, education, and protection. Although tertiary care is associated with specialized diagnostic and therapeutic care generally delivered in the acute-care setting, it also includes specialized services such as rehabilitation and hospice services, which are most often delivered in community settings.**

2. Although primary health-care activities generally take place in the community setting, secondary health-care activities take place in the acute-care setting and generally not in the community setting.

3. Although tertiary care is associated with specialized services such as rehabilitation, rehabilitation is not a category of health-care delivery. Rehabilitation is a specialized service provided in acute-care and community settings. Activities that help people maintain or restore function after an illness are in the tertiary prevention, not primary prevention, category.

4. Rehabilitation is not considered a category of health care but rather a type of service provided in acute and community settings. Secondary health care is associated with hospital-based service (e.g., critical, emergency, and acute care).

10. 1. Assuming the sick role (passivity, social and psychological regression, and submission to treatment regimens) is adaptive and beneficial if not taken to the extreme. Because illness is a modification in the ability to function, there is always a concurrent need to modify behavior in an attempt to rest and recover, which is adaptive. Assumption of the sick role becomes maladaptive and harmful when a person is unable to move on physically and emotionally after the crisis is resolved.

2. **Where people place themselves on the health–illness continuum is a highly individual perception based on personal expectations and values. People generally fulfill numerous roles. In the role performance model of health and wellness, people who are disabled or** ill but are able to carry out their role according to personal expectations tend to view themselves as closer to the high-level wellness end of the health–illness continuum. When role performance becomes impaired, people are more likely to view themselves as disabled.

3. People react in diversified ways to illness and disability. Every person is an individual, and how an individual reacts depends on many factors, such as age, gender, cultural/ethnic background, religious beliefs, economic status, previous experiences, role in the family, and available support systems.

4. How people anticipate the future has a significant impact on their ability to understand their health. The nurse should assess what people believe and feel about their future life. The nurse must work within the context of the person's situation to best assist with the development of coping mechanisms.

11. **TEST-TAKING TIP** The word "most" in the stem sets a priority.

1. The number of people living in poverty is increasing, not decreasing, in the United States.

2. Although this is a true statement, it does not have the same impact on the health-care needs of the society as the individuals mentioned in another option.

3. **By 2020, the number of people older than the age of 65 will increase to 50 million individuals in the United States; this is the fastest-growing segment of the population. These individuals tend to have multiple chronic health problems.**

4. Diversity is increasing, not decreasing, in the United States.

12. **TEST-TAKING TIP** The word "most" in the stem sets a priority. The word "coalition" is the key word in the stem because it is related to words such as *partnership*, *alliance*, and *unification*. The definition of the word "coalition" should lead you to the word "share" in option 3.

1. A "wellness program" and a "community coalition" are two different concepts. A wellness program is a type of health promotion program that focuses on the reduction of risks and the development of positive health habits.

2. Growing diversity speaks to the increasing differences in culture and ethnicity in the population. People of different cultures maintain cultural values, traditions, and beliefs that contribute to the texture and complexity of a community. Although a group of people from one cultural or ethnic group may share a common purpose, this concept is different from community coalition.

3. **Synonyms for the word "coalition" include** *alliance, unification*, **and** *combination*. **A community coalition is the unification of individuals and groups to address issues related to a shared purpose.**

4. "Home care" and "community coalition" are two different concepts. Home care is associated with providing services for a patient in the individual's place of residence.

13. **TEST-TAKING TIP The word "different" is the key word in the stem that directs attention to content. The word "every" in option 3 is a specific determiner.**

1. Pressure ulcers should be measured at least weekly whether the patient is in the hospital or in the home. It may be done more frequently depending on the needs of the individual.

2. **Sterile technique is used when a hospitalized person requires a wound dressing change to prevent the occurrence of a hospital-acquired infection. The risk of infection for a hospitalized person is increased at several stages of the chain of infection. Medical aseptic technique often is used when changing a wound dressing in the home. People usually are further along in recovery and less susceptible to infection and have built up a resistance to the "familiar microorganisms" in the home environment.**

3. The frequency of changing the dressing on a wound is individualized depending on the patient's needs. The setting is irrelevant.

4. Both bulb and piston syringes can be used in either home or acute-care settings.

14. **TEST-TAKING TIP The words "lowest-level need" and "Maslow" are key words in the stem that direct attention to content.**

1. Identifying hazards in the environment is a health promotion activity that supports

the safety of employees. The needs for safety and security are second-level needs according to Maslow's Hierarchy of Needs.

2. **Assessing the health of an employee includes identifying the physical status of the individual, which addresses first-level needs, such as air, food, water, shelter, rest, sleep, and activity, necessary for survival.**

3. An immunization program is a specific health protection activity that helps to keep a person safe from a specific disease. The needs for safety and security are second-level needs according to Maslow's Hierarchy of Needs.

4. Promoting social adaptation addresses people's love and belonging needs. The need to feel loved and the need to attain a place within a group are third-level (love and belonging) needs according to Maslow's Hierarchy of Needs.

15. 1. The size of a community is the total number of people in the community.

2. **Density refers to the number of people who live within a square mile. High- and low-density areas have their own commonalities (e.g., high-density areas are usually more stressful; low-density areas may have a decreased availability of health services).**

3. Mobility refers to how frequently people move in and out of the community.

4. The composition of a community includes factors such as the age, gender, marital status, and occupations of people in the community.

16. **TEST-TAKING TIP The word "most" in the stem sets a priority. Options 2 and 4 are equally plausible because they both relate to respiratory assessments.**

1. **The leading cause of death in older adults is heart disease. Assessments of rate and rhythm of heartbeats are essential.**

2. Although breath sounds should be assessed, they are not the priority. Although chronic obstructive pulmonary disease is a major health problem in older adults, it is not the leading cause of death.

3. Chronic liver disease is a common cause of death in adults 45 to 64 years of age.

4. Although respiratory rates should be assessed, they are not the priority. Chronic

obstructive pulmonary disease is a major health problem in older adults, but it is not the leading cause of death.

17. **TEST-TAKING TIP** The word "most" in the stem sets a priority. The concept "activities of daily living" is associated with the concept of "assisted living" and is an obscure clang association.

    1. Group homes are for specific populations, such as people who are developmentally disabled, mentally ill, or recovering from alcohol or drug abuse.
    2. A nursing home provides skilled nursing care, which this patient does not need.
    3. This patient needs more care than can be provided in a day-care center. This person needs assistance with toileting, grooming, dressing, and eating, which all occur before arrival at a day-care center.
    4. **Assisted-living facilities help with activities of daily living, prepare meals, and dispense medications as prescribed.**

18. **TEST-TAKING TIP** The words "maturational/developmental" are key words in the stem that direct attention to content.

    1. ____ A recent divorce is a situational, not a maturational, crisis. A situational crisis is an external event that is not part of everyday living. It causes a high degree of anxiety and generally requires learning new coping mechanisms.
    2. **X Maturational crises are changes that occur during a period of growth that often require the assumption of a new role. Adolescents experience rapid bodily changes, have a need to be accepted and to be part of a group, and attempt to become independent. Most important, adolescents strive to establish sexual identity. This maturational crisis is compounded in adolescents who recognize that they are homosexual. Many schools and parents are unprepared to deal with this situation, which can often have lifelong emotional effects on the individual.**
    3. ____ Being critically ill is not an expected part of normal growth and development. It is a situational crisis for the child and parents.
    4. ____ Unemployment is a situational crisis.
    5. **X New parents experience a maturational/developmental crisis**

because they are assuming a new role and must provide total care for another human being.

19. **TEST-TAKING TIP** The word "most" in the stem sets a priority. The words "basic" and "Maslow's Hierarchy of Needs" are key words in the stem that direct attention to content.

    1. **X Meals on Wheels delivers meals daily to those at home who need assistance with preparing nutritious meals. Adequate nutrition (food) is essential for survival and is a first-level (physiological) need according to Maslow's Hierarchy of Needs.**
    2. ____ Exploring the meaning of one's life relates to self-actualization, which is the highest level in Maslow's Hierarchy of Needs.
    3. ____ Encouraging socialization helps to support the need to belong to a group, which is a third-level need according to Maslow's Hierarchy of Needs. When people feel that they belong and are appreciated for who they are, love and belonging needs are being met.
    4. ____ Removing throw rugs protects a person from falls. According to Maslow's Hierarchy of Needs, safety and security needs become significant after basic physiological needs are met.
    5. **X Performing a colostomy irrigation is a skill related to the basic need for fecal elimination. Meeting elimination needs is a basic physiological need identified by Maslow.**

20. Answer: 11
    Knowledge: The patient received a score of 4 for having adequate knowledge about diabetes, self-monitoring of blood glucose, and injection of insulin. *Behavior:* The patient received a score of 3 because the patient is inconsistent in monitoring blood glucose levels before lunch. *Status:* The patient received a score of 4 because the patient exhibited minimal signs and symptoms associated with the condition of diabetes mellitus. The patient's total score is 11.

21. 1. ____ This is providing care after a person has a disease, such as diabetes, which reflects "downstream thinking."
    2. ____ This is providing care after a person has a disease, such as hypertension, which reflects "downstream thinking."

3. <u>X</u> "Upstream thinking" challenges providers to look "upstream" to identify the etiology of disease and intervene to prevent illness rather than to provide care "downstream," when the person is in the "river of illness."

4. <u>X</u> A vaccine contains attenuated or killed microorganisms or antigen proteins derived from them to prevent an infectious disease. Preventing disease is associated with "upstream" thinking.

5. <u>X</u> Cigarette smoke is a known carcinogen. By eliminating smoking a person reduces the risk of developing oral cancer and lung cancer.

22. **TEST-TAKING TIP** The word "first" in the stem sets a priority.

1. Administering insulin coverage as prescribed is the first thing the nurse should do based on the information presented in the scenario. The blood glucose level is too high and the patient needs to have insulin immediately.

2. Implementing the dressing change as per the order is the last action the nurse should implement of the options presented. The wound is not as serious a concern at this time as is the hyperglycemia and the need for the patient to be in a protected environment.

3. Immediately calling 911 for an ambulance to transport the patient to the hospital is the second action that the nurse should implement because the patient demonstrates an inability to manage self-care and is unsafe at home. The patient's vital signs support the conclusion that the patient is most likely dehydrated and needs medical intervention more than just the administration of insulin.

4. Once actions are implemented to ensure that the patient's immediate metabolic needs are met, the primary health-care provider should be notified.

23. **TEST-TAKING TIP** The word "most" in the stem sets a priority. The word "adolescents" is the key word in the stem that directs attention to content.

1. ____ Mumps occurs most often in toddlers and young school-age children. With the measles, mumps, and rubella (MMR) vaccine, the incidence of this disease has declined considerably.

2. ____ Measles occurs most often in toddlers and young school-age children.

With the measles, mumps, and rubella (MMR) vaccine, the incidence of this disease has declined considerably.

3. <u>X</u> Scoliosis is identified most often during the growth spurt associated with puberty/adolescence. It occurs more frequently in girls, and its actual etiology is unknown. Screening for scoliosis usually is performed in the school setting.

4. ____ Although child abuse occurs in teenagers, it is most commonly identified in toddlers and young school-age children.

5. <u>X</u> Substance abuse (e.g., alcohol, cigarettes, illegal drugs, inhalants) is a health problem commonly associated with adolescents. Complex physical, emotional, cognitive, and social changes, along with the desire to take risks and the need to develop a self-identity, all influence behavior.

6. <u>X</u> Motor vehicle accidents are the leading cause of death in adolescents; this is followed by homicide and suicide. Driver education is often provided in the school setting.

24. **TEST-TAKING TIP** The word "situational" is the key word in the stem that directs attention to content.

1. ____ Counseling a parent experiencing "empty nest" syndrome is an intervention that supports a person experiencing a maturational, not situational, stress. Maturational stresses are situations that occur during a period of growth. Maturational growth requires the mastery of tasks in a relatively predictable order and includes the assumption of new roles, according to Erikson.

2. <u>X</u> A situational stress is an external event that is not associated with growth and development. Although the abuse of a child occurs during a developmental level, the reporting of the person to the authorities constitutes a situational crisis. Child abuse is not an expectation of growth and development.

3. ____ Counseling an older adult to visit the senior center is an intervention supporting a person experiencing a maturational, not situational, stress.

4. ____ Providing sex education to an adolescent is an intervention that supports a

person experiencing a maturational, not situational stress.

5. <u>X</u> A situational stress is an external event that is not associated with growth and development. Physical illness is always a situational stress because it is a physical and emotional assault on the "self," requires the sudden assumption of new roles, triggers behaviors that reflect an attempt to cope, and requires the learning of new coping skills to deal with the stress.

25. **Answer: 2, 3, 1, 5, 4**

2. Examine own beliefs and values. Nurses must explore their own beliefs and values before caring for others. This activity supports the advice, "Know Thyself."

3. Remain open to other peoples' views. Nurses must remain open to the thoughts, beliefs, and values of patients; a nonjudgmental attitude is essential for patients to feel accepted.

1. Listen attentively. Once the nurse has a self-awareness and conveys an openness to others, then the nurse must actively listen to hear the content and feeling tone of messages from others.

5. Assist patients and family members to problem-solve. After complete collection of data is accomplished, then identifying problems and exploring possible solutions to the problems should be performed.

4. Elicit the support of community resources. Once potential solutions are identified, appropriate community resources can be explored and selected to assist with the resolution of the problem.

PHARMACOLOGY

This section encompasses questions related to how drugs physiologically and biochemically affect the body (pharmacodynamics) and how drugs are absorbed, distributed, metabolized, and eliminated from the body (pharmacokinetics). The questions include topics such as the therapeutic and side effects of classifications of drugs, medication toxicity, peak and trough values, factors affecting drug action, common assessments before and after drug administration, use of the nursing process in drug therapy, and the role of the nurse in patient teaching and adherence to the medication regimen.

QUESTIONS

1. Which medication acts as a wetting agent to soften stool and is **most** effective in preventing straining during defecation?
   1. Magnesium hydroxide
   2. Docusate sodium
   3. Bisacodyl
   4. Senna

   TEST-TAKING TIP Identify the word in the stem that sets a priority.

2. Which drug should the nurse identify as being **most** effective in the immediate treatment of anaphylaxis?
   1. Epinephrine HCl
   2. Methylprednisolone acetate
   3. Hydrocortisone sodium succinate
   4. Methylprednisolone sodium succinate

   TEST-TAKING TIP Identify the word in the stem that sets a priority. Identify the key word in the stem that directs attention to content. Identify equally plausible options. Identify the unique option.

3. Which classification of drugs does the nurse anticipate is **most** likely to be prescribed when a patient has difficulty sleeping?
   1. Benzodiazepines
   2. Barbiturates
   3. Analgesics
   4. Opioids

   TEST-TAKING TIP Identify the word in the stem that sets a priority. Identify equally plausible options.

4. A patient is receiving prednisone, a glucocorticoid. For which responses should the nurse monitor the patient's electrolytes?
   1. Hypokalemia and hyponatremia
   2. Hypokalemia and hypernatremia
   3. Hyperkalemia and hyponatremia
   4. Hyperkalemia and hypernatremia

   TEST-TAKING TIP Identify duplicate facts among options. Identify opposites in options.

5. Which classification of medications is at risk for a drug interaction with digoxin?
   1. Glucocorticoids
   2. Sulfonamides
   3. Antibiotics
   4. Antacids

   TEST-TAKING TIP Identify equally plausible options.

6. Which patient response indicates a therapeutic outcome after receiving a cathartic?
   1. Has a bowel movement
   2. Describes pain relief
   3. Falls asleep
   4. Voids urine

7. A nurse is administering heparin to a patient daily. For which undesirable clinical response that indicates the need to discontinue the heparin sodium therapy should the nurse assess the patient?
   1. International normalized ratio of 2.5
   2. Platelet count of 100,000/mm³
   3. Hematuria
   4. Gastritis

   TEST-TAKING TIP Identify the word in the stem that indicates negative polarity.

8. A nurse is caring for a group of patients receiving drugs in the following classifications. Which classification of drug may precipitate a superinfection?
   1. Diuretic
   2. Antibiotic
   3. Antiemetic
   4. Thrombolytic

9. An antibiotic to be administered via intravenous piggyback (IVPB) every 12 hours is prescribed for a patient. At which time should the nurse schedule a blood sample to be drawn to determine a trough level when the drug is administered at 2:00 p.m.?
   1. 1:30 a.m.
   2. 2:30 a.m.
   3. 3:00 p.m.
   4. 8:00 p.m.

   TEST-TAKING TIP Identify opposites in options.

10. A nurse is evaluating a patient's response to an antitussive. A decrease in which clinical finding indicates that the antitussive was effective?
    1. Fever
    2. Mucous viscosity
    3. Nasal congestion
    4. Frequency of coughing

11. When performing a health history a patient states, "I take 1 package of psyllium every day no matter what." Which drug effect should the nurse **most** likely expect to occur?
    1. Tolerance
    2. Synergistic
    3. Habituation
    4. Idiosyncratic

    TEST-TAKING TIP Identify the word in the stem that sets a priority.

12. A patient is receiving an antibiotic that has a 4 to 10 µg/mL therapeutic range, an optimum peak value of 8 to 10 µg/mL, and a minimum trough level of 0.5 µg/mL. Which value requires the nurse to notify the primary health-care provider?
    1. Peak value of 5 µg/mL
    2. Peak value of 9 µg/mL
    3. Trough value of 0.7 µg/mL
    4. Trough value of 0.3 µg/mL

    TEST-TAKING TIP Identify the words in the stem that indicate negative polarity.

13. A nurse administers an expectorant to a patient. Which result indicates that the patient is experiencing a therapeutic response?
1. Reduced fever
2. Productive cough
3. Relieved nasal congestion
4. Dilation of respiratory airways

14. The therapeutic blood level range for an antibiotic is 4 to 10 μg/mL. Which should the nurse conclude when the laboratory test indicates a peak level of 12 μg/mL?
1. Drug dose is safe.
2. Drug dose is subtherapeutic.
3. Patient is at risk for drug accumulation.
4. Patient's next dose of the drug should be given over a longer period of time.

TEST-TAKING TIP Identify opposites in options. Identify the unique option.

15. A patient is receiving a neuroleptic antipsychotic medication. For which extrapyramidal reactions should the nurse assess the patient?
1. Respiratory depression and diarrhea
2. Akathisia and respiratory depression
3. Diarrhea and spasms of the muscles of the face
4. Spasms of the muscles of the face and akathisia

TEST-TAKING TIP Identify duplicate facts among options.

16. A nurse administers an analgesic to a patient. For which therapeutic response should the nurse monitor the patient?
1. Pain is tolerable.
2. Nausea has subsided.
3. Breathing is less labored.
4. Temperature is in the expected range.

17. Which statement by a patient receiving digoxin 0.25 mg every day indicates that the nurse should provide further teaching?
1. "I should not take antacids with this medication."
2. "I will not take the digoxin if my pulse is less than 60."
3. "I should call the doctor if I have nausea, vomiting, or weakness."
4. "If I forget to take my digoxin, I should take 2 pills the next day."

TEST-TAKING TIP Identify the word in the stem that indicates negative polarity.

18. A nurse is caring for a patient receiving an opioid (narcotic) analgesic for pain. Which information about how opioid (narcotic) analgesics work in the body should the nurse consider before administering this medication?
1. Diminishes peripheral pain reception
2. Modifies the patient's perception of pain
3. Competes with receptors for sensory input
4. Closes the gating mechanism for impulse transmission

TEST-TAKING TIP Identify clang associations.

19. A nurse is collecting a health history from a patient who will be receiving intravenous heparin sodium therapy. Which statement by the patient requires further exploration by the nurse?
1. "I may be pregnant."
2. "I eat a lot of green, leafy vegetables."
3. "I always experience heavy menstrual periods."
4. "I stopped taking my daily aspirin tablet about 5 days ago."

TEST-TAKING TIP Identify the words in the stem that indicate negative polarity.

20. A patient who had an antidepressant prescribed for depression asks the nurse, "How long will it take before I feel better?" Which length of time should the nurse include in the response to the patient's question?
    1. 2 hours
    2. 2 days
    3. 2 weeks
    4. 2 months

    TEST-TAKING TIP Identify key words in the stem that direct attention to content.

21. A nurse is caring for a patient who experienced fluid volume excess exhibited by lower extremity edema, increased blood pressure, dyspnea, and distended neck veins. Furosemide is prescribed. The nurse is monitoring the patient's daily potassium level. On which day should the nurse inform the primary health-care provider of the patient's potassium level and seek an order for potassium supplementation?
    1. Day 1 – Serum potasium: 5.5 mEq/L
    2. Day 2 – Serum potasium: 4.2 mEq/L
    3. Day 3 – Serum potasium: 3.6 mEq/L
    4. Day 4 – Serum potasium: 3.2 mEq/L

22. Codeine for pain is prescribed for a patient of Asian descent. Which element of pharmacokinetics does the nurse understand is critical when assessing this patient's response to the medication?
    1. Excretion
    2. Absorption
    3. Distribution
    4. Biotransformation

23. A primary health-care provider prescribes montelukast 10 mg PO daily for a patient with asthma. Which should the nurse teach this patient?
    1. Take the medication before lunch.
    2. Report behavioral changes to the doctor immediately.
    3. Discontinue taking the drug when symptoms subside.
    4. Understand that this drug is used to treat an acute respiratory episode.

24. A patient at the health clinic, receiving a diuretic for treatment for an elevated blood pressure, asks the nurse if it is all right to take over-the-counter glucosamine sulfate to reduce the discomfort of osteoarthritis. Which should the nurse teach the patient about taking this herbal product?
    1. You can expect a therapeutic response with glucosamine within two weeks of initiating therapy.
    2. Take chondroitin along with glucosamine for an enhanced therapeutic effect.
    3. Seek guidance from your doctor before taking the glucosamine.
    4. Do not take glucosamine if you are allergic to shellfish.

25. A patient is receiving a medication that has a narrow therapeutic window. The medication is administered every 6 hours at 12 a.m., 6 a.m., 12 p.m., and 6 p.m. There is an order for the nurse to assess the peak plasma level of the medication. At what time should the nurse obtain a blood specimen for this test?
    1. 0500 hr (6 a.m.)
    2. 0800 hr (8 a.m.)
    3. 1200 hr (12 p.m.)
    4. 1900 hr (7 p.m.)

26. A nurse is caring for a patient receiving an oral hypoglycemic agent. Which age-related alterations in older adults that may affect the absorption of this drug should the nurse recognize? **Select all that apply.**
1. ____ Decrease in hydrochloric acid production
2. ____ Increase in length of gastric emptying
3. ____ Decrease in mesenteric blood flow
4. ____ Decrease in subcutaneous fat
5. ____ Increase in cardiac output

TEST-TAKING TIP Identify key words in the stem that direct attention to content.

27. The illustration represents a comparison of drug onsets and duration of action by route of administration (e.g., PO, IM, and IV). Which line represents a medication administered via the intramuscular route?
1. Black
2. Gray
3. Blue

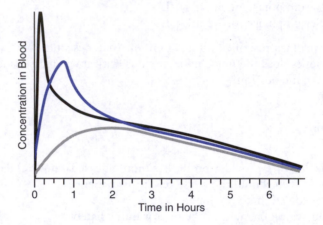

28. Which drugs are palliative in their therapeutic action? **Select all that apply.**
1. ____ oxycodone
2. ____ ondansetron
3. ____ calcium chloride
4. ____ penicillin G procaine
5. ____ levothyroxine sodium

29. Clorazepate 7.5 mg PO twice a day was prescribed for a patient. This sedative/hypnotic was prescribed for its skeletal muscle relaxant effect. The medication is supplied as 3.75 mg/tablet. How many tablets should the nurse administer? **Record your answer using a whole number.**

Answer: _____

30. A nurse has been administering a diuretic to a patient. Which clinical findings should the nurse assess that reflect the patient is having a therapeutic response to the diuretic? **Select all that apply.**
1. ____ Decreased weight
2. ____ Increased appetite
3. ____ Increased urinary output
4. ____ Decreased blood pressure
5. ____ Decreased white blood cells

31. The home care nurse reviews the transfer information and the primary health-care provider's orders and takes the patient's vital signs. Based on the information collected, which nursing action is the priority?

1. Discuss the appropriateness of the ibuprofen prescription with the primary health-care provider.
2. Notify the primary health-care provider regarding the patient's stage I hypertensive status.
3. Assess for other signs of infection besides the increased temperature.
4. Complete a thorough skin assessment for the clinical record.

PATIENT'S HOME CARE CLINICAL RECORD

Transfer Information From Hospital to Home Care Agency

Patient transferred to home care with a diagnosis of lower extremity arterial disease with 1-cm ulcer on the distal end of the right large toe. Patient also has asthma, hypothyroidism, and osteoarthritis and reports intermittent joint pain on a level 5. Daily wound irrigation with NS and wet-to-moist dressings to right large toe as well as health teaching regarding drug therapy ordered by the primary health-care provider.

Vital Signs During Home Visit

Blood pressure: 145/90 mm Hg
Pulse: 100 beats/min, regular
Respirations: 22 breaths/min, unlabored
Temperature: 100°F

Primary Health-Care Provider's Orders

Mometasone (Asmanex Twisthaler) 220 mcg per dose, 2 puffs daily
Triamcinolone (Nasacort Nasal Spray) 2 sprays in each nostril daily
Levothyroxine (Synthroid) 125 mcg, PO, once daily
Clopidogrel (Plavix) 75 mg once daily
Ibutrofen (Motrin IB) 2 caplets every 6 hours for joint discomfort
Cleanse right large toe wound with NS and apply wet-to-moist dressing daily.

TEST-TAKING TIP Identify clang associations.

32. A nurse is administering an antineoplastic drug that is neurotoxic. For which side effects should the nurse assess this patient? **Select all that apply.**

1. _____ Diarrhea
2. _____ Renal failure
3. _____ Paralytic ileus
4. _____ Electrolyte imbalances
5. _____ Peripheral neuropathies
6. _____ Decreased red blood cells

TEST-TAKING TIP Identify the key word in the stem that directs attention to content. Identify the clang association.

33. A nurse is caring for a patient with a history of falls and who is receiving multiple medications. Which classifications of medication may increase this patient's risk for falls?
    1. ____ Antibiotic
    2. ____ Antiemetic
    3. ____ Antihistamine
    4. ____ Antihypertensive
    5. ____ Antidysrhythmic

    TEST-TAKING TIP Identify the key word in the stem that directs attention to content.

34. A nurse is caring for several patients who are receiving an antipsychotic medication as well as another medication. The nurse plans to assess these patients for signs of drug interactions. Which classifications of drugs can the action of antipsychotic medication potentiate? **Select all that apply.**
    1. ____ Amphetamines
    2. ____ Anticoagulants
    3. ____ Opioid analgesics
    4. ____ Antihypertensives
    5. ____ Oral hypoglycemic agents

35. A patient has a prescription for the administration of NPH insulin. The nurse must understand the pharmacokinetics of this medication to assess the patient's response to the medication especially when the patient is at risk for developing hypoglycemia. Which time action profile reflects the onset, peak, and duration pharmacokinetics of NPH insulin?
    1.

Onset	Peak	Duration
1 to 1.5 hrs	No peak action	20 to 24 hrs

    2.

Onset	Peak	Duration
1.5 to 4 hrs	4 to 12 hrs	18 to 24 hrs

    3.

Onset	Peak	Duration
30 to 60 min	2 to 5 hrs	5 to 8 hrs

    4.

Onset	Peak	Duration
10 to 20 min	1 to 3 hrs	3 to 5 hrs

36. A patient who has a history of sensitivity reactions to new drugs is being cared for in a primary health-care provider's office. A new medication is prescribed. The office nurse administers the first dose from a sample pack of the drug provided by a pharmaceutical representative. List the nurse's actions in order of priority.
    1. Give the patient the drug according to the prescription.
    2. Ask the patient if this drug was ever received in the past.
    3. Instruct the patient to remain in the waiting room for at least 30 minutes.
    4. Ask the patient if this drug has ever caused a sensitivity reaction in the past.
    5. Instruct the patient to notify the primary health-care provider immediately if any sensitivity reactions occur.

    Answer: _____

37. A primary health-care provider prescribes hydrochlorothiazide (HCTZ) for a patient with hypertension. What should the nurse teach the patient to do while taking this medication? **Select all that apply.**
   1. _____ Avoid drinking alcohol.
   2. _____ Limit salt intake to 4 g daily.
   3. _____ Take it in the evening before going to sleep.
   4. _____ Monitor for signs of hypernatremia such as thirst, dry mouth, and confusion.
   5. _____ Report muscle weakness, cramps, nausea, vomiting, diarrhea, dizziness or irregular heartbeats if they occur.

38. A nurse is caring for a patient receiving hydrocodone/acetaminophen for back pain. For which effects should the nurse monitor the patient? **Select all that apply.**
   1. _____ Nausea
   2. _____ Diplopia
   3. _____ Euphoria
   4. _____ Irritability
   5. _____ Hypotension

39. A patient with panic disorder has been taking alprazolam 0.5 mg by mouth three times a day. After a week of therapy the prescription is increased to 1 mg by mouth three times a day. The patient has leftover alprazolam tablets 0.25 mg. How many tablets should the nurse instruct the patient to take for each dose? **Record your answer using a whole number.**

   Answer: _____ **tablets**

40. Which physiological changes in the older adult should the nurse consider that contribute to prolonged drug half-life? **Select all that apply.**
   1. _____ Decreased liver function
   2. _____ Reduced subcutaneous tissue
   3. _____ Reduced glomerular filtration rate
   4. _____ Decreased hydrochloric acid production
   5. _____ Decreased gastrointestinal absorptive surface

   TEST-TAKING TIP Identify key words in the stem that direct attention to content.

1. **TEST-TAKING TIP** The word "most" in the stem sets a priority.
   1. Magnesium hydroxide (Milk of Magnesia) is a saline or osmotic agent that draws water into the fecal mass.
   2. **Docusate sodium (Colace) is a detergent that lowers the surface tension of feces, allowing penetration by water and fat, which soften stool.**
   3. Bisacodyl (Dulcolax) is a stimulant cathartic because it irritates the intestinal mucosa, increasing intestinal motility.
   4. Senna (Senokot) is a stimulant laxative. It irritates the intestinal mucosa, increasing intestinal motility.

2. **TEST-TAKING TIP** The word "most" in the stem sets a priority. The word "immediate" is the key word in the stem that directs attention to content. Options 2, 3, and 4 are equally plausible because they are all corticosteroids. Option 1 is unique because it is the only option that is not a corticosteroid. It is the only option with capital letters (HCl) in the generic name.
   1. **Epinephrine HCl (Adrenalin Chloride) is administered as soon as possible after a person demonstrates clinical findings of systemic anaphylaxis or as a preventive measure in a person who is highly allergic and has been exposed to an allergen. Epinephrine quickly stimulates alpha- and beta-adrenergic receptors of the autonomic nervous system, causing vasoconstriction and bronchodilation.**
   2. Methylprednisolone acetate (Depo-Medrol) is a corticosteroid. Corticosteroids, which have an anti-inflammatory action, generally are administered to prevent the recurrence of symptoms.
   3. Methylprednisolone sodium (Solu-Cortef) is a corticosteroid.
   4. Methylprednisolone sodium succinate (Solu-Medrol) is a corticosteroid.

3. **TEST-TAKING TIP** The word "most" in the stem sets a priority. Options 3 and 4 are equally plausible because they are both categories of drugs that relieve pain.
   1. **Benzodiazepines, such as temazepam (Restoril) and zolpidem (Ambien),** are a group of nonbarbiturate sedative-hypnotics. They influence the neurons in the central nervous system that suppress responsiveness to stimuli, thereby decreasing levels of arousal.
   2. Barbiturates, such as pentobarbital sodium (Nembutal sodium), have many side effects and have been replaced by benzodiazepines as the first drugs of choice to induce sleep.
   3. Analgesics are primarily administered to reduce pain, not to induce sleep.
   4. Opioids are primarily administered to reduce pain, not to induce sleep.

4. **TEST-TAKING TIP** The question is asking about potassium and sodium imbalances as a result of glucocorticoid therapy. If you know at least one electrolyte imbalance that can occur, two options can be eliminated from consideration. Options 2 and 3 are opposites and options 1 and 4 are opposites. The test-taking tip "identify opposites in options" is not helpful in this question because there are two sets of opposites. It is better to use the test-taking tip "identify duplicate facts among the options" to eliminate options.
   1. Although hypokalemia may occur, hypernatremia, not hyponatremia, may occur.
   2. **Prednisone, a glucocorticoid, has significant water- and sodium-retaining (mineralocorticoid) activities. As sodium is retained, potassium is depleted.**
   3. The opposite may occur. The patient may experience hypokalemia and hypernatremia.
   4. Although hypernatremia may occur, hypokalemia, not hyperkalemia, may occur.

5. **TEST-TAKING TIP** Options 2 and 3 are equally plausible. Sulfa drugs are antibiotics.
   1. **Prednisone, a glucocorticoid with mineralocorticoid activity, can precipitate hypokalemia. Hypokalemia increases the sensitivity of the myocardium to digitalis. Hypokalemia can precipitate digitalis toxicity, even if digoxin serum levels are in the therapeutic range of 0.5 to 2.0 ng/mL.**
   2. Sulfonamides do not interact with digoxin.
   3. Antibiotics do not interact with digoxin.
   4. Antacids do not interact with digoxin.

6. 1. **Cathartics, also called laxatives, induce defecation.**
  2. Analgesics relieve pain. Also, some cathartics may cause slight abdominal discomfort due to increased intestinal peristalsis.
  3. Sedatives and hypnotics promote sleep.
  4. Diuretics increase urinary output.

7. **TEST-TAKING TIP** The word "undesirable" in the stem indicates negative polarity.
  1. An international normalized ratio (INR) value is obtained to assess the effectiveness of warfarin sodium (Coumadin) therapy, not heparin therapy. An activated partial thromboplastin time (APTT) is one test that is performed to assess the effects of heparin therapy.
  2. A low platelet count (thrombocytopenia) occurs in 5% to 10% of patients receiving heparin therapy. Platelets can decrease to 100,000 units from the expected range of 195,000 to 400,000/mm³. This often resolves without intervention even with continued heparin therapy.
  3. **Hematuria (blood in the urine) is a serious side effect of heparin therapy that requires the temporary termination of therapy. If severe bleeding is identified, protamine sulfate is administered as an antidote.**
  4. Heparin is administered parenterally, not by mouth, and does not cause gastritis.

8. 1. Diuretics increase the formation and excretion of urine. They can cause dehydration and electrolyte imbalance, but they do not precipitate a superinfection.
  2. **Prolonged or inappropriate use of antibiotics can stimulate bacterial growth as normal flora of the gastrointestinal tract and skin are destroyed. Infections that occur while a patient is receiving antimicrobial therapy are called *superinfections*.**
  3. Antiemetics are used to prevent nausea and vomiting. They may cause side effects such as headache, dizziness, fatigue, and diarrhea, not superinfections.
  4. Thrombolytics dissolve thrombi or emboli; they also prolong the coagulation processes, which may increase the risk of bleeding. Thrombolytics do not precipitate superinfections.

9. **TEST-TAKING TIP** Options 1 and 2 are opposites. One is 30 minutes before the drug is administered and the other is 30 minutes after the drug is administered.
  1. **The blood level of an antibiotic is at its lowest level just before the next scheduled dose.**
  2. After the drug is administered, the blood level of the drug increases. A value taken 30 minutes after the drug is administered does not reflect the lowest serum level, which is the purpose of identifying a trough level.
  3. This is too soon for a trough level. This time is appropriate for a peak level.
  4. This is too soon for a trough level. This time is halfway between two doses.

10. 1. Antipyretics reduce a fever; antitussives do not.
  2. Mucolytics reduce mucus viscosity; antitussives do not.
  3. Nasal decongestants reduce nasal congestion; antitussives do not.
  4. **Antitussives reduce the frequency and intensity of a cough. They act on the central or peripheral nervous system or on the local mucosa.**

11. **TEST-TAKING TIP** The word "most" in the stem sets a priority.
  1. Tolerance occurs when an individual requires increases in the dosage of a drug to maintain its therapeutic effect.
  2. A synergistic effect occurs when the effect of two medications given together is greater than the effect of the medications when given individually.
  3. **Drug habituation occurs when an individual develops a mild form of psychological dependence and relies on the use of a substance such as psyllium (Metamucil).**
  4. An idiosyncratic effect occurs when a person's response to a drug is an underresponse, an overresponse, or a different response from that which is expected.

12. **TEST-TAKING TIP** "Notify the primary health-care provider" are words that reflect negative polarity. The question is asking, "Which blood level result is unacceptable?"
  1. Although this is below the optimal peak value of 8 to 10 μg/mL, it is within the

therapeutic window of 4 to 10 µg/mL, which is acceptable.

2. This falls within the optimal peak value range of 8 to 10 µg/mL, which is acceptable.

3. A value of 0.7 µg/mL is higher than 0.5 µg/mL, which is the minimum trough value necessary for a dose to be effective.

4. **The primary health-care provider should be notified because the dose of the antibiotic should be increased. A value of 0.3 µg/mL is below 0.5 µg/mL, which is the lowest trough value of the antibiotic necessary to inhibit bacterial growth.**

13. 1. An antipyretic reduces a fever; an expectorant does not.

2. **Expectorants cause a cough to be more productive by decreasing viscosity of mucus and increasing the flow of respiratory tract secretions.**

3. A nasal decongestant relieves nasal edema and congestion; an expectorant does not.

4. A bronchodilator dilates airways of the respiratory tract; an expectorant does not.

14. **TEST-TAKING TIP Options 2 and 3 are opposites. Option 3 is unique. It is the only option that does not include the word "dose."**

1. The drug dose is not safe. A peak level of 12 µg/mL indicates that the drug dose is too high and needs to be reduced by the primary health-care provider. The optimum peak value should be between 8 to 10 µg/mL.

2. The drug level will be less than 4 µg/mL if the dose is subtherapeutic.

3. **A value of 12 µg/mL is 2 µg/mL more than is necessary to be effective and contributes to drug accumulation and toxicity if it continues for 3 to 5 days.**

4. The dose needs to be adjusted by the primary health-care provider and not just given at a slower rate.

15. **TEST-TAKING TIP This question is associating four possible effects of neuroleptics: respiratory depression, diarrhea, akathisia, and spasms of the muscles of the face. If you know just one effect, unrelated or related to neuroleptics, you can delete two options from consideration.**

1. Respiratory depression is associated with opioid analgesics, not neuroleptics. Constipation, not diarrhea, is a common anticholinergic effect of neuroleptics.

2. Although akathisia can occur with neuroleptics, respiratory depression is often seen with opioid analgesics, not neuroleptics.

3. Although tardive dyskinesia occurs with neuroleptics, constipation, not diarrhea, is a common anticholinergic effect of neuroleptics.

4. **Spasms of the muscles of the face (tardive dyskinesia) and restlessness/ agitation (akathisia) occur in response to dopamine blockage or depletion in the basal ganglia. These undesirable responses are common to most neuroleptic drugs and occur within the first few days of therapy.**

16. 1. **Analgesics are given mainly to reduce pain and discomfort. There are various types of analgesics: non-narcotic and nonsteroidal anti-inflammatory drugs (NSAIDs), narcotic analgesics or opioids, and adjuvants or co-analgesics.**

2. Antiemetics are designed to minimize nausea and vomiting.

3. Bronchodilators dilate respiratory airways, facilitating breathing.

4. Antipyretics are a group of drugs designed to reduce fever. Although some analgesics also may have an antipyretic effect, when given as analgesics they reduce pain.

17. **TEST-TAKING TIP The word "further" in the stem indicates negative polarity.**

1. Antacids can interfere with the absorption of digoxin and should not be taken at the same time.

2. Digoxin slows the heart rate and strengthens cardiac contractions. If the apical pulse is below a predetermined parameter set by the primary health-care provider (frequently between 50 to 60 beats per minute), the dose should be withheld.

3. Nausea, vomiting, and weakness are signs of toxicity. The patient needs a test to determine the digoxin serum blood level.

4. **This action is unsafe and may lead to toxicity. If a dose is missed, it should be taken within 12 hours of the scheduled dose.**

18. **TEST-TAKING TIP The word "pain" in the stem and option 1 and 2 comprise clang associations.**

1. Local anesthetics, not narcotics, diminish localized sensation and the perception of pain by inhibiting nerve conduction.

2. **Opioids act on the higher centers of the brain to modify pain perception.**

3. Competing with receptors for sensory input is the theory related to using distracting sensory input to inhibit pain perception.

4. Opioids do not close synaptic gates; stimulation of large nerve fibers, via methods such as transcutaneous electrical stimulation, closes synaptic gates.

19. **TEST-TAKING TIP** The words "requires further exploration" in the stem indicate negative polarity. The question is asking, "Which situation is unsafe when a person is receiving intravenous heparin?"

    1. Heparin does not cross the placental barrier and has no effects on the fetus or newborn.

    2. Eating a lot of green, leafy vegetables can contribute to the ineffectiveness of warfarin sodium (Coumadin), not heparin sodium.

    3. **Heavy menstrual periods is a contraindication for the use of heparin because of an increased risk of prolonged bleeding during menstruation.**

    4. Although aspirin can prolong bleeding time when given with heparin, 5 days is sufficient time to be aspirin free for safe administration of heparin.

20. **TEST-TAKING TIP** The words "how long" and "feel better" are key words in the stem that direct attention to content.

    1. Two hours is too short a time to achieve a therapeutic response to an antidepressant.

    2. Two days is too short a time to experience a therapeutic response to antidepressants.

    3. **Generally patients demonstrate an initial response 1 to 3 weeks after the start of antidepressant therapy; it takes this long to establish a therapeutic plasma level.**

    4. One or two months may be necessary to achieve a maximal, not initial, response to antidepressant therapy.

21. 1. The patient's serum potassium level of 5.5 mEq/L is higher than the expected range of 3.5 to 5.0 mEq/L and therefore supplemental potassium is unnecessary and inappropriate.

    2. The patient's serum potassium level of 4.2 mEq/L is within the expected range

of 3.5 to 5.0 mEq/L and therefore supplemental potassium is unnecessary and inappropriate.

3. **Although the patient's serum potassium level of 3.6 mEq/L is within the expected range of 3.5 to 5.0 mEq/L, the level has progressively decreased over the last 72 hours. Furosemide (Lasix), a loop diuretic, decreases sodium and chloride resorption in the ascending loop of Henle and distal renal tubule. This in turn inhibits potassium reabsorption mechanisms. If the patient continues to receive furosemide without potassium supplementation, the potassium level will continue to decrease, placing the patient at risk for a cardiac dysrhythmia and other signs and symptoms associated with a low serum potassium level (hypokalemia).**

4. When a patient is receiving furosemide, potassium supplementation should begin when the patient's serum potassium level is in the low expected range, not when it decreases below the expected range. A low potassium level (hypokalemia) can result in cardiac dysrhythmias, muscle weakaness, fatigue, nausea and vomiting, decreased gastric motility, decreased reflecxes, and abdominal distention, which can be avoided with prophylactic potassium supplementation.

22. 1. Another element of pharmacokinetics is of more concern than elimination of an opioid from the body (excretion) by a person of Asian descent.

    2. Another element of pharmacokinetics is of more concern than the process of movement of a medication into the bloodstream (absorption) by a person of Asian descent.

    3. Another element of pharmacokinetics is of more concern than transport of a medication from the site of absorption to the site of medication action (distribution) by a person of Asian descent.

    4. **Genes can cause liver metabolism to be slower in individuals of Asian descent. Because conversion of a medication to a less active form (biotransformation) in preparation for excretion from the body occurs in the liver, toxic levels of a medication may occur when liver metabolism is slowed in a patient of Asian**

descent. **Nurses must assess patients of Asian descent for drug toxicity when they receive an opioid that includes clinical manifestations such as decreased respiratory rate and depth, drowsiness, sedation, confusion, and hypotension. A person of Asian descent may require a lower dose of an opioid to achieve a therapeutic effect.**

23. 1. Montelukast should be taken in the evening, not before lunch. Most people with asthma experience worsening of symptoms at night. By taking montelukast at night its peak action (3 to 4 hours after ingestion) will be optimal when asthma symptoms generally peak.

2. **Agitation, aggression, depression, irritability, hallucinations, and thoughts of hurting oneself are serious adverse reactions to montelukast (Singulair) that should be reported immediately to the primary health-care provider. Montelukast may need to be discontinued if these responses occur.**

3. Montelukast is used for the maintenance treatment of asthma and should not be discontinued when symptoms subside without consulting the primary health-care provider.

4. Montelukast is not used to treat an acute asthma attack; it is used to prevent and treat chronic asthma and seasonal allergic rhinitis and to prevent exercise-induced bronchoconstriction.

24. 1. It takes at least 4 weeks of therapy before noticeable improvement of symptoms in individuals who state that glucosamine sulfate is helpful in reducing symptoms of osteoarthritis. Most research demonstrates no improvement when compared with a placebo. Glucosamine should be discontinued if no improvement is noted within 12 weeks of therapy.

2. Glucosamine is a molecule used in the formation and repair of cartilage. Chondroitin, a structural component of cartilage, is responsible for the resiliency of cartilage. However, research demonstrates that there is no benefit in taking chondroitin concurrently with glucosamine; therefore, its use is discouraged.

3. **Discussing herbal products with the primary health-care provider is advisable because the primary health-care provider understands the risks, benefits, and interactions of herbal**

products in light of the other medications a patient is receiving.

4. Glucosamine sulfate is produced from the shells of shrimp, lobster, and crabs. Research demonstrates that it is the protein in the shellfish that causes a shellfish allergy, not the shells themselves. Because a small amount of shellfish protein may be included during the manufacture of the product, there may be some risk of an allergic reaction. To avoid any risk of a shellfish allergic reaction, a patient should take a synthetic form of glucosamine.

25. 1. Five a.m. (0500 hr) is an appropriate time to obtain a blood specimen to test the lowest, not highest, plasma concentration of the medication for this patient. Trough levels are assessed via a blood specimen obtained 30 to 60 minutes before the next dose.

2. Eight a.m. (0800 hr) is an inappropriate time to assess either a peak or trough level of the medication for this patient. It is approximately halfway between two doses.

3. Twelve p.m. (1200 hr) is an inappropriate time to assess either a peak or trough level of the medication for this patient.

4. **Seven p.m. (1900 hr) is an appropriate time to obtain a blood specimen to assess the peak level of the medication for this patient. Blood specimens for assessing the peak level of the medication should be obtained 30 to 60 minutes after a dose is administered. Additional acceptable times to obtain a blood specimen to measure a peak plasma concentration of the medication in this patient are 0100 hr (1 a.m.), 0700 hr (7 a.m.), and 1300 hr (1 p.m.).**

26. TEST-TAKING TIP The words "older adults" are the key words in the stem direct attention to content.

1. X Hydrochloric acid production decreases as the body ages; this may influence the way a tablet or capsule dissolves in gastric fluids and affect the stability of the drug in the gastrointestinal system.

2. X Gastric emptying time is prolonged in older adults. Because absorption of drugs primarily takes place in the intestine, delayed gastric emptying results in delayed absorption.

3. __X__ Mesenteric blood blow decreases as the body ages which can interfere with absorption of oral medication.
4. ____ As the body ages, there is a decrease in subcutaneous fat. However, this does not influence the absorption of oral medications; it may influence the absorption of subcutaneous injections.
5. ____ Cardiac output decreases as the body ages.

27. 1. The black line represents the onset and duration of a medication administered via the intravenous route. It produces the fastest pharmacological response because the medication is administered directly into the intravascular compartment.
2. The gray line represents the onset and duration of a medication administered via the oral route. The oral route is the slowest route because the medication must reach the small intestine for the majority of absorption to take place. Absorption of oral medications is influenced by a variety of factors such as the presence of food, emotions, physical activity, and concurrent diseases.
3. **The blue line represents the onset and duration of a medication administered via the intramuscular route. An intramuscular injection inserts medication directly into skeletal muscle. Skeletal muscles contain a rich blood supply that promotes transport of the medication into the intravascular compartment.**

28. 1. __X__ **Oxycodone (Oxycontin), an opioid analgesic, relieves the symptoms of a disease (palliative action) but does not alter the disease process itself.**
2. __X__ **Ondansetron (Zofran), an antiemetic, is used to prevent or treat nausea and vomiting associated with chemotherapy, surgery, and radiation therapy.**
3. ____ Mineral supplements are considered restorative, not palliative; they return the body to health.
4. ____ Penicillin G procaine is an antibiotic that kills pathogenic organisms; a drug that kills an organism is considered to have a curative, not palliative, action.
5. ____ Levothyroxine sodium (Synthroid) replaces the thyroxine that is deficient in hypothyroidism. When a drug replaces

body fluids or substances, it is substitutive, not palliative, in its therapeutic action.

29. **Answer: 2 tablets**
Solve the problem using a formula for ratio and proportion.

$$\frac{\text{Desire}}{\text{Have}} \quad \frac{7.5 \text{ mg}}{3.75 \text{ mg}} = \frac{x \text{ tablets}}{1 \text{ tablet}}$$

3.75 x = 7.5

x = 7.5 ÷ 3.75

x = 2 tablets

30. 1. __X__ **A diuretic enhances the selective excretion of water and various electrolytes. One liter of fluid is equal to 2.2 pounds. A rapid decrease in weight indicates fluid loss.**
2. ____ A diuretic does not increase appetite.
3. __X__ **A diuretic enhances the selective excretion of water and various electrolytes by affecting renal mechanisms for tubular secretion and reabsorption, thereby increasing urinary output.**
4. __X__ **The blood pressure will decrease as excess fluid is excreted from the body because there is less fluid in the intravascular compartment.**
5. ____ Diuretics are not antibiotics and therefore will not destroy microorganisms resulting in a decrease in the white blood cell count.

31. **TEST-TAKING TIP** The words "primary health-care provider's" in the stem and "primary health-care provider" in options 1 and 2 comprise clang associations.

1. Ibuprofen (Motrin IB) can cause an increased risk of bleeding when the patient is concurrently taking clopidogrel (Plavix). The inappropriateness of this prescription must be discussed with the primary health-care provider.
2. Although the primary health-care provider should be notified of the increased blood pressure, it is not the priority of the options presented.
3. The temperature of 100°F is within the expected range of 96.8°F to 100°F for an adult. The temperature may be increased slightly because of inflammation associated with the patient's wound.
4. Although a thorough skin assessment should be completed by the nurse, it is not the most important initial concern.

32. **TEST-TAKING TIP** The word "neurotoxic" is the key word in the stem that directs attention to content. The word "neurotoxic" in the stem and the word "neuropathies" in option 5 are closely related and comprises an obscure clang association. Consider option 5 carefully. In this question, it is one of the correct answers.

1. ____ Constipation, not diarrhea, can occur.
2. ____ Renal failure is related to the urinary, not neurological, system.
3. **X Decreased innervation of the bowel causes a decrease or absence of intestinal peristalsis (paralytic ileus), resulting in constipation or obstipation.**
4. ____ Electrolyte imbalances are not related to the neurological system.
5. **X A peripheral neuropathy occurs in almost every patient, particularly depression of the Achilles tendon reflex.**
6. ____ Red blood cells are part of the hematopoietic, not neurological, system.

33. **TEST-TAKING TIP** The word "falls" is the key word in the stem that directs attention to content.

1. ____ Postural hypotension is not a common side effect of antibiotics.
2. ____ Postural hypotension is not a common side effect of antiemetics.
3. ____ Postural hypotension is not a common side effect of antihistamines.
4. **X Most antihypertensives contribute to postural hypotension because of actions such as peripheral vasodilation, decreased peripheral resistance, decreased heart rate, and decreased cardiac contraction.**
5. **X Antidysrhythmics affect the conduction system of the heart. Common side effects are decreased blood pressure (hypotension) and decreased heart rate (bradycardia), both of which may predispose a person to falls.**

34. 1. ____ Antipsychotics decrease, not potentiate, the effectiveness of amphetamines.
2. ____ Antipsychotics decrease the effectiveness of anticoagulants.
3. **X Antipsychotics potentiate the effects of other central nervous system depressants such as opioid analgesics.**
4. **X Antipsychotics potentiate the effects of antihypertensives, increasing the risk of hypotension.**
5. ____ Antipsychotics decrease the effectiveness of oral hypoglycemic agents.

35. 1. This time action profile reflects the pharmacokinetics of glargine (Lantus), a long-acting insulin.
2. **This time action profile reflects the pharmacokinetics of NPH insulin, an intermediate-acting insulin.**
3. This time action profile reflects the pharmacokinetics of regular insulin, a short-acting insulin.
4. This time action profile reflects the pharmacokinetics of aspart (Novolog) insulin, a rapid-acting insulin.

36. Answer: 2, 4, 1, 3, 5
2. **The first step involves identifying if the patient has ever received the drug in the past.**
4. **The second step is to determine whether the patient has ever had a sensitivity reaction to the drug.**
1. **Once a prior sensitivity reaction to the drug in the past is eliminated, the medication can be administered.**
3. **Once the drug is administered the patient should be monitored for at least 30 minutes to ensure that an immediate anaphylactic reaction does not occur.**
5. **After 30 minutes without a sensitivity reaction, the patient can be sent home with the instructions to notify the primary health-care provider immediately if a sensitivity reaction occurs.**

37. 1. **X Alcohol taken concurrently with hydrochlorothiazide (HCTZ), a thiazide diuretic, can increase the medication's side effects.**
2. ____ A 2-g, not 4-g, sodium diet limits the retention of fluid, which should lower the blood pressure. Excessive salt intake contributes to fluid retention, which in turn increases blood pressure.
3. ____ Patients should take hydrochlorothiazide (HCTZ) in the morning to avoid nocturia and interruption of sleep.
4. ____ Hyponatremia, not hypernatremia, is associated with thiazide diuretic therapy. Hyponatremia occurs when the serum level of sodium falls below the normal range of 135 and 145 mEq/L. The signs and symptoms of hyponatremia include nausea, vomiting; headache; confusion; lethargy; fatigue; loss of appetite; restlessness; irritability; and muscle weakness, spasms, or cramps and can lead to decreased consciousness and coma.

5. <u>X</u> A thiazide diuretic inhibits sodium reabsorption in the distal tubule of the kidney, thereby increasing the excretion of sodium and water. It also promotes the excretion of potassium, chloride, magnesium, and bicarbonate, resulting in electrolyte imbalances.

38. 1. <u>X</u> Hydrocodone/acetaminophen (Vicodin) is an opioid/nonopioid analgesic combination. The acetaminophen in Vicodin may weaken the ability of the stomach lining to resist stomach acid contributing to nontherapeutic gastrointestinal responses such as nausea.
2. ____ Diplopia (double vision) is not an expected response to Vicodin.
3. <u>X</u> Vicodin contains hydrocodone and acetaminophen, which comprise an opioid/nonopioid analgesic combination. The hydrocodone in Vicodin is a central nervous system depressant that can cause an exaggerated sense of well-being in the physical and mental realm.
4. ____ Vicodin contains hydrocodone and acetaminophen, which comprise an opioid/nonopioid analgesic combination. The hydrocodone in Vicodin is a central nervous system depressant that causes drowsiness, not irritability.
5. <u>X</u> Vicodin contains hydrocodone and acetaminophen, which comprise an opioid/nonopioid analgesic combination.

The hydrocodone in Vicodin is a central nervous system depressant, which relaxes the neurovascular system contributing to hypotension.

39. **Answer: 4 tablets**
Solve the problem using a formula for ratio and proportion.

$$\frac{\text{Desire}}{\text{Have}} \quad \frac{1 \text{ mg}}{0.25 \text{ mg}} = \frac{x \text{ tablets}}{1 \text{ tablet}}$$

$$0.25 \, x = 1$$
$$x = 1 \div 0.25$$
$$x = 4 \text{ tablets}$$

40. **TEST-TAKING TIP The words "older adult" are key words in the stem that direct attention to content.**

1. <u>X</u> The hepatic microsomal enzyme system causes biotransformation of drugs within the body. Aging decreases the effectiveness of this system.
2. ____ Reduced subcutaneous tissue is unrelated to drug accumulation.
3. <u>X</u> A reduced glomerular filtration rate contributes to reduced excretion of a drug, thereby prolonging drug half-life.
4. ____ Drugs that rely on gastric acid for absorption are less effective when there is a reduction in hydrochloric acid production in older adults.
5. ____ Diminished absorptive surface reduces the absorption of drugs.

This test is provided to give you an opportunity to practice your test-taking skills. It is designed to measure your knowledge of nursing content and motivate you to continue with your efforts to succeed in testing situations.

When self-administering this 100-question practice test, set aside 2 hours of uninterrupted time. This will allow approximately 1 minute per question with 20 minutes for review. To simulate a testing environment, you should sit at a table and select a time when you will not be disturbed. If you spend less than 1 minute on a question, you can use this time for the questions you find more difficult or add it to the time you have reserved for your review at the end of the test. Use the full 2 hours to complete this practice test. If your school allots more or less time than 1 minute per question, adjust your time accordingly. If your examinations are not timed, use all the time you need to complete the test.

Answer every question. If you do not know the answer to a question, attempt to eliminate as many options as you can by using test-taking skills and then make an educated guess. If you are preparing for a computer-administered test that does not permit you to return to previous questions, answer each question before moving on to the next question. Do not go back to answer or change the answer to a previous question.

After you complete this practice test, compare your answers with the answers and rationales provided at the end of the chapter. Evaluate your performance by following the directions in Chapter 10, Analyze Your Test Performance. This will help you diagnose information processing errors and identify knowledge deficits; suggestions for corrective actions are also provided. Do not be tempted to avoid this important step in taking a practice test. In addition, see if you were able to identify the test-taking techniques presented at the end of the rationales for each question. The ability to use test-taking techniques to eliminate distractors and focus on potential correct answers should improve your success when taking a nursing examination. It is through this self-analysis that you can eventually maximize your strengths and address your educational needs in preparation for your next test.

Two Comprehensive Course Exit Exams appear on the enclosed disk. Each examination consists of 75 questions and includes the correct answers and rationales for all the options as well as the identification of test-taking tips when applicable. These exams provide additional opportunities for applying your test-taking skills and simulating taking a test on a computer.

QUESTIONS

1. A debilitated patient is admitted to the hospital with the diagnoses of heart failure and osteoporosis. Which should the nurse do to help prevent injury to this patient who has bone demineralization?
   1. Apply emollients to the skin every day.
   2. Encourage walking in the hall once daily.
   3. Have the patient drink several liters of fluid daily.
   4. Support joints when changing the patient's position.

2. A primary health-care provider prescribes 40 mg of a medication to be delivered IV push. The medication vial is labeled 50 mg/mL. The nurse decides to use a tuberculin syringe to ensure accuracy. How much medication should the nurse draw up into the tuberculin syringe?

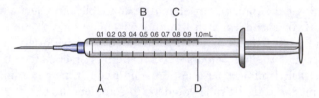

   1. A
   2. B
   3. C
   4. D

3. A patient has a progressive, debilitating disease. Although usually pleasant, the patient begins to report that the doctor is incompetent, the nurses are uncaring, the room is too cold, and the food is terrible. Which defense mechanism is the patient using to cope?
   1. Displacement
   2. Projection
   3. Denial
   4. Anger

4. A nurse is routinely monitoring a patient's blood pressure. Which should the nurse do **first** when an assessment reveals an increase in the patient's blood pressure?
   1. Notify the primary health-care provider.
   2. Report the change to the charge nurse.
   3. Document the observed change.
   4. Obtain the other vital signs.

5. Which action by a patient should the nurse report to the primary health-care provider, because the patient may need a restraint?
   1. Pulling out an intravenous catheter line
   2. Climbing off the end of the bed at night
   3. Wandering into other rooms
   4. Picking at lint on bed linens

6. A comatose patient begins to vomit while lying in bed. In which position should the nurse immediately place the patient?
   1. Lateral
   2. Supine
   3. High-Fowler
   4. Dorsal recumbent

7. A patient whose spouse recently died begins to cry. Which is the nurse's **best** response?
   1. Arrange for grief counseling.
   2. Explain that being sad is normal.
   3. Look away when the patient becomes upset.
   4. Sit down while touching the patient's hand.

8. A nurse is assessing a patient who is having difficulty sleeping. Which patient response **best** supports the nurse's conclusion that an adequate night's sleep was attained?
   1. Has the ability to remember dreams
   2. Does not awaken during the night
   3. Demonstrates renewed strength
   4. Slept seven hours

9. Differentiating among facts, inferences, and opinions is essential for critical thinking when providing nursing care. Which statements are inferences? **Select all that apply.**
   1. _____ The patient weighs 265 pounds.
   2. _____ The patient will lose weight when eating fewer calories.
   3. _____ The patient needs to lose weight because of being too heavy.
   4. _____ The patient will lose 2 pounds a week over the next 6 weeks.
   5. _____ The patient is not following the diet because 4 pounds were gained.

10. A patient is admitted to the postanesthesia care unit after abdominal surgery. The patient's vital signs are blood pressure, 150/90 mm Hg; pulse, 88 beats per minute and bounding; and respirations, 24 breaths per minute with some crackles. Which response does the nurse conclude that the patient **most** likely is experiencing?
   1. Hypoglycemia
   2. Hyponatremia
   3. Hyperkalemia
   4. Hypervolemia

11. A patient has left-sided hemiplegia as the result of a brain attack (cerebrovascular accident). While being dressed, the patient states in a disgusted tone of voice, "I feel like a 2-year-old. I can't even get dressed by myself." Which is the nurse's **best** response?
   1. "It's hard to feel dependent on others."
   2. "Most people who have had a stroke feel this way."
   3. "It must be terrible not being able to move your arm."
   4. "You are feeling down today, but things will get better."

12. A newly admitted patient reports not having had a good bowel movement in 10 days. Which questions should the nurse ask the patient to identify the possibility of a fecal impaction? **Select all that apply.**
   1. _____ "How long has it been since you had a formed stool?"
   2. _____ "Have you had small amounts of liquid stool?"
   3. _____ "Do you notice a bad odor to your breath?"
   4. _____ "Have you been eating food with fiber?"
   5. _____ "Are you having any vomiting?"

13. A patient is receiving Droplet Precautions. Which is the **most** effective way to reduce the transmission of microorganisms at meal times for patients who are receiving Droplet Precautions?
   1. Washing and rinsing the dishes with hot water
   2. Isolating used trays in the dirty utility room
   3. Implementing hand hygiene after eating
   4. Using disposable dishes and utensils

14. A nurse is caring for a patient who is actively dying. What do people generally do according to Kübler-Ross's theory on death and dying that the nurse should consider when caring for this patient?
1. Pass through the stages smoothly
2. Finally reach the stage of acceptance
3. Move back and forth between stages
4. Always move progressively forward through stages

15. A nurse is caring for a patient who is on contact precautions and is having temperatures taken with a non-mercury thermometer. Which temperature is indicated in the illustration?
1. 100.4°F
2. 100.8°F
3. 101.4°F
4. 101.8°F

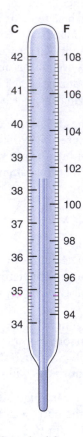

16. A nurse is providing a bed bath for a bed-bound patient. Which area of the patient should the nurse wash last?
1. Feet
2. Legs
3. Axillae
4. Perianal

17. A bed-bound older adult has a stage I pressure ulcer in the sacral area. In which position should the nurse place the patient to relieve pressure and promote circulation to the sacral area?
1. Dorsal recumbent
2. Semi-Fowler
3. Lateral
4. Supine

18. Ampicillin 250 mg every 6 hours is prescribed for a patient. An oral suspension is obtained because the patient has difficulty swallowing pills as a result of a brain attack (stroke). The bottle of ampicillin (Omnipen) indicates there are 125 mg/5 mL. How much oral suspension should the nurse administer? **Record your answer using a whole number.**

Answer: _____ mL

19. The bed of a patient who has an indwelling urinary retention (Foley) catheter is found wet with urine. Which should the nurse do next after determining that the catheter is patent?
1. Insert a larger-size catheter.
2. Provide perineal care whenever necessary.
3. Position a waterproof pad under the patient's buttocks.
4. Tell the patient to use the bedpan when there is an urge to void.

20. A nurse is assessing a patient in pain. Which information about pain does the nurse anticipate eliciting when exploring its location and description?
1. Etiology
2. Intensity
3. Duration
4. Threshold

21. With which type of fire should the nurse use a class A fire extinguisher?
1. Toaster oven
2. Wastepaper basket
3. Stove in the pantry
4. Maintenance closet

22. A nurse is caring for a patient in a coma because of a traumatic brain injury. Which should the nurse do when providing mouth care for this patient?
1. Explain to the patient what will be done.
2. Apply petroleum jelly to the tongue and lips.
3. Use glycerin and lemon swabs to cleanse the mouth.
4. Position the patient in the dorsal recumbent position.

23. A nurse is considering the principles associated with the spectrum of wellness and illness when caring for an older adult. Which word do **most** older adults use to describe themselves?
1. Frail
2. Tired
3. Healthy
4. Dependent

24. A patient's therapeutic serum level for a prescribed antibiotic should be between 4 and 10 µg/mL (micrograms per milliliter). Which should the nurse conclude about a peak level that is 11 µg/mL?
1. The drug dose is appropriate.
2. The drug dose is subtherapeutic.
3. The patient's next dose should be given over a longer period of time.
4. Another dose will further increase the patient's risk for drug accumulation.

25. A 1,000 mL daily fluid restriction is ordered for a patient with kidney failure. Which should the nurse do?
1. Eliminate liquids between meal times.
2. Indicate the order for clear liquids in the patient's plan of care.
3. Divide the fluids equally among the hours the patient is awake.
4. Give proportionally more fluids during the day than during the night.

26. A nurse is making patient rounds at the beginning of a shift. Which patient assessment requires immediate intervention?
  1. Ten respirations per minute by a sleeping patient
  2. Slight shortness of breath after walking to the bathroom
  3. Rattling sounds in the pharynx of an unconscious patient
  4. Expectorating large amounts of thick mucus from the mouth

27. Which actions by a nurse support a patient's right to privacy? **Select all that apply.**
  1. _____ Leaving a crying patient alone
  2. _____ Addressing a patient by the last name
  3. _____ Closing the door when interviewing the patient
  4. _____ Positioning a bath blanket over the patient during a bath
  5. _____ Pulling a curtain closed when changing a sterile dressing

28. Identify the range of motion being performed in the following illustration.

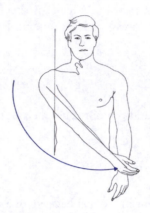

  1. Flexion
  2. Inversion
  3. Adduction
  4. Circumduction

29. Which should the nurse do when washing the genitals of an uncircumcised patient? **Select all that apply.**
  1. _____ Use a circular motion to clean the head of the penis.
  2. _____ Retract the patient's foreskin completely.
  3. _____ Wash down the shaft toward the meatus.
  4. _____ Always employ a very light touch.
  5. _____ Use a rubbing motion.

30. An older adult who received 4 weeks of rehabilitation after a brain attack (cerebrovascular accident, stroke), is preparing for discharge to a daughter's home. Which recommendations concerning safety in the home should the nurse discuss with the patient and daughter? **Select all that apply.**
  1. _____ Mount safety bars around the toilet.
  2. _____ Position a shower chair in the shower.
  3. _____ Install a higher toilet seat in the bathroom.
  4. _____ Limit scatter rugs to those with a rubber backing.
  5. _____ Use an overbed table for support when getting out of bed.

31. Which piece of information documented in the clinical record of an adult male patient should the nurse consider problematic?
1. Temperature 99.2°F
2. Potassium 3.0 mEq/L
3. Pulse 62 beats per minute
4. Ibuprofen 400 mg, PO, qid for joint pain

PATIENT'S CLINICAL RECORD

Laboratory Results
Calcium: 5.4 mEq/L
Sodium: 137 mEq/L
Potassium: 3.0 mEq/L

Physical Assessment
Temperature (oral): 99.2°F
Pulse: 62 beats per minute
Respirations: 20 breaths per minute
Blood pressure: 110/76 mm Hg

Medication Reconciliation Form
Ibuprofen 300 mg, PO, qid for joint pain
Digoxin 0.125 mg, PO, daily

32. A nurse administers an antiemetic to a patient. A decrease in which patient responses indicates to the nurse that the patient is experiencing a therapeutic response?
1. Nausea and anxiety
2. Vomiting and nausea
3. Coughing and anxiety
4. Vomiting and coughing

33. Daily weights are ordered for the purpose of evaluating a patient's fluid loss or gain. When should the nurse weigh the patient?
1. Twice a day
2. One hour before meals
3. At the same time each day
4. Before urinating in the morning

34. A nurse identifies reactive hyperemia over a patient's bony prominence. Which **most** likely is the cause of this response?
1. Applying a warm soak
2. Using the effleurage massage technique
3. Pulling the patient up in bed without using a pull sheet
4. Turning a patient who was in one position for several hours

35. A nurse is assessing a variety of patients with respiratory problems. Which patient response should cause the **most** concern?
1. Inspiratory stridor
2. Pleural friction rub
3. Expiratory wheezing
4. Nonproductive cough

36. A nursing student graduates from an educational program that prepares people to be registered professional nurses. Which is responsible for the authorization of licensure of registered nurses in the United States?
1. Federal law
2. Individual states
3. Constitutional law
4. American Nurses Association

37. A primary nurse is responsible for a group of patients. Which two patients should the nurse attend to before the others? **Select the two options that apply.**
1. _____ A patient who is awaiting to be escorted to the lobby after being discharged
2. _____ A patient admitted for hypertension who wants pain medication for a headache
3. _____ A patient who five days after surgery states, "Something feels very strange in my belly"
4. _____ A patient who got dizzy when the nursing assistant was transferring the patient from a wheelchair to the bed
5. _____ A patient who is anxious to have an IV line removed after being informed by the primary health-care provider that it can be discontinued

38. A nurse is caring for a patient who is diagnosed with hypernatremia caused by excessive watery diarrhea. For which additional clinical indicators should the nurse assess the patient? **Select all that apply.**
1. _____ Muscle twitches
2. _____ Bradycardia
3. _____ Confusion
4. _____ Agitation
5. _____ Thirst

39. Which action is associated with the correct administration of medication delivered by the Z-track method? **Select all that apply.**
1. _____ Using a special syringe designed for Z-track injections
2. _____ Pulling laterally and downward on the skin before inserting the needle
3. _____ Giving the injection in the muscle on the anterior lateral aspect of the thigh
4. _____ Waiting 5 to 10 seconds after instilling the solution before removing the needle
5. _____ Inserting the needle in a separate spot for each dose on a Z-shaped grid on the abdomen

40. A nurse is caring for a patient with a hearing deficit. Which is the **most** significant intervention to ensure that the patient heard what the nurse said?
1. Speak distinctly.
2. Face the patient.
3. Obtain feedback.
4. Raise the volume of speech.

41. How much fluid should the nurse use when preparing a soapsuds enema to effectively stimulate the bowel of an adult?
1. 250 mL
2. 500 mL
3. 700 mL
4. 900 mL

42. A nursing assistant informs the nurse that a patient's pulse seems irregular. How should the nurse monitor this patient's pulse?
1. Via two different sites
2. At the carotid artery
3. For a full minute
4. With a Doppler

43. A nurse is recording the fluid intake for a postoperative patient who just ingested a 4 ounce container of Italian ice and 150 mL of ginger ale. How many milliliters of fluid should the nurse document on the intake section of the patient's Intake and Output Sheet? **Record your answer using a whole number.**

Answer: _____ mL

44. A nurse is teaching oral care to a patient with a history of gingivitis and dental plaque. Which should the nurse teach the patient to do to **best** prevent dental plaque?
    1. Rinse the mouth with diluted hydrogen peroxide.
    2. Have the teeth cleaned by a licensed hygienist once a year.
    3. Brush the biting surface of the teeth using a forward and backward motion.
    4. Vibrate the toothbrush holding it at an angle where the teeth meet the gums.

45. A nurse reviews a patient's admission note and laboratory findings as well as obtains the patient's vital signs. Which question will provide the **most** useful information related to the patient's problem?
    1. "Do you feel very tired?"
    2. "What is your normal blood pressure?"
    3. "When was your last bowel movement?"
    4. "Are you having any difficulty breathing?"

PATIENT'S CLINICAL RECORD

Admission Note:
A female patient was admitted to the hospital directly from the office of a primary health-care provider because of stabbing abdominal pain of unknown origin on a level 8 when using a pain scale of 0 to 10. The patient has a history of diverticulosis. The patient was medicated for pain in the primary health-care provider's office 30 minutes before admission.

Vital Signs:
Blood pressure: 145/90 mm Hg
Pulse: 110 beats/min, regular rhythm
Respirations: 24 breaths per minute; rapid, unlabored
Temperature: 100.6°F

Laboratory Findings:
Hb: 10 g/dL
Hct: 36%
WBC: 16,000/μL (mm³)

46. Which action associated with restraint use can the nurse delegate to an unlicensed nursing team member?
    1. Assessment of a patient's safety needs
    2. Evaluation of a patient's response to restraint use
    3. Selection of the appropriate type restraint to meet a patient's needs
    4. Performance of range-of-motion exercises to a patient's joints after release of a restraint

47. A patient on a bladder-retraining program is incontinent at 1:00 AM every day. Which should the nurse do to promote continence?
    1. Toilet the patient at 1:30 AM.
    2. Toilet the patient at 12:30 AM.
    3. Limit the patient's intake of fluid after dinner.
    4. Position the patient's call bell within easy reach.

48. A nurse is implementing tracheal suctioning for an adult. Which should the nurse do?
    1. Always suction the trachea after the oropharyngeal area.
    2. Apply intermittent suction during removal of the catheter.
    3. Use wall suction with a pressure setting below 90 mm Hg.
    4. Employ continuous suction for 20 seconds during insertion of the catheter.

49. A nurse is caring for patients from culturally diverse populations. Which is the **best** action by the nurse to facilitate communication?
  1. Honor cultural differences when communicating.
  2. Facilitate communication by asking family members to interpret.
  3. Convey the meaning of nursing interventions by using a picture book.
  4. Learn important phrases in different languages of cultural groups in the community.

50. A patient has dysphagia because of a stroke (brain attack). Which should the nurse do when feeding this patient? **Select all that apply.**
  1. _____ Insert food on the strong side of the patient's mouth
  2. _____ Provide small amounts of food with each forkful
  3. _____ Offer fluids to assist with swallowing
  4. _____ Allow adequate time between bites
  5. _____ Place in a low-Fowler position

51. Medicated eye drops are prescribed for a patient. Place the following steps in the order in which they should be implemented after donning clean gloves.
  1. Apply gentle pressure over the inner canthus.
  2. Release the lower lid and instruct the patient to close the eyes gently.
  3. Tilt the patient's head slightly back and toward the eye being medicated.
  4. Clean the eyelid and lashes with sterile normal saline–soaked cotton balls from the inner to outer canthus.
  5. Place a finger just below the lower eyelashes and exert gentle downward pressure over the boney prominence of the cheek.
  6. Hold the dropper close to the eye without touching the eye and administer the prescribed number of drops so they fall into the conjunctival sac.

  Answer: _____

52. A woman who has dependent edema is shopping for a jar of prepared pasta sauce. Which ingredient that appears on the Nutrition Facts label is of **most** concern for this person?
  1. Cholesterol
  2. Calories
  3. Sodium
  4. Protein

53. A nurse is preparing an intradermal injection that is prescribed for a patient. Which factor is related to an intradermal injection?
  1. 3-mL syringe
  2. 26-gauge needle
  3. 1-inch needle length
  4. 30-degree angle of insertion

54. Which action by law is a nurse required to do?
  1. Stop at the scene of an accident.
  2. Report all situations concerning rape.
  3. Notify authorities about instances of child abuse.
  4. Obtain parental consent if an adolescent seeks an abortion.

55. A patient who was in an automobile collision is at risk for internal hemorrhage. For which signs should the nurse monitor this patient? **Select all that apply.**
  1. _____ Increasing abdominal girth
  2. _____ Decreased respiratory rate
  3. _____ Thready pulse
  4. _____ Hypotension
  5. _____ Warm skin
  6. _____ Bradypnea

56. A nurse is transferring a patient from the bed to a chair and sits the patient on the side of the bed for several minutes. Which is the primary rationale for this action?
1. Provides the heart rate time to return to the expected range
2. Enables the body to adapt to a drop in blood pressure
3. Permits the patient to take several deep breaths
4. Allows the patient to regain energy expended

57. Sublingual nitroglycerin is prescribed for a patient with the diagnosis of angina pectoris (chest pain related to transient cardiac ischemia). Which should the nurse teach the patient about this medication?
1. "Take only 1 dose of nitroglycerin. If the pain continues, get immediate help."
2. "Double the dose of nitroglycerin 5 minutes after the first dose if there is no pain relief."
3. "Take 1 dose of nitroglycerin every 3 minutes as often as is necessary until the pain is relieved."
4. "Repeat the dose of nitroglycerin every 5 minutes for 3 doses. If pain is unrelieved, immediately call 911."

58. Which should the nurse do when auscultating a patient's breath sounds?
1. Move the stethoscope systematically from the apices to the bases of the lungs.
2. Place the stethoscope over the ribs along the midclavicular line.
3. Instruct the patient to inhale deeply through the nose.
4. Position the patient in a low-Fowler position.

59. A terminally ill patient appears sad and withdrawn. Which word **best** describes how the nurse should respond?
1. Animated
2. Cheerful
3. Present
4. Aloof

60. A nurse is withdrawing a liquid medication from an ampule. Place the following steps in the order in which they should be implemented.
1. Use a filtered needle.
2. Draw up the desired volume of solution.
3. Shake the ampule with a rapid snap of the wrist.
4. Place an ampule opener over the neck of the ampule.
5. Snap the head of the ampule away from the caregiver.
6. Replace the filtered needle with an appropriate needle.

Answer: _____

61. A nurse is assessing a patient for a systemic response to an inflammatory process. For which responses should the nurse monitor the patient? **Select all that apply.**
1. _____ Pain
2. _____ Fever
3. _____ Edema
4. _____ Erythema
5. _____ Leukocytosis

62. A medication that is to be administered via the buccal route is prescribed for a patient. Which illustration reflects the medication being administered via the buccal route?

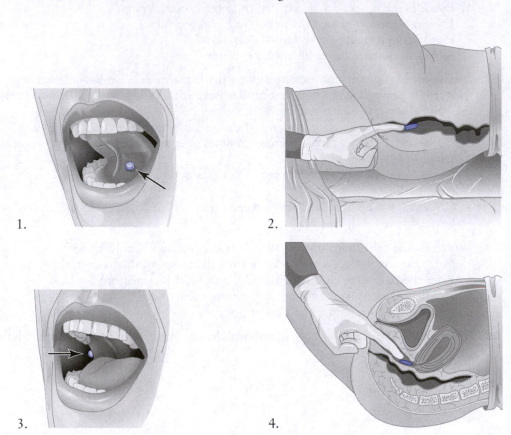

1.

2.

3.

4.

63. A patient tells the nurse, "What fruit should I eat because I have such problems with constipation?" Which of the following fruits is the **best** source of fiber that the nurse should include in the teaching plan to address the patient's constipation?
1. Apples
2. Cherries
3. Apricots
4. Pineapples

64. A nurse identifies an excoriated perineal area in a patient with diarrhea. Which step of the nursing process has the nurse performed?
1. Analysis
2. Evaluation
3. Assessment
4. Implementation

65. Which should the nurse do **first** when caring for patients in a culturally competent manner?
1. Learn what people of common cultures believe about health and illness practices.
2. Behave in an ethnocentric manner when interacting with people of other cultures.
3. Recognize beliefs and attitudes about one's own culture and the culture of others.
4. Focus on the cultural aspects that are similar rather than those that are different.

66. On the third day of hospitalization, a patient communicates a preference to shower at night. Which should the nurse do to **best** promote continuity of care?
1. Orally inform the other health-care team members.
2. Indicate this preference on the patient's plan of care.
3. Explain that hygiene care always is provided in the morning.
4. Initially encourage a modification of personal routines while hospitalized.

67. A nurse is planning care to relieve a patient's pain. Which nursing intervention is based on the gate-control theory of pain relief?
1. Promoting rest
2. Encouraging activity
3. Administering a narcotic
4. Applying a warm compress

68. A nurse is teaching a preoperative patient about leg exercises. The patient asks the nurse why these exercises are necessary. Which primary reason for these exercises should the nurse include in a response to the patient's question?
1. Promote venous return.
2. Prevent muscle atrophy.
3. Limit joint contractures.
4. Increase muscle strength.

69. A patient with a large pressure ulcer is being cared for in the home by a spouse. To promote wound healing, the nurse teaches the spouse about foods high in vitamin C. Which foods selected by the spouse indicates that the teaching is understood?
Select all that apply.
1. _____ Sunflower seeds
2. _____ Green peppers
3. _____ Fresh broccoli
4. _____ Orange juice
5. _____ Black beans

70. Rosuvastatin 10 mg PO once daily is prescribed for a patient. Which should the nurse teach the patient in relation to this lipid-lowering drug? **Select all that apply.**
1. _____ Follow a low-cholesterol diet.
2. _____ Avoid drinking grapefruit juice.
3. _____ Ingest this medication with food.
4. _____ Take this medication in the evening.
5. _____ Call the clinic if you experience muscle weakness.

71. A nurse is assessing a patient's urinary status. Which clinical manifestations indicate urinary retention? **Select all that apply.**
1. _____ Absence of urine
2. _____ Wet undergarments
3. _____ Distended suprapubic area
4. _____ Burning sensation when voiding
5. _____ Sudden, overwhelming urge to void

72. A nurse is making rounds at the beginning of a shift and assesses a patient who has an IV infusion in progress. Which does the nurse need to know to ensure that the correct IV solution is running? **Select all that apply.**
1. _____ Tubing drop factor
2. _____ Drip rate per minute
3. _____ Solution indicated on the IV bag
4. _____ Volume of solution in the IV bag
5. _____ Solution ordered by the primary health-care provider

73. Which is the **best** way that a nurse should remove a soiled sheet from an unoccupied bed?
1. Push the sheet together on the bed.
2. Roll the sheet into itself on the bed.
3. Slide the sheet to the side of the bed.
4. Fanfold the sheet to the foot of the bed.

74. A nurse is assessing a patient for an emotional response to stress. For which response should the nurse monitor the patient?
1. Headache
2. Irritability
3. Heartburn
4. Hypertension

75. A nurse is teaching a patient to perform self-breast examination. The nurse understands that there are 3 patterns for breast examination. Which pattern should the nurse teach the patient because it is considered **most** effective?

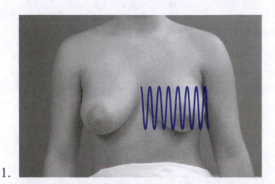

1.

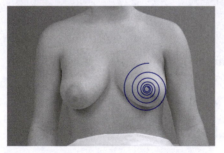

2.

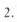

3.

76. Which statement indicates that a patient understands the teaching about diaphragmatic breathing?
1. "I should feel my abdomen flatten on inspiration."
2. "I should raise my shoulders and chest when I inhale."
3. "I should hold my breath for several seconds at the height of inspiration."
4. "I should use my hands to put pressure against the abdomen when I inhale."

77. An obese patient who has a history of heart failure is prescribed metoprolol 50 mg PO twice a day. Which should the nurse teach the patient regarding self-administration of this antihypertensive? **Select all that apply.**
1. _____ Weigh yourself twice a week.
2. _____ Check your pulse before taking the medication.
3. _____ Stop taking the medication when you feel better.
4. _____ Take the medication at the same times every day.
5. _____ Move from a sitting to a standing position slowly.
6. _____ Monitor your blood pressure before taking each dose of the medication.

78. A nurse is caring for a patient who is nauseated and vomiting. Which should the nurse do after the patient is done vomiting?
1. Always contain the vomitus in a medical waste container.
2. Pour the vomitus down the sink in the dirty utility room.
3. Save a specimen of the vomitus for testing.
4. Discard the vomitus in the toilet.

79. A nurse must obtain a urine specimen from an indwelling urinary catheter. The nurse identifies the patient, explains the procedure, and clamps the drainage tubing below the port 20 minutes before performing the procedure. The nurse then washes the hands and collects the necessary equipment. Place the following steps in the order in which they should be performed.
1. Remove the clamp and allow urine to drain
2. Provide for patient privacy and expose the port
3. Don gloves and wipe the port with an alcohol swab
4. Remove the syringe and wipe the port with an alcohol swab
5. Insert the syringe and aspirate a minimum of five mL of urine
6. Transfer urine into a sterile specimen cup and discard the syringe and gloves into appropriate containers

Answer: _____

80. A nurse is administering heparin intravenously to a patient with a deep vein thrombosis. Which is **most** important for the nurse to have readily available on the unit when a patient is receiving heparin intravenously?
1. Potassium chloride
2. Protamine sulfate
3. Prothrombin
4. Plasma

81. Which nursing actions interfere with the chain of infection at the level of transmission? **Select all that apply.**
1. _____ Covering the nose when sneezing
2. _____ Placing used linen into a linen hamper
3. _____ Repositioning a patient every two hours
4. _____ Disposing of an item that touches the floor
5. _____ Applying a sterile dressing over a contaminated wound

82. A nurse is supervising the activities of a nursing assistant. Which actions observed by the nurse reflect inappropriate body mechanics on the part of the nursing assistant? **Select all that apply.**
1. _____ Standing on a patient's weak side when assisting with ambulation
2. _____ Holding clean equipment close to the body when walking
3. _____ Flexing the knees when lifting an object from the floor
4. _____ Placing the feet apart when transferring a patient
5. _____ Bending from the waist when making a bed

83. A patient tells the nurse about problems with constipation. Which should the nurse teach the patient to avoid eating?
1. Cheese and broccoli
2. Yogurt and cheese
3. Broccoli and peas
4. Peas and yogurt

84. A nurse is caring for a patient who is on intake and output. During the 11 to 7 shift the patient voids a total of 700 mL of dark yellow urine and vomits 200 mL of greenish-yellow fluid at 0300 hr and 150 mL of greenish-yellow fluid at 0600 hr. Place an X where the nurse should record the total amount the patient vomited during the 11 to 7 shift.

Intake and Output

INTAKE	11-7	7-3	3-11	24 HR	11-
Oral/Tube					
Blood/Plasma					
I.V.					
Other					
Other					
TOTAL					
OUTPUT	11-7	7-3	3-11	24 HR	11-
Liquid Stool					
Urine					
G.I. Suction					
Emesis					
Bowel Movement					
Other					
TOTAL					
INITIALS					

85. A nurse is planning care for an older adult. When does the frequency of falls increase for hospitalized older adults that the nurse must consider when planning care for this patient?
1. At night
2. Before meals
3. After surgery
4. During visiting hours

86. A nurse instills 2 medicated drops into a patient's ear as prescribed. Place an X over the site the nurse should compress to help disperse the medication throughout the external auditory canal.

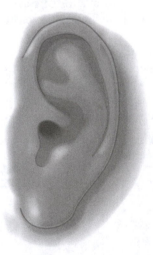

87. A patient ingests a 2,000-calorie meal consisting of 60 grams of fat. Which percentage of calories came from fat? **Record your answer using a whole number.**

Answer: _____%

88. A day nurse gives a change of shift report to the evening nurse who just arrived on duty. Place the following 4 patients in the order in which they should be attended to by the evening nurse.
  1. A 25-year-old alert patient returned from the postanesthesia care unit 15 minutes ago after surgery on the left knee. The patient is receiving continuous passive range-of-motion exercises via a mechanical device.
  2. A 60-year-old woman who had a temporary colostomy 3 days ago and who arranged for her spouse to be present for a teaching session on how to care for the colostomy.
  3. A 75-year-old adult who was admitted for observation after a fall, has a history of dementia, and is restless and rubbing the right hip.
  4. A 65-year-old man who was a victim of an assault who request medication to relieve epigastric pain after having lunch.

  Answer: _____

89. Which action violates a principle of surgical asepsis?
  1. Recapping a syringe after withdrawing medication from a vial
  2. Holding a wet sterile gauze with sterile forceps while the handle is higher than the tip
  3. Failing to wipe the rubber port of a newly opened sterile multiple-dose vial with an alcohol swab
  4. Pouring normal saline on gauze that is lying in its opened sterile paper wrapper while on an overbed table

90. Which should the nurse assess to **best** evaluate peripheral circulation in the lower extremities?
  1. Pedal pulses and excessive hair on the toes
  2. Excessive hair on the toes and blood pressure
  3. Speed of capillary refill in the toenails and pedal pulses
  4. Blood pressure and speed of capillary refill in the toenails

91. A patient, who had a brain attack (stroke, cerebrovascular accident), has hemiparesis. Which should the nurse do to **best** prevent this patient from developing contractures?
  1. Teach the patient to perform range-of-motion exercises.
  2. Transfer the patient to a chair 2 times a day.
  3. Support the patient's joints with pillows.
  4. Reposition the patient every 2 hours.

92. A nurse is teaching a female patient with a urinary tract infection about why women have a higher incidence of urinary tract infections than men. Which is the primary reason for this increased risk in women?
  1. Urine flows toward the rectum via gravity when women void.
  2. The anus is closer to the urinary meatus in women.
  3. Women use bedpans, which harbor microorganisms.
  4. Women must sit, rather than stand, when toileting.

93. A confused patient is incontinent of urine and stool. Which should the nurse do to **best** prevent skin breakdown in this patient?
  1. Instruct the patient to always call the nurse when soiled.
  2. Check for soiling frequently and wash if necessary.
  3. Place sheepskin on the bed and apply a diaper.
  4. Reposition the patient frequently.

94. A patient has a prescription for an opioid every 4 hours prn for pain after abdominal surgery. Which patient outcome **best** indicates that the medication is effective?
  1. Is able to cough with a tolerable level of discomfort
  2. Is able to maintain the semi-Fowler position
  3. Requests another tablet in three hours
  4. Has a decrease in the respiratory rate

95. A school-age child is to be hospitalized for several weeks. Which should the nurse encourage the parents to do to enhance achievement of the developmental task associated with this age group?
    1. Have siblings visit several times a week.
    2. Bring a favorite stuffed animal from home.
    3. Plan for schoolwork to be brought to the hospital.
    4. Arrange for the television to be turned on in the room.

96. A nurse is caring for a patient who has a history of urge incontinence. Which should the nurse do to **best** provide for the elimination needs of this patient?
    1. Toilet the patient every 4 hours.
    2. Toilet the patient as soon as requested.
    3. Encourage the patient to stay near the bathroom.
    4. Ask the patient to limit fluid intake after 6:00 in the evening.

97. A nurse is evaluating a patient's use of a liquid metered-dose inhaler. Which behaviors indicate that the patient is using the inhaler appropriately? **Select all that apply.**
    1. _____ Holding the breath at the height of inhalation when using the inhaler
    2. _____ Shaking the container before pressing down on the inhaler
    3. _____ Using tap water to rinse the mouth after the procedure
    4. _____ Pressing down on the device while inhaling quickly
    5. _____ Tilting the head back slightly during the procedure

98. Where should the nurse stand when assisting a blind patient to walk?
    1. In front of the patient while the patient uses the corridor handrail
    2. Next to the patient while the patient holds the nurse's arm
    3. In front of the patient while providing verbal directions
    4. Next to the patient while holding the patient's elbow

99. A nurse is caring for a patient with a nasogastric tube. Which should the nurse do to **best** assess for correct placement of the tube?
    1. Auscultate the lungs.
    2. Place the end of the tube in water.
    3. Instill a small amount of normal saline.
    4. Aspirate stomach contents through the tube.

100. A patient has metastatic lung cancer and the primary health-care provider discusses the diagnosis and prognosis in detail with the patient. After a severe episode of coughing and shortness of breath later in the day, the patient says to the nurse, "This is just a cold. I'll be fine once I get over it." Which is the nurse's **best** response?
    1. "Tell me more about your illness."
    2. "It's really not a cold; it's lung cancer."
    3. "I understand that you had some bad news this morning."
    4. "Remember what you were told about your condition earlier today."

1. 1. Emollients hold moisture in the skin, making it supple; they do not prevent bone injury.
2. Weight bearing helps limit bone demineralization, but it will not prevent bone injury.
3. An intake of 2500 mL of fluid daily flushes the kidneys and limits calculi formation, which can occur because of the high level of calcium salts in the urine as a result of demineralization. It does not prevent bone injury.
4. **Bone demineralization (osteoporosis) causes the bones to become weak, brittle, and fragile; supporting joints when turning or moving limits the stress that may cause a fracture.**

TEST-TAKING TIP The word "demineralization" is the key word in the stem that directs attention to content. Option 4 is unique because it is the only option that does not say "daily" or "day."

2. 1. This is an incorrect calculation; it is not enough of the prescribed medication.
2. This is an incorrect calculation; it is not enough of the prescribed medication.
3. **0.8 mL is the desired dose. Solve the problem using ratio and proportion.**

$$\frac{\text{Desire}}{\text{Have}} \quad \frac{40 \text{ mg}}{50 \text{ mg}} = \frac{x \text{ mL}}{1 \text{ mL}}$$

Cross-multiply: $50x = 40$

Divide both sides by 50: $x = 40 \div 50$
$$x = 0.8 \text{ mL}$$

4. This is an incorrect calculation; it will result in an overdose.

3. 1. **The patient is anxious and is reducing anxiety by transferring emotions from something stressful to substitutes that are less anxiety producing.**
2. Projection is the attribution of unacceptable thoughts or actions to another.
3. Denial is a defense mechanism used to avoid emotional conflicts and to refuse to cope with unpleasant realities by keeping them out of conscious awareness.
4. Anger is a behavior that is an adaptive response; it defends the individual but is not known as a defense mechanism.

4. 1. Notifying the primary health-care provider may be done later; it is not the priority at this time.
2. Reporting the change to the charge nurse may be done later; it is not the priority at this time.
3. Documenting the observed change may be done later; it is not the priority at this time.
4. **Because of the interrelationships among the circulatory system, respiratory system, and the basal metabolic rate, all the vital signs should be obtained for an accurate assessment.**

TEST-TAKING TIP The word "first" in the stem sets a priority. Option 4 is unique. It is the only option that indicates additional assessment. Options 1, 2, and 3 all refer to communicating the event in some way.

5. 1. **Physical or chemical restraints may be necessary to protect the patient from self-harm. Pulling out an IV line can cause tissue injury and will interrupt medical therapy.**
2. Climbing off the end of the bed at night can be addressed by interventions other than a restraint.
3. Wandering should be controlled by observation, not a restraint.
4. Picking at the gown and bed linens is not an unsafe behavior that requires application of a restraint.

6. 1. **The lateral position prevents aspiration because it allows vomitus to drain out of the mouth via gravity.**
2. The supine position is contraindicated because it promotes aspiration by allowing vomitus to flow to the posterior oral pharynx and enter the trachea.
3. A high-Fowler position provides inadequate support for an unconscious patient.
4. The dorsal recumbent position is contraindicated because it promotes aspiration by allowing vomitus to flow to the posterior oral pharynx and enter the trachea.

TEST-TAKING TIP The word "immediately" in the stem sets a priority. Options 2 and 4 are equally plausible because both positions are back-lying positions that promote aspiration of vomitus.

7. 1. Grief counseling may be done later; it is not the priority at this time.
   2. Although feeling sad is a common response to a loss, the nurse is making an assumption the patient is sad without knowing the patient-spouse relationship; the tears may indicate other feelings, such as relief or joy.
   3. Avoiding eye contact may give the patient the message that it is not acceptable to cry.
   4. **Sitting down and touching the patient's hand communicate acceptance and caring.**

   TEST-TAKING TIP The word "best" in the stem sets a priority. Option 4 is patient centered. Option 1 is premature and abdicates the nurse's responsibility to another. Option 2 minimizes the patient's feelings. Option 3 ignores the patient's feelings.

8. 1. Remembering dreams is unrelated to adequate sleep.
   2. Although a person sleeps at night without waking, the length of the sleep or the length of rapid-eye-movement sleep may be insufficient to restore or renew the body.
   3. **The purpose of sleep is to rest and restore the body, which generally is evidenced by renewed strength.**
   4. Seven hours may or may not be enough sleep because each person has unique needs and a biological clock for determining sleeping intervals.

   TEST-TAKING TIP The word "best" in the stem sets a priority.

9. 1. ____ "The patient weighs 265 pounds" is a fact. A fact can be confirmed and verified through investigation.
   2. **X "If the patient eats fewer calories, the patient will lose weight" is an inference. An inference is a conclusion drawn from logic derived from deductive or inductive reasoning.**
   3. ____ "The patient needs to lose weight because he is too heavy" is an opinion. An opinion reflects the beliefs of the speaker and may fit the facts but can also be a miscalculation or error.
   4. ____ This is a patient goal, not an inference. It is patient focused, measurable, specific, and has a time frame.
   5. **X "The patient is not following the diet because 4 pounds were gained is"**

an inference. An inference is a conclusion drawn from logic derived from deductive or inductive reasoning.

10. 1. Hypoglycemia is indicated by fatigue, dizziness, restlessness, hunger, sweating, palpitations, tremors, nausea, and a capillary blood glucose level of less than 70 mg/dL.
    2. Hyponatremia is indicated by lethargy, confusion, apprehension, muscle cramps, anorexia, nausea, vomiting, and a serum sodium level less than 135 mEq/L.
    3. Hyperkalemia is indicated by muscle weakness, areflexia, decreased heart rate, irregular pulse, irritability, apathy, confusion, and a serum potassium level more than 5.0 mEq/L.
    4. **These are signs of fluid volume excess; fluids are administered during surgery to maintain an adequate circulating blood volume. Occasionally, intraoperative IV fluids may be excessive and is a complication that must be monitored by the nurse in the postanesthesia care unit.**

    TEST-TAKING TIP The word "most" in the stem sets a priority.

11. 1. **This statement identifies the patient's feelings and provides an opportunity for further discussion.**
    2. This statement is a generalization that may not be true; also, it cuts off communication.
    3. This statement focuses on the inability to move rather than feelings of helplessness, dependence, and regression.
    4. This statement is false reassurance because the nurse does not know if things will get better.

    TEST-TAKING TIP The word "best" in the stem sets a priority. The word "most" in option 2 is a specific determiner. Option 4 is false reassurance and denies the patient's feelings. Option 1 is patient centered.

12. 1. **X There are no formed stools with a fecal impaction. Knowing how long ago the patient had a formed stool provides additional information for identifying if the patient has a fecal impaction.**

    2. **X A fecal impaction is an obstruction in the large intestine; peristalsis behind the obstruction initially increases in an attempt to move the mass, causing liquid stool to pass around the area of the impaction.**

3. _____ A bad odor to the breath is unrelated to a fecal impaction in the large intestine. A bad odor to the breath may be related to a small bowel obstruction.

4. _____ This question is not significant at this time; foods with fiber promote intestinal peristalsis, which prevents constipation.

5. _____ People with a fecal impaction may experience rectal pressure, bloating, and nausea, but rarely do they vomit; nausea and vomiting occur more frequently with small bowel obstructions.

TEST-TAKING TIP The words "fecal impaction" are key words in the stem that direct attention to content. The words "bowel movement" in the stem and the word "stool" in options 1 and 2 are obscure clang associations.

13. 1. Washing and rinsing dishes with hot water are not effective in reducing the transmission of microorganisms.

2. Used trays from an isolation room will contaminate the dirty utility room.

3. The hands should be washed before eating.

4. **Contaminated disposable articles can be bagged and discarded, which prevents the spread of microorganisms.**

TEST-TAKING TIP The words "Droplet Precautions" are key words in the stem that direct attention to content. The word "most" in the stem sets a priority.

14. 1. Although passing through the stages may be smooth for some people, it is not smooth for most individuals; the intensity and speed of progression depend on many factors such as extent of loss, level of growth and development, cultural and spiritual beliefs, gender roles, and relationships with significant others.

2. Some people never progress past denial, the first step in Kübler-Ross's theory of grieving.

3. **The stages are not concrete, and the patient's behavior changes as different levels of awareness and/or coping occur. Kübler-Ross's theory of grieving is behaviorally oriented.**

4. Progression is not always forward. Patients tend to move back and forth among stages or may remain in one stage.

TEST-TAKING TIP Options 3 and 4 are opposites. The word "always" in option 4 is a specific determiner.

15. 1. The illustration does not indicate a temperature of 100.4°F.

2. The illustration does not indicate a temperature of 100.8°F.

3. **The illustration indicates a temperature of 101.4°F. Each line represents 0.2 of a degree of temperature.**

4. The illustration does not indicate a temperature of 101.8°F.

16. 1. The feet are cleaner than the perianal area, and if washed last they will become more contaminated from microorganisms and fecal material from the rectum.

2. The legs are cleaner than the perianal area, and if washed last they will become more contaminated from microorganisms and fecal material from the rectum.

3. The axillae are cleaner than the perianal area, and if washed last they will become more contaminated from microorganisms and fecal material from the rectum.

4. **The perianal area has fecal material and microorganisms that can contaminate other parts of the body; therefore, the perianal area should be washed last.**

TEST-TAKING TIP The word "last" indicates the need to identify the order in which the options should be implemented. Once the three options that must come first are identified, then the remaining option is "last." Option 4 is unique because there is only 1 perianal area. In options 1, 2, and 3 human anatomy includes two of each; an individual has two legs, two feet, and two axillae.

17. 1. In the dorsal recumbent position, pressure will still be on the sacrum because it is a back-lying position.

2. In the semi-Fowler position, pressure will still be on the sacrum; and with the head elevated, shearing force to the back and sacral areas may occur if the patient slides down in bed.

3. **In the lateral position, the iliac crest and greater trochanter, not the sacrum, bear the body's weight.**

4. In the supine position, pressure will still be on the sacrum because it is a back-lying position.

TEST-TAKING TIP Options 1 and 4 are equally plausible because both positions are horizontal, back-lying positions.

18. **Answer: 10 mL. Solve the problem using ratio and proportion.**

$$\frac{\text{Desire}}{\text{Have}} \quad \frac{250 \text{ mg}}{125 \text{ mg}} = \frac{\text{x mL}}{5 \text{ mL}}$$

125x = 250 × 5

125x = 1250

x = 1250 ÷ 125

x = 10 mL

19. 1. **Urine is leaking around the urinary retention catheter and a larger-size catheter is required; once ordered, it is within the role of the nurse to select the appropriate size catheter and perform the insertion.**
    2. With a urinary retention catheter in place, the patient should not be wet with urine because it is a closed system from the bladder to the collection bag.
    3. A waterproof pad should be unnecessary because there should be no leaking of urine with an indwelling urinary retention catheter.
    4. The presence of a retention catheter negates the need to void.

    TEST-TAKING TIP The word "next" in the stem sets a priority. The word "catheter" in the stem and option 1 is a clang association.

20. 1. **The location of pain is often related to the underlying disease or illness; the quality or subjective description of pain often have commonalities related to specific illness, such as burning epigastric pain associated with gastric ulcers and crushing chest pain associated with myocardial infarctions.**
    2. The intensity of pain is totally individual and unreliable for determining relationships among location and description of pain.
    3. The location and the description of pain are not significant in determining the duration of pain.
    4. Pain threshold is totally individual and unreliable for determining relationships among location and description of pain.
21. 1. A Class A fire extinguisher contains water and is contraindicated in an electrical fire because water conducts electricity. A Class C fire extinguisher should be used.
    2. **A Class A fire extinguisher contains water, which safely and effectively puts out fires composed of burning wood, paper, or cloth.**

3. Water should not be used because it causes grease to spatter; also the stove might be an electric stove. A Class C fire extinguisher should be used.
4. A maintenance closet usually contains flammable materials; water is contraindicated because it dilutes flammable liquids, which spreads the fire. A Class B fire extinguisher should be used.

TEST-TAKING TIP The words "class A fire extinguisher" are key words in the stem that direct attention to content. Option 2 is unique because it is the only option that is related to ordinary rubbish such as paper, wood, or fabric. Options 1 and 3 are equally plausible because stoves in health-care agencies generally are electric, as are toasters.

22. 1. **Hearing is the last sense to deteriorate, and the patient may hear the nurse; all patients have a right to know what will be done and why.**
    2. A petrolatum-based lubricant is for external, not internal, use.
    3. Glycerin and lemon swabs, if used, should be applied after the mouth is cleansed. Many nurses no longer use lemon and glycerin swabs because they cause drying of the mucous membranes.
    4. The dorsal recumbent position will promote aspiration and is contraindicated. A side-lying position is appropriate.

    TEST-TAKING TIP Options 2 and 3 are equally plausible; both focus on cleaning the mouth. Option 1 is unique because it is the only option that addresses the patient's emotional needs. Options 2, 3, and 4 are interventions that provide physical care. Option 1 is a patient-centered option.

23. 1. The majority of older adults rarely see themselves as frail. They perceive themselves as being independent and active even if they have several chronic illnesses.
    2. Although people lead more sedentary lifestyles as they age, they are still active; most older adults do not view themselves as tired.
    3. **Most older adults perceive themselves as healthy because they measure their health in relation to how well they function, rather than by the absence or presence of disease.**
    4. Most older adults view themselves as independent, not dependent.

TEST-TAKING TIP The word "most" in the stem sets a priority. Option 3 is unique. Option 3 is the only option that has a positive connotation (healthy). Options 1, 2 and 4 have negative connotations (frail, tired, and dependent).

24. 1. The drug dose is too high because the peak serum level of 11 µg/mL (micrograms per milliliter) is higher than the therapeutic serum peak level of 10 µg/mL.
    2. The peak serum level is too high, not too low. If either the peak or trough level decreases below 4 µg/mL, the drug dose is subtherapeutic.
    3. The dose is too high because 11 µg/mL is more than the therapeutic level of 10 µg/mL. The dose should be reduced, not just administered at a slower rate.
    4. **11 µg/mL is higher than the therapeutic peak serum level range. Another dose will further increase the already excessive level of the drug.**

25. 1. Liquid intake should be dispersed over the hours when the patient is awake and not just ingested with meals.
    2. Fluid restriction is concerned with limiting the volume of fluid, not the type of fluid.
    3. Consuming an equal amount of fluids at night is unrealistic because the patient will be sleeping.
    4. **The patient and nurse should make a fluid schedule, taking into consideration factors such as periods of wakefulness, number of meals, oral medications, personal preferences, and so on. An appropriate schedule might be 500 mL between 8 AM and 4 PM, 400 mL between 4 PM and 11 PM, and the remainder of the fluid, 100 mL, during the night.**

TEST-TAKING TIP The words "fluid restriction" are key words in the stem that direct attention to content. The word "fluid" in the stem and the word "fluids" in option 3 and 4 are clang associations. Seriously consider these options.

26. 1. While a person is awake, expected respiratory rates usually are between 12 and 20 per minute; when a person is asleep, the need for oxygen declines, resulting in a slight decrease in the respiratory rate and an increase in the depth of respirations.

2. Slight shortness of breath is an expected response to activity.
3. **Rattling sounds in the pharynx indicate mucus is in the airway; suctioning may be necessary to maintain a patent airway because an unconscious patient cannot cough voluntarily.**
4. Coughing and expectorating are actions that maintain a patent airway.

TEST-TAKING TIP The word "immediate" in the stem sets a priority.

27. 1. ____ Leaving abandons the patient; a crying patient needs support, not isolation.
    2. ____ Calling the patient by name supports the patient's need for identity, dignity, and respect, not privacy.
    3. **X This provides a personal, secluded environment for a confidential discussion.**
    4. **X Placing a bath blanket over the patient during a bath prevents unnecessary exposure of the patient. The bath blanket allows the nurse to expose just the areas being washed, which provides for patient privacy.**
    5. **X This provides privacy when performing a physically invasive procedure.**

TEST-TAKING TIP The words "right to privacy" are key words in the stem that direct attention to content. Option 1 denies the needs of the patient.

28. 1. Flexion is the decrease in the angle between the bones forming a joint.
    2. Inversion is turning the sole of the foot medially.
    3. **Adduction of the shoulder occurs when the arm and hand are brought across the midline in the front of the body with the elbow straight.**
    4. Circumduction is movement of a ball-and-socket joint in a full circle.

29. 1. **X Using a circular motion to clean the head of the penis follows the principle of "clean" to "dirty". The urinary meatus is considered cleaner than the rest of the head of the penis or the shaft of the penis.**
    2. **X Smegma collects under the foreskin, which must be retracted to permit thorough cleaning.**
    3. ____ Washing should move secretions and debris away from the urinary meatus, preventing infection.
    4. ____ A light touch may be too stimulating; a gentle but firm touch is more effective.

5. _____ A rubbing motion may injure delicate perineal tissue and be too stimulating.

TEST-TAKING TIP Option 2 is unique because it is the only option with the word "patient." The word "always" in option 4 is a specific determiner.

30. Answer: 1, 2, 3
    1. X Safety bars provide a stationary support around the toilet; this facilitates patient safety and requires less exertion to sit and stand when using the toilet.
    2. X A shower chair helps to prevent falls when taking a shower. Also, it conserves energy and minimizes the fear of falling.
    3. X A higher toilet seat facilitates sitting and rising when using the toilet, which requires less exertion.
    4. _____ All scatter rugs regardless of backing should be avoided to prevent falls. A scatter rug can cause a person to trip on the edge of the rug, resulting in a fall.
    5. _____ This action is unsafe. An over bed table has wheels and does not provide firm, stationary support for changing position or ambulating.

31. 1. A temperature of 99.2°F is within the expected range of 96.6°F to 99.3°F for an adult and is not a cause for concern.
    2. **A potassium level of 3.0 mEq/L is below the expected range of 3.5 to 5.3 mEq/L and is a cause for concern. In addition, a low serum potassium level (hypokalemia) enhances the action of digoxin. Classic clinical indicators of hypokalemia include dizziness, cardiac dysrhythmias, nausea and vomiting, abdominal distention, diarrhea, muscle weakness, leg cramps, confusion, irritability, and hypotension.**
    3. A pulse rate of 62 beats per minute is within the expected range of 60 to 100 beats per minute for an adult and is not a cause for concern.
    4. Three hundred milligrams of ibuprofen by mouth 4 times a day is within the over-the-counter maximum daily dose of 1,200 milligrams daily and is not a cause for concern.

32. 1. Although antiemetics reduce nausea, anxiolytics reduce anxiety.
    2. **Antiemetics block the emetogenic receptors to prevent or treat nausea or vomiting.**

3. Antitussives reduce the frequency and intensity of coughing. Anxiolytics reduce anxiety.
4. Although antiemetics reduce vomiting, antitussives reduce coughing.

TEST-TAKING TIP The word "antiemetic" is the key word in the stem that directs attention to content. There are duplicate facts in options. The question presents four responses: nausea, anxiety, vomiting, and coughing. If you can identify one response unrelated to an antiemetic, you can eliminate two options. If you can identify one response related to an antiemetic, you can focus on two options. You have increased your chances of selecting the correct answer to 50%.

33. 1. Weighing a patient twice a day is unnecessary. Weight varies over the course of the day depending on food and fluids ingested and the weight of clothing being worn. These factors produce information that is not comparable.
    2. Weighing a patient 1 hour before meals is unnecessary. Meal times may vary from day to day, and the information collected will not be comparable.
    3. **To obtain the most accurate comparable data, patients should be weighed at the same time every day (preferably first thing in the morning), after toileting, wearing the same clothing, and using the same scale. This controls as many variables as possible to make the daily measurements an accurate reflection of the patient's weight.**
    4. Weighing the patient before urinating in the morning collects information influenced by the volume of urine in the urinary bladder. Weights should always be measured after, not before, voiding to obtain the most accurate, comparable measurements. One liter of fluid is equal to 2.2 pounds.

34. 1. Heat causes vasodilation that increases circulation to the area and results in erythema, not reactive hyperemia.
    2. Effleurage, light stroking of the skin, simulates the peripheral nerves and should not change skin coloration.
    3. Pulling a patient up in bed without using a pull sheet exerts a shearing force that can injure blood vessels and tissues, resulting in a friction burn.
    4. **Compressed skin appears pale because circulation to the area is impaired. When pressure is relieved, the skin**

takes on a bright red flush as extra blood flows to the area to compensate for the period of impeded blood flow (reactive hyperemia).

TEST-TAKING TIP The word "most" in the stem sets a priority. The words "reactive hyperemia" are key words in the stem that direct attention to content.

35. 1. Inspiratory stridor is an obvious audible shrill, harsh sound caused by laryngeal obstruction. Obstruction of the larynx is life threatening because it prevents the exchange of gases between the lungs and atmospheric air.
    2. Although pleural friction rub reflects a problem, it is not as life threatening as a condition in another option. A pleural friction rub is a grating, rubbing sound that is heard by auscultating over the base of the lung. It is caused by inflamed pleura (pleurisy) rubbing together.
    3. Although expiratory wheezing reflects a problem, it is not as life threatening as a condition in another option. Expiratory wheezing is the presence of high-pitched musical sounds caused by high-velocity movement of air through narrowed airways. It is associated with asthma, bronchitis, and pneumonia.
    4. Although a nonproductive cough reflects a problem, it is not as life threatening as a condition in another option. A nonproductive cough is coughing without mobilizing or expectorating sputum.

TEST-TAKING TIP The word "most" in the stem sets a priority. The word "inspiratory" in option 1 is opposite to the word "expiratory" in option 3. Carefully examine options that are opposites; often one of them is the correct answer. In this question option 1 is the correct answer.

36. 1. Nurse Practice Acts, not federal law, govern the practice of nursing and licensure.
    2. **The power to grant nursing licenses is reserved for the states through their Nurse Practice Acts. An individual must meet minimum proficiency standards to receive a nursing license, thus protecting the public.**
    3. Nurse Practice Acts, not constitutional law, govern the practice of nursing and licensure.
    4. The American Nurses Association (ANA) is the national professional organization

for nursing in the United States. It fosters high standards of nursing practice; it does not grant licensure.

37. 1. ____ Escorting a patient to the lobby after being discharged is not a priority.
    2. **X The headache may indicate that the blood pressure is too high, which may precipitate a brain attack (stroke, cerebrovascular accident).**
    3. **X A patient saying that something feels funny about the incision may indicate separation of surgical wound edges (dehiscence) and/or protrusion of viscera through separated wound edges (evisceration); these need immediate action to prevent extension of the wound separation and to limit invasion of microorganisms.**
    4. ____ Orthostatic hypotension is a common occurrence when moving from a sitting to standing position. The patient is safe in bed at this time. This concern can be addressed later after patients who need immediate attention receive care.
    5. ____ Although this needs to be done, it is not life threatening and can wait.

38. 1. **X With hypernatremia the nervous system is stimulated causing muscle twitches. Fluid moves from the intracellular compartment to the extracellular compartment with excessive watery diarrhea.**
    2. ____ Tachycardia, not bradycardia, is associated with hypernatremia, not hyponatremia.
    3. **X With hypernatremia excitable tissue, such as cerebral cells, becomes stimulated, causing confusion.**
    4. **X With hypernatremia excitable tissue, such as cerebral cells, becomes stimulated, causing agitation. Fluid moves from the intracellular compartment to the extracellular compartment with excessive watery diarrhea.**
    5. **X Marked thirst is a clinical indicator of hypernatremia because of cellular dehydration. Fluid moves from the intracellular compartment to the extracellular compartment with excessive watery diarrhea.**

39. 1. ____ A special syringe is not required for administering a medication via Z-track. The barrel of the syringe must be large enough to accommodate the volume of

solution to be injected (usually 1 to 3 mL) and the needle long enough to enter a muscle (usually 1½-inch needle).

2. **X Pulling laterally and downward on the skin before inserting the needle creates a zigzag track through the various tissue layers that prevents backflow of medication up the needle track when simultaneously removing the needle and releasing the traction on the skin.**

3. _____ The use of the vastus lateralis muscle for a Z-track injection may cause discomfort for the patient. Z-track injections are tolerated better when the well-developed gluteal muscles are used.

4. **X Waiting 5 to 10 seconds allows time for the medication to disperse before withdrawing the needle and hand holding the skin in a lateral position. This limits the risk of solution leaking up the needle track.**

5. _____ The needle is inserted into a large muscle, not the abdomen, for a Z-track injection. The Z represents the zigzag pattern of the needle track that results when the skin traction and the needle are simultaneously removed.

TEST-TAKING TIP The word "correct" in the stem indicates positive polarity. Options 1 and 5 both have the letter "Z" which are clang associations with the letter "Z" in the stem. Consider these options carefully; however, neither of these options is the correct answer.

40. 1. Although clear, accurate articulation allows the patient to decode the combination of vowels and consonants, it does not determine if the message was heard.

2. Although facing the patient allows the speaker's lips and facial expression to be seen, which helps the patient to receive and decode the message, it does not determine if the message was heard.

3. **A patient is the only person who can tell the nurse whether the message was heard and understood.**

4. Raising the voice does not make the message clearer; it may actually make it more difficult to understand. In addition, shouting can be demeaning.

TEST-TAKING TIP The word "most" in the stem sets a priority. Options 1, 2, and 4 are equally plausible. They explain what the nurse should do when speaking. Option 3 is unique because it is an action that occurs

after the message is sent and is the only option that seeks information on which an evaluation can be made.

41. 1. 250 mL is too little fluid; this is the recommended amount for a toddler.

2. 500 mL is too little fluid; this is the recommended amount for a large school-age child or small adolescent.

3. 700 mL is too little fluid for an adult. 700 mL is the recommended volume for an average-sized adolescent.

4. **The range of 750 to 1000 mL, with an average of 900 mL, is the suggested volume of solution for a soapsuds or tap water enema administered to an adult to stimulate effective evacuation of the bowel. It provides enough fluid to fill the bowel and apply pressure to the intestinal mucosa to stimulate defecation.**

TEST-TAKING TIP The words "adult" and "soapsuds enema" are key words in the stem that direct attention to content.

42. 1. Initially the response should be to obtain an apical rate. Ultimately, the apical and radial rates are compared to determine if there is a pulse deficit.

2. The apical, not the carotid, pulse should be obtained when the pulse is irregular.

3. **Taking the pulse for a full minute is necessary to obtain an accurate count. Taking the pulse for 15 seconds and multiplying by 4 or taking the pulse for 30 seconds and multiplying by 2 may result in inaccurate readings and is unsafe.**

4. A Doppler is unnecessary; palpation and the use of a stethoscope are adequate.

TEST-TAKING TIP The word "irregular" is the key word in the stem that directs attention to content.

43. **Answer: 270 mL**
One ounce equals 30 mL.
4 ounces × 30 mL = 120 mL
120 mL + 150 mL = 270 mL

44. 1. Rinsing the mouth with diluted hydrogen peroxide does not provide the necessary friction needed to remove debris that contributes to the formation of plaque.

2. A dental hygienist will use various dental instruments to remove tartar, which is hardened plaque.

3. Although brushing the biting surface of the teeth using a forward and backward motion is an integral part of dental hygiene, it removes debris from the biting

surface of the teeth, not plaque where the teeth and gums meet.

4. **Plaque, composed of bacteria and saliva, forms on the teeth primarily at the gum line. Vibrating a toothbrush at a 45° angle where the teeth meet the gums provides friction that helps to dislodge plaque from the teeth.**

TEST-TAKING TIP The word "best" in the stem sets a priority. The words "prevent dental plaque" are key words in the stem that direct attention to content.

45. 1. This question assesses the hematologic status of the patient, not the gastrointestinal system which should be the concern. Although the hemoglobin (Hb) is below the expected range of 12 to 15 g/dL for an adult female and the hematocrit (Hct) is on the low end of the expected range of 36% to 46%, and may indicate anemia, it is not information that is most significant at this time. Although, the white blood cell count of 16,000 μL (mm³) is significant for the presence of inflammation, infection, tissue necrosis, stress, and hemolytic and other diseases, it is not an assessment of the gastrointestinal system.

2. Although knowing the blood pressure is important because the patient's blood pressure is higher than the expected range of equal to or less than 120 mm Hg systolic over a diastolic of equal to or less than 80 mm Hg, the blood pressure is often increased with anxiety associated with pain.

3. **This is the most important question at this time. The abdominal pain may be associated with a problem with the gastrointestinal system such as diverticulitis or bowel obstruction.**

4. Although the patient's respirations are more than the expected range of 12 to 20 breaths per minute for an adult, they are unlabored. The increased respiratory rate most likely is a response to anxiety associated with pain. In addition, assessing for shortness of breath or difficulty breathing assesses the respiratory, not the gastrointestinal, system which should be the concern.

46. 1. Assessment of patient needs requires the knowledge and judgment of a registered nurse. This task has great potential for harm if the caregiver incorrectly assesses the patient's condition. In addition, it requires an assessment of numerous

systems and risk factors, a complex level of interaction with the patient, problem solving, and innovation in the form of an individually designed plan of care that provides for the patient's safety.

2. The skill of evaluation requires the knowledge and judgment of a registered nurse. This task has great potential for harm if the caregiver incorrectly evaluates the patient's response.

3. The choice of the type of restraint is based on the primary health-care provider's order.

4. **Performing range-of-motion exercises is not complex, requires simple problem-solving skills, and employs a simple level of interaction with the patient. It is within the scope of practice of an unlicensed nursing assistant and does not require the more advanced competencies of a registered nurse.**

TEST-TAKING TIP The word "delegate" is the key word in the stem that directs attention to content.

47 1. Toileting the patient at 1:30 AM is too late. The patient will probably have already voided.

2. **Toileting the patient at 12:30 AM provides the patient with the opportunity to void before becoming incontinent; if effective, it contributes to self-esteem and personal hygiene.**

3. Limiting the amount of fluid intake after dinner decreases the volume of urine voided; it does not prevent incontinence.

4. The patient may not have time to communicate the need to void or may be unaware of the need to void before being incontinent.

TEST-TAKING TIP The stem contains a time indicated numerically. The student should examine options 1 and 2 carefully because they also both contain a time indicated numerically. This is a type of clang association. An option with a clang association often is a correct answer, although, not always. In this question, one of the options with a clang association is the correct answer. Options 1 and 2 also are opposites— a half hour on either side of 1:00 a.m.

48. 1. The opposite is the acceptable technique. The trachea is considered sterile and is suctioned before the oropharyngeal area, which is considered clean; this minimizes contamination of the sterile area.

2. Intermittent suctioning prevents trauma to any one section of the respiratory mucosa because it avoids prolonged suction pressure.
3. For wall suctioning to be effective when suctioning an adult, it should be maintained at 100 to 120 mm Hg.
4. Suction is applied on removal, not insertion, of the catheter. Continuous suctioning is too traumatic to the mucous membranes of the respiratory tract.

TEST-TAKING TIP Options 2 and 4 are opposites. The word "tracheal" in the stem and "trachea" in option 1 is a clang association. However, option 1 contains a specific determiner (always). Eliminate option 1.

49. 1. The nurse must interact with individuals from different cultures in a way that respects cultural differences. For example, the nurse needs to be aware of the impact of eye contact, touch, and invasion of personal space because they have different meanings in different cultures.
2. The question does not indicate that the patient does not speak English. However, if the patient does not speak English, the nurse should use a nonpartisan interpreter. The patient may not be willing to share delicate information with the nurse in the presence of family members.
3. The question does not indicate that the patient does not speak English. Although this may be helpful if the patient does not speak English, it is not the best answer for this question.
4. The question does not indicate that the patient does not speak English. Although this may be helpful if the patient does not speak English, it is not the best answer for this question.

TEST-TAKING TIP The word "best" in the stem sets a priority. Option 1 is global in nature. Options 2, 3, and 4 are specific interventions. Although options 2 and 4 each have a word that is a clang association with a word in the stem, option 1, which is the correct answer, has two clang associations.

50. 1. X Placing food on the strong side of the mouth allows the unaffected muscles to control chewing, moves the bolus of food to the posterior oral cavity, and facilitates swallowing.

2. X Small amounts of food allow the patient to chew (masticate) a manageable mass of food (bolus) safely.
3. ____ Offering fluids to assist with swallowing will promote aspiration and is contraindicated. Fluids should be taken after a mouthful of food is swallowed.
4. X Allowing adequate time between bites permits the patient to chew (masticate) and swallow food.
5. ____ A low-Fowler position may promote aspiration; the patient should be placed in a high-Fowler position to allow gravity to facilitate swallowing.

51. Answer: 4, 3, 5, 6, 2, 1
4. Cleaning the eyelid and eyelashes removes debris and minimizes the presence of microorganisms. Swiping from the inner to outer canthus moves microorganisms and debris away from the lacrimal duct.
3. Tilting the head slightly back and toward the eye being medicated prevents solution from flowing toward the other eye.
5. This action exposes the conjunctival sac, where the drops should be placed to avoid trauma to the cornea.
6. These actions prevent injury to the eyeball and contamination of the dropper.
2. Instructing the patient to gently close the eyes prevents the medication from being squeezed out of the eye.
1. Applying gentle pressure over the inner canthus prevents medication from flowing into the lacrimal duct.

52. 1. Cholesterol intake is not directly related to an increase in interstitial edema.
2. Calories are not directly related to an increase in interstitial edema.
3. An increase in dietary sodium will increase interstitial edema in this patient. This patient should identify the number of milligrams of sodium contained in a serving of the pasta sauce and determine if this amount of sodium is acceptable on the ordered diet.
4. Protein intake is not directly related to an increase in interstitial edema.

TEST-TAKING TIP The word "most" in the stem sets a priority. The words

"Nutritional Facts label" and "dependent edema" are key words in the stem that direct attention to content.

53. 1. An intradermal injection usually involves a small volume of fluid (e.g., 0.1 mL). A 1-mL syringe, rather than a syringe that can accommodate larger volumes, permits a more precise measurement of a small volume of fluid.

2. A 26-gauge needle has a narrow diameter and short bevel that is conducive to the formation of the wheal associated with an intradermal injection.

3. An intradermal injection usually is administered with a needle that is ½ inch in length.

4. This angle is too extreme and results in an injection that is too deep to form a wheal. An intradermal injection uses a 15-degree angle of needle insertion.

TEST-TAKING TIP The word "intradermal" is the key word in the stem that directs attention to content.

54. 1. Stopping at the scene of an accident is an ethical responsibility, not a legal requirement.

2. Competent adults who are raped are personally responsible for reporting an incident of rape. The nurse is responsible for reporting incidents of rape when a minor or a developmentally or emotionally impaired adult is involved.

3. The law requires professionals, such as teachers, certain health-care professionals, and social workers, to report suspicions of child abuse to authorities.

4. In June 1992, the Supreme Court of the United States upheld the constitutional right of a woman to control her own body to the extent that she can abort a fetus in the early stages of pregnancy. However, the decision stipulated that each state may legislate its own reasonable restrictions. It is likely that some states require parental notification if the woman seeking an abortion is a minor. Notification should not be confused with consent.

TEST-TAKING TIP The word "required" is the key word in the stem that directs attention to content. The word "all" in option 2 is a specific determiner.

55. 1. **X The abdominal girth will increase as blood accumulates within the abdominal cavity. Abdominal girth should be measured using a centimeter tape placed around the body over the umbilicus.**

2. _____ The respiratory rate will increase, not decrease, in an effort to bring more oxygen to body cells.

3. **X With hemorrhage there is a decrease in the circulating blood volume resulting in a pulse that can easily be obliterated when using palpation to assess a peripheral pulse.**

4. **X With hemorrhage there is a decrease in the circulating blood volume resulting in a decrease in the systolic blood pressure below the expected rate of 100 mm Hg (hypotension). Hypotension is reflected in a thready pulse.**

5. _____ The skin will be cool and clammy because of the sympathetic nervous system response.

6. _____ The heart rate will increase, not decrease, in an effort to increase cardiac output and bring more oxygen to body cells.

TEST-TAKING TIP Options 2 and 6 are equally plausible. They both are a decreased respiratory rate.

56. 1. Providing time for the heart rate to return to its expected range is not the primary reason for sitting on the side of the bed before transfer.

2. Orthostatic hypotension is a condition that contributes to impaired stability. When moving to a sitting or standing position from lying or sitting, cerebral circulation is reduced, resulting in light-headedness and dizziness; sitting on the side of the bed allows the peripheral blood vessels to constrict in response to the vertical position.

3. Although the patient might take several deep breaths, it is not the primary reason for sitting on the side of the bed before transfer.

4. Allowing the patient to regain energy is not the primary reason for sitting on the side of the bed before transfer.

TEST-TAKING TIP The word "primary" in the stem sets a priority.

57. 1. Sublingual nitroglycerin has a rapid onset and a relatively short duration of action. One dose may not be enough.
2. Doubling the dose may precipitate severe or even life-threatening hypotension.
3. Excessive administration of nitroglycerin can cause severe hypotension and death; when a therapeutic response does not occur after following the prescribed nitroglycerin protocol, medical attention is necessary because the person may be experiencing a cardiac event.
4. **Sublingual nitroglycerin has a rapid onset and a relatively short duration of action. Three doses may be necessary to achieve a desired therapeutic response. However, if pain persists beyond 15 minutes, it may indicate the presence of an acute cardiac event that requires immediate emergency medical intervention.**

TEST-TAKING TIP The word "only" in option 1 is a specific determiner.

58. 1. **The systematic sequence for assessment of breath sounds facilitates a thorough assessment that allows for comparison of similar lung fields on the right and left sides of the thorax.**
2. Bone interferes with the transmission of breath sounds. Placing the stethoscope over intercostal spaces enhances the volume and quality of breath sounds.
3. Inhaling through the nose can cause turbulence that can imitate adventitious breath sounds. Mouth breathing can augment the volume of breath sounds.
4. A low-Fowler position interferes with placement of the stethoscope over the lung fields on the back. An upright position, such as the sitting or high-Fowler position, is preferred because it promotes thoracic excursion and permits placement of the stethoscope.

59. 1. An animated demeanor may be overwhelming for the patient. The patient is in the fourth stage of grieving—depression; during this stage people become quiet and withdrawn.
2. Cheerfulness denies the patient's feelings and cuts off communication.
3. **The patient is developing a full awareness of the impact of dying and is expressing sorrow; this stage of coping should be supported by the quiet presence of the nurse.**

4. Being aloof is a form of abandonment; the nurse must be present and accessible.

TEST-TAKING TIP The word "best" in the stem sets a priority. The word "animated" in option 1 and the word "cheerful" in option 2 are equally plausible. Options 3 and 4 are opposites.

60. Answer: 3, 4, 5, 1, 2, 6
3. **Shaking the ampule with a rapid snap of the wrist moves medication trapped in the top of the ampule into the body of the ampule. This permits all of the medication to be available for withdrawal, ensuring an accurate dose.**
4. **Using an ampule opener over the neck of the ampule protects the nurse's hand from shattered glass when the neck of the ampule is snapped off.**
5. **Snapping the head of the ampule away from the nurse propels any shattered glass away from the nurse.**
1. **Using a filtered needle when solution is withdrawn from the ampule prevents glass shards from entering the syringe.**
2. **Withdrawing the volume of solution prescribed by the primary health-care provider ensures that the patient receives the desired dose.**
6. **Replacing the filtered needle ensures that a sterile needle free of glass shards is used to administer the mediation.**

61. 1. _____ Pain is a local response to stimulation of nerve endings at the site of an injury.
2. **X The inflammatory response is stimulated by trauma or infection, which increases the basal metabolic rate; with infection, fever results from the effect of pyrogens on the temperature-regulating center in the hypothalamus.**
3. _____ Edema is a local response resulting from local vasodilation and increased vessel permeability.
4. _____ Erythema is a local response resulting from increased circulation and local vasodilation in the involved area.
5. **X An increase in white blood cells (leukocytosis) more than the expected range of 4,500 to 11,000 per cubic millimeter of blood can increase to 20,000 or more when there is an inflammatory process. Leukocytes protect the body from pathogens.**

TEST-TAKING TIP The words "systemic" and "inflammatory process" are the key words in the stem that direct attention to content.

62. 1. This illustration reflects the administration of medication via the sublingual route. The medication is placed under the tongue, where it dissolves quickly and is absorbed via the mucous membranes. The sublingual route is used for a systemic effect.
2. This illustration reflects the administration of medication via the rectal route. The rectum is the last 7 to 8 inches of the large intestine. The medication is inserted through the anus and anal canal to reach the rectum. The rectal route is used for either a local or systemic effect.
3. This illustration reflects the administration of medication via the buccal route. The medication is placed in the mouth between the cheek and gum, where it dissolves slowly and is absorbed via the mucous membranes. The buccal route is used for a local effect.
4. This illustration reflects the administration of medication via the vaginal route. The medication is inserted through the vaginal introitus and advanced deep within the vaginal canal. The vaginal route is used for a local effect.

63. **1. Apples are an excellent source of fiber. One medium apple supplies approximately 3.5 grams of dietary fiber.**
2. Ten cherries provide approximately 1.2 grams of dietary fiber.
3. Five halves of dried apricots provide approximately 1.2 grams of dietary fiber.
4. A ½ cup of pineapple provides approximately 1.1 gram of dietary fiber.

TEST-TAKING TIP The word "best" in the stem sets a priority. The words "source of fiber" are key words in the stem that direct attention to content.

64. 1. In the analysis step of the nursing process, the nurse interprets data, determines the significance of data, and formulates a nursing diagnosis.
2. Evaluation involves determining patient responses to nursing interventions, identifying whether goals and outcomes are met, and revising the plan of care when necessary.
3. Observation of human responses is part of the assessment phase of the nursing process; assessment involves collecting, verifying, clustering, and documenting objective and subjective data.
4. Implementation involves carrying out the plan of care and documenting the care provided.

65. 1. Although learning about what people of common cultures believe about health and illness practices may be helpful, the nurse must understand that each person is an individual who may or may not embrace some or all of the values and beliefs identified with one's cultural heritage. Stereotyping (the assigning of a trait existing in some members of the group to all members of the group) must be avoided if care is to be culturally competent.
2. An ethnocentric manner interferes with the nurse's ability to be culturally competent. Ethnocentrism is the view that one's own attitudes, beliefs, customs, and culture are better than those of another.
3. The nurse has to clarify personal values and beliefs before understanding and accepting nonjudgmentally the cultural beliefs and practices of others.
4. Although different cultures share common elements, they may be demonstrated through different behaviors and customs. Recognizing only the similarities denies the differences that make cultures unique.

TEST-TAKING TIP The word "first" in the stem sets a priority.

66. 1. Oral instructions may not reach all members of the nursing team.
2. Indicating the patient's preference on the patient's plan of care provides written documentation of what should be done for the patient; it supports communication among health-care team members, contributes to continuity, and individualizes care.
3. Hygiene care is not done only in the morning.
4. Encouraging a modification of personal routines is not necessary; care should be individualized.

TEST-TAKING TIP The word "best" in the stem sets a priority. The word "always" in option 3 is a specific determiner. Options 3 and 4 deny the patient's preference. The word "preference" in the stem and in option 2 is a clang association. Option 2 is patient centered, and it is the best intervention because it communicates the patient's preferences to other nursing team members in writing.

67. 1. Rest, sleep, and relaxation associated with pain relief are not based on the gate-control theory.
2. Activity uses distraction to focus attention on stimuli other than the pain. When in pain, patients often do not have the physical or emotional energy to concentrate on activities.
3. Narcotics act on the higher centers of the brain to modify the perception of pain.
4. **The gate-control theory assumes that pain fibers that originate in the peripheral areas of the body have synapses in the gray matter of the dorsal horns of the spinal cord. Large nerve fibers stimulated by heat, cold, and touch transmit impulses through the same synapses as those that transmit pain. When larger fibers are stimulated, they close the gate to painful stimuli and thus reduce pain.**

68. 1. **Circulatory stasis occurs after surgery because postoperative patients are not as active as they were before surgery; leg exercises promote venous return and prevent the formation of thrombi and thrombophlebitis.**
2. Although leg exercises prevent muscle atrophy, it is not the primary reason for performing leg exercises postoperatively.
3. Although leg exercises may prevent contractures, it is not the primary reason for performing leg exercises postoperatively.
4. Although active leg exercises increase muscle strength, it is not the primary reason for postoperative leg exercises.

TEST-TAKING TIP The word "primary" in the stem sets a priority.

69. 1. _____ Sunflower seeds contain only trace amounts of vitamin C.
2. **X Green peppers are an excellent source of vitamin C (ascorbic acid). One pepper contains approximately 95 mg of vitamin C.**
3. **X One cup of fresh boiled broccoli contains approximately 116 mg of vitamin C.**
4. **X Citrus fruits such as oranges and grapefruit are excellent sources of vitamin C. One cup of orange juice contains approximately 124 mg of vitamin C.**
5. _____ Black beans contain no vitamin C.

70. 1. **X Patients receiving an HMG-CoA reductase inhibitor (statin) usually have several risk factors for cardiovascular**
disease including high serum cholesterol, LDL, and triglyceride levels. These patients usually are prescribed a diet low in fat and cholesterol.
2. **X Patients should not drink more than 200 mL of grapefruit juice while taking this drug because it potentiates the action of the medication, which can result in toxicity.**
3. _____ It is not necessary to take rosuvastatin with food. It does not cause gastric irritation.
4. _____ Rosuvastatin can be taken at any time of the day because it remains in the body longer than other statins. Other statins such as fluvastatin (Lescol), pravastatin (Pravachol), and simvastatin (Zocor) should be taken in the evening because they are shorter acting. The body produces its cholesterol mostly at night.
5. **X Common side effects of rosuvastatin (Crestor) are muscle aches, weakness, nausea, and headache. However, rhabdomyolysis, a rare serious effect, can occur. It is the accumulation of the byproducts of skeletal muscle destruction in the renal tubules; it can result in renal failure and death. Rhabdomyolysis is manifested by muscle pain, weakness, fever, and dark urine.**

71. 1. **X With urinary retention urine is kept in the bladder and there is a lack of voiding.**
2. _____ Urine is being passed from, not retained in, the bladder when voiding occurs. Wet undergarments may indicate urinary incontinence.
3. **X With urinary retention urine accumulates in the bladder, with resulting bladder fullness. When the bladder is full it expands and appears as suprapubic distention.**
4. _____ Painful or difficult urination is called dysuria, not urinary retention.
5. _____ A sudden, overwhelming need to void is called urgency, which is not related to urinary retention.

TEST-TAKING TIP The word "urinary" in the stem and the word "urine" in option 1 comprise a clang association.

72. 1. _____ This is necessary to know to calculate the IV drip rate, not to determine if the correct IV solution is running.
2. _____ The drip rate per minute indicates the current rate at which the IV is running, not whether the correct IV solution is running.

3. <u>X</u> The nurse needs to have two pieces of data to determine if the correct IV solution is running. One piece of information is identifying what solution is in the IV bag. When this is compared with another piece of data the nurse can make a determination of whether the correct IV solution is running.

4. ____ This is necessary to know to calculate the IV drip rate.

5. <u>X</u> The nurse needs to have two pieces of data to determine if the correct IV solution is running. One piece of information is verifying the solution ordered by the primary health-care provider. When this is compared with another piece of data the nurse can make a determination of whether the correct IV solution is running. The administration of IV fluids is a dependent function of the nurse. The solution ordered by the primary health-care provider must be verified.

TEST-TAKING TIP The word "solution" in the stem and in options 3, 4, and 5 are clang associations. Consider these options carefully.

73. 1. Pushing a sheet together will not secure loose ends; debris may fall on the floor.
    2. **Rolling a sheet into itself secures loose ends and keeps debris contained within the center of the sheet.**
    3. Sliding a sheet to the side of the bed will not secure loose ends; debris may fall on the floor.
    4. Fanfolding the sheet to the foot of the bed will not secure loose ends; debris may fall on the floor.

TEST-TAKING TIP The word "best" in the stem sets a priority.

74. 1. Headache is a physiological response to pain.
    2. **Irritability is a behavioral-emotional response; the body is using physical and emotional energy to reduce stress.**
    3. Heartburn (epigastric pain associated with gastric reflux) can be a physiological response to stress.
    4. An increase in blood pressure (hypertension) is a physiological response to stress.

TEST-TAKING TIP The word "emotional" is the key word in the stem that directs attention to content. Option 2 is unique because it is the only option that does not start with a word that begins with the letter "H."

75. 1. **This is the vertical strip method of breast palpation. The vertical strip method is preferred because it ensures that all breast tissue is examined. The examiner is better able to track which areas have been examined and the entire nipple/areolar complex is included.**
    2. This is the pie wedge (radial spoke) method of breast palpation. This method is difficult to ensure that all breast tissue is examined, especially the areas around and under the nipple and areola, as well as the area in the upper outer quadrant into the axilla (tail of Spence).
    3. This is the concentric circles method. This method is difficult to ensure that all breast tissue is examined, especially the areas around and under the nipple and areola, as well as the area in the upper outer quadrant into the axilla (tail of Spence).

TEST-TAKING TIP The word "most" in the stem sets a priority.

76. 1. The abdomen rises on inspiration.
    2. These accessory muscles should not be involved consciously with diaphragmatic breathing. The abdomen should rise and fall rather than the shoulders; the chest naturally expands and recoils.
    3. **Diaphragmatic breathing involves a pattern of a slow deep inhalation followed by a slow exhalation with a tightening of the abdominal muscles to aid exhalation; the patient should hold the breath for 2 to 3 seconds at the height of inhalation, just before exhalation.**
    4. Pressure against the abdomen will interfere with the amount of air that is drawn into the lungs on inspiration.

TEST-TAKING TIP The word "breathing" in the stem and the word "breath" in option 3 is a clang association.

77. 1. <u>X</u> An increase in weight may indicate that the patient is retaining fluid because the heart is not efficiently circulating blood to the kidneys. A decrease in renal perfusion stimulates the renin-angiotensin response that causes vasoconstriction and the release of aldosterone. Aldosterone causes sodium and water retention. One liter of fluid weighs 2.2 pounds.
    2. <u>X</u> Metoprolol (Lopressor) blocks the stimulation of beta1 (myocardial)

adrenergic receptors that can result in an irregular or slow (bradycardia) heart rate.

3. _____ Metoprolol should not be stopped abruptly because it can precipitate life-threatening dysrhythmias, hypertension, or myocardial ischemia.

4. X Taking the medication at the same times every day maintains a therapeutic blood level of the drug.

5. X Metoprolol (Lopressor) can cause orthostatic hypotension, a vasomotor response. Therefore, the patient should be cautioned to change from horizontal to vertical positions slowly to allow the cardiovascular system to adjust to the change in position.

6. _____ Obtaining the blood pressure before taking each dose is unnecessary. It is sufficient to monitor the blood pressure twice a week.

78. 1. Vomitus should be flushed down a toilet, not contained in a medical waste container.

2. It is unnecessary to remove vomitus from the room; vomitus should be poured down a toilet rather than a sink.

3. Saving vomitus for a specimen generally is unnecessary. Although a primary health-care provider may request that vomitus be assessed, it is rarely sent for laboratory analysis.

4. Discarding vomitus in the toilet represents the most practical action when disposing of vomitus; the toilet contains it, dilutes it, and removes the vomitus from the environment.

TEST-TAKING TIP The word "always" in option 1 is a specific determiner.

79. Answer: 2, 3, 5, 4, 1, 6

2. The port is close to the perineal area and privacy provides for emotional comfort. Exposing the port permits adequate visualization of the port and tubing during the procedure.

3. Gloves protect the nurse from the patient's body excretions. Wiping the port removes microorganisms before insertion of the syringe.

5. Inserting the syringe (via a needle or needleless system) accesses the lumen of the urinary catheter; 5 mL of urine usually is adequate for most urine specimens.

4. Wiping the port after removal of the syringe removes microorganisms from the port.

1. Removing the clamp allows urine to flow down into the collection chamber, which prevents a backflow of urine into the bladder.

6. Urine collected via a sterile procedure should be placed in a sterile specimen cup to prevent extraneous microorganisms from contaminating the specimen. Syringes should be placed into a hard-sided sharps container to prevent injury to and contamination of others. Contaminated gloves can be placed into a plastic-lined garbage container.

80. 1. Potassium chloride is used for the treatment or prevention of potassium deficiency and is unrelated to heparin therapy.

2. Protamine sulfate can chemically combine with heparin, neutralizing its anticoagulant action; it should be kept readily available for the treatment of heparin overdose.

3. Prothrombin is a plasma protein coagulation factor synthesized by the liver, not a drug that should be used as an antidote to heparin.

4. If a heparin overdose occurs plasma may be ordered after the antidote is given. Packed red blood cells will more likely be ordered than plasma.

TEST-TAKING TIP The word "most" in the stem sets a priority.

81. 1. _____ Covering the nose when sneezing interferes with the chain of infection at the portal of exit stage, not at the transmission stage.

2. X Placing used linen in a linen hamper contains microorganisms in an appropriate receptacle, which prevents cross contamination.

3. _____ Turning and positioning contribute to maintaining skin integrity. An intact skin interrupts the chain of infection at the portal of entry stage, not the transmission stage, of the chain of infection.

4. X Disposing of any item that touches the floor is an action that interferes with the transmission of microorganisms in the chain of infection. Items that touch the floor are contaminated and must be disposed of in a manner that contains the spread of microorganisms.

5. _____ Applying a sterile dressing over a contaminated wound interferes with the chain of infection at the reservoir or source of the infection. It interrupts the chain of infection at the portal of exit stage.

82. **1.** **X The nursing assistant should stand on the patient's strong side when assisting with ambulation. This maximizes the patient's strengths and provides firm support. If a client is extremely weak and unstable, then two health-care personnel should ambulate the patient, one on each side of the patient.**

   2. ____ Weight carried close to the center of gravity helps maintain balance.

   3. ____ Using the strong muscles of the legs to carry a load helps prevent back strain.

   4. ____ The wider the base of support and the lower the center of gravity, the greater the stability of the individual.

   5. **X Bending from the waist puts stress on the vertebrae and muscles of the back because it does not distribute the work among the largest and strongest muscle groups of the legs.**

TEST-TAKING TIP The word "inappropriate" in the stem indicates negative polarity. The question is asking, "Which action violates principles of body mechanics?"

83. 1. Although cheese can contribute to constipation, broccoli facilitates defecation.

   2. **Dairy products are low in roughage and lack bulk; they produce too little waste to stimulate the defecation reflex. Low-residue foods move more slowly through the intestinal tract, permitting increased fluid uptake from stool, resulting in hard-formed stools and constipation.**

   3. Both broccoli and peas provide bulk that increases peristalsis, which facilitates defecation.

   4. Although yogurt contributes to constipation, peas provide bulk (undigested residue), which facilitates fecal elimination.

TEST-TAKING TIP The word "avoid" in the stem indicates negative polarity. The question is asking, "What foods should the patient not eat because they can contribute to constipation?" The options in this question contain duplicate facts. Four nutrients are presented: cheese, broccoli, yogurt, and peas. If you know that broccoli contains fiber that helps to increase peristalsis, you can eliminate options 1 and 3. If you know that peas contain fiber that helps to increase peristalsis, you can eliminate options 3 and 4. In either event, you have increased your chances of choosing the correct answer to 50%. If you know that cheese is low in roughage resulting in hard-formed stools and constipation, you

can focus on options 1 and 2. If you know that yogurt is low in roughage, you can focus on options 2 and 4. In any event, you have increased your chances of choosing the correct answer to 50%.

84. The patient vomited a total of 350 mL of greenish-yellow fluid during the 11 to 7 shift. This total amount should be recorded in the first column (11-7) next to Emesis.

Intake and Output

INTAKE	11-7	7-3	3-11	24 HR	11-
Oral/Tube					
Blood/Plasma					
I.V.					
Other					
Other					
TOTAL					
OUTPUT	11-7	7-3	3-11	24 HR	11-
Liquid Stool					
Urine					
G.I. Suction					
Emesis	X				
Bowel Movement					
Other					
TOTAL					
INITIALS					

85. **1.** **Because of a dark, unfamiliar environment at night older adults may become confused and disoriented, which contributes to the occurrence of falls.**

   2. The time before meals generally is unrelated to falls. The incidence of falls may increase after meals because the gastrocolic reflex increases peristalsis, causing a need to defecate. Walking to the bathroom may result in a fall.

   3. All patients, including postoperative patients, should be assisted when ambulating until they are able to ambulate safely on their own; therefore, these patients should not fall.

   4. Visiting hours generally are unrelated to falls.

TEST-TAKING TIP The words "older adult" are key words in the stem that direct attention to content.

86. **Compressing the tragus disperses the medication throughout the external auditory canal (see illustration on page 448).**

87. **Answer: 27%. Each gram of fat equals 9 calories. 60 grams of fat × 9 = 540 calories. 540 ÷ 2000 = 0.27, or 27%.**

88. **Answer: 4, 3, 1, 2**

   4. **A patient reporting epigastric pain may be experiencing a cardiac event that**

could be life-threatening. The nurse should obtain the patient's vital signs and determine whether this situation requires initiation of the rapid response team or a cardiac event can be ruled out and the prescribed antacid administered.

3. **This patient should be scheduled second to be attended to by the evening nurse. The patient may be experiencing pain that is unable to be communicated because of the dementia. Although patients with pain should have their needs attended to quickly, a patient in another option may be experiencing a life-threatening event that requires immediate attention.**

1. **This patient should be scheduled third to be attended to by the evening nurse. Two other patients with more serious potential problems require more immediate attention by the nurse. A patient with continuous passive range of motion generally is assessed every 30 minutes. An alert patient receiving continuous passive range-of-motion exercises via a mechanical devise has a turn off button if a problem should arise or the patient is unable to tolerate the procedure. The patient can activate the alarm button and receive immediate assistance at any time.**

2. **This patient should be scheduled fourth to be attended to by the evening nurse. Although it may be inconvenient for the patient and spouse to have to wait for the teaching session to begin, three other patients have more serious potential problems that require attention first.**

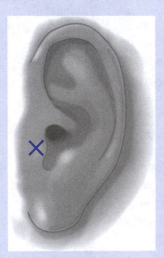

89. 1. Recapping a sterile syringe that has not had contact with a patient or a nonsterile surface does not violate surgical asepsis; the needle of a syringe and the area inside the needle cap are both sterile and pose no microbiological risk of contamination.

2. This is correct technique. Fluids flow in the direction of gravity. When the tip is held lower than the handle, fluid remains at the level of the gauze and the tip of the forceps; this area is considered sterile.

3. When the metal protective ring and cap are removed from around the top of a multiple-dose vial, the rubber port surface is sterile until it is touched by something nonsterile. The rubber stopper does not have to be wiped with alcohol the first time the vial is accessed with a sterile syringe.

4. **Although the inside of a sterile gauze wrapper is sterile, when the paper wrapper becomes wet, capillary action transfers microorganisms from the nonsterile surface of the table to the inside of the wrapper; the gauze then becomes contaminated, which violates sterile technique.**

TEST-TAKING TIP The word "violates" in the stem indicates negative polarity. The question is asking, "Which action is not based on a principle of surgical asepsis?"

90. 1. Pedal pulses are assessed to determine circulation to the feet. A lack of, not presence of, excessive hair on the feet and lower legs may be caused by prolonged hypoxia. In addition, other factors such as genetic endowment may cause a lack of hair in the lower extremities.

2. Lack of hair on the feet and lower legs may indicate prolonged hypoxia. A blood pressure does not evaluate peripheral circulation in the lower extremities as does inspection and palpation.

3. **Applying pressure causes blanching, and when the pressure is released, the normal color should return quickly (within 1 to 2 seconds), indicating adequate arterial perfusion. Assessing pedal pulses measures the adequacy of circulation to the feet.**

4. Although capillary refill assesses adequacy of peripheral circulation, blood pressure does not evaluate peripheral circulation in the lower extremities as does inspection and palpation.

TEST-TAKING TIP The word "best" in the stem sets a priority. Use the technique of duplicate facts to arrive at the correct answer. This question presents four assessments: pedal pulses, excessive hair on the toes, blood pressure, and speed of capillary refill in the toenails. If you know that assessing pedal pulses is a way to evaluate peripheral circulation, then you should focus on options 1 and 3. If you know that the speed of capillary refill of the toenails is a way to evaluate peripheral circulation to the feet then you should focus on options 3 and 4. If you know that there is less hair on the toes as a result of hypoxia, then you can eliminate options 1 and 2. You have thus increased your chances of identifying the correct answer.

91. 1. **Range-of-motion exercises maximally stretch all muscle groups; this prevents shortening of muscles, which can result in contractures.**
2. Although movement of joints experienced during activity will contribute to preventing contractures, it will not move all joints through their full range; also, prolonged sitting can cause flexion contractures of the hips and knees.
3. Although supporting joints contributes to maintaining functional alignment, which helps prevent contractures, it is not the best intervention.
4. Turning and repositioning a patient every 2 hours will reduce pressure, not prevent contractures.

TEST-TAKING TIP The word "best" in the stem sets a priority.

92. 1. Urine that flows toward the anus rarely causes infection; however, bacteria from the large intestine that enter the urinary meatus can cause urinary tract infections.
2. **Stool wiped toward the urinary meatus can cause urinary tract infections; *Escherichia coli*, a common bacterium in stool, causes urinary tract infections.**
3. If properly cleaned after use, bedpans are not a source of infection.
4. The act of sitting when toileting should not increase the incidence of infection.

TEST-TAKING TIP The word "primary" in the stem sets a priority.

93. 1. Instructing a confused patient to call the nurse when incontinent of urine and stool is an unrealistic instruction for this patient; a cognitively impaired patient will have difficulty with this task.
2. **When patients are incontinent, they should be checked frequently and cleaned immediately; feces contain digestive enzymes and urine contains ammonia and other irritating substances that cause skin breakdown.**
3. Sheepskin and an incontinence pad (the word "diaper" should be avoided because it is demeaning) hold moisture next to the skin, and their use should be avoided.
4. Although repositioning the patient frequently should be done, it is more significant to remove urine and feces from the skin.

TEST-TAKING TIP The word "best" in the stem sets a priority. The word "always" in option 1 is a specific determiner. The words "incontinent" in the stem and "soiled" in option 1 and "soiling" in option 2 are obscure clang associations. Consider options 1 and 2 carefully. More often than not an option with a clang association is the correct answer.

94. 1. **The main purpose of pain relief medication is to enable the patient to comfortably engage in necessary activity.**
2. If patients remain perfectly still in the semi-Fowler position, they may be able to tolerate pain. However, being sedentary can precipitate complications such as atelectasis, venous stasis, and muscle atrophy.
3. The patient is experiencing pain before the next scheduled dose; this indicates that the patient is in pain and the intervention was ineffective.
4. A decrease in the respiratory rate is a side effect, not a therapeutic effect, of an opioid; opioids decrease respiration by depressing the respiratory center in the brainstem.

TEST-TAKING TIP The word "best" in the stem sets a priority.

95. 1. Although visits by siblings are appropriate, it does not address the task of initiative versus guilt.
2. A stuffed animal is appropriate for an infant or a toddler.
3. **Completing homework is an appropriate activity for a school-age child. School-age children are interested in doing and producing.**
4. Watching television does not support the developmental tasks of a school-age child.

TEST-TAKING TIP The word "hospitalized" in the stem and the word "hospital" in option 3 is a clang association.

96. 1. A patient with urge incontinence generally is unable to wait 4 hours between voidings.
2. **Toileting the patient immediately upon request supports continence because the person with urge incontinence must immediately void or lose control of urine.**
3. Encouraging the patient to stay near the bathroom promotes isolation and should be avoided.
4. Limiting fluid intake during the early evening and night may be part of a toileting program to provide uninterrupted sleep; however, it does not address the patient's need to urinate immediately when feeling the urge to void.

TEST-TAKING TIP The word "best" in the stem sets a priority. Option 2 is patient centered.

97. 1. X **Holding the breath at the height of inhalation is desirable because it allows tiny drops of aerosol spray to reach deeper branches of the airway.**
2. X **Shaking the canister for 3 to 5 seconds before administration is an acceptable practice because it mixes the medication within the solution so that the aerosol drug concentration is even.**
3. X **Rinsing the mouth removes remaining medication, which reduces mucosal irritation.**
4. _____ When using a metered-dose inhaler, inhalation should be slow; this limits bronchial constriction and promotes

a more even distribution of the aerosolized medication.
5. X **Tilting the head back slightly while using a metered-dose inhaler is desirable because it maximizes airway exposure to medication from the inhaler. Tilting the head backward moves the tongue away from the back of the throat, moves the epiglottis away from the trachea, and straightens the passage from the mouth to the trachea.**

TEST-TAKING TIP The word "inhaler" in the stem and in options 1 and 2 are clang associations.

98. 1. Standing in front of the patient is unsafe and does not support confidence. Corridor rails are not continuous, and standing in front does not position the nurse in a way that will protect the patient.
2. **Instructing the blind patient to hold onto the nurse's arm allows the nurse to guide and the patient to follow; it supports the patient's comfort and promotes confidence.**
3. Verbal directions do not provide for the patient's safety; also, it will not promote comfort and confidence.
4. Walking on the side while holding the patient's elbow is one method used to assist a patient who has a mobility, not visual, deficit.

99. 1. The tube is in the stomach, not the lungs.
2. Placing the end of the tube in water is unsafe; if the tube is in the respiratory system rather than the stomach, a deep inhalation may cause an aspiration of fluid.
3. Instilling a small amount of normal saline is unsafe; if the tube is in the wrong place (e.g., esophagus, trachea), it may result in aspiration of the fluid.
4. **The tube is in the stomach, and application of negative pressure to the tube will cause gastric contents to be pulled up the tube and into the syringe.**

TEST-TAKING TIP The word "best" in the stem sets a priority. The word "tube" in the stem and options 2 and 4 are clang associations. You should examine these two options carefully. Option 4 is the correct answer.

100. 1. This provides an opportunity to discuss the illness; eventually, a developing awareness occurs, and the patient probably will move on to other coping mechanisms.

2. This blunt response is confrontational. It may take away the patient's coping mechanism, is demeaning, and cuts off communication; the patient is using denial to cope with the diagnosis.

3. This response may take away the patient's coping mechanism, is demeaning, and cuts off communication; the patient is using denial to cope with the diagnosis.

4. This response is demeaning and may cut off communication; the patient is using denial to cope with the diagnosis.

TEST-TAKING TIP The word "best" in the stem sets a priority. Option 2, 3, and 4 deny the patient's feelings; confronting the patient with reality when in denial takes away the patient's coping mechanism. Although the word "cancer" in the stem and option 2 is a clang association, this option denies the patient's feelings and can be eliminated. Option 1 is patient-centered.

Bibliography

Ackley BJ, Ladwig GB: Nursing Diagnosis Handbook: An Evidence-Based Guide to Planning Care. ed. 10. Mosby Elsevier, St. Louis, 2014.

Adams AK: The Home Book of Humorous Quotations. Dodd, Mead & Company, New York, 1969.

Aexaitus I, Broome B: Implementation of a nurse-driven protocol to prevent catheter-associated urinary tract infections. Journal of Nursing Care Quality 29(3):245–252, 2014.

Ahern J, and Kumar C: Caring for a patient with mental illness in the acute care setting. Nursing Made Incredibly Easy! 11(3):18–23, 2013.

Alexander-Magalee MA: Patient safety: addressing pharmacology challenges in order adults. Nursing 2013 43(10):58–60, 2012.

Alfaro-LeFevre R: Critical Thinking and Clinical Judgment: A Practical Approach to Outcome-Focused Thinking, ed. 4. Philadelphia, W. B. Saunders, 2009.

Alfaro-LeFevre R: Critical Thinking, Clinical Reasoning, and Clinical Judgment: A Practical Approach. ed. 5. Elsevier, St. Louis, 2011.

American Association of Colleges of Nursing, AACN White Paper: Distance Technology in Nursing Education. http://eric.ed.gov/?id=ED446494, accessed 8/29/2014.

American Philosophical Association: Critical thinking: A Statement of Expert Consensus for Purposes of Educational Assessment and Instruction. The Delphi Report: Research Findings and Recommendations Prepared for the Committee on Pre-college Philosophy. (ERIC Document Reproduction Service No. ED 315–423). 1990.

Aschenbrenner DS: Drug watch: preventing injuries from OTC eyedrops and nasal sprays. American Journal of Nursing 113(2):23, 2013.

Aschenbrenner DS: Overuse of certain OTC laxatives may be dangerous. American Journal of Nursing 114(5):25, 2014.

Association for Professionals in Infection Control and Epidemiology, Greene L (ed.), Felix K (lead author): APIC Guide to Prevent Catheter-Associated Urinary Tract Infections. http://bit.ly/1syFer5, accessed 9/15/2014.

Association for the Advancement of Wound Care (AAWC). Education for the Generalist. http://aawconline.org/education-for-the-generalist/, accessed 9/1/2014.

Association for the Advancement of Wound Care (AAWC). The ABC's of Skin and Wound Care. http://aawconline.org/wp-content/uploads/2011/04/ABCsPublic.pdf, accessed 9/1/2014.

Association for the Advancement of Wound Care (AAWC). The Skin You're In. http://aawconline.org/wp-content/uploads/2011/04/Skin-Brochure.pdf, accessed 9/1/2014.

Association for the Advancement of Wound Care (AAWC). Take the Pressure Off. http://aawconline.org/wp-content/uploads/2012/04/Take-the-Pressure-Off.pdf, accessed 9/1/2014.

Babine RL, Farrington S, Wierman HR: Inspiring change: HELP© prevent falls by preventing delirium. Nursing 43(5):17–20, 2013.

Black BP: Professional Nursing: Concepts & Challenges. ed. 7. Elsevier, St. Louis, 2013.

Bowers B, McCarthy D: Developing analytic thinking skills in early undergraduate education. Journal of Nursing Education 32(3):107–113, 1993.

Bradshaw M, Lowenstein A: Innovative Teaching Strategies in Nursing and Related Health Professions. Jones & Bartlett Learning, Burlington, MA, 2014.

Brookfield DD: Developing Critical Thinkers: Challenging Adults to Explore Alternate Ways of Thinking and Acting. Jossey-Bass, San Francisco, 1991.

Brous E: Lessons learned from litigation: maintaining professional boundaries. American Journal of Nursing 114(7):60–63, 2014.

Bryant R, Nix D: Acute and Chronic Wounds: Current Management Concepts. ed. 4. Elsevier/Mosby, St. Louis, 2012.

Buck HG: Transitions: help patients and families choose end-of-life care "wisely." Nursing 43(7):16–17, 2013.

Buck HG: Transitions: The Joint Commission "speaks up" for palliative care. Nursing 43(5):14, 2013.

Buck HG: Transitions: when we speak, what do families really hear? Nursing 43(1): 14–15, 2013.

Bulechek G, Butcher H, Dochterman J, Wagner C (eds.): Nursing Interventions Classification (NIC). ed. 6. Elsevier, St. Louis, 2012.

Burton MA, Ludwig LJ: Fundamentals of Nursing Care: Concepts, Connections & Skills. ed. 2. FA Davis, Philadelphia, 2015.

Carter D: In the news: the right balance between hand sanitizers and handwashing. American Journal of Nursing 113(7)13, 2013.

Case B: Walking around the elephant: a critical-thinking strategy for decision making. Journal of Continuing Education in Nursing 25(3):101–109, 1994.

Castillo SLM, Werner-McCullough M: Calculating Drug Dosages: A Patient-Safe Approach to Nursing and Math. FA Davis, Philadelphia, 2015.

Catalano JT: Nursing Now! ed. 7. FA Davis, Philadelphia, 2014.

Center for Nursing Classification and Clinical Effectiveness. Center for Nursing Classification and Clinical Effectiveness (CNC). www.nursing.uiowa.edu/center-for-nursing-classification-and-clinical-effectiveness, accessed 8/29/2014.

Chaffee J: Thinking Critically, ed. 11. Cengage Learning, Stamford, CT, 2015.

Chancellor J: Student voices: effective study habits for nursing students. Nursing 43(4):68–69, 2013.

Cherry B, Jacob SR: Contemporary Nursing: Issues, Trends, & Management. ed. 6. Elsevier, St. Louis, 2014.

Cohen H: Patient safety: prevent adverse drug events from topical medications. Nursing 43(7):68–69, 2013.

Cohen MR: Medication errors. Nursing 44(9):72, 2014.

Cohen NL: Patient safety: using the ABCs of situational awareness for patient safety. Nursing 43(4):64-65, 2013.

Colancecco EM, Moriarty S, Litak L: Inspiring change: none shall pass...without answering the call bell. Nursing 44(1):16–17, 2014.

Costedio E, Powers J, Stuart TL: Student voices: Change-of-shift report: from hallways to the bedside. Nursing 43(8):18–19, 2013.

Cross HH: Obtaining a wound swab culture specimen. Nursing 44(7):68–69, 2014.

Crusse EP, Kent VP: Making SENSE of sensory changes in older adults. Nursing Made Incredibly Easy! 11(5):20–30, 2013.

Daly W: Critical thinking as an outcome of nursing education. What is it? Why is it important to nursing practice? Journal of Advanced Nursing 28(2):323–331, 1998.

Davis C: Critical thinking skills for back to school. Nursing Made Incredibly Easy! 12(5):11–13, 2014.

Davis C: The importance of professional standards. Nursing Made Incredibly Easy! 12(5):4, 2014.

Davis C, Stone AM: Ask an expert: refusal of life-sustaining treatment. Nursing Made Incredibly Easy! 11(3):54–55, 2013.

Davis D, Shuss S, Lockhart L: Assessing suicide risk. Nursing Made Incredibly Easy! 12(1):22–29, 2014.

de Castillo MLM: Strategies, Techniques, & Approaches to Critical Thinking: A Clinical Reasoning Workbook for Nurses. ed. 5. Elsevier, St. Louis, 2014.

Delamont A: On the horizon: how to avoid the top seven nursing errors. Nursing Made Incredibly Easy! 11(2):8–10, 2013.

Dillon P: Nursing Health Assessment: A Critical Thinking Case Studies Approach. ed. 3. FA Davis, Philadelphia, 2015.

Dillon P: Nursing Health Assessment: Clinical Pocket Guide. ed. 2. FA Davis, Philadelphia, 2007.

Doenges ME: Nursing Care Plans. ed. 9. FA Davis, Philadelphia, 2014.

Doenges ME, Moorhouse MF, Murr AC: Nurse's Pocket Guide: Diagnoses, Prioritized Interventions, and Rationales. ed. 13. FA Davis, Philadelphia, 2013.

Elsevier (author). Clinical Key: Urinary Incontinence. http://www.cliniclkey.com/topics/urology/urinary-incontinence.html, accessed 9/2/2014.

Erikson EH: Childhood and Society. Norton, New York, 1993.

Evans V: Recognizing and managing concussion in school sport. Journal of Neuroscience Nursing 46(4):E25–E32, 2014.

Facione PA: The Executive Summary "Delphi Report." California Academic Press, Millbrae, CA, 1990.

Fahlberg B: Promoting patient dignity in nursing care. Nursing 44(7):14, 2014.

Farinde A: Drug challenge: Antidepressants. Nursing 43(9):64, 2013.

Farmilo K: Quitting smoking also improves mental health. American Journal of Nursing 114(5):19, 2014.

Federewisch M, Ramos H, Adams SC: The sterile cockpit: an effective approach to reducing medication errors. American Journal of Nursing 114(2):47–55, 2014.

Fowler C: Caring for the caregiver. Nursing 44(5):60–64, 2014.

Fronczek M: Physical restraints: to use or not to use? Nursing Made Incredibly Easy! 12(2):5455, 2014.

George RP: Patient safety: how nurses can encourage shared decision making. Nursing 43(8):65-66, 2013.

Gibson M, Keeling A: Shaping family and community health: a historical perspective. Family & Community Health 37(3):168–169, 2014.

Glennon R: It's about quality of life, not quantity. Nursing 44(8):18, 2014.

Goldsack J, Cunningham J, Mascioli S: Patient falls: searching for the elusive "silver bullet." Nursing 44(7):61–62, 2014.

Gordon M: Assess Notes. FA Davis, Philadelphia, 2008.

Grobecker P: Ask an expert: improve communication with non–English-speaking patients. Nursing Made Incredibly Easy! 11(4):55, 2013.

Grossman SC: The New Leadership Challenge, ed. 4. FA Davis, Philadelphia, 2012.

Hale A, Hovey J: Fluid and Electrolyte Notes. FA Davis, Philadelphia, 2013.

Hargrove-Huttel RA, Colgrove KC: Client Management and Leadership Success. FA Davis, Philadelphia, 2008.

Hargrove-Huttel RA, Colgrove KC: Pharmacology Success. ed. 2. FA Davis, Philadelphia, 2014.

Hargrove-Huttel RA, Colgrove KC: Prioritization, Delegation, & Management of Care for the NCLEX-RN® Exam. FA Davis, Philadelphia, 2014.

Harper D: Infusion therapy: much more than a simple task. Nursing 44(7):66–67, 2014.

Harris CD: Physician-assisted suicide: a nurse's perspective. Nursing 44(3):55–58, 2014.

Herrmann EK: Remembering Mrs. Chase. Imprint 55(2):52–55, 2008.

Hislop JO: Fighting frailty in older patients. Nursing 44(2):64–66, 2014.

Holloway BW: Physical Assessment Check-Off Notes. FA Davis, Philadelphia, 2013.

Holmes TH, Rahe RH: The social readjustment rating scale. Journal of Psychosomatic Research 11(2):213–218, 1967.

Hopp L: Introduction to Evidence-Based Practice. FA Davis, Philadelphia, 2012.

Horntvedt R: Calculating Dosages Safely. FA Davis, Philadelphia, 2012.

Huber D: Leadership and Nursing Care Management. ed. 5. St. Louis: Elsevier, 2014.

Huston CJ: Professional Issues in Nursing: Challenges and Opportunities. ed. 3. Lippincott Williams & Wilkins, Baltimore, 2014.

Julian MK: I.V. essentials: caring for your patient receiving TPN. Nursing Made Incredibly Easy! 11(1):8–11, 2013.

Jones J: Misread labels as a cause of medication errors. American Journal of Nursing 114(3):11, 2014.

Jones SA: Pocket Anatomy and Physiology. ed. 2. FA Davis, Philadelphia, 2013.

Kaakinen JR, Coehlo DP, Steele R, Tabacco A, Harmon Hanson SM: Family Health Care Nursing. ed. 5. FA Davis, Philadelphia, 2014.

Kataoka-Yahiro M, Saylor C: A critical thinking model for nursing judgment. Journal of Nursing Education 33(8):351–356, 1994.

Kelly P, Marthaler M: Nursing Delegation, Setting Priorities, and Making Patient Care Assignments. ed. 2. Delmar Cengage Learning, Clifton Park, NY, 2011.

Kelton D, Davis C: Ask an expert: the art of effective communication. Nursing Made Incredibly Easy! 11(1):55–56, 2013.

Kenneley I: *Clostridium difficile* infection is on the rise. American Journal of Nursing 114(3):62–67, 2014.

Kilburn FL, Bailey P, Price D: Inspiring change: Sepsis: recognizing the next event. Nursing 43(10):14–16, 2013.

Kirchner RB: Introducing nursing informatics. Nursing 44(9):22–23, 2014.

Klever S: Sharing: Reminiscence therapy: finding meaning in memories. Nursing 43(4): 36–37, 2013.

Kübler-Ross E: On Death and Dying. Macmillan, New York, 1969.

Landon D, Dickens M, Davis C: Peak technique: 12 ways to take a temperature. Nursing Made Incredibly Easy! 11(5):13–19, 2013.

Lange JW: The Nurse's Role in Promoting Optimal Health of Older Adults. FA Davis, Philadelphia, 2011.

Laskowski-Jones L: Communication: the good, the bad, and the ugly. Nursing 44(6): 6, 2014.

Laskowski-Jones L: Editorial: the devil's in the details. Nursing 43(8):6, 2013.

Laskowski-Jones L: The art of harmonious delegation. Nursing 44(5):6, 2014.

Lee A: The role of informatics in nursing. Nursing Made Incredibly Easy! 12(4):55, 2014.

Leeuwen AM, Bladh ML: Davis's Comprehensive Handbook of Laboratory Tests With Nursing Implications. ed. 6. FA Davis, Philadelphia, 2015.

Loving GL: Competence validation and cognitive flexibility: a theoretical model grounded in nursing education. Journal of Nursing Education 32(9):415–421, 1993.

Lutz CA: Nutrition and Diet Therapy. ed. 6. FA Davis, Philadelphia, 2014.

Maslow AH: Hierarchy of Needs: A Theory of Human Motivation. Martino Fine Books Publishers, Eastford, CT, 2013.

Maslow AH: Motivation and Personality. ed. 3. Harper & Row, New York, 1987.

Mason J, Leavitt JK, Chaffee MW (eds.): Policy and Politics in Nursing and Healthcare. Revised reprint. ed. 6. Elsevier/Saunders, St. Louis, 2014.

McCarron K: Blood essentials. Nursing Made Incredibly Easy! 11(2):16–24, 2013.

McCarron K: Med check: routine labs for common meds. Nursing Made Incredibly Easy! 11(2):50–53, 2013.

McKenry LM, Tessier E, Hogan MA (eds.): Mosby's Pharmacology in Nursing. ed. 22. Mosby/Elsevier. St. Louis, 2006.

Meyers E, Hale A: RN Pocket Pro. FA Davis, Philadelphia, 2013.

Mills S: Clinical queries: performing a clinical breast exam. Nursing 43(9):68, 2013.

Moorhead S, Johnson M, Maas M, Swanson E: Nursing Outcomes Classification (NOC). ed. 5. Elsevier, St. Louis, 2012.

Morton JA: Nurses week tribute: notes on noise. Nursing 43(5):37–40, 2013.

Murdock A, Griffin B: How is patient education linked to patient satisfaction? Nursing 43(6):43–45, 2013.

Murphy K: Recognizing depression across the lifespan. Nursing Made Incredibly Easy! 11(3):26–32, 2013.

National Council of State Board of Nursing: Innovations in Education Regulation Report: Background and Literature Review. www.ncsbn.org/Innovations_Report.pdf, accessed 8/29/2014.

National Council of State Board of Nursing: Nursing Pathways for Patient Safety. Mosby/Elsevier, St. Louis, 2010.

Nugent PM, Vitale BA: Fundamentals Success: A Course Review Applying Critical Thinking to Test Taking. ed. 4. FA Davis, Philadelphia, 2016.

Nugent PM, Vitale BA: Fundamentals of Nursing: Content Review PLUS Practice Questions. FA Davis, Philadelphia, 2014.

Nursing 2013 (author). Infobytes: online resources for managing chronic pain. Nursing 43(5):65, 2013.

O'Keeffe M, Saver C (contributors): Communication, Collaboration & You: Tools, Tips, and Techniques for Nursing Practice. American Nurses Association, Silver Spring, MD, 2014.

The Omaha System: Solving Clinical Data-Information: Problem Rating Scale for Outcomes. 2013 (updated 5/11/2009). http://www.omahasystem.org/problemratingscaleforoutcomes.html, accessed 8/29/2014.

Ortega L, Parash B: Clinical queries: Improving change-of-shift report. Nursing 43(2): 68, 2013.

Paul RW, Heaslip PH: Critical thinking and intuitive nursing practice. Journal of Advanced Nursing 22(1):40–47, 1995.

Perry AG, Potter, PA, Ostendorf, W: Clinical Nursing Skills and Techniques. ed. 8. Mosby, St. Louis, 2013.

Perry SE: Hard of hearing. American Journal of Nursing 114(8):13, 2014.

Pfeifer GM: Health care reform expands many services for woman. American Journal of Nursing 114(6):14, 2014.

Pfeifer GM: In the news: The top nursing news story of 2012: health care reform goes hand in hand with expanded nursing roles. American Journal of Nursing 113(1):15, 2013.

Phillips J, Stinson K, Strickler J: Avoiding eruptions: de-escalating agitated patients. Nursing 2014 44(4):60–63, 2014.

Phillips LD, Gorski L: Manual of I.V. Therapeutics. ed. 6. FA Davis, Philadelphia, 2014.

Pless BS, Clayton GM: Clarifying the concept of critical thinking in nursing. Journal of Nursing Education 32(9):425–428, 1993.

Pond EE, Bradshaw MJ: Teaching strategies for critical thinking. Nurse Educator 16(3): 18–22, 1991.

Primeau MS, Frith KH: Clinical queries: teaching patients with an intellectual disability. Nursing 43(6):68–69, 2013.

Purnell LD: Guide to Culturally Competent Health Care, ed. 3. FA Davis, Philadelphia, 2014.

Purnell LD: Transcultural Health Care. ed. 4. FA Davis, Philadelphia, 2012.

Quinlan-Colwell A: Controlling pain: making an ethical plan for treating patients in pain. Nursing 43(10):64–68, 2013.

Quinn S: Home healthcare from a student nurse's perspective. Home Healthcare Nurse 32(7):444, 2014.

Raines V: Davis's Basic Math Review for Nurses. FA Davis, Philadelphia, 2009.

Rank W: Performing a focused neurologic assessment. Nursing 43(12):37–40, 2013.

Roe E: Using evidence-based practice to prevent hospital-acquired pressure ulcers and promote wound healing. American Journal of Nursing 114(8):61–65, 2014.

Rogers TL, Darden CD: How clinical nurse leaders can improve rural healthcare. Nursing 44(9):52–55, 2014.

Rosenberg K: Updated guidelines on hepatitis B protection for health care personnel. American Journal of Nursing 114(4):19, 2014.

Rosini JM, Srivastava N: Patient safety: understanding vancomycin levels. Nursing 43(11):66–67, 2013.

Saathoff A, Turnham N: Stick it to me: the complexities of glucose testing. Nursing Made Incredibly Easy 12(5):50–53, 2014.

Saba V, McCormick K: Essentials of Nursing Informatics. ed. 5. McGraw-Hill, New York, 2011.

Sabella D: Mental health matters: mental illness and violence. American Journal of Nursing 114(1):49–53, 2014.

Safire W: Good Advice. Times Books, New York, 1982.

Said AA, Kautz DD: Patient safety: reducing restrint use for older adults in acute care. Nursing 43(12):59–61, 2013.

Salladay SA: Ethical problems. Nursing 44(8):12–13, 2014.

Savage C, Kub J, Groves S: Public Health Science and Nursing Practice: Caring for Populations. FA Davis, Philadelphia, 2015.

Scanlon VC, Sanders T: Essentials of Anatomy and Physiology. ed. 7. FA Davis, Philadelphia, 2014.

Schuster PM: Communication for Nurses. FA Davis, Philadelphia, 2010.

Seay AN: A child's story. American Journal of Nursing 114(7):72, 2014.

Seckel MA: Patient safety: Maintaining urinary catheters: what does the evidence say? Nursing 2013 43(2):63–65, 2013.

Segobiano A, Waters J, Davis C: All about acetaminophen – I.V.!. Nursing Made Incredibly Easy! 12(2):50–52, 2014.

Selye H: The Stress of Life. rev ed. McGraw Hill, New York, 1976.

Simpson E, Courtney M: Critical thinking in nursing education: literature review. International Journal of Nursing Practice 8(2):89–98, 2002.

Snyder M: Critical thinking: a foundation for consumer-focused care. Journal of Continuing Education in Nursing 24(5):206–210, 1993.

Stanhope M, Lancaster J: Foundations of Nursing in the Community: Community-Oriented Practice. ed. 4. Elsevier/Mosby, St. Louis, 2014.

Stanhope M, Lancaster J: Public Health Nursing – Revised Reprint: Population-Centered Health Care in the Community. ed. 8. Elsevier/Mosby, St. Louis, 2014.

Starr KT: Whistleblower liability: are you ready to put your job on the line? Nursing 44(2):16–17, 2014.

Stuart B: Pocket Guide to Culturally Sensitive Health Care. FA Davis, Philadelphia, 2011.

Taggart W, Torrance PE: Administrator's Manual for the Human Information Processing and Survey. Scholastic Testing Service, Bensenville, IL, 1984.

Teasdale G, Jennett B: Assessment of coma and impaired consciousness: a practical scale. Lancet. 1974;304:81–84.

The Regents of the University of Michigan. FLACC Behavioral Scale. 2002.

Tompson GS: Understanding Anatomy & Physiology: A Visual, Auditory, Interactive Approach. ed. 2. FA Davis, Philadelphia, 2015.

Townsend MC: Psychiatric Nursing. ed. 9. FA Davis, Philadelphia, 2014.

Treas LS, Wilkinson JM: Basic Nursing: Concepts, Skills & Reasoning. FA Davis, Philadelphia, 2014.

Ulbricht C: Davis's Pocket Guide to Herbs and Suppolements. FA Davis, Philadelphia, 2010.

Vacca VM, McMahon-Bowen E: Time critical: anaphylaxis. Nursing 43(11):16–17, 2013.

Vacca VM: Time critical: vesicant extravasation. Nursing 43(9):21–22, 2013.

Vallerand AH, Sanoski CA: Davis's Drug Guide for Nurses. ed.14. FA Davis, Philadelphia, 2014.

Venes D (ed.): Taber's Cyclopedic Medical Dictionary. ed. 22. FA Davis, Philadelphia, 2013.

Vitale BA: NCLEX-RN: Core Review and Exam Prep. ed. 2. FA Davis, Philadelphia, 2013.

Weiss SA, Tappen RM: Essentials of Nursing Leadership & Management. ed. 6. FA Davis, Philadelphia, 2014.

Widner-Kolberg M: Hard of hearing is not deaf. American Journal of Nursing 114(2):11, 2014.

Wilkinson JM: Nursing Process and Critical Thinking. ed. 5. Prentice Hall, Upper Saddle River, NJ, 2011.

Wilkinson JM, Treas LS, el al: Fundamentals of Nursing. ed. 3. FA Davis, Philadelphia, 2015.

Williams LS, Hopper PD: Understanding Medical Surgical Nursing. ed. 5. FA Davis, Philadelphia, 2015.

Williams W, Davis C, Brothers K: I.V. essentials: fluid management basics. Nursing Made Incredibly Easy! 11(4):48–51, 2013.

Winstanley HD: How to bring caring to the high-tech bedside. Nursing 44(2):60–63, 2014.

Woods AD: Implementing evidence into practice. Nursing 43(1-Supplement: Lippincott's 2013 Nursing Career & Education Directory):4–6, 2013.

Zerwekh JA, Garneau AZ: Nursing Today: Transition and Trends. ed. 8. Elsevier/Saunders, St. Louis, 2015.

Illustration Credits

Chapter 6

Figure 6-1: Maslow, AH: Motivation and Personality, ed 3. Harper & Row, New York, 1987.

Chapter 8

Sample Item 8-31: Reproduced with permission from Merck Sharp & Dohme Corp, a subsidiary of Merck & Co., Inc., Whitehouse Station, NJ. All rights reserved., Whitehouse Station, NJ.

Chapter 11

THE WORLD OF THE PATIENT AND THE NURSE

Questions 27 and 39: Burton M, Ludwig L: Fundamentals of Nursing Care: Concepts, Connections & Skills. ed. 2. FA Davis, Philadelphia, 2015. Reprinted with permission.

COMMON THEORIES RELATED TO MEETING PATIENTS' BASIC HUMAN NEEDS

Question 20: Wilkinson JM, Treas LS: Fundamentals of Nursing. ed. 2, vol. 1. FA Davis, Philadelphia, 2011. Reprinted with permission.

Questions 24, 32, and 34: Burton M, Ludwig L: Fundamentals of Nursing Care: Concepts, Connections & Skills. ed. 2. FA Davis, Philadelphia, 2015. Reprinted with permission.

COMMUNICATION AND MEETING PATIENTS' EMOTIONAL NEEDS

Questions 18, 26, and 31: Dillon P: Nursing Health Assessment: A Critical Thinking, Case Studies Approach. ed. 3. FA Davis, Philadelphia, 2015. Reprinted with permission.

PHYSICAL ASSESSMENT OF PATIENTS

Questions 18, 26, and 31: Dillon P: Nursing Health Assessment: A Critical Thinking, Case Studies Approach. ed. 3. FA Davis, Philadelphia, 2015. Reprinted with permission.

Questions 20, 25, 27, and 32: Burton M, Ludwig L: Fundamentals of Nursing Care: Concepts, Connections & Skills. ed. 2. FA Davis, Philadelphia, 2015. Reprinted with permission.

Question 29: Thompson G: Understanding Anatomy and Physiology: A Visual, Auditory, Interactive Approach. ed. 2. FA Davis, Philadelphia, 2015. Reprinted with permission.

Question 35: Teasdale G, Jennett B: Assessment of coma and impaired consciousness: a practical scale. Lancet. 1974; 304: 81-84. Reprinted with permission from Elsevier.

Question 37: Scanlon VC, Sanders T: Essentials of Anatomy and Physiology. ed. 7. FA Davis, Philadelphia, 2014. Reprinted with permission.

MEETING PATIENTS' PHYSICAL SAFETY AND MOBILITY NEEDS

Question 20: Dillon P: Nursing Health Assessment: A Critical Thinking, Case Studies Approach. ed. 3. FA Davis, Philadelphia, 2015. Reprinted with permission.

Question 25: Scanlon VC, Sanders T: Essentials of Anatomy and Physiology. ed. 7. FA Davis, Philadelphia, 2014. Reprinted with permission.

Question 30: Burton M, Ludwig L: Fundamentals of Nursing Care: Concepts, Connections & Skills. ed. 2. FA Davis, Philadelphia, 2015. Reprinted with permission.

Question 33: Myers E, Hale A: RN Pocket Pro. FA Davis, Philadelphia, 2013. Reprinted with permission.

MEETING PATIENTS' HYGIENE, PAIN, COMFORT, REST, AND SLEEP NEEDS

Question 31: FLACC Behavioral Scale. 2002. The regents of the University of Michigan. All Rights Reserved. Reprinted with permission.

Questions 33 and 35: Wilkinson JM, Treas LS: Fundamentals of Nursing. ed. 2, vol. 1. FA Davis, Philadelphia, 2011. Reprinted with permission.

MEETING PATIENTS' FLUID AND NUTRITIONAL NEEDS

Question 36: Phillips LD: Manual of I.V. Therapeutics: Evidence-Based Infusion Therapy. ed. 6. FA Davis, Philadelphia, 2014. Reprinted with permission.

Question 38: Wilkinson JM, Treas LS: Fundamentals of Nursing. ed. 3, vol. 1. FA Davis, Philadelphia, 2015. Reprinted with permission.

Question 40: Scanlon VC, Sanders T: Essentials of Anatomy and Physiology. ed. 7. FA Davis, Philadelphia, 2014. Reprinted with permission.

MEETING PATIENTS' ELIMINATION NEEDS

Questions 20, 32, and 34: Burton M, Ludwig L: Fundamentals of Nursing Care: Concepts, Connections & Skills. ed. 2. FA Davis, Philadelphia, 2015. Reprinted with permission.

Question 21: Dillon P: Nursing Health Assessment: A Critical Thinking, Case Studies Approach. ed. 3. FA Davis, Philadelphia, 2015. Reprinted with permission.

Question 25: Scanlon VC, Sanders T: Essentials of Anatomy and Physiology. ed. 7. FA Davis, Philadelphia, 2014. Reprinted with permission.

Question 27: Myers E, Hale A: RN Pocket Pro. FA Davis, Philadelphia, 2013. Reprinted with permission.

MEETING PATIENTS' OXYGEN NEEDS

Question 22: Wilkinson JM, Treas LS: Fundamentals of Nursing. ed. 3, vol. 1. FA Davis, Philadelphia, 2015. Reprinted with permission.

Question 24: Burton M, Ludwig L: Fundamentals of Nursing Care: Concepts, Connections & Skills. ed. 2. FA Davis, Philadelphia, 2015. Reprinted with permission.

Questions 28 and 29: Williams LS, Hopper PD: Understanding Medical Surgical Nursing. ed. 5. FA Davis, Philadelphia, 2015. Reprinted with permission.

Question 33: Wilkinson JM, Treas LS: Fundamentals of Nursing. ed. 3, vol. 1. FA Davis, Philadelphia, 2015. Reprinted with permission.

ADMINISTRATION OF MEDICATIONS

Questions 26 and 35: Phillips LD: Manual of I.V. Therapeutics: Evidence-Based Infusion Therapy. ed. 6. FA Davis, Philadelphia, 2014. Reprinted with permission.

Questions 31 and 39: Burton M, Ludwig L: Fundamentals of Nursing Care: Concepts, Connections & Skills. ed. 2. FA Davis, Philadelphia, 2015. Reprinted with permission.

MEETING THE NEEDS OF PERIOPERATIVE PATIENTS

Questions 23, 31, and 32: Burton M, Ludwig L: Fundamentals of Nursing Care: Concepts, Connections & Skills. ed. 2. FA Davis, Philadelphia, 2015. Reprinted with permission.

Questions 29 and 34: Wilkinson JM, Treas LS: Fundamentals of Nursing. ed. 3, vol. 1. FA Davis, Philadelphia, 2015. Reprinted with permission.

Question 35: Myers E, Hale A: RN Pocket Pro. FA Davis, Philadelphia, 2013. Reprinted with permission.

MEETING PATIENTS MICROBIOLOGICAL SAFETY NEEDS

Questions 19, 24, and 26: Burton M, Ludwig L: Fundamentals of Nursing Care: Concepts, Connections & Skills. ed. 2. FA Davis, Philadelphia, 2015. Reprinted with permission.

MEETING THE NEEDS OF PATIENTS IN THE COMMUNITY SETTING

Question 20: The Omaha System: Solving Clinical Data-Information: Problem Rating Scale for Outcomes, 2013 (updated 5/11/2009), accessed 7/23/14. http://www.omahasystem.org/problemratingscaleforoutcomes.html

PHARMACOLOGY

Question 27: Adapted from McKenry LM, Tessier E, Hogan MA (eds.): Mosby's Pharmacology in Nursing. ed. 22. Mosby/Elsevier, St. Louis, 2006, page 42.

Chapter 12

Question 15: Adapted from Wilkinson JM, Treas LS: Fundamentals of Nursing. ed. 3, vol. 1. FA Davis, Philadelphia, 2015.

Question 28: Adapted from Dillon P: Nursing Health Assessment: Clinical Pocket Guide. ed. 2. FA Davis, Philadelphia, 2007. Reprinted with permission.

Question 62: Burton M, Ludwig L: Fundamentals of Nursing Care: Concepts, Connections & Skills. ed. 2. FA Davis, Philadelphia, 2015. Reprinted with permission.

Questions 75 and 86: Dillon P: Nursing Health Assessment: A Critical Thinking, Case Studies Approach. ed. 3. FA Davis, Philadelphia, 2015. Reprinted with permission.

Index